Frontiers in Viral Hepatitis

Frontiers in Viral Hepatitis

Edited by
Raymond F. Schinazi
Emory University/Veterans Affairs Medical Center
USA

Jean-Pierre Sommadossi
Idenix Pharmaceuticals, Inc.
USA

Charles M. Rice
The Rockefeller University
USA

2003

ELSEVIER
Amsterdam-Boston-Heidelberg-London-New York-Oxford-Paris
San Diego-San Francisco-Singapore-Sydney-Tokyo

ELSEVIER B.V.
Sara Burgerhartstraat 25
P.O. Box 211, 1000 AE Amsterdam
The Netherlands

ELSEVIER Inc.
525 B Street, Suite 1900
San Diego, CA 92101-4495
USA

ELSEVIER Ltd
The Boulevard, Langford Lane
Kidlington, Oxford OX5 1GB
UK

ELSEVIER Ltd
84 Theobalds Road
London WC1X 8RR
UK

First edition 2003

Library of Congress Cataloging in Publication Data
A catalog record is available from the Library of Congress.

British Library Cataloguing in Publication Data
A catalogue record is available from the British Library.

ISBN: 0 444 50986 0

⊗ The paper used in this publication meets the requirements of ANSI/NISO Z39.48-1992 (Permanence of Paper).
Printed in The Netherlands.

CONTENTS

Frontiers in Viral Hepatitis Ed. by RF Schinazi, J-P Sommadossi and CM Rice. v — x

PREFACE

Viral hepatitis is one of the most common infectious diseases in the world, causing significant morbidity and mortality. It is estimated that over 300 million people are persistently infected with viral hepatitis; as a result many will develop associated liver pathologies such as chronic hepatic insufficiency, cirrhosis, and hepatocellular carcinoma. More than two billion people worldwide have evidence of past or current hepatitis B virus (HBV) infection, while 350 million people are chronic carriers. The World Health Organization (WHO) reports that HBV is the ninth leading cause of mortality in the world, accounting for more than a million deaths every year. Alarmingly, HBV is 50 to 100 times more infectious than human immunodeficiency virus (HIV). Hepatitis C virus (HCV) is also widespread; approximately 3% of the world's population is infected with this virus, and up to 170 million are chronic carriers, with three to four million persons newly infected each year. A recent estimate by the Centers for Disease Control and Prevention (CDC) places the number of chronically infected Americans at approximately 2.7 million, making HCV infection approximately two times more prevalent than HIV infection.

HBV is spread through contact with blood or bodily fluids from an infected person and, in the adult population, is most often transmitted by sexual contact, unsafe injections, or transfusions. The CDC reports that persons chronically infected with HBV are at an increased risk of death from cirrhosis and liver cancer, predicting that 15-25% will die from chronic liver disease. While HCV is primarily spread through direct contact with the blood of an infected person, adults usually acquire the disease through needle sharing, transfusions, or percutaneous procedures. CDC data suggest that 75-80% of HCV-infected persons will develop chronic infection, potentially leading to cirrhosis, liver failure, and/or hepatocellular carcinoma over a period of 10 to 20 years.

Pediatric HBV and HCV cases are on the rise, especially in developing countries where these infectious diseases are endemic. Worldwide, HBV and HCV are most frequently transmitted from infected mother to child during childbirth or the early childhood years. Unfortunately, many times these infections go undiagnosed. According to the latest CDC report, 90% of infants infected at birth and 30% of children infected between the ages of one and five will develop chronic HBV infection, while only 6% of persons infected after age five will become chronically infected. The HBV vaccine, although 95% effective in immunizing against the virus, is not a treatment or a cure for chronic hepatitis. The vaccine has played a vital role in the prevention of new pediatric HBV cases in the US; however, it is not readily accessible on a global level, and, in fact, is not currently available to the poorest countries that have the greatest need. Scientific research is currently in progress for an HCV vaccine, yet the high mutability of the HCV genome complicates the process. Internationally, there is a great need for safe, effective, and inexpensive treatments for pediatric HBV and HCV cases.

With antiretroviral therapies leading to increased survival rates in HIV-infected patients, coinfection with HBV/HCV has emerged as a significant clinical problem

Frontiers in Viral Hepatitis Ed. by RF Schinazi, J-P Sommadossi and CM Rice. xi — xiii

in the global population. Long-term HIV survivors coinfected with HBV can expect to develop chronic active hepatitis and cirrhosis. Studies have demonstrated that HIV infection results in a higher rate of HBV replication as well as an increased risk for cirrhosis in HBV/HIV coinfected homosexual males. Additionally, cohort studies in HCV/HIV coinfected patients confirmed earlier findings that although HIV is not strongly affected by HCV infection, HCV progresses at an accelerated rate. A significant increase in mortality was observed in HCV/HIV coinfected patients: death occurred in 7% of the HIV-study population and in 11% of the coinfected-study population, over a mean follow-up period of two years and 10 months. In the future, many HIV-infected patients will outlive their disease only to battle the complications of viral hepatitis.

A major milestone was achieved with the approval of lamivudine and the development of promising new nucleoside analogs, although the emergence of HBV-resistant virus remains a confounding issue for all of these. Clinical studies show that lamivudine can suppress the levels of HBV viral load, while reducing liver inflammation. Additionally, the CDC estimates that lamivudine is effective in up to only 40% of patients.

The treatment options for HCV are widening and include various formulations of interferon (IFN), IFN in combination with ribivarin, aggressive IFN dosing regimens, and novel antiviral drugs. This combination therapy results in sustained virologic response in up to 30 to 40% of patients; yet, it also causes significant toxicities and is usually more efficacious in patients who have HCV subtypes 2 and 3. Pegylated IFN, which has a longer half-life and a more favorable pharmacokinetic profile than IFN alpha, has surfaced as a promising new treatment for chronic HCV infection. Recent clinical trials demonstrated that pegylated IFN in combination with ribavirin leads to sustained response rates of about 50%, with minimal side effects.

To be effective, today's antiviral agents must aim to completely inhibit viral replication or to reduce viral burden to a level where the immune system can take over. HBV and HCV are characterized by high levels of replication and turnover, which results in an increase in resistant viruses and chronic progressive disease. With the emergence of antiviral-resistant mutations in hepatitis, the scientific community will recommend combination chemotherapy as the treatment of choice once new drugs become available. Thus, the need to develop safe and effective combined modalities that completely inhibit viral replication and the development of resistance is essential to the treatment of infected and coinfected patients.

Frontiers in Viral Hepatitis focuses on the latest advances in the search for new, more effective therapeutic options as well as related topics in viral hepatitis. These include regulatory issues, epidemiology, and emerging viruses; immunology and vaccines; viral hepatitis B and C infections in children; genetics, pathology and viral diagnosis; cell systems and animal models; novel therapeutics for hepatitis B and C; resistance and therapeutic strategies in humans; and prevention and treatment options for hepatocellular carcinoma.

The breadth of information published in this book provides insight into current prevention and treatment options. Recent advances in our understanding of the molecular biology, immunology and pathogenesis of hepatitis viruses have accelerated at a remarkable rate, offering a more comprehensive perspective on hepatitis. *Frontiers in Viral Hepatitis* provides a compilation of the latest research on this important group of viruses, and ultimately serves as a catalyst for interdisciplinary dialogue. It is our intention to open the doors for a global discussion on viral hepatitis, in hopes of laying the foundation for eradicating these infectious diseases, which lead to so much pain and suffering worldwide.

Raymond F Schinazi
Jean-Pierre Sommadossi
Charles M Rice

ACKNOWLEDGMENTS

This book is dedicated to our wives and children for their unwavering support of our research endeavors and our passion for science, and to the millions who have suffered or are currently suffering from viral hepatitis and its complications.

BIOGRAPHIES

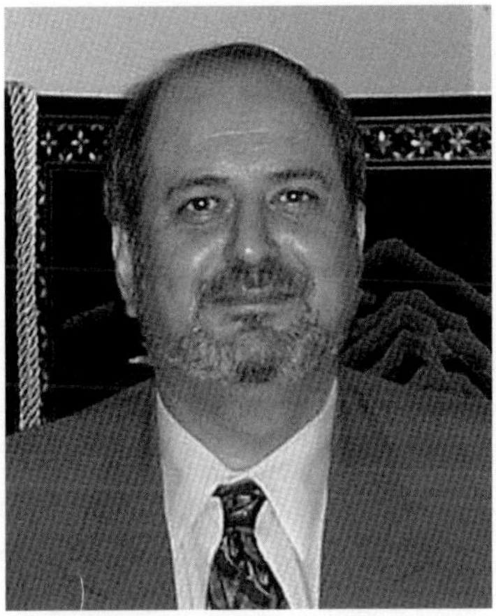

Raymond F Schinazi, PhD

Dr. Schinazi is Professor of Pediatrics and Chemistry and Director of the Laboratory of Biochemical Pharmacology at Emory University School of Medicine. He serves as the Senior Research Career Scientist and Scientific Director at the Georgia Veterans Affairs (VA) Research Center on AIDS and HIV Infections. He is currently Director of the Pharmacology/Virology Core for the NIH-sponsored Emory University Center for AIDS Research (CFAR). Dr. Schinazi is the principal founder of several biotech companies including Pharmasset, Inc., Tucker, GA, Idenix, Inc., Boston, MA, QuadPharma, Inc., Atlanta, GA, and Triangle Pharmaceuticals, Inc., Durham, NC. He currently serves on the Board of Director of Pharmasset Ltd.

Dr. Schinazi received his Ph.D. in Chemistry from the University of Bath, UK in 1976. He secured a postdoctoral position in pharmacology at Yale University. After his postdoctoral training, he joined the Department of Pediatrics at the Emory University School of Medicine in 1978. He has served on study sessions for the NIH and various other funding agencies and is currently on the editorial board of five journals dealing with anti-infective agents, including *Antimicrobial Agents and Chemotherapy, Antiviral Research, Antiviral Chemistry and Chemotherapy, Antiviral Therapy,* and *International Antiviral News.* Dr. Schinazi has published over 260 original papers and has contributed to the development of several HIV and hepatitis drugs, including stavudine (D4T), lamivudine (3TC), emtricitabine (FTC), amdoxovir (DAPD) and clevudine (L-FMAU). Dr. Schinazi has co-authored three books and numerous chapters on viral diseases. He is listed as an inventor on more than 60 issued US patents.

In 1996, Dr. Schinazi served on the Presidential Commission on AIDS. In 2000 he received the prestigious Bruce Witte Annual Distinguished Award from the Hepatitis B Foundation. Dr. Schinazi is also the recipient of two NIH Merit Awards. His research continues to be focused on the discovery of novel antiviral agents and anticancer agents and on the development of combined modalities to combat drug resistance.

Frontiers in Viral Hepatitis Ed. by RF Schinazi, J-P Sommadossi and CM Rice. xv — xvii

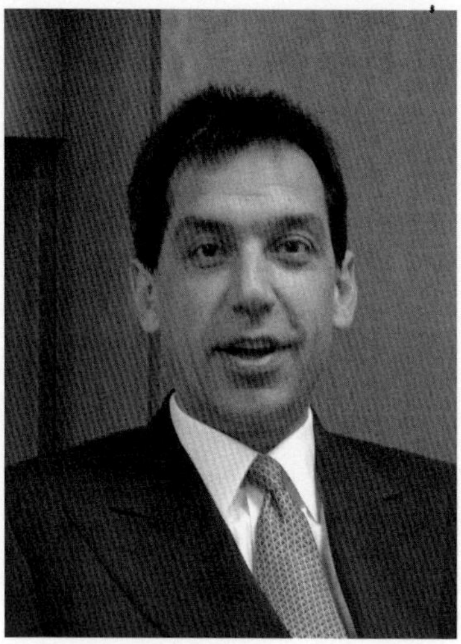

Jean-Pierre Sommadossi, PhD

Dr. Sommadossi is the Founder, Chairman and Chief Executive Officer of Idenix, based in Cambridge, Massachusetts and Montpellier, France. Until 2000, Dr. Sommadossi was a Professor of Clinical Pharmacology, Pharmacology and Toxicology; Associate Director, The Liver Center and Associate Director, The Center for AIDS Research at the University of Alabama at Birmingham School of Medicine.

He received his Ph.D. in pharmacology in 1984 from the University of Marseilles in France. In 1985, after a postdoctoral fellowship at the Medical College of Virginia in Richmond, he was appointed Assistant Professor at the University of Alabama at Birmingham; he was made a full Professor in 1992.

Dr. Sommadossi's research into the development of nucleoside analogs for the treatment of AIDS and hepatitis has led to a better understanding of the molecular pharmacology of these drugs and to the elucidation of their full mechanisms of action and toxicity, including the detailed molecular mechanism(s) involved in the lethal toxicity of FIAU observed in HBV-infected patients. Using *in vitro* and cell-based assays, his work has led to the discovery of novel inhibitors of HBV and HCV replications. Dr. Sommadossi's work on antiviral drug development has attracted national and international attention, and he has given over 70 major presentations as an invited speaker during the past five years. He is the author of more than 150 peer-reviewed publications.

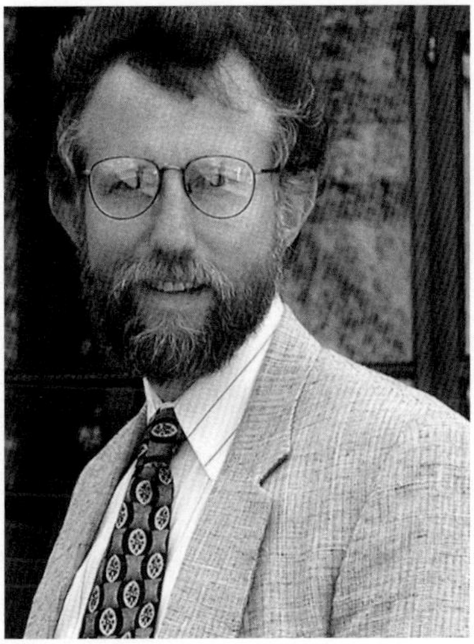

Charles Rice, PhD

Dr. Rice is the Maurice R. and Corinne P. Greenberg Professor and the Head of the Laboratory of Virology and Infectious Disease at The Rockefeller University. He also serves as the Scientific and Executive Director of the Center for the Study of Hepatitis C, a multi-institutional center jointly established in 2000 by The Rockefeller University, New York-Presbyterian Hospital, and Weill Medical College of Cornell University.

Dr. Rice received his Ph.D. in biochemistry in 1981 from the California Institute of Technology. From 1981 to 1985, he was a postdoctoral research fellow at the Institute. In 1986, Dr. Rice was appointed Assistant Professor of the Department of Molecular Microbiology at Washington University's School of Medicine. He was promoted to Professor in 1995. In 1997, his research team was the first to demonstrate that HCV alone is sufficient to cause the disease, a revelation that should help scientists determine the best strategy for developing an effective vaccine. Rice joined The Rockefeller University in 2000 from Washington University in St. Louis, where he is regarded as one of the world's most accomplished virologists and a prominent figure in research on HCV. Dr. Rice founded Apath, LLC, a company primarily devoted to HCV research and development.

Dr. Rice's research focuses on several different aspects of molecular virology, viral pathogenesis, and vaccine development. Currently, his laboratory team is involved in animal model studies of RNA viruses, including Sindbis virus (a togavirus), yellow fever virus (type flavivirus), bovine viral diarrhea virus (pestivirus), and HCV. Dr. Rice's work on the development of innovative approaches to fighting these viruses will serve to re-establish Rockefeller's preeminence in the field of virology as well to globally benefit the field of hepatitis research.

CONTRIBUTORS

Janice Albrecht, PhD
Schering-Plough Research Institute
Kenilworth, NJ, USA

Harvey J Alter, MD
Chief Infectious Diseases Section
Associate Director for Research
Department of Transfusion Medicine
Warren Grant Magnuson Clinical Center,
NIH, Bethesda, MD, USA

Angeline Bartholomeusz, PhD
Victorian Infectious Diseases Reference
Laboratory, 10 Wreckyn Street, North
Melbourne, Victoria, 3051, Australia

Pierre Bedossa, PhD
Service d'Anatomie Pathologique
Hôpital de Bicètre
94275 Kremlin Bicêtre, France

L Bellon, PhD
Ribozyme Pharmaceuticals, Inc
2950 Wilderness Place
Boulder, CO 80301, USA

Samira Benzaria, PhD
Idenix, SARL
Immeuble "La Vigie",
170 Rue Leon Blum,
34000, Montpellier, France

Paul Black, PhD
QuadPharma, Inc., 1860 Montreal Road,
Suite 217, Tucker, GA 30084, USA

Larry M Blatt, PhD
Ribozyme Pharmaceuticals, Inc
2950 Wilderness Place
Boulder CO 80301, USA

Timothy M Block, PhD
Department of Biochemistry and
Molecular Pharmacology
Thomas Jefferson University College of
Medicine
Philadelphia, PA, 19107, USA

Hubert E. Blum, PhD
Department of Medicine II
University of Freiburg
D-79106 Freiburg, Germany

M Robert Blum, PhD
Triangle Pharmaceuticals
4611 University Drive
Durham, NC 27717-0530, USA

Baruch S Blumberg, PhD
Fox Chase Cancer Center
Philadelphia, PA, USA

BB Bordier, PhD
Stanford University
Stanford, CA, USA

Edward G Bridges
Idenix, Inc.,
125 CambridgePark Dr
Cambridge, MA 02140, USA

Nathaniel A Brown, MD
Idenix, Inc.,
125 CambridgePark Drive
Cambridge, MA 02476, USA

Martin L Bryant, MD, PhD
Idenix, Inc.,
125 CambridgePark Dr
Cambridge, MA 02140, USA

Frontiers in Viral Hepatitis Ed. by RF Schinazi, J-P Sommadossi and CM Rice. xix — xxviii

Nigel Burroughs, PhD
University of Warwick
Coventry, UK

Pat Cane, PhD
PHLS Antiviral Susceptibility Reference
Unit, Division of Immunity and Infection
University of Birmingham Medical
School, UK

William F Carman, PhD
Massachusetts General Hospital
and the Department of Medicine
Harvard Medical School
Boston, MA 02114, USA

Andreas Cerny, PhD
Clinica Medica, Ospedale Civico
CH-6903 Lugano, Switzerland

Wei Ning Chen, PhD
Hepatitis and Liver Cancer Research
Unit, Department of Clinical Research
Singapore General Hospital, Singapore
169608, Republic of Singapore

L Cionca, PhD
University of Medicine Timisoara,
III-rd Pediatric Clinic Timisoara,
1900 Romania

Marcia M Clayton
Department of Pathology
Anatomy and Cell Biology
Thomas Jefferson University
Philadelphia, PA 19107, USA

Alessandra Colantoni, MD
Division of Gastroenterology and
Hepatology, Loyola University Medical
Center, Building 114, Room 48
2160 South 1st Ave
Maywood, IL 60153, USA

AD Cooper, PhD
Palo Alto Medical Foundation
Palo Alto, CA, USA

David Cooper, MD, DSc
National Centre in HIV Epidemiology
and Clinical Research
University of New South Wales
Darlinghurst, New South Wales,
Australia

Markus Cornberg, PhD
Department of Gastroenterology
and Hepatology,
Medizinische Hochschule Hannover
Hannover, Germany

R Costa, PhD
University of Medicine Timisoara,
III-rd Pediatric Clinic Timisoara,
1900 Romania

Paul Cote, PhD
Division of Molecular Virology
and Immunology
Georgetown University College
of Medicine
Rockville, MD 20852, USA

Erika Cretton-Scott, PhD
Idenix, Inc
125 CambridgePark Dr
Cambridge, MA 02140, USA

JM Cullen, PhD
North Carolina State University
Raleigh, NC, USA

Gary L Davis, PhD
Section of Hepatobiliary Diseases
PO Box 100214, University of Florida,
Gainesville, FL 32610-0214, USA

Nicola De Maria, MD
Division of Gastroenterology
and Hepatology,
Loyola University at Chicago
Maywood, IL 60153, USA

Erik Depla, PhD
Innogenetics, Inc.
Industriepark Zwijnaarde 7, Box 4
Ghent B-9052, Belgium

Adrian M Di Bisceglie, PhD
Department of Internal Medicine
Saint Louis University School of
Medicine, 1402 South Grand Boulevard
St Louis, MO 63124, USA

Jules L Dienstag, PhD
Massachusetts General Hospital
and the Department of Medicine
Harvard Medical School
Boston, MA 02114, USA

József Dudás, PhD
First Institute of Pathology and
Experimental Cancer Research
Semmelweis University,
Budapest, Hungary

David Dukhan, PhD
Idenix, SARL,
Immeuble "La Vigie",
170 Rue Leon Blum,
34000, Montpellier, France

Geoffrey M Dusheiko, PhD
Centre for Hepatology,
Royal Free Campus
Royal Free and University College
Medical School
Rowland Hill Street,
London, UK, NW3 2PF

Raymond A Dwek, PhD
University of Oxford,
Oxford, OX1-3QU, UK

Gerald Eder, PhD
Hans Popper Primate Center
Orth/Donau, Austria

Martha M. Eibl, PhD
Immunology Outpatient Clinic
Vienna, Austria

Rafael Esteban-Mur, PhD
Servei de Medicine Interna-Hepatologia
Valle Hebron Hospital, 119
08035 Barcelona, Spain

Xiaofeng Fan, PhD
Department of Internal Medicine
Saint Louis University School of
Medicine, 1402 South Grand Boulevard
St Louis, MO 63124, USA

Abdesslem Faraj, PhD
Idenix, SARL
Immeuble "La Vigie",
170 Rue Leon Blum,
34000, Montpellier, France

Mark Feitelson, PhD
Department of Pathology
Anatomy and Cell Biology
Thomas Jefferson University
1020 Locust Street
Philadelphia, PA 19107, USA

Eric B Ferrari, PhD
Department of Structural Chemistry,
Schering-Plough Research Institute
2015 Galloping Hill Road,
Kenilworth, NJ 07033-0539, USA

Russell Fleischer
Division of Antiviral Drug Products
Center for Drug Evaluation and Research
U.S. Food and Drug Administration
Rockville, MD, USA

Phillip Furman, PhD
Triangle Pharmaceuticals
4611 University Drive
4 University Place
Durham, NC 27717-0530, USA

Zachary Goodman, PhD
Department of Hepatic and
Gastrointestinal Pathology
Armed Forces Institute of Pathology
Washington, DC 20306-6000, USA

Gilles Gosselin, PhD
Laboratoire de Chimie Bioorganique
CNRS UMR 5625,
Universite de Montpellier II,
Place Eugene Bataillon
34095 Cedex 5 Montpellier, France

Jenny Heathcote, MD
University of Toronto
Division of Gastroenterology
Toronto M5T 258, Canada

Markus H Heim, PhD
Department of Research
University Hospital Basel
CH-4031 Basel, Switzerland

Brenda Hernandez, PhD
Department of Pharmacology and
Toxicology,
Division of Clinical Pharmacology
The Liver Center, University of Alabama
at Birmingham
Birmingham, AL 35294, USA

Craig L. Hill, PhD
Emory University
Department of Chemistry
Atlanta, GA 30322, USA

Hirohito Honda, PhD
Second Department of Internal Medicine
Tokushima University School of
Medicine
Tokushima 770-8503, Japan

Zhi Hong, PhD
Ribapharm
3300 Hyland Avenue
Costa Mesa, CA, 92626, USA

Chiyo Horie, PhD
Second Department of Internal Medicine,
Tokushima University School of
Medicine, Tokushima 770-8503, Japan

Takahiro Horie, PhD
Second Department of Internal Medicine
Tokushima University School of
Medicine, Tokushima 770-8503, Japan

Shiro Iino, PhD
Division of Gastroenterology and
Hepatology,
Department of Internal Medicine
St. Marianna University School of
Medicine
2-16-1 Sugao, Miyamae-Ku, Kawasaki,
Kanagawa
216-8511, Japan

Jean-Louis Imbach, PhD
Laboratoire de Chimie Bioorganique
CNRS UMR 5625, Universite de
Montpellier II, Place Eugene Bataillon,
34095 Cedex 5 Montpellier, France

Susumu Ito, PhD
Second Department of Internal Medicine
Tokushima University
School of Medicine,
Tokushima 770-8503, Japan

Mina Itonaga, PhD
Second Department of Internal Medicine
Tokushima University School of
Medicine, Tokushima 770-8503, Japan

Gary Jacob, PhD
Synergy Pharmaceuticals, Inc
Edison, NJ 08837, USA

KL Jensen, PhD
Ribozyme Pharmaceuticals, Inc
2950 Wilderness Place
Boulder, CO 80301, USA

SF Jamison, PhD
Ribozyme Pharmaceuticals, Inc
2950 Wilderness Place
Boulder, CO 80301, USA

Katalin Jármay, PhD
First Department of Internal Medicine
Albert Szent-Györgyi Medical University
Szeged, Hungary

C Jinca, PhD
University of Medicine Timisoara,
III-rd Pediatric Clinic Timisoara,
1900 Romania

Heidi M. Jolson
Division of Antiviral Drug Products
Center for Drug Evaluation and Research
U.S. Food and Drug Administration
Rockville, MD, USA

Robert Jordan, PhD
Department of Biochemistry and
Molecular Pharmacology
Thomas Jefferson University
College of Medicine
Philadelphia, PA, 19107, USA

Amy Juodawlkis, PhD
Idenix, Inc
125 CambridgePark Dr
Cambridge, MA 02140, USA

T Kalinina, PhD
Heinrich Pette Institute
Martinistr. 52 20246 Hamburg, Germany

Milind Kamkolkar
Department of Pathology
Anatomy and Cell Biology
Thomas Jefferson University
Philadelphia, PA 19107, USA

Brent Korba, PhD
Division of Molecular Virology
and Immunology
Georgetown University College of
Medicine
Rockville, MD 20852, USA

Ilona Kovalszky, PhD
First Institute of Pathology and
Experimental Cancer Research
Semmelweis University Budapest
H-1085 Budapest, Üllöi street 26
Hungary

Fritz Kury, PhD
Vienna Lab Labordiagnostika GmbH
Vienna, Austria

Ching-Lung Lai, PhD
Chief of Division of Hepatology
Department of Medicine, Queen Mary
Hospital, The University of Hong Kong
Hong Kong

Charles Lesburg, PhD
Department of Structural Chemistry,
Schering-Plough Research Institute
2015 Galloping Hill Road
Kenilworth, NJ 07033-0539, USA

K Liittschwager, PhD
Stanford University
Stanford, CA, USA

Dennis Liotta, PhD
Emory University School of Medicine
Decatur, GA, 30033, USA

Xuefeng Liu, PhD
Lab of Biochemical Pharmacology
Medical Research 151
Veterans Affairs Medical Center/
Department of Pediatrics
Emory University School of Medicine
Decatur, GA 30033, USA

Stephen Locarnini, PhD
Victorian Infectious Diseases Reference
Laboratory, 10 Wreckyn Street,
North Melbourne, Victoria, 3051,
Australia

Anna-Giulia Loi, PhD
Idenix, SARL
Immeuble "La Vigie", 170 Rue Leon
Blum, 34000, Montpellier, France

Anna Lok, PhD
University of Michigan Medical Center
Ann Arbor, MI 48109, USA

Gabor Lotz, PhD
2nd Department of Pathology
Semmelweis Medical University
Budapest, Hungary, H-1091

Xuanyong Lu, PhD
Department of Biochemistry and
Molecular Pharmacology
Thomas Jefferson University College
of Medicine
Philadelphia, PA 19107, USA

Andre Castro Lyra, PhD
Department of Internal Medicine
Saint Louis University School of
Medicine, 1402 South Grand Boulevard
St Louis, MO 63124, USA

D G Macejak, PhD
Ribozyme Pharmaceuticals, Inc
2950 Wilderness Place
Boulder, CO 80301, USA

Patricia L Marion, PhD
Divisions of Gastroenterology and
Infectious Disesease
Stanford University School of Medicine
Stanford, CA 94305-5107, USA

Michael Manns, PhD
Department of Gastroenterology and
Hepatology
Medizinische Hochschule Hannover
Carl-Neuberg-Straße 1
D-30623 Hannover, Germany

Bruce McCreedy, PhD
Intelligent Therapeutic Solutions Inc.
2505 Meridian Parkway Suite 200
Durham, NC 27713, USA

John G McHutchison, PhD
Scripps Clinic and Research Foundation,
Division of Gastroenterology/Hepatology,
10666 N Torrey Pines Road
La Jolla, CA 92037, USA

Anand Mehta, PhD
Department of Biochemistry and
Molecular Pharmacology
Thomas Jefferson University
College of Medicine, Philadelphia,
PA 19107, USA

Yuzo Miyakawa, PhD
Miyakawa Memorial Research Foundation
2-19-8 Minami-Aoyama
Minato-Ku, Tokyo 107-0062, Japan

Darius Moradpour, PhD
Department of Medicine II
University of Freiburg
D-79106 Freiburg, Germany

David Mutimer, PhD
Liver and Hepatobiliary Unit
University Hospital NHS Trust
(Queen Elizabeth Hospital)
Birmingham, UK

Maureen Myers, PhD
Idenix, Inc
125 CambridgePark Dr
Cambridge, MA 02140, USA

Florence Myrick, PhD
Triangle Pharmaceuticals, Inc
4611 University Drive
P.O. Box 50530
Durham, NC 27717-0530, USA

Yoshihiro Okamura, PhD
General Laboratory for Medical Research
Tokushima University School of Medicine
Tokushima 770-8503, Japan

Masao Omata, MD
Department of Gastroenterology
University of Tokyo, 7-3-1 Hongo,
Bunkyo-ku, Tokyo 113, Japan

Toshihiro Omoya, PhD
Second Department of Internal Medicine
Tokushima University
School of Medicine,
Tokushima 770-8503, Japan

Chong Jin Oon, PhD
Hepatitis and Liver Cancer
Research Unit,
Department of Clinical Research
Singapore General Hospital
Singapore 169608, Republic of Singapore

Victor Ovsiannikov, PhD
D V Efremov Scientific Research
Institute of Electrophysical Apparatus
Saint Petersburg, Russia

George R Painter, PhD
Triangle Pharmaceuticals
4611 University Dr
Durham, NC 27717, USA

PA Pavco, PhD
Ribozyme Pharmaceuticals, Inc
2950 Wilderness Place
Boulder, CO 80301, USA

Borislava G Pavlova, PhD
Ludwig Boltzmann Institute for
Leukemia Research and Hematology
Hanusch Hospital
Pav. 4/4, H. Collinstr. 30
Vienna, Austria

Donald Picker, PhD
Synergy Pharmaceuticals, Inc.
Edison, NJ 08837, USA

Claire Pierra, PhD
Idenix, SARL
Immeuble “La Vigie”, 170 Rue Leon
Blum, 34000, Montpellier, France

Deenan Pillay, PhD
PHLS Antiviral Susceptibility Reference
Unit, Division of Immunity and Infection
University of Birmingham Medical
School
Edgbaston, Birmingham B15 2TT, UK

Laurent Placidi, PhD
Department of Pharmacology and Toxicology, Division of Clinical Pharmacology
The Liver Center,
University of Alabama at Birmingham
Birmingham, AL 35294, USA

Maria Pop, PhD
University of Medicine Timisoara,
III-rd Pediatric Clinic Timisoara,
1900 Romania

Thierry Poynard, PhD
Service d'Hépato-Gastroentérologie
Groupe Hospitalier Pitié-Salpêtrière
47 Boulevard de l'Hôpital
75651 Paris Cedex 13, France

Joseph B Quinn
Triangle Pharmaceuticals
4611 University Dr
Durham, NC 27717, USA

Birgit Reipert, PhD
Baxter Hyland Immuno AG
Vienna, Austria

Charles M Rice, PhD
Scientific & Executive Director,
Center for the Study of Hepatitis C
The Rockefeller University
New York-Presbyterian Hospital
Weill Medical College of Cornell University, 1230 York Avenue
New York, NY 10021, USA

Douglas D Richman, PhD
San Diego Veterans Affairs
Medical Center and University of California San Diego
La Jolla, CA 92093-00679, USA

Laurence T Rimsky
Triangle Pharmaceuticals
4611 University Dr
Durham, NC 27717, USA

FH Salazar, PhD
Hepadnavirus Testing, Inc
Mountain View, CA, USA

Zsuzsa Schaff, PhD
2nd Department of Pathology
Semmelweis Medical University
Budapest, Hungary, H-1091

Raymond F Schinazi, PhD
Emory University/Veterans Affairs
Medical Center/Department of Pediatrics
1670 Clairmont Road, Room 5A197
Medical Research 151-H
Decatur, GA 30033, USA

Richard A Schreiber, MD
Associate Professor of Pediatrics
University of British Columbia
Division of Pediatric Gastroenterology
BC Children's Hospital
Vancouver BC Canada, V6H 3V4

C Seeger, PhD
Fox Chase Cancer Center
Philadelphia, PA, USA

M Serban, PhD
University of Medicine Timisoara,
III-rd Pediatric Clinic Timisoara,
1900 Romania

Ichiro Shimizu, MD
Second Department of Internal Medicine
Tokushima University
School of Medicine
Tokushima 770-8503, Japan

Yasushi Shiratori, MD
Department of Gastroenterology
Faculty of Medicine
University of Tokyo
7-3-1 Hongo, Bunkyo-ku
Tokyo 113, Japan

Daniel Shouval, MD
Liver Unit, Division of Medicine
Hadassah University Hospital
P.O. Box 12000
Jerusalem, Israel

Susan Simon, PhD
2nd Department of Pathology
Semmelweis Medical University
Budapest, Hungary, H-1091

Angela Skelton, PhD
Department of Structural Chemistry,
Schering-Plough Research Institute 2015
Galloping Hill Road
Kenilworth, NJ 07033-0539, USA

Jean-Pierre Sommadossi, PhD
Idenix Pharmaceuticals, Inc
125 CambridgePark Drive, 3rd Floor
Cambridge, MA 02140, USA

H.C. Spangenberg, PhD
Liver Research Center
Rhode Island Hospital and
Brown University School of Medicine
55 Claverick Street, 4th floor
Providence, RI 02903

Alexander Steinkasserer, PhD
Immunology Outpatient Clinic
Vienna, Austria

Martina Sterneck, PhD
Department of Liver Transplant Surgery
University Hospital Hamburg Eppendorf
Hamburg D-20246, Germany

Lieven Stuyver, PhD
Pharmasset, Inc.
1860 Montreal Rd,
Tucker, GA 30084, USA

Barbara Styrt
Division of Antiviral Drug Products,
Center for Drug Evaluation and Research
U.S. Food and Drug Administration
Rockville, Maryland, USA

Andrea Snow, PhD
Triangle Pharmaceuticals, Inc.
4611 University Drive
P.O. Box 50530
Durham, NC 27717-0530, USA

George M. Szczech, PhD
Triangle Pharmaceuticals
4611 University Drive
4 University Place
Durham, NC 27717-0530, USA

Bud Tennant, PhD
Department of Clinical Sciences
College of Veterinary Medicine,
Cornell University
Ithaca, NY 14853, USA

Phillip M Tharnish, PhD
Emory University School of Medicine
VA Medical Center
Atlanta, GA 30033, USA

Lawrence C Trost, PhD
Triangle Pharmaceuticals
4611 University Drive
Durham, NC 27717-0530, USA

David H Van Thiel, MD
Division of Gastroenterology and
Hepatology
Loyola University at Chicago
Maywood, IL 60153, USA

Charles Wakeford, PhD
Triangle Pharmaceuticals, Inc
4611 University Drive
P.O. Box 50530
Durham, NC 27717-0530, USA

Christopher M Walker, PhD
Department of Pediatrics, Division of Molecular Medicine
The Children's Research Institute and Ohio State University
Columbus, OH, 43205, USA

Jack Wands, PhD
Liver Research Center
Rhode Island Hospital and Brown University School of Medicine
55 Claverick Street, 4th floor
Providence, RI 02903

George JM Webster, PhD
Centre for Hepatology,
Royal Free Campus
Royal Free and University College Medical School, Rowland Hill Street,
London, UK, NW3 2PF

M A Winters, PhD
Hepadnavirus Testing, Inc.
Mountain View, CA, USA

Jacquelyn Wright-Minogue, PhD
Department of Structural Chemistry,
Schering-Plough Research Institute
2015 Galloping Hill Road,
Kenilworth, NJ 07033-0539, USA

Teresa Wu
Division of Antiviral Drug Products,
Center for Drug Evaluation and Research
U.S. Food and Drug Administration
Rockville, Maryland, USA

Deng-Fu Yao, PhD
Nantong Medical College, Nantong,
Jiangsu Province, China

Haruhiko Yoshida, MD
Department of Gastroenterology
University of Tokyo
7-3-1 Hongo, Bunkyo-ku
Tokyo 113, Japan

Hiroshi Yotsuyanagi, PhD
Division of Gastroenterology and Hepatology, Department of Internal Medicine
St. Marianna University School of Medicine
2-16-1 Sugao,
Miyamae-Ku, Kawasaki
Kanagawa 216-8511, Japan

Man-Fung Yuen, PhD
Division of Hepatology,
Department of Medicine,
Queen Mary Hospital
The University of Hong Kong
Hong Kong

Shu Min Zhang
Department of Pathology
Anatomy and Cell Biology
Thomas Jefferson University
Philadelphia, PA 19107, USA

Weidong Zhong, PhD
Department of Structural Chemistry,
Schering-Plough Research Institute
2015 Galloping Hill Road,
Kenilworth, NJ 07033-0539, USA

REGULATORY ISSUES, EPIDEMIOLOGY, AND EMERGING VIRUSES

Current issues in the regulation and approval of antiviral drugs for hepatitis [a]

BARBARA A. STYRT [b], RUSSELL FLEISCHER [b], TERESA WU [b] and HEIDI M. JOLSON [b]

Division of Antiviral Drug Products, Center for Drug Evaluation and Research, U.S. Food and Drug Administration, Rockville, Maryland, USA

Introduction

This brief overview describes general features of drug development in the United States, emphasizing regulatory issues applicable to hepatitis. Examples from published literature will be cited to illustrate complexities in this field, but are not intended as exhaustive and do not imply endorsement of any product or experimental approach. Current status of U.S. drug approvals for hepatitis will be summarized, and ongoing issues will be outlined.

General considerations in drug development

Allocation of review

This overview is written from the perspective of the FDA Center for Drug Evaluation and Research (CDER), responsible for review and approval of drugs for treatment of human disease. The Center for Biologics Evaluation and Research licenses biologic

[a] The views expressed are those of the authors and do not necessarily represent those of nor imply endorsement from the US Food and Drug Administration (FDA) or the US government. This paper is an August 2000 expanded and updated version of a talk delivered at the Third International Conference on Therapies for Viral Hepatitis, December 1999. FDA scheduled an August 2002 advisory committee meeting for further discussion of additional drug studies and study design issues (Federal Register 2002; 67(143):48664-5).

[b] All of the authors were employees of the US government at the time this work was prepared. Manuscripts produced by US government employees are excepted from requirements of the Copyright Revision Act of 1976 if they constitute works of the US government. Under copyright law, a work of authorship prepared by an officer or employee of the US government as part of that person's official duties is in the public domain and is not subject to copyright protection. The submitted writing is work of authorship prepared as part of the authors' official duties as officers or employees of the US government, and therefore is in the public domain.

Frontiers in Viral Hepatitis Ed. by RF Schinazi, J-P Sommadossi and CM Rice. 3 — 13

therapies. Diagnostic tests may be reviewed in the Center for Biologics Evaluation and Research or the Center for Devices and Radiologic Health. Internal consultations between Centers are frequent in areas of common interest, but specific procedures may differ.

Stages of development

Development of drugs for human use begins with identification of a compound with therapeutic promise by a research sponsor. When an Investigational New Drug (IND) application is submitted proposing pilot studies in humans, prominent preclinical data components include Chemistry, Manufacturing, and Controls information to characterize the drug, and Pharmacology/Toxicology information from animal studies [1, 2]. IND applications should include a "rationale for the drug or the research study" [3]; for drugs to treat infectious diseases, this might arise in part from data indicating activity of the drug against the microbe. If there are not appropriate animal models or *in vitro* assay systems, or the postulated mechanism of action is not direct antiviral activity, additional information regarding rationale for studies should contribute to their assessment. FDA reviews the documentation of safety for initiation of proposed human studies; if this is inadequate, and if acceptable modifications cannot be agreed upon [4], administration of the drug to humans under the IND may be prohibited from proceeding.

Human studies have several sequential phases [5]. Phase 1 trials generally are small safety, tolerability, and pharmacokinetic studies. Phase 2 studies typically constitute the first small therapeutic trials in patients with the target disease, and may provide dose-finding information in addition to preliminary short-term safety and initial effectiveness data. The principal basis for marketing approval is the conduct of statistically powered controlled Phase 3 trials confirming safety and efficacy. Phase 4 studies, after marketing, may provide increased information on safety, or on efficacy for additional populations or indications.

A New Drug Application (NDA) for marketing approval should contain "substantial evidence" for effectiveness [6, 7], including adequate and well-controlled trials conducted by qualified experts. Evaluation of submitted evidence includes judgment of whether claimed effects have been adequately shown, and whether there is sufficient information to develop directions for use; thus, the nature and amount of evidence required for marketing approval may be broader than for some individual treatment decisions. FDA does not regulate individual practice of medicine (as in off-label use of drugs).

Viral hepatitis and the drug approval process

Development of drugs for chronic viral hepatitis has posed challenges arising from attributes of the viruses and the diseases. Preclinical information that will reasonably predict activity in human disease is far more limited for hepatitis viruses at present than for many other infectious diseases, and there is no fully standardized approach to preclinical assessment of activity. Submissions should make a maximal effort to present clearly the rationale and supporting evidence for initiation of human studies.

So far, treatment studies and indications for drugs for viral hepatitis have focused on chronic hepatitis B or C infection associated with manifestations of chronic hepatic disease. Outcomes of greatest concern (for example, hepatoma or decompensated cirrhosis) may not occur for years or decades, so that selection and reassessment of markers of clinical benefit continue to pose challenges. Variations in disease course over time and variations among individuals in disease progression (as illustrated, for example, by references 8-12] reinforce the importance of controlled studies of substantial size and duration in relevant populations.

Prior experience with treatment alternatives for hepatitis is limited, especially for antiviral drug products (as distinct from biologic products, which may have different mechanisms of action and different procedural approaches to evaluation). The drugs approved recently for chronic viral hepatitis represent a stage in the refinement of the information base, but do not necessarily provide a comprehensive system of precedents.

Regulatory means for facilitating development

General issues

The FDA has a number of provisions for cooperative efforts to facilitate development. Pre-IND consultations can identify problems in preclinical data and initial human protocols prior to submission of an IND. In addition, several types of formal expedited processes can be applied when appropriate.

Fast track designation

The "fast track" program [13] provides for facilitating development of new drugs for serious life-threatening conditions through frequent FDA-industry interactions, and for submitting certain portions of an NDA before the complete application. "Fast track" designation requires that a new drug meet criteria, such as offering advantages over already available therapy [14], and can be rescinded if this promise is not borne out. "Fast track" drugs are not held to any lesser standard of evidence than any other drug. In many ways, "fast track" designation could be considered as formalization of the interactive process of review that is normally applied to new options in treatment of serious and life-threatening diseases (and might result in timelines similar to "fast track" even without this designation). "Fast track" drugs may receive accelerated approval or may receive priority review, if submitted materials meet qualifications for those processes.

Accelerated approval

Traditional approval involves demonstration of an effect on clinically meaningful endpoints, whereas accelerated approval [15] may be granted based on surrogate endpoints reasonably likely to predict clinical benefit, in serious and life-threatening conditions where a new drug offers benefit over existing treatments. Continued studies post-approval are required to verify clinical benefit and maintain approval: these are generally designed during development and are in progress when accelerated approval takes place. If a sponsor were to propose an application for accelerated approval for a chronic hepatitis indication, initial discussion would likely include selection of endpoints and identification of subsequent studies to verify clinical benefit.

Priority review

Priority review may be given to fast track drugs, and may be given to drugs considered for accelerated approval, but does not depend on these other designations. Review priority is based on criteria such as meaningful advantages in efficacy and safety, and extension of efficacy and safety to new populations. Public health considerations can enter into this determination in addition to results applicable to decisions for individual patients. Drugs currently approved for hepatitis have received priority review.

Pre-approval individual use of drugs under development

In discussions of facilitating drug development, the FDA sometimes receives questions regarding pre-approval use of a drug by individuals. For example, under certain circumstances on a case-by-case basis, emergency IND applications may be made for individual use of a drug not yet approved for marketing [16]. Open-label research protocols proposed by IND sponsors may also allow such use. These provisions have been employed at times in the hepatitis field, but had little or no effect on overall development.

Current status of drug approvals for viral hepatitis

Lessons from history

The history of drug development for hepatitis contains some reminders of the complexity of safety and efficacy evaluation in this area. In 1993 development was halted for safety reasons for fialuridine (FIAU), which initially appeared promising in its effects on certain markers of hepatitis B, but proved to have catastrophic toxicity not apparent in preclinical animal studies or the first few short-term human exposures [17]. Efficacy issues arose in ribavirin monotherapy for hepatitis C: prior to the approval of ribavirin for use in combination with interferon alfa, there were several publications suggesting that ribavirin was associated with decreases in transaminases during treatment, without a consistently beneficial effect on circulating viral RNA, on histology, or on post-treatment sustained response [see, for example, references 18-19]. Upon approval of ribavirin for use in combination with interferon, the package insert [20] carried a warning regarding lack of efficacy of the ribavirin component alone. Given these experiences and the limited overall history of drug therapy for hepatitis, safety and efficacy assumptions must be approached carefully and reevaluated frequently.

Currently approved drugs

Thus far, two drugs have U.S. FDA approval for treatment of chronic viral hepatitis. Ribavirin for use with interferon is approved for treatment of chronic hepatitis C – the proprietary name for the ribavirin capsules being Rebetol®, studied in combination with the interferon preparation Intron® A (which like other interferons is a biologic product licensed through the Center for Biologics Evaluation and Research); combination therapy having the proprietary name Rebetron®. This product was approved in June 1998 for treatment of patients with chronic hepatitis C who relapse after responding to an initial course of interferon, and in December 1998 for previously untreated patients. Approval was based on improvement in histology and suppression of circulating HCV RNA, sustained for six months after stopping treatment. Lamivudine was approved in December 1998 at 100 mg daily, under the proprietary name Epivir®-HBV™, for treatment of chronic hepatitis B. This approval was based on placebo-controlled studies in which the primary endpoint was histologic improvement, and the principal secondary endpoint was e antigen seroconversion, defined as the combination of e antigen loss, appearance of antibody to e antigen, and suppression of circulating HBV DNA below the limits of the research assay.

Common characteristics of approved drugs

For each of these two approvals, the new drug had previously been marketed for a non-hepatitis indication. Ribavirin is used in an aerosol formulation for respiratory syncytial virus infection, and the oral formulation was studied in combination with a previously marketed interferon preparation, while lamivudine had been on the market in a higher-dose form for HIV infection. Therefore, safety profiles had been partly worked out through usage more extensive than the hepatitis studies. For both drugs, principal studies were performed in adults with documented, chronic active liver disease without decompensation. Active drug was compared to placebo and showed superiority: Rebetron studies compared ribavirin plus interferon to placebo plus interferon, while lamivudine was compared to placebo in the Epivir-HBV studies on which efficacy determination was based. Histologic improvement was important in both approvals: other outcome measures generally showed effects compatible with histologic measures for overall ranking of treatment groups, but were not shown fully predictive of either histologic endpoints or longer-term clinical outcomes, and did not necessarily provide the same strength of evidence for efficacy.

Evolving issues

Study design

There are numerous active issues in the design of hepatitis studies. For example: when is it appropriate to use placebo controls, when active controls, and what is the impact on interpretation? When combination therapies are proposed, how will the contribution of each therapeutic component be evaluated, and how will optimal dose and timing be determined? How can optimal treatment duration be defined, when is it appropriate to have primary endpoints measured on treatment or after a period of time off treatment, and how will durability of treatment effect be ascertained? It is useful to discuss the laboratory values and assays intended for use well in advance of study initiation, if possible, to minimize questions arising later. Studies in special populations may be important to initial development and to study of new indications following approval.

Outcome measures

As part of evolution of study design, accumulation of information to refine outcome measures is desirable. Histology has been used as a principal marker of events in the liver, contributing to long-term sequelae with major morbidity and mortality; while histology has not been shown to be a perfect predictor, there also has not been solid evidence that other markers are better, or as good. For drugs approved thus far, multiple markers have been examined along with histology, including virologic, serologic, and biochemical outcomes. In both the ribavirin/interferon review and Advisory Committee discussion [21] and the lamivudine review and Advisory Committee discussion [22], virologic or serologic markers were only partially predictive of histologic outcome. In the lamivudine studies in chronic hepatitis B, seroconversion markers were not as convincing for efficacy as the histologic endpoint, and some subjects had reversion of serologic markers; some Advisory Committee panelists expressed disappointment that study results did not support use of non-histologic markers as the sole outcome.

NDA reviews and Advisory Committee discussions for the two approved drugs for chronic hepatitis also highlighted uncertainties surrounding use of viral nucleic acid assays. In both applications, reductions of viral nucleic acid measurements below the limits of the study assay (HCV RNA or HBV DNA, using investigational assays) were used in composite endpoints, but classification of a subject as a treatment success did not depend on the nucleic acid assay alone. In the lamivudine studies, a substantial minority of lamivudine recipients had reduction in HBV DNA below the assay limit, followed by re-emergence of HBV DNA while continuing therapy, related both to detection of viral mutations associated with reduced susceptibility and to less favorable results on other outcome measures compared to subjects without re-emergence of HBV DNA. Thus, ability to achieve initial suppression did not reliably predict outcome.

In addition to the difficulty in predicting longer-term outcome based on systemically circulating viral nucleic acid markers alone in these studies, interpretation is complicated by the lack of FDA-approved assays. Multiple different research assays have been used, which may not perform predictably in different settings, and may not provide equivalent or readily interconvertible results [see for example references 23-25]. There is little information regarding clinically meaningful thresholds for prognostic conclusions based on quantitative measurements of circulating viral nucleic acid levels or partial changes in these levels.

At present, it may be that no available endpoint for studies of chronic hepatitis is entirely satisfactory. Outcomes such as decompensated cirrhosis and hepatocellular carcinoma are unlikely to show meaningful treatment effects in studies of feasible size and duration. Liver biopsy as an indicator of liver damage has problems, including procedure complications, variability in biopsy readings, and sampling error, so it is important to minimize risk through appropriate subject selection and clinical care, to ensure adequate blinding and randomization, and to design studies with adequate power and standardization to avoid obscuring meaningful differences between treatment groups through variability in sampling and interpretation. The use of less invasive measurements is an important adjunct, such that serologic or virologic outcomes may, when appropriate, be considered as co-primary endpoints or in composite endpoints, and development of information to support better validated use of such measurements is desirable.

Some of the issues in endpoint selection include the following: How well standardized is the marker, and how reproducibly can it be measured in different settings? How reliably and precisely has the marker been shown to reflect or predict liver damage? Do changes in the marker during therapy, persistent changes after therapy, and changes during natural history of untreated hepatitis have comparable implications? Has the proposed marker been shown to have a consistent relationship to other markers, and can evaluation of clinical benefit be improved by combining several markers? In the evolving history of hepatitis studies, information about relationships between measurements has accumulated gradually, and results have not been uniform [see, for example, references 26-35]. Different studies may lead to differing conclusions about the absolute or relative ability of circulating markers to predict histologic activity; studies suggesting prognostic significance of specified tests may not be generalizable when assay methods change; and the relative importance of different predictors may need to be defined separately for different viruses and different long-term outcomes. A treatment effect on many different markers is helpful in decisions regarding drug efficacy, but does not prove that any of these markers would serve equally well to demonstrate efficacy.

Pediatric studies

Labeling of drugs as safe and effective for use in children should ordinarily be based on results of applicable studies. There are circumstances in which drugs may be labeled for pediatric use based on adequate and well-controlled studies in adults, plus supporting pediatric information, when the Agency has made a determination that the course of the disease and its response to treatment are sufficiently similar in adults and children to justify extrapolation of adult-study results to children [36]. Marketing exclusivity provisions have been introduced as an incentive for performance of pediatric studies [37]. For situations in which this incentive is not applicable or sufficient, a 1998 Final Pediatric Rule [38] provides that FDA may require pediatric studies under certain circumstances. This establishes a presumption that all new products will be studied in children during usual drug development.

In the study of drugs for hepatitis in children, there has not been a determination that the disease and response to treatment are sufficiently similar to permit direct extrapolation of adult results. For example, although specified outcomes such as clearance of viral markers, development of cirrhosis, and hepatocellular carcinoma can of course occur both in adults and in children, some studies suggest that disease progression is rare or slow in children and conversion to reduced levels of viral replication relatively common, other studies suggest that persistence of infection and evidence of active liver disease are common, and there is little information to provide direct comparative estimates of the risks of different outcomes over time, or the effects of treatment on these risks, in pediatric as compared to adult patients [see, for example, references 39-49]. Proposals for studies to document efficacy in children are encouraged.

Viral resistance

Information on viral resistance can be important to development of adequate directions for use of drugs for hepatitis, and therefore to substantial evidence in support of approval. Improvements in the knowledge base are needed in many areas including definition of resistance, assays, *in vitro/in vivo* correlations, understanding of clinical implications, risks of resistance in different populations, and effect on optimal drug use. Partly because of emergence of resistance-related concerns in hepatitis and other chronic viral diseases, FDA has encouraged research sponsors to develop plans for study of combination therapies. Design of such studies for optimal interpretability poses special challenges.

Conclusion

The complex and variable natural history of chronic disease caused by hepatitis viruses, and the ongoing development of diagnostic and prognostic approaches, contribute to the distinctive challenges to research sponsors and to regulatory personnel in this area of drug development. Consultation and dialogue at all stages can be valuable, in expediting processes where feasible and in contributing to shared understanding of potential obstacles. Recent and ongoing advances in this area should contribute over time to the evolution of development plans utilizing focused and updated information to guide assessment of activity, effectiveness, and safety for new therapeutic agents.

References

1. Code of Federal Regulations (CFR), 21 CFR 312.23
2. Guidance for Industry: Content and Format of Investigational New Drug Applications (INDs) for Phase 1 Studies of Drugs, Including Well-Characterized, Therapeutic, Biotechnology-derived Products, available on the FDA website under CDER Regulatory Guidance
3. 21 CFR 312.23(a)(3)(iv)(*a*)
4. 21 CFR 312.42
5. 21 CFR 312.21
6. Food, Drug, and Cosmetic Act, Section 505(d)
7. Guidance for Industry, Providing Clinical Evidence of Effectiveness for Human Drug and Biological Products, on the FDA website

8. Davis GL, Hoofnagle JH, Waggoner JG, "Spontaneous reactivation of chronic hepatitis B virus infection, " Gastroenterology 1994;86:230-235
9. Lok ASF, Lai CL, "Acute exacerbations in Chinese patients with chronic hepatitis B virus (HBV) infection, " J Hepatol 1990;10:29-34
10. Evans AA, Fine M, London WT, "Spontaneous seroconversion in hepatitis B e antigen-positive chronic hepatitis B: implications for interferon therapy, " J Infect Dis 1997;176:845-850
11. Seeff LB, Miller RN, Rabkin CS, Buskell-Bales A, Straley-Eason KD, Smoak BL, Johnson LK, Lee SR, Kaplan EL, "45-year follow-up of hepatitis C virus infection in healthy young adults", Ann Intern Med 2000;132:105-111
12. Fanning L, Kenny-Walsh E, Levis J, Choudhury KR, Cannon B, Sheehan M, Whelton M, Shanahan F, "Natural fluctuations of hepatitis C viral load in a homogeneous patient population: a prospective study, " Hepatology 2000;31:225-229
13. Food and Drug Administration Modernization Act of 1997, subtitle B, Section 112
14. Guidance for Industry, Fast Track Drug Development Programs – Designation, Development, and Application Review, on the CDER website
15. 21 CFR 314.510
16. 21 CFR 312.36
17. Transcript, Antiviral Drugs Advisory Committee Meeting, "Mitochondrial damage associated with nucleoside analogues, " Food and Drug Administration, Rockville, MD, September 21, 1993
18. Di Bisceglie AM, Conjeevaram HS, Fried MW, Sallie R, Park Y, Yurdaydi C, Swain M, Kleiner DE, Mahaney K, Hoofnagle JH, "Ribavirin as therapy for chronic hepatitis C. A randomized, double blind, placebo-controlled trial. Ann Intern Med 1995;123:897-903
19. Dusheiko G, Main J, Thomas H, Reichard O, Lee C, Dhillon A, Rassam S, Fryden A, Reesink H, Bassendine M, Norkrans G, Cuypers T, Lelie N, Telf P, Watson J, Weegink C, Sillidens P, Weiland O, "Ribavirin treatment for patients with chronic hepatitis C: results of a placebo-controlled study, " J Hepatol 1996;25:591-598
20. Rebetron® package insert, June 1998
21. Transcript, Antiviral Drugs Advisory Committee Meeting, May 4, 1998
22. Transcript, Antiviral Drugs Advisory Committee Meeting, October 6, 1998
23. Butterworth LA, Prior AL, Buda PJ, Faoagali JL, Cooksley WGE, "Comparison of four methods for quantitative measurement of hepatitis B viral DNA, " J Hepatol 1996;24:686-691
24. Pawlotsky JM, Bastie A, Lonjon I, Remire J, Darthuy F, Soussy CJ, Dhumeaux D, "What technique should be used for routine detection and quantification of HBV DNA in clinical samples?" J Virol Meth 1997;65:245-253
25. Olaso V, Cordoba J, Lopez B, Arguello L, Molina J, Lainez B, Ortiz V, Pastor M, Prieto M, Berenguer J, "Comparative analysis of quantification of viral load in patients infected with hepatitis C virus: quantiplex HCV RNA assay and amplicor monitor assay, " Rev Esp Enferm Dig 1999;91:569-582
26. Chu CM, Karayiannis P, Fowler MJF, Monjardino J, Liaw YJ, Thomas HC, "Natural history of chronic hepatitis B virus infection in Taiwan: studies of hepatitis B virus DNA in serum", Hepatology 1985;5:431-434
27. Brechot C, Degos F, Lugassy C, Thiers V, Zafrani S, Franco D, Bismuth H, Trepo C, Benhamou JP, Wands J, Isselbacher K, Tiollais P, Berthelot P, "Hepatitis B virus DNA in patients with chronic liver disease and negative tests for hepatitis B surface antigen, " N Engl J Med 1985;312:270-276
28. Fattovich G, Biustina G, Schalm SW, Hadziyannis S, Sanchez-Tapias J, Almasio P, Christensen E, Krogsgaard K, Degos F, Carneiro de Moura M, Solinas A, Noventa F, Realdi G, and the EUROHEP

Study Group on Hepatitis B Virus and Cirrhosis, "Occurrence of hepatocellular carcinoma and decompensation in Western European patients with cirrhosis type B, " Hepatology 1995;21:77-82

29. Sato A, Kato Y, Nakata K, Makao K, Daikoku M, Ishii N, Matsumoto T, Iseki K, Mazume H, Nagataki S, "Aetiopathogenesis of hepatocellular carcinoma. Relationship between sustained elevation of serum alanine aminotransferase and progression from cirrhosis to hepatocellular carcinoma: Comparison in patients with hepatitis B virus- and hepatitis C virus-associated cirrhosis, " J Gastroenterol Hepatol 1996;11:944-948
30. Heijtink RA, Kruining J, Honkoop P, Kuhns MC, Hop WCJ, Osterhaus ADME, Schalm SW, "Serum HB e Ag quantitation during antiviral therapy for chronic hepatitis B, " J Med Virol 1997;53:282-287
31. Niitsuma H, Ishii M, Miura M, Kobayashi K, Toyota T, "Low level hepatitis B viremia detected by polymerase chain reaction accompanies the absence of HB e antigenemia and hepatitis in hepatitis B virus carriers, " Am J Gastroenterol 1997;92:119-123
32. Zavaglia C, Mondazzi Lm Maggi G, Iamoni G, Gelosa F, Bellati G, Colloredo G, Bottelli R, Ideo G, "Are alanine aminotransferase, hepatitis B virus DNA or IgM antibody to hepatitis B core antigen serum levels predictors of histological grading in chronic hepatitis B?" Liver 1997;17:83-87
33. ter Borg F, ten Kate FJW, Cuypers HTM, Leentvaar-Kuijpers A, Oosting J, Wertheim-van Dillen PME, Honkoop P, Rasch MC, de Man RA, van Hattum J, Chamuleau RAFM, Reesink HW, Jones EA, "Relation between laboratory test results and histological hepatitis activity in individuals positive for hepatitis B surface antigen and antibodies to hepatitis B e antigen, " Lancet 1998;351:1914-1918
34. Puchhammer-Stockl E, Mandl CW, Kletzmayr J, Holzmann H, Hofmann A, Aberle SW, Heinz FX, Watschinger B, Hofmann H, "Monitoring the virus load can predict the emergence of drug-resistant hepatitis B virus strains in renal transplantation patients during lamivudine therapy, " J Infect Dis 2000;181:2063-2066
35. Hayashi J, Furusyo N, Ariyama I, Sawayama Y, Etoh Y, Kashiwagi S, "A relationship between the evolution of hepatitis C virus variants, liver damage, and hepatocellular carcinoma in patients with hepatitis C viremia, " J Infect Dis 2000;181:1523-1527
36. 21 CFR 201.57(f)(9)
37. Food and Drug Administration Modernization Act of 1997, subtitle B, Section 111
38. Federal Register notice, "Regulations Requiring Manufacturers to Assess the Safety and Effectiveness of New Drugs and Biologic Products in Pediatric Patients; Final Rule, " 63 FR 66632, December 2, 1998
39. Chang MH, Hwang LY, Hsu HC, Lee CY, Beasley RP, "Prospective study of asymptomatic HB s Ag carrier children infected in the perinatal period: clinical and liver histologic studies, " Hepatology 1988;8:374-377
40. Zancan L, Chiaramonte M, Ferrarese N, Zacchello F, "Pediatric HB s Ag chronic liver disease and adult asymptomatic carrier status: two stages of the same entity, " J Pediatr Gastroenterol Nutr 1990;11:380-384
41. Whittle H, Inskip H, Bradley AK, McLaughlan K, Shenton F, Lamb W, Eccles J, Baker BA, Hall AJ, "The pattern of childhood hepatitis B infection in two Gambian villages, " J Infect Dis 1990;161:1112-1115
42. Bortolotti F, Calzia R, Cadrobbi P, Crivellaro C, Alberti A, Marazzi MG, "Long-term evolution of chronic hepatitis B in children with antibody to hepatitis B e antigen, " J Pediatr 1990;116:552-555
43. Bortolotti F, Cadrobbi P, Crivellaro C, Guido M, Rugge M, Noventa F, Calzia R, Realdi G, "Long-term outcome of chronic type B hepatitis in patients who acquire hepatitis B virus infection in childhood, " Gastroenterology 1990;99:805-810

44. Hsu HY, Chang MH, Lee CY, Chen JS, Hsu HC, Chen DS, "Spontaneous loss of HB s Ag in children with chronic hepatitis B virus infection, " Hepatology 1992;15:382-386
45. Chang MH, Hsu HY, Hsu HC, Ni YH, Chen JS, Chen DS, "The significance of spontaneous hepatitis B e antigen seroconversion in childhood: with special emphasis on the clearance of hepatitis B e antigen before 3 years of age, " Hepatology 1995;22:1387-1392
46. Bortolotti F, Wirth S, Crivellaro C, Alberti A, Martine U, de Moliner L, "Long-term persistence of hepatitis B virus DNA in the serum of children with chronic hepatitis B after hepatitis B e antigen to antibody seroconversion, " J Pediatr Gastroenterol Nutr 1996;22:270-274
47. Bortolotti F, Faggion S, Con P, "Natural history of chronic viral hepatitis in childhood, " Acta Gastro-Enterologic Belgica 1998;61:198-201
48. Vogt M, Lang T, Frosner G, Klingler C, Sendl AF, Zeller A, Wiebecke B, Langer B, Meisner H, Hess J, "Prevalence and clinical outcome of hepatitis C infection in children who underwent cardiac surgery before the implementation of blood-donor screening, " N Engl J Med 1999;341:866-870
49. European Paediatric Hepatitis C Virus Infection Network, Tovo PA, Pembrey LJ, Newell ML, "Persistence rate and progression of vertically acquired hepatitis C infection, " J Infect Dis 2000;181:419-424

Molecular and serum epidemiology of HBV and HCV infection and the impact of antiviral agents in China

XUEFENG LIU[1, 2] and RAYMOND F. SCHINAZI[1*]

[1] *Lab of Biochemical Pharmacology, Veterans Affairs Medical Center and Department of Pediatrics, Emory University School of Medicine, Decatur, GA 30033, USA*
[2] *Virus Research Institute, Wuhan University, school of Medicine Wuhan, Hubei 430071, P.R. China*

Introduction

Human hepatitis B virus infection is a major public health problem worldwide. There are over 250 million people around the world carrying the virus in their blood, nearly 100 million persons in China alone, and just 1-1.25 million persons in the USA. In some Chinese provinces the HBV infection rate is as high as 50-70%. The persistent infection causes serious liver diseases, including liver cirrhosis and primary hepatocellular carcinoma (HCC). To date, there is no effective cure for this disease, making HBV infection one of the most important health problems in China.

Hepatitis C virus (HCV) is the major etiology of parenteral non-A, non-B hepatitis. Before it was discovered, there was little awareness worldwide that HCV was a serious, progressive liver disease. Since diagnostic reagents became available to detect HCV antibody (anti-HCV) and HCV RNA, the epidemiology of HCV infection has been investigated around the world, and basic and clinical studies on HCV have progressed rapidly. As with HBV, HCV was also recognized as another major cause of liver cirrhosis and HCC.

Hepatitis B virus infection

Some of the distinct epidemiological characteristics for HBV infection in China include: high prevalence of HBV infection, high rate of asymptomatic carriers, high risk of maternal-infant transmission, high ratio of chronic to acute disease, high risk of developing liver cirrhosis and primary HCC, high rate of HBV genetic mutation and poor response to interferon treatment.

Frontiers in Viral Hepatitis Ed. by RF Schinazi, J-P Sommadossi and CM Rice. 15 — 33

Prevalence of HBV infection

The prevalence of HBV markers (HBsAg, anti-HBs, HBeAg, anti-HBe, anti-HBc) is estimated at 50-70% in China, and it increases with age. The lifetime risk of HBV infection, as judged by the peak prevalence of HBV markers in elderly people, is approximately 80%. The annual incidence of HBV infection varies between two percent and five percent according to age. Thus, Chinese people have a high level of exposure to HBV throughout life [1, 2].

Asymptomatic HBV carrier rate and chronic HBV

The asymptomatic HBsAg carrier rate in China is as high as eight to 20% (Table 1), and a rapid increase in asymptomatic carrier rate was observed solely in children under five years of age. In spite of the continuous increase of HBV infection with age, in both school children and adults, the asymptomatic carrier rate in these age groups remains stable. Only neonates and children are at a high risk of acquiring chronic HBV after acute infection. This chronic infection can be reactivated in adulthood, usually between 20-40 years of age, and can result in clinical, chronic liver diseases [1, 2]. In a 10-year follow-up study, chronic liver diseases were observed in 28% of chronic HBV asymptomatic carriers [3].

Table 1. Prevalence of HBsAg in different sexes and regions of China

Sex or Region	Population	No. of sera	%	Survey done in:	Reference
Male	General	61,702	11.3	1992	1
Female	General	61,702	8.2	1992	1
Rural	General		10.5	1992	1
Urban	General		8.1	1992	1
Mainland	General	61,702	9.8	1992	1
Northern China	General		8.5	1992	1
Southern China			10.9	1992	1
Eastern China			11.1	1992	1
Western China			8.7	1992	1
Taiwan	Children*	1,515	9.8	1984	48
			1.3	1994	48

* under 12 years of age.

HBV transmission, maternal-infant transmission and chronic HBV

HBV is transmitted efficiently, primarily by percutaneous and mucous membrane exposure to infectious body fluids. Percutaneous exposures that have resulted in HBV transmission include: transfusion of blood or blood products, sharing contaminated equipment during intravenous drug use, hemodialysis, acupuncture, and needle stick or other injuries from sharp instruments sustained by hospital personnel. Sexual (both heterosexual and homosexual) and perinatal transmission of HBV usually result from mucous membrane exposure to infectious blood or body fluids. In China, HBV transmission is associated with the use of reusable syringes and needles for injection, toothbrush sharing, towel and cup sharing, and personal contact, including maternal-infant transmission and sexual activities. The incidence of HBV in some high-risk groups are summarized in Table 2.

Table 2. Incidence of HBV in some high-risk groups in China

Group	No. of Cases	HBV positive, %	Reference
IVDAs*	92	68.0	50
Prostitutes	55	52.7	53
Hemodialysis	199	78.4	55
Barbers	316	86.1	58

IVDAs: intravenous drug abusers

A high prevalence of HBsAg (8-15%) and HBeAg (2.0-6.5%) has been observed in pregnant women in China. Infants born to HBV-carrier mothers have a 20-40% chance of becoming chronic carriers, and this risk increases to 70-90% for those born to HBeAg-positive mothers. In the absence of universal vaccination, efficient maternal-infant transmission may play a role in perpetuating the virus from generation to generation. This transmission may occur in perinatal as well as in postnatal periods. Maternal-infant transmission might be one of the main reasons for the high ratio of chronic to acute HBV infection. The rates of maternal-infant transmission and chronic infection in China are probably higher than those in western countries [1, 2, 4].

Severe liver disease

Chronic HBV infection has been known as a major cause of liver cirrhosis and primary HCC [1, 5]. In a population and hospital-based, case-control study [6], the prevalence rates of HBsAg in 359 pairs of HCC cases and controls were 66.3% and 23.4%, respectively; the prevalence of anti-HCV in 340 pairs of HCC cases and controls was 17.9% and 6.5%, respectively. When both markers were positive, the odds ratio (OR) was higher than their multiple effects of HBsAg and anti-HCV. In the Haimen case-control study, serum HGV RNA was detected in 22% of HCC cases, compared with 10% of controls matched with age and sex. These data suggested that HBV might play a more important role than HCV and HGV in the development of HCC in China. Several molecular epidemiological reports on the relationship between chronic HBV infection and HCC would support this conclusion [5-9].

HBV genotypes and mutations

HBV is the prototype member of the *Hepadnaviridae* and is the etiological agent of a widespread form of acute and chronic liver disease, which is distributed throughout the world. The genome of HBV consists of four open reading frames — S, C, P and X — encoding the envelope [pre-S1, pre-S2 and surface antigen (HBsAg)], core (precore precursor protein and HBeAg and HBcAg), polymerase (HBV pol), and X proteins, respectively. Historically, HBV variability has been assessed by means of monoclonal antibodies against HBsAg and classified into serological subtypes. Two mutually exclusive determinant pairs, d/y, w/r and a common "a" determinant, define the latter. By further subdivision of the four major subtypes, a total of nine different subtypes have been identified: adw1, ayw1, ayw2, ayw3, ayw4, adwyp-, adrq+, adrq- and ayr. It has been known that the main serological subtypes of HBV in China are adr (72.4%), and adw (16.2%). Based on the entire nucleotide sequence of HBV genomes, a genetic classification system has been established. Seven genomic groups were described: A, B, C, D, E, F and G, each having intergroup divergence of 8% or more, with reference to the complete nucleotide sequence were described [10].

Guo et al. [11] analyzed the whole gene sequences of HBV from seven Chinese asymptomatic HBV carriers. Two strains were of genotype B, and the others were of genotype C, with serotype adr and adw in 4 and 3 strains, respectively. To study the relationship between focal variation of HBV S gene and seronegative HBV, Fan et al. [12] conducted sequencing and comparative analysis of the 52nd to 512th nucleotide of the S-gene in HBV, in 43 cases of seropositive and 52 cases of seronegative HBV from eight cities, including Changchun, Datong, Hangzhou, Shenzhen, Qingtao, Xi'an, Kunming and Lahsa. It was found that sequences of HBV S gene fragment in the same genotype were most conserved, with mutations happening randomly, and no detectable insertion, deletion or null mutations. There were three and five hyper-variable nucleotide points in HBV isolated from two different HB groups with identical genotype and serotype (C genotype/adr serotype and C genotype/ayw1 serotype), respectively, and there were five hypervariable nucleotide points in HBV of D genotype/ayw1 serotype (five strains of seropositive HBV) and D genotype/ayw3 serotype (ten strains of seronegative HBV), respectively. This suggests that most cases of seronegative HBV may correlate with a low level of HBV in their blood, and a small number of cases may be caused by HBV S-gene mutation.

To investigate if the concomitant presence of HBV DNA and antibodies to hepatitis B surface antigen (anti-HBs) is associated with mutations in the HBV envelope gene, Zhang et al. [13] applied PCR and sequencing to determine selected sequences of the HBV genome in 54 patients with chronic liver disease, collected from the Wuhan district. The part of the S gene coding for the 'a' determinant of HBsAg was found to be prone to diversity. A total of 19 aberrations occurring at 11 of the 69 nucleotide positions of this part of the genome were found in sera from 15 HBsAg-negative but anti-HBs-positive patients. One of 13 HBsAg/HBeAg-positive and eight of 17 HBsAg/anti-HBe-positive samples also showed point mutations in this gene sequence. Most prevalent was a point mutation from A-to-G at nucleotide 530, resulting in a change from threonine to alanine at amino acid position 126. This study highlighted that the long duration of chronic HBV infection could favor a selection of escape mutants.

The occurrence of such HBV variants in patients with chronic liver disease is not detected by conventional HBV serology, and the patients may be misdiagnosed. If viral mutants like those described here can be transmitted to other patients, there will be difficulties in identifying these infections, and conventional HBV vaccination will presumably not be protective. In another study, He et al. [14] studied 24 infants who became positive for the surface antigen of HBV (HBsAg), despite a complete course of active post-exposure immunization with plasma-derived hepatitis B vaccine. The PCR amplified products of the common neutralizing epitope 'a' determinant of HBsAg (nucleotide 419-598) from serum samples were sequenced and analyzed for nucleotide mutations. Four cases (16.7%) had mutations that led to amino acid substitutions between codons 124 and 147. Only one case (N1) showed a substitution at codon 145 (from glycine to arginine, 145R), the other three were at codons 126-129. The mother of N1 was co-infected with the wild type and mutant virus. Five years later, serum of N1 showed only the wild type virus. There was no significant relationship between the mutation rate and the anti-HBs response to hepatitis B vaccination. Results suggest that without immune selective pressure, 145R variant was not frequently observed, and was not stable. Furthermore, mutation in the 'a' determinant was not an important cause of failure to prevent maternal-infant transmission of HBV despite active post-exposure HBV immunization in Chinese children.

Seroconversion from HBeAg to anti-HBe is frequently seen in the course of chronic HBV infection. This phenomenon is closely related to mutation of the precore region; a G-to-A substitution of nucleotide position 1896 replaces tryptophan with a translational stop codon. Several papers support the finding that this mutant is responsible for the fulminant hepatitis or acute exacerbation of chronic HB. Tu et al. [15] collected 446 serum samples from HBsAg-positive, chronic HB patients from five areas in China (eastern coastal city, Shanghai; southwestern inland city, Chengdu; mid-inland city, Wuhan; southern island city, Haikou; and northeastern city, Changchun). Precore stop-codon variants (e-minus mutants) were screened using a rapid PCR amplification of a precore and partial core gene fragment (nucleotides 1785-2172), followed by dot-blot hybridization with specific oligonucleotide probes (M0, and M1 + M2). The sequence of the M0 probe covered the distal precore region of wild-type virus (nucleotides 1887-1908), and the sequences of the M1 and M2 probes were from sequences mutated at nt.1898 (TGG to TAG), with or without additional change at nt.1901. A significantly lower incidence of the precore stop codon was found in anti-HBe-positive serum samples from Haikou (17.6%), whereas in other areas the percentages of this mutation in anti-HBe-positive sera ranged from 47.4% to 78.9%. In HBeAg-positive samples, the rate of e-minus mutant in coexistence with wild-type virus was low in specimens from Haikou (9.5%) and Changchun (2.9%) compared to other areas in China. In contrast, coexistence of mutant and wild-type virus was frequently detected in half the samples from Wuhan. These mutations might be related to the poor response of chronic HB patients to interferon treatment.

The effect of interferon and lamivudine treatment in chronic HB

Chinese patients with CHB differ from Caucasian patients because they are immunologically tolerant to HBV, having acquired HBV infection perinatally or in early childhood. In the treatment of CHB, the short-term aims of loss of HBV early antigen (HBeAg) and HBV DNA need to be reassessed. In 1,296 Chinese CHB patients, 67.7% of those who developed complications of cirrhosis or hepatocellular carcinoma were anti-HBe positive. Therefore, longer follow-up of patients is required to assess the efficacy of a treatment regimen. After long-term follow up (median 90 months) of 206 Chinese CHB patients treated with interferon alpha (IFN-alpha) compared with 203 untreated subjects, IFN-alpha conferred no benefit in cumulative HBeAg seroconversion or in HBV DNA negativity, as determined by PCR assays or in decreasing long-term complications of cirrhosis and HCC [16].

Lamivudine is a nucleoside analogue with potent and selective anti-HBV activity. In a recent one-year study of 358 Chinese CHB patients in Hong Kong and Taiwan, Lai et al. [17] conducted a one-year, double-blind trial of lamivudine in 358 Chinese patients with CHB. The patients were randomly assigned to receive 25 mg of lamivudine (142 patients), 100 mg of lamivudine (143), or placebo (73) orally once daily. The patients underwent liver biopsies before entering the study and after completing the assigned treatment regimen. The primary endpoint was a reduction of at least two points in the Knodell necro-inflammatory score. Hepatic necro-inflammatory activity improved by two points or more in 56 percent of the patients receiving 100 mg of lamivudine, 49 percent of those receiving 25 mg of lamivudine, and 25 percent of those receiving placebo ($p < 0.001$ and $p = 0.001$, respectively, for the comparisons of lamivudine treatment with placebo). Necro-inflammatory activity worsened in seven percent of the patients receiving 100 mg of lamivudine, eight percent of those receiving 25 mg, and 26 percent of those receiving placebo. The 100 mg dose of lamivudine was associated with a reduced progression of fibrosis ($p = 0.01$ for the comparison with placebo) and with the highest rate of HBeAg seroconversion (loss of HBeAg, development of antibody to HBeAg, and undetectable HBV DNA) (16 percent), the greatest suppression of HBV DNA (98 percent reduction at week 52 as compared with the baseline value), and the highest rate of sustained normalization of alanine aminotransferase (ALT) levels (72 percent). Ninety-six percent of the patients completed the study. The incidence of adverse events was similar in all groups, and there were few serious events. These results indicate that lamivudine was associated with substantial histological improvement in many patients with chronic hepatitis B (including a reduction in fibrosis), with HBV DNA suppression and normalization of ALT levels, and that a daily dose of 100 mg was more effective than a daily dose of 25 mg. However, lamivudine may have to be given on a long-term basis, as withdrawal of lamivudine results in rebound of HBV DNA to pretreatment levels.

In another study in mainland of China, 429 patients with chronic HBV infection as defined by positive HBsAg, HBeAg and HBV DNA, were enrolled and randomized into lamivudine and placebo groups [18]. In this study, 322 patients received 100 mg lamivudine daily and 107 patients received placebo treatment for 12 weeks. Then, all patients were offered a further 40 weeks of open label lamivudine treatment. The efficacy and safety were evaluated with clinical, biochemical, hematological and virological parameters. After 12 weeks treatment, HBV DNA response (serum HBV DNA < 1.6 ng/L) rate in the lamivudine group was higher than in the placebo group (92.2% *versus* 14.1%, $p < 0.01$); but at week 52, there was no difference between lamivudine and placebo/lamivudine groups (71.0% *versus* 77.7%, $p > 0.05$). The rate of HBV DNA breakthrough in the lamivudine group was higher than in the placebo/lamivudine group (24.4% *versus* 8.5%, $p < 0.01$). The proportion of HBeAg/anti-HBe seroconversion was not different in the two groups (7.5% *versus* 5.2%, $p > 0.05$). By week 12, the ALT normalization rate in the lamivudine group was higher than in the placebo group (60.3% *versus* 27.5%, $p < 0.01$); but after 52 weeks treatment, there was no difference between the two groups (70.9% *versus* 74.5%, $p > 0.05$). At week 48, HBV drug-induced mutation rate in the lamivudine group was higher than in the placebo/lamivudine group (14.6% *versus* 5.0%, $p < 0.05$). The incidence of adverse events was similar for both the lamivudine and placebo/lamivudine groups up to week 12 and 52. There were few severe drug-related adverse events. Sustained HBV replication suppression was attained with long-term treatment with 100 mg lamivudine daily, accompanied by good tolerance and safety, although resistant virus was detected in a significant number of patients.

Lamivudine is effective in suppressing replication of HBV, however, the emergence of HBV variants resistant to lamivudine is a major concern [17, 18, 59-66]. Lamivudine resistance has been attributed mainly to a change from methionine to isoleucine or valine at codon 550 in the catalytic site of the virus polymerase (genotype B). The incidence and its evolution of lamivudine-selected HBV resistance is summarized in Table 3.

Hepatitis C infection

HCV infects approximately 200 million individuals worldwide. In about 20% of cases, chronic HCV infection leads to cirrhosis, which predisposes the patient to HCC.

Prevalence of HCV infection

In China, the prevalence of HCV infection in the general population is low, ranging from one to five percent (Table 4). There is a significant difference in the rates of anti-HCV in the different populations [1-2, 19-20]. In Western Europe and the USA, the prevalence rates range from 0.2 to two percent, and in most African countries, over five percent of the general population is infected with HCV [38, 74].

In a study of anti-HCV in the sera of different populations [21], out of the general population, 2.1% (9/438) were anti-HCV-positive, and of the patients that underwent blood transfusion, 11.1% (6/54) were anti-HCV-positive. Among patients with chronic liver diseases, anti-HCV was positive in 10.5% (36/342) of patients with chronic persistent hepatitis (CPH), 12.1% (13/107) of those with chronic active hepatitis (CAH), 42.6% (63/148) of those with liver cirrhosis (LC) and 38.4% (20/52) of those with HCC.

It is noteworthy that the anti-HCV-positive rate significantly increased with disease progression from CPH to CAH, LC and HCC.

Table 3. Sequence evolution of lamivudine-selected HBV resistance in humans

Treatment Time (Weeks)	Type of Trial	Patients	Number of cases	Dose (mg/d)	Resistance (%)	Method	Area	Reference
26 52	DB, PC, R	CHB	60	100	1.9 27	PCR-RFLP	Greece, Italy, UK, Spain, Canada	63
36 48	DB, PC, R	CHB	107 429	100	5.0 14.6	PCR-sequencing	Mainland China	18
24 36 52	DB, PC, R	CHB	267 267 133 134	25 or 100 25 100	0 4 14 14	RFLP	Hong Kong, Taiwan	17, 72
38 52 77 104	—	CHB	37	100	11 32 56 66	PCR-RFLP		60
52 104 456	DB, PC, R	CHB	58	100	17 40 55	PCR-RFLP	Hong Kong, Taiwan Singapore	73

Note: CHB, chronic hepatitis B; DB, double blind; PC, placebo control; R, randomized; PCR, polymerase chain reaction; RFLP, restricted fragment length polymorphism.

Table 4. Prevalence of anti-HCV in the general population of China

Region	No. of sera	HCV positive, %	Survey done in:	Reference
Mainland	67,185	3.2	1992	1
Northern China		3.6	1992	1
Southern China		2.9	1992	1
Taiwan	275	2.9	1993	49

HCV transmission

Like HBV, the most efficient transmission of HCV is through direct percutaneous exposure to infectious blood, such as through transfusion of blood or blood products or transplantation of organs or tissues from infectious donors, and sharing of contaminated equipment among intravenous drug users [1-2]. The incidence rates of post-transfusion HC in several cities of China were in excess of 10% before 1997. The high risk associated with blood transfusion for surgical patients was a result of the lack of sensitive and reliable reagents for blood screening and the spread of HCV infection among blood donors. In several areas of China, plasma donation was performed with reusable and contaminated equipment before 1996. HCV infection was found in 10.8% of the professional donors who gave one donation, and 56.5% and 94.8% in those who gave 10-19 and 20-29 donations, respectively. HCV may also be transmitted by vertical, sexual and intrafamilial parenteral or non-parenteral routes. As the economy of China improves and Chinese lifestyles change, the patients infected by HCV through sexual route and illicit intravenous drug abuse is likely to increase (Table 5) [22-23]. Therefore, HCV infection, as with HBV, is not only a public health problem, but also a social problem.

Table 5. Incidence of anti-HCV in some high-risk groups in China

Group	Cases	Anti-HCV, %	Reference
IVDAs	92	92	50
	158	86	51
	703	82.2	52
Prostitutes	223	10.3	52
	55	3.64	53
	431	9.51	54
Haemodialysis	63	36.5	52
	144	24.3	57
HIV infected	63	25.4	52
Tattooed	87	12.6	56

IVDAs: intravenous drug abusers

HCV genotypes and subtypes

HCV comprise a group of highly variable isolates or strains. Currently, HCV has been classified into at least 11 major genotypes and over 70 subtypes, based on analysis of complete or partial HCV genomic sequences. It has been found that the genotypes and subtypes differ in their geographical distribution, the resulting severity of disease and in the responsiveness to interferon treatment. For instance, interferon-alpha (IFN-alpha) treatment of genotypes 1a, 2, 3, and 5 appears to be more effective than when used for genotype 1b and 4 infections. Therefore, there is a need for routine diagnosis of HCV types and subtypes prior to treatment. There are many reports concerning HCV genotype in China [24-36]. Genotype 1b (50-80%) and 2a (10-40%) predominate in mainland China and Taiwan, whilst approximately 10-30% of patients from Hong Kong are infected with genotype 6a [28, 29, 70, 71]. Genotype 1a and 1b infections accounted for 37% and 31% in the USA, respectively [38, 75]. The genotypes found in different regions of China are summarized in Table 6.

HCV genotypes in Northeastern China

Huang et al. [24] evaluated 3,902 serum samples in the Shenyang area of Northeastern China for anti-HCV by ELISA, and 100 samples were genotyped. HCV genotypes were detected by PCR with type-specific primers. The results indicated that anti-HCV-positive rates in general populations were 0.42% to 1.66%. Anti-HCV-positive rates in the group of post-transfusion hepatitis and sporadic hepatitis (excluding HAV, HBV, EBV, CMV infection), hepatitis B post-hepatitis cirrhosis (excluding HBV infection) and HCC were significantly higher than the group of patients without liver diseases or the group of patients without transfusion ($p < 0.01$). The incidence of HCV-1b, HCV-2a, and 1b/2a mixed type were 58%, 27%, 14%, respectively. The rate of infection with HCV-2a was 80% in the normal population, but 91.7% with type 1b HCV in the group of patients with cirrhosis. These results suggested that patients with different liver diseases were at high risk of HCV infection, and that HCV 2a type was predominant, followed by HCV 1b as well as 1b/2a mixed in HCV genotype distribution in the Shenyang area.

HCV genotypes in Southwestern China

Ding et al. [25] studied 206 serum samples in the Guizhou area of Southwestern China. Thirty-five serum samples were anti-HCV-positive, and only 30 samples were positive for HCV RNA by nested PCR at 5'-noncoding region. The 30 patients consisted of 18 patients with chronic hepatitis and 12 blood recipients with hemopathy. Subtype 1b and 2a infections were found in 90% and 10% of the samples, respectively.

HCV genotypes in Eastern China

There are two interesting reports from Eastern China, specifically Shanghai. The first conducted by Jiang et al. [26] investigated the distribution and frequency of various genotypes in different populations in Shanghai using second generation HCV line probe assay. Among 81 HCV isolates from patients with HC, there were 71 (87.6%) genotype 1b, 4 (4.9%) 2a, 2 (2.5%) 3b, 1 (1.2%) 6a, 2 (2.5%) mixed genotypes (1 for 2a or 2c+2b+1, 1 for 1b+6a) and 1 (1.2%) indeterminate, respectively. Among seven isolates from blood donors, there were 5 1b and 2 genotype 2a, and among 21 from intravenous drug abusers (IVDAs), there were 8 (38.1%) genotype 1a, 5 (23.8%)1b, 2 (9.5%) 2a or 2c, 2 (9.5%) 3a, 1 (4.8%) 3b and 3 (14.3%) mixed genotypes (1 for 1a+2a or 2c, 1 for 1b+2a or 2c+6a, and 1 for 1a+1b+3b), respectively. The results showed that

Table 6. HCV genotypes in different regions of China

Region	Patients	No. of cases	HCV Genotype, % 1a	1b	2a	2b	2a or 2c	3a	3b	6a	Mixed	Unclassified	Method	Reference
Shenyang	CH	100		58	27						14		Type-specific PCR	24
Guizhou	CH	30		90	10								PCR-RFLP	25
Shanghai	CH	81		87.6	4.9				2.5	1.2	2.5	1.2	LiPA	26
	BD	7		71.4	28.6								LiPA	26
	IVDAs	17	38.1	23.8			9.5	9.5	4.8		14.3		LiPA	26
	CO	17		41.2			29.4				29.4		LiPA	27
Shanxi	CH	94		85.1	12.8						2.1		PCR-RFLP	31
Beijing	CH	49		67.3	32.7								PCR-Sequencing	32
Jilin	CH	24	20.8	66.7	12.5								PCR-Sequencing	33
Anhui	CH, BD	531	0.5	75.7	12.3	0.5					6.4		PCR-RFLP	67
Nanjing	CH	16	62.5		31.3							6.5	Sequencing	34
Taiwan	BD	562	0.4	60.1	15.5	11.9		2			6.6	3.5	Type-specific PCR	68
	CH	56		44.6	41.1	3.6					7.2	3.6	Type-specific PCR	69
	CH	100		60	15.6	8.2					15.3 (with unclassified)		PCR bDNA	30
Hong Kong	unknown	unknown		70						14			PCR-Sequencing	28
	RT	76		78	10					8			PCR-RFLP	29
	CH, CRF	172		69.6						18.8			PCR-RFLP	70
	BD	212	6.2	58.8	1.4	1.4		1.9		27			PCR-RFLP	71

Note: CH: chronic hepatitis; BD: blood donors; IVDAs: intravenous drug abusers; CO: coinfection of HIV and HCV; RT: renal transplantation; CRF: chronic renal failure.

seven HCV subtypes (1a, 1b, 2a, 2b, 3a, 3b and 6a) belonging to four HCV genotypes (1, 2, 3, 6) were present in different populations in Shanghai. Of these, 2b, 3a, 3b and 6a were first found in China, and HCV genotype 1b was most commonly found in patients with HC and blood donors. Genotype 1a and 3a were only found in IVDAs. The second report by Zhong et al. [27] focused on genotyping of HCV in the HCV and HIV-1 co-infected samples, using second-generation HCV LiPA kits. A reverse-hybridization technique was used for genotyping HCV from seventeen HCV and HIV-1 co-infected samples derived from six different high-risk geographic areas in China. The results indicated that seven (41.2%) of the samples were found to be of 1b genotype, five (29.4%) were 2a/2c genotype and five (29.4%) were mixed-genotype with 1b and 2a/2c. Notably, HCV 1b genotype, which usually fails to respond to IFN-alpha and is apt to proceed much faster to severe chronic hepatitis, cirrhosis and HCC, had a significantly higher prevalence of 12/17 (70.6%) than other subtypes in this study.

HCV genotypes in Hong Kong and Taiwan

A greater diversity of HCV genotypes was found in Hong Kong than in mainland China [28]. Although the Hong Kong Chinese patients had predominantly genotype 1b (70%), it was noteworthy that 6a was the second most common genotype (14%). Three other HCV genotypes, 1a, 2a and 2b, were also present. In contrast, HCV infection in mainland China was confined to genotypes 1b and 2a. Chan et al. [29] conducted HCV genotypes in renal transplant patients, and found that the most prevalent HCV genotype among these patients was 1b (78%), followed by 1a (10%) and 6a (8%). This result implied that in addition to viral characteristics, host factors such as the immunosuppressed state play an important role in the pathogenesis of liver disease in these patients. Chan et al. [30] detected 60% HCV 1b, 16.5% HCV 2a, 8.2% 2b and 15.2% mixed or underdetermined types in Taiwan.

HCV genotypes and interferon treatment

To study the genotypes of HCV infection in Shanxi Province and the response of HCV genotypes to interferon therapy, Zhao et al. [31] analyzed the genotypes of HCV by restriction fragment length polymorphism in 94 chronic HC patients who were positive for HCV RNA by RT-PCR. They reported that 80 patients (85.1%) were genotype 1b infection, 12 (12.8%) were genotype 2a infection and 2 (2.1%) were 1b/2a co-infection. The 45 chronic HC patients with different genotypes (35 with HCV 1b, 10 with HCV 2a) received rIFN α-1b 3 million units (MU) three times a week for six months and were followed up after 12-34 months. As expected, the response rate was significantly higher in patients with HCV 2a infection (80%) than that in patients infected with genotype 1b (37.1%) ($p < 0.05$). Sustained response was observed in 60% for 2a and in 17.1% for 1b ($p < 0.025$). The data indicated that HCV 1b is the major type of HCV infection in Shanxi Province, and HCV genotype seems to be an important factor in determining the response rate to interferon treatment in patients with chronic HCV infection.

Chronic HCV infection and interferon treatment

IFN-α is the only drug approved for the treatment of HCV infection in many countries. Its effectiveness appears to be related to dose and duration of therapy. Yao et al. [37] reported that IFN-α 2a is effective in the treatment of Chinese patients with chronic HCV infection, and the sustained response rates and adverse drug reactions between two schedules (a dose of 3 MU of IFN-α 2a three time times per week for six months, and a starting dose of 6 MU for three months and subsequent reduction to 3 MU three times per week for a further 3 months) are similar. However, the degrees of response to IFN treatment [interferon responses were defined as: (1) prolonged response during the period of treatment is referred to as sustained response, SR; (2) a future response of at least six months after cessation of therapy is regarded as long-term response, LTR; (3) if there are only minor or no changes in some parameters, such as serum levels of ALT and clearance of HCV RNA, in some treated cases, it should be defined as nonresponse or poor response, NR or PR] seem to be associated with HCV genotypes or subtypes and genomic diversity. Among patients treated with 3 MU of IFN-α three times per week for six months, overall LTRs are only 15-25%, only 4-8% of cases infected with HCV subtype 1b are LTR, while genotype 1a (15-20% LTR), 2a/2b (30-40% LTR) and 3a (35-50% LTR) respond more favorably [38]. In patients with HCV genotype 1b infection, a substantial correlation between the ALT response and genomic diversity was suggested [31, 39-42], but this correlation was not shown in other studies [37, 43]. Since HCV genotype 1b is the most common genotype in China, there are many patients with HCV 1b infection who cannot respond to IFN-α treatment, although the efficacy of IFN-alpha in the treatment of Chinese patients with chronic HCV infection has been reported [37]. The combination of ribavirin with interferon is being evaluated in Chinese patients.

Coinfection of hepatotropic viruses

Since HBV and HCV share similar routes of transmission, coinfection by hepatotropic viruses and/or HIV or HGV can occur. This situation is of special clinical significance.

Superinfection of HBV and HCV

In a recent study of 712 patients with HBV infection, anti-HCV-positive rates were 3.3%, 14.3%, 49.0% and 15.4% in patients with acute, chronic, and severe hepatitis and liver cirrhosis, respectively [44]. There were markedly different anti-HCV-positive rates ($p < 0.0001$) in patients of different clinical stages. Of 103 patients with superinfection of HBV and HCV, serum HBsAg, HBeAg and anti-HBcIgM-positive rates were statistically significantly lower than those in patients with hepatitis B, but the anti-HBe positive rates were higher.

HIV and hepatitis virus infection in Chinese drug addicts [45]

The prevalence of antibody against HCV (anti-HCV) and five HBV markers were measured in 176 Chinese drug addicts, of whom 23 were AIDS patients. Of 176 drug addicts, 147 were members of ethnic minorities, while 29 were Han, the majority ethnic group. The total prevalence rates of anti-HCV and HBV markers were 35.8% and 50.6%, respectively ($p < 0.01$). Both anti-HCV and HBV markers were found in 22.7% of the samples. Similar prevalence rates were found among the different ethnic groups. Among the ethnic minorities, there was a significantly higher prevalence rate of anti-HCV in IVDAs (51.1%) than in oral drug addicts (20.3%). Furthermore, the prevalence of anti-HCV was significantly higher in needle-sharing abusers (60.4%) than in non-needle sharing ones (37.1%, $p < 0.05$). The prevalence of HBV markers was also significantly higher in needle-sharing abusers (69.8%) than in non-needle sharing ones (34.3%). Prevalence of HBsAg was significantly higher in drug abusers with HIV (47.8%) than in IVDAs only (16.1%). The anti-HCV-positive rates among ethnic minority people were: for the Yi, 69.2%, the Hui, 55.6%, the Bai, 53.9%, the Dai, 26.8% and the Wa, 23.1%. No obvious difference was identified for HBV markers. The prevalence rates of HCV, HBV and HCV + HBV in IVDAs showed no significant difference between the two regions. HIV, HCV and HBV infections may be related to needle-sharing behavior in drug abuse and to different subcultures and living habits.

Multiple infection with hepatitis B, C and G viruses

To study the possibility of superinfection and multiple infection in patients with hepatitis G virus (HGV) infection, Du et al. [46] applied an RT-PCR technique in the non-structural gene 3 (NS3) region of HGV to detect HGV RNA in serially-diluted, quality-control sera and an HGV-C reference panel of samples. These samples included 90 that were positive for HCV RNA, and 12 samples were from blood donors with superinfection of HBV and HCV. Serially-diluted, quality-control sera were positive for HGV RNA at dilutions of 10^{-1} to 10^{-5}, but were negative at dilutions of 10^{-6} to 10^{-8}. HGV RNA was positive in two samples of control HGV-C serum. HGV RNA was positive in eight of the 90 HCV samples and in four of the 12 cases with superinfection with HCV and HBV. These are not only superinfections of HBV and HCV, but also multiple infections.

Precore stop codon mutation and coinfection of HBV and HCV [47]

In order to study the mutation of HBV precore gene in patients with dual infections of HBV and HCV, and its possible clinical significance, the precore stop codon mutation (stop 28) was analyzed by PCR and restriction fragment length polymorphism (RFLP) in patients with chronic liver disease. These included 25 cases with HBV DNA and HCV RNA positive (group A) and 31 cases with HBsAg and HBV DNA positive, but anti-HCV and HCV RNA negative (group B). The results demonstrated that the serum HBV DNA-positive rate by the first PCR in patients with dual infections (group A, 16%) was significantly lower than that in patients with HBV infection alone (group B, 65%).

The stop codon-positive rate was also significantly lower (28% *versus* 68%). The results suggest that the low frequency of precore stop codon mutants in patients with HBV and HCV dual infections was possibly due to low replication of HBV.

Conclusion

Viral hepatitis A, B, C, D, and E are important public health problems in China. However, HBV and HCV overshadow the other viruses because of their severe and frequent sequelae, such as chronic hepatitis, cirrhosis and primary hepatocellular carcinoma, which can seriously imperil the health and life of infected individuals. Epidemiological patterns for HBV and HCV infection in China are different from those in other advanced countries in several ways, such as high prevalence of infection, high ratio of chronic to acute infection, high risk of maternal-infant transmission, high rate of mutation of viral genes and poor response to IFN treatment. In the absence of combination treatment with powerful anti-HBV drugs, resistant HBV is likely to occur. Thus, it may be preferable to use monotherapy approaches such as lamivudine sparingly. There is a critical need for effective and safe therapies for HCV. Clearly, Interferon is usually ineffective in Chinese patients, because genotype 1b predominates in this population. Orally bioavailable, powerful HCV drugs are desperately needed. The need to continue prevention programs and childhood vaccination for HBV are essential. Education and improved social services will decrease the rate of infection for both HBV and HCV in China. Further studies on sera and the molecular epidemiology of HBV and HCV infections should contribute to improved vaccination control and provide the basis for the development of specific therapies for these infections.

Acknowledgement

This work was supported in part by Emory University Center for AIDS Research, and NIH grant AI-41980.

References

1 Liu C. Study on epidemiological characterization and epidemical factors of viral hepatitis population in China. *Chin J Hepatol* 1998; 6(2):67-700

2 Xu Z, Zhao S, Mahoney RT, Deng X, Lin X, Xu J and Ding D. Epidemiology and control of hepatitis B and C in eastern Asian. In *Therapies for Viral Hepatitis*, 1998; pp. 13-18. Edited by RF Schinazi, JP Sommadossi and H Thomas. International Medical Press.

3 Wu SM. Ten year follow-up study of 52 chronic HBsAg carriers. *Chin J Infect Dis* 1984; 2:36-39

4 Jiang Y. Approaches in Viral Hepatitis. *Progress in Epidemiology*. Beijing: People's Press, 1988: 122-123

5 Ye B, Shen J, Xu Y. Etiologic study on the relationship between HBV, HCV and HCC. *Chin J Epidemiol* 1994; 15(3):131-134

6 Yu SZ, Zi XL, Chen G. The relationship between viral hepatitis and primary liver cancer in four areas of China. *Chin J Epidemiol* 1997; 18(4):214-216

7 Zhang JY, Wang X, Han SG, Lu WQ, Zhang MX, Wang KJ, Han SG, Zhou YF and Zhuang H. A case-control study of risk factors for hepatocellular carcinoma in Henan, China. *Am J Trop Med Hyg* 1998; 59(6):947-951

8 Luo TY, Pan NQ. A study on the multiple factorial causation of hepatoma among young patients. *Chin J Epidemiol* 1997; 18(1):37-39

9 Wang SS, Jian PL, Pang HX. An epidemiological study on the etiology of primary hepatocellular carcinoma in Guangzhou, Guangdong Province. *Chin J Epidemiol* 1997; 18(1):33-36

10 Stuyver L, Gendt SD, Van Geyt C, Zoulim F, Fried M, Schinazi RF and Rossau R. A new genotype of hepatitis B virus: Complete genome and phylogenetic relatedness. *J Gen Virol* 2000; 81(1):67-74

11 Guo Y, Hou J, and Dai W. Establishment of the consensus sequence of hepatitis B virus prevailing in the mainland of China. *Chin J Microbiol Immunol* 1999; 19(3):197-200

12 Fan J, Zhuang H, and Li Y. Comparison of sequences of hepatitis B virus S gene fragment in eight cities of China. *Chin J Pre Med* 1997; 31(3):140-143

13 Zhang YY, Nordenfelt E, Hansson BG. Increasing heterogeneity of the 'a' determinant of HBsAg found in the presumed late phase of chronic hepatitis B virus infection. *Scand J Infect Dis* 1996; 28(1):9-15

14 He JW, Lu Q, Zhu QR, Duan SC and Wen YM. Mutations in the 'a' determinant of hepatitis B surface antigen among Chinese infants receiving active post-exposure hepatitis B immunization. *Vaccine* 1998; 16(2-3):170-173

15 Tu H, Xiong SD, Trepo C and Wen YM. Frequency of hepatitis virus e-minus mutants varies among patients from different area of China. *J Med Virol* 1997; 51(2):85-89

16 Lai CL. Antiviral therapy for hepatitis B and C in Asians. *J Gastroenterol Hepatol* 1999; 14(Suppl):S19-21

17 Lai CL, Chien RN, Leung NW, Chang TT, Guan R, Tai DI, Ng KY, Wu PC, Dent JC, Barber J, Stephenson SL and Gray DF. A one-year trial of lamivudine for chronic hepatitis B. Asia Hepatitis Lamivudine Study Group. *N Engl J Med* 1998; 339(2):61-68

18 Yao G, Wang B and Cui Z. Long-term effect of Lamivudine treatment in chronic hepatitis B virus infection. *Chin J Hepatol* 1999; 7(2):80-83

19 Tao QM, Wang Y, Wang H. Preliminary report on seroepidemiology of HCV and HBV infection in northern China. *Chin Med J* 1992; 105(3):209-211

20 Lee SD, Chan CY and Wang YJ. Seroepidemiology of hepatitis C virus infection in Taiwan. *Hepatology* 1991; 13:830-833

21 Tao Q. Investigation of anti-hepatitis C virus in the sera of different population of Beijing. *Natl Med J Chin* 1992; 72(1):18-20, 62-63

22 Zhang GQ, Chen SD, Lian JH. Seroepidemiological study of HBV and HCV infection in sexually promiscuous group. *Chin J Epidemiol* 1995; 16(4):213-216

23 Tang B, Tong L and Yan Q. A survey on HIV and HV infection of heroin addicts in Linchang and Kunming. *Chin J Pre Med* 1995; 29(4):228-230

24 Huang F, Cai C and Zhao G. Study on HCV genotypes in different clinical types of hepatitis C patients in Shenyang area. *Chin J Exp Clin Virol* 1999; 13(1):64-67

25 Ding J, Akira T, Noriko Y, Mikihiro T and Takayasu D. Study of hepatitis C genotype in Guizhou area of southwestern China. *Chin Med J* 1998; 111(2):128-132

26 Jiang W, Gu S and Hu Y. Genotyping of HCV isolates from different population in Shanghai by using second-generation line probe assay. *Chin J Hepatol* 1999; 7(1):29-31

27 Zhong P, Duan J and Liu G. Genotyping of HCV in the HCV and HIV-1 co-infected samples. *Chin J Infect Dis* 1998; 16(4):209-211

28 Zhang YY, Lok AS, Chan DT and Widell A. Greater diversity of hepatitis C virus genotypes found in Hong Kong than in mainland China. *J Clin Microbiol* 1995; 33(11):2931-2934

29 Chan TM, Lau JY, Wu PC, Lai LC, Lok AS and Cheng IK. Hepatitis C virus genotypes in patients on renal replacement therapy. *Nephro Dial Transplant* 1998; 13(3):731-734

30 Chan CY, Lee SD, Hwang SJ, Lu RH, Lu CL and Lo KJ. Quantitative branched DNA assay and genotyping for hepatitis C virus RNA in Chinese patients with acute and chronic hepatitis C. *J Infect Dis* 1995; 171(2):443-446

31 Zhao H, Cheng B, Guo H. Genotypic analysis of hepatitis C viruses and its significance in interferon treatment. *Chin J Exp Clin Virol* 1998; 12(1):15-17

32 Wei L, Wang Y, Du S, Wang H and Tao Q. Genetic variability and characterization of non-structural region 5 of hepatitis C virus genome from Chinese patients. *J Gastroenterol* 1998; 33(1):62-72

33 Niu J, Kumar U, Pan Y, Liu Y, Zhan Q, Thomas H and Monjardino J. Hepatitis C virus type I (1a) in northern China. *J Med Virol* 1995; 46(1):56-60

34 Suzuki K, Mizokami M, Cao K, Wu XS, Wu RR, Hata A, Sasaki M, Fang ZX, Zhang LY, Lau JY and Iino S. Prevalence of hepatitis C virus infection in Nanjing, southern China. *Eur J Epidemiol* 1997; 13(5):511-515

35 Wu RR, Mizokami M Lau JY, Ohno T, Fang ZX, Wu XS, Hata A, Sasaki M and Iino S. Seroprevalence of hepatitis C virus infection and its genotype in Lanzhou, western China. *J Med Virol* 1995; 45(2):174-178

36 Cui XH, Pan W and Qi ZT. Genotyping of hepatitis C virus in patients with hepatocellular carcinoma. *Chin Med J* 1995; 75(2):92-93, 126-127

37 Yao G, Ji Y, Yang M, Xu D, Gao J, Wu X, Zhang Q and Hu D. Long-term efficacy of recombinant interferon alpha 2a in the treatment of chronic hepatitis C: a randomized prospective study comparing schedules in Chinese patients. *Chin Med J* 1998; 111(10):922-926

38 Maertens G and Stuyver L. Genotypes and genetic variation of hepatitis C virus. In *The Molecular Medicine of Viral Hepatitis*. Edited by Harrison TJ and Zucerman AJ. John Wiley & Sons Ltd 1997:183-233

39 Martinot-Peignoux M, Marcellin P, Pouteau M, Castelnau C, Boyer N, Poliquin M, Degott C, Descombes I, Le Breton V, Milotova V, Benhamou JP and Erlinger S. Pretreatment serum hepatitis C virus genotype are the main and independent prognostic factors of sustained response to interferon alpha therapy in chronic hepatitis C. *Hepatology* 1995; 22:1050-1056

40 Enomoto N, Sakuma I, Asahina Y, Kurosaki M, Murakami T, Yamamoto C, Ogura Y, Izumi N, Marumo F and Sato C. Mutations in the nonstructural protein 5A gene and response to interferon in patients with chronic hepatitis C virus 1b infection. *N Eng J Med* 1996; 334:77-81

41 Kurosaki M, Enomoto N, Murakami T, Sakuma I, Asahina Y, Yamamoto C, Ikeda T, Tozuka S, Izumi N, Marumo F and Sato C. Analysis of genotypes and amino acid residues 2209 to 2248 of theNS5A region of hepatitis C virus in relation to the response to interferon-beta therapy. *Hepatology* 1997; 25(3):750-3

42 Wei L, Tao Q, Sun Y, Wang H. Interaction between variability of nonstructural gene 5b of hepatitis C virus and interferon therapy. *Chin J Microbiol Immunol* 1999; 19(4):330-333

43 Chung RT, Monto A, Dienstag JL and Kaplan LM. NS5A mutations do not predict response to interferon in American patients infected with genotype 1 hepatitis C virus. *Gastroenterology* 1997; 112:A1244

44 Chen X, Wu D, and Yin Y. Study of superinfection of HBV and HCV. *Chin J Epidemiol* 1999; 20(3):141-143

45 Baozhang T, Kaining Z, Jinxing K, Ming L, Caixia Z and Li T. Infection with human immunodeficiency virus and hepatitis viruses in Chinese drug addicts. *Epidemiol Infect* 1997; 119(3):343-347

46 Du S, Tao Q, Chang J. Studies on multiple infection with hepatitis B, C and G viruses. *Chin J Pre Med* 1998; 32(1):11-13

47 Qiu W, Hou J and Lou K. Low frequency of precore stop mutation in patients with dual infection of hepatitis B and C viruses. *Chin J Exp Clin Virol* 1998; 12(2):123-125

48 Chen HL, Chang MH, Ni YH, Hsu HY, Lee PI, Lee CY and Chen DS. Seroepidemiology of hepatitis B virus infection in children: Ten years of mass vaccination in Taiwan. *JAMA* 1996; 276(11):906-908

49 Chuang WL, Chang WY, Lu SN, Lin ZY, Chen SC, Hsieh MY, Wang LY, You SL and Chen CJ. The role of hepatitis C virus in chronic hepatitis B virus infection. *Gastroenterol Jpn* 1993; 28(Suppl 5):23-27

50 Cheng H. Epidemiologic studies on HCV and HBV infections among intravenous drug users in the area with HIV infection. *Chin J Epidemiol* 1993; 14(5):275-278

51 Cao K, Mizokami M, Orito E, Ding X, Ge XM, Huang GY and Ueda R. TT virus infection among IVDUs in south western China. *Scand J Infect Dis* 1999; 31(1):21-25

52 Wu JS, Lu CF, Liu WT and Lin SY. Prevalence of antibodies to hepatitis C virus (anti-HCV) in different populations in Taiwan. *Chung Hua Min Kuo Wei Sheng Wu Chi Mien I Husueh Tsa Chih* 1991; 24(1):55-60

53 Pang Z, Chu Q, and Xu Y. Research on risk factors of 5 types of viral hepatitises among population with high-risk behaviors. *Chin J Epidemiol* 1998; 19(3):141-143

54 Zhang GQ, Chen SD and Lian JH. Seroepidemiological study of HBV and HCV infection in sexually promiscuous groups. *Chin J Epidemiol* 1995; 16(4):213-216

55 Xie Z. Hepatitis B virus infection in hemodialysis patients. *Chin J Epidemiol* 1992; 13(1):12-15

56 Ko YC, Ho MS, Chiang TA, Chang ST and Chang PY. Tattooing as a risk of hepatitis C infection. *J Med Virol* 1992; 38(4):288-291

57 Chen LJ, Yang DL and Yu ZQ. A prevalence study on HBV and HCV infection status in patients with hemopathy. *Chin J Epidemiol* 1996; 17(2):74-76

58 She SL, Shi LY, Wu YJ, Li ZZ, Zheng CZ, Wu YP and Yu XH. A seroepidemiologic study of hepatitis B virus infection among barbers in Huangshi City, Hubei, China. *Microbiol Immunol* 1998; 32(2):229-233

59 Honkoop P, Niesters HG, de Man RA, Osterhaus AD and Schalm SW. Lamivudine resistance in immunocompetent chronic hepatitis B. *J Hepatol* 1997; 26(6):1393 -1395

60 Buti M, Rosendo J, Francisco R, Montse C, Xose C, Carles P, Rafael E, Jaume G. Rapid detection of lamivudine-resistant hepatitis B virus polymerase gene variants. *Hepatology* 1999; 30(4, Pt. 2):444A

61 Perrillo R, Rakela J, Dienstag J, Levy G, Martin P, Wright T, Caldwell S, Schiff E, Gish R, Villeneuve JP, Farr G, Anschuetz G, Crowther L, Brown N and the Lamivudine Transplant Group. Multicenter study of lamivudine therapy for hepatitis B after liver transplantation. *Hepatology* 1999; 29(5):1581-1586

62 Dienstag JL, Schiff ER, Wright TL, Perrillo RP, Hann HL, Goodman Z, Crowther L, Condreay LD, Woessner M, Rubin M and Brown NA. Lamivudine as initial treatment for chronic hepatitis B in the United States. *New Engl J Med* 1999; 341(17):1256-1263

63 Tassopoulos NC, Volpes R, Pastore G, Heathcote J, Buti M, Goldin RD, Hawley S, Barber J, Condreay L, Gray DF and the Lamivudine Precore Mutant study Group. Efficacy of lamivudine in patients with hepatitis B e antigen-negative/hepatitis B virus DNA-positive (precore mutant) chronic hepatitis B.

Hepatology 1999; 29(3):889-896

64 Dienstag JL, Schiff ER, Mitchell M, Casey Jr DE, Gitlin N, Lissoos T, Gelb LD, Condreay L, Crowther L, Rubin M and Brown N. Extended lamivudine retreatment for chronic hepatitis B: maintenance of viral suppression after discontinuation of therapy. *Hepatology* 1999; 30(4):1082-1087

65 Benhamou Y, Bochet M, Thibault V, Di Martino V, Caumes E, Bricaire F, Opolon P, Katlama C and Poynard T. Long-term incidence of hepatitis B virus resistance to lamivudine in human immunodeficiency virus-infected patients. *Hepatology* 1999; 30(5):1302-1306

66 Liaw YF, Chien RN, Yeh CT, Tsai SL and Chu CM. Acute exacerbation and hepatitis B virus clearance after emergence of YMDD motif mutation during lamivudine therapy. *Hepatology* 1999; 30(2):567-572

67 Su H, Wu XK, Ni JF. An investigation on genotypes of hepatitis C virus in Anhui province. *Chin J Epidemiol* 1997; 18(4):205-207

68 Wu CH, Lee MF, Kuo HS. Distribution of hepatitis C virus genotypes among blood donors in Taiwan. *J Gastroenterol Hepatol* 1997; 12(9-10):625-628

69 Yu ML, Chuang WL, Lu SN, Chen SC, Wang JH, Lin ZY, Hsieh MY, Wang LY and Chang WY. The genotypes of hepatitis C virus in patients with chronic hepatitis C virus infection in southern Taiwan. *Kao Hsiung J Med Sci* 1996; 12(11)605-612

70 Wong DA, Tong TK, Lim W. High prevalence of hepatitis C genotype 6 among certain risk groups in Hong Kong. *Eur J Epidemiol* 1998; 14(5):421-426

71 Prescott LE, Simmonds P, Lai CL, Chan NK, Pike I, Yap PL and Lin CK. Detection and clinical features of hepatitis C virus type 6 infections in blood donors from Hong Kong. *J Med Viol* 1996; 50(2):168-175

72 Lai CL, Liaw YF, Leung NWY, Deslauries M, Barnard J, Sanathanan L, Gray DF and Condreay LD. Genotypic resistance to lamivudine in a prospective, placebo-controlled multicenter study in Asia of lamivudine therapy for chronic hepatitis B infection: incidence, kinetics of emergence, and correlation with disease parameters. *Hepatology* 1997; 26(Suppl 4):259A

73 Leung NWY, Lai CL, Chang TT. Three years lamivudine in chronic HBV. *J Hepatol* 1999; 30(Suppl 1):59

74 Alter MJ and Shapiro CN. Epidemiology and prevention of chronic hepatitis B and C in North and South America. In *Therapies for Viral Hepatitis*, 1998; pp. 7-12. Edited by RF Schinazi, JP Sommadossi and H Thomas. International Medical Press.

75 Mahaney K, Tedeschi V, Maerten G, Di Bisceglie AM, Vergalla J, Hoofnagle JH and Sallie R. Genotypic analysis of hepatitis C virus in American patients. *Hepatology* 1994; 20(6):1405-1411

New viruses and their relationship to hepatitis

HARVEY J. ALTER

Chief Infectious Diseases Section,
Associate Director for Research, Department of Transfusion Medicine,
Warren Grant Magnuson Clinical Center, NIH, Bethesda, MD

Abstract

Ten to 20% of community-acquired and transfusion-associated hepatitis cases, 20%-30% of chronic hepatitis cases and perhaps 50% of fulminant hepatitis cases have no defined etiology. Because these cases have similar characteristics to hepatitis cases of established viral origin, there has been an intensive effort to discover new viral agents utilizing molecular technology. This has led to the discovery of the GB virus and its variant, the hepatitis G virus (HGV), and more recently to discovery of the TT virus family that includes the SEN virus. The GB agent and the hepatitis G virus (HGV) are RNA viruses in the flaviviridae family. Extensive investigations have failed to show that these agents play a causal role in cases of acute or chronic liver disease.

The TT Virus (TTV) has been shown to be a small, non-enveloped, single-stranded, circular DNA virus in the family of circoviridae. Circoviruses are classically animal viruses, and they have not previously been known to cause human disease. It is now clear that TTV is a heterogeneous group of agents that can be transmitted to humans by both parenteral and non-parenteral routes. The agent is found throughout the world, but in particularly high prevalence in Japan, where TTV has been detected in from 12% to 93% of healthy persons. Although initially implicated in fulminant hepatitis and cryptogenic chronic liver disease, these associations have not been confirmed, and presently there are no proven disease associations for this agent.

Continued molecular studies on TTV revealed increasing diversity, and new members of the family have been identified that differ from the prototype strain by as much as 50% in nucleotide sequence and as much as 70% in amino acid content. The SEN virus (SEN-V), which like TTV was named after the initials of the patient in whom it was found, was discovered independently using amplification strategies with highly degenerate TTV primers. Two SEN-V variants (SEN-D and SEN-C/H) have been studied extensively and have been found as acute infections in 11 of 12 (93%) of transfusion-transmitted, non-A to E hepatitis cases. This proportion is significantly different from the 24% prevalence in patients without hepatitis ($p < 0.001$), but extrapolation shows that no more than 6% of SEN-V infections are associated with hepatitis. Whether this strong statistical association indicates a causal role for this agent in the development of transfusion-associated hepatitis is uncertain at this time. There is

Frontiers in Viral Hepatitis Ed. by RF Schinazi, J-P Sommadossi and CM Rice. 35 — 46

no current evidence that SEN-V is a cause of fulminant hepatitis, hepatitis-associated aplastic anemia or cryptogenic chronic liver disease.

Thus there appears to be a new complex super-family of non-enveloped single-stranded, circular DNA viruses whose clinical relevance is uncertain. There is a need to confirm intrahepatic localization and replication, to define optimal primer sets and to do large, systematic, controlled investigations to determine if any of these agents play an etiologic role in liver disease or disease of other organ systems.

Introduction

Cloning of the hepatitis C virus (HCV) [8] dramatically changed the paradigm for viral discovery. HCV was discovered in the absence of a tissue culture system, an observed particle, a serologic assay or a means to measure *in vitro* or *in-vivo* replication. Substituting for these classic virologic methods was blind cloning, immuno-screening of expressed proteins and the detection of novel nucleic acid sequences. A novel sequence and/or a gene product observed in the majority of patients with non-A, non-B hepatitis, and rarely in controls without hepatitis, proved sufficient to establish causality and to develop sensitive diagnostic assays that have virtually eliminated transmission by blood transfusion. The new paradigm of viral discovery bypasses tissue culture, electron microscopy and small animal models and advances directly to molecular virology. Hence, in search of non-A-E agents, the hepatitis G virus was discovered by sequence independent single primer amplification (SISPA) [9], the GB group of viruses (GBV-A, GBV-B, GBV-C) [18] by representational difference analysis (RDA), a form of subtractive cloning, the TTV family, including TT virus [13], Sanban [6], and Yonban, by RDA, and the SEN virus by using highly degenerate TTV primers followed by amplification and sequencing. None of these more recent molecular discoveries have been proven to have clinical relevance, but most are still under investigation. It is probable that these advanced techniques will lead to a continuing series of "new agents", each of which will be extensively investigated for clinical associations and causal linkage. The commercial success of the hepatitis C virus discovery will continue to drive these investigations, and the critical issue will remain, when does a novel sequence become a relevant infectious agent? In this chapter, I will address the evidence that there might be a hepatitis agent beyond hepatitis virus E (HEV) and describe the candidate agents thus far reported, particularly TTV, Sanban, Yonban and SEN.

Evidence for additional hepatitis agents

One of the remarkable features of the HCV discovery (Kuo G, et al., 1989) was that this agent accounted for the vast majority of previously unexplained hepatitis cases. Nonetheless, a retrospective analysis of prospectively-followed transfusion recipients in the NIH series [1] revealed that 12% of non-A, non-B hepatitis cases were unrelated to HCV infection. The majority of non-A, non-B, non-C (non-ABC) cases had asymptomatic infection and mild biochemical abnormalities, but more marked ALT elevations were noted in some, and approximately 20% appeared to develop chronic hepatitis. More severe non-ABC hepatitis cases were observed in the CDC Sentinel Counties studies [3] that focused on overt, community-acquired hepatitis. In the CDC studies, 18% of cases were serologically and molecularly unrelated to hepatitis viruses A, B, or C. Hence, although the established hepatitis viruses, HAV, HBV and HCV accounted for the majority of both transfusion-related and community-acquired hepatitis, approximately 10%-20% of such cases might be due to additional, unrecognized hepatitis agents. In addition, as sensitive tests for HCV were applied to patients with non-A, non-B fulminant hepatitis, it became apparent that HCV was rarely implicated in these cases. It was thus speculated that novel hepatitis agents might be responsible for fulminant hepatitis cases that did not have an established viral or toxic etiology. Additional clinical evidence for a non-ABC hepatitis agent derived from studies of hepatitis-associated aplastic anemia [5]. In these cases, often occurring in children, a classic case of clinical hepatitis was followed in one to two months by severe aplastic anemia that was otherwise indistinguishable from idiopathic aplastic anemia. Lastly, up to 30% of cases of chronic hepatitis and cirrhosis have no identified etiology and are designated cryptogenic [2]. Thus, in five different settings (transfusion-associated hepatitis, community-acquired hepatitis, fulminant hepatitis, hepatitis-associated aplastic anemia and cryptogenic chronic hepatitis), an argument could be made for the existence of at least one additional human hepatitis agent. Conversely, the possibility exists that these cases represent cryptic manifestations of known hepatitis agents, particularly HBV and HCV, or represent noninfectious causes of hepatitis, such as unrecognized drug-toxicity. Indeed, in some of these cases, HBV and HCV have been found in liver tissue in the absence of serologic or molecular markers in the blood.

Paradoxically, as efforts to discover the agent of non-A to E hepatitis intensified, the incidence of such infections declined. Testing donors for antibody to HCV has not only reduced the incidence of transfusion-associated hepatitis C to near zero, but has also resulted in a marked decline in non-A to E hepatitis. Similarly, in recent analyses of the CDC Sentinel Counties studies, there has been an absolute decline in non-A to E cases, as well as those due to HCV. It thus appears that measures, such as needle exchange programs, that result in a decline of hepatitis C also diminish cases of non-A to E hepatitis. It is probable that HCV and the postulated non A to E virus traverse the same epidemiologic routes and reside in the same individuals, such that exclusion/prevention of the known agent simultaneously impacts on the unknown agent. Whatever, the relationship between the known and the unknown, the possibility that a clinically significant non-A to E agent(s) exists incited interest in both the academic and commercial scientific community and spurred the establishment of several viral discovery programs. These programs sequentially led to the discoveries of GB virus (types A, B and C) [18], the hepatitis G virus (HGV) [9], the TT virus (TTV) [13], the TTV-related viruses Sanban [6] and Yonban, the TTV-Like Mini Virus (TLMV) [19] and the SEN virus (SEN-V) [20]. These viruses and their interrelationships are discussed below.

GB agents and hepatitis G virus

In the 1950s, a surgeon whose initials were G.B. developed acute icteric hepatitis. In that decade, prior to the discovery of any hepatitis agent, the GB serum was extensively investigated for the presence of a transmissible hepatitis virus. There was initial success when the GB serum was inoculated into marmosets and reproducibly caused hepatitis in that animal model. Serial passage in marmosets was achieved and the GB agent seemingly fulfilled criteria for a transmissible hepatitis virus. However, after initial enthusiasm, debate ensued as to whether this represented a human hepatitis agent or the reactivation of a marmoset hepatitis agent. The debate was never fully resolved, and no additional data came forth to prove that the GB agent was a human hepatitis virus. Interest in this agent then waned, especially after the discovery of hepatitis viruses A, B and C. However, in the 1990s, following the recognition that there might be a non-ABC human hepatitis agent, investigators at Abbott Laboratories resurrected the GB story. Using frozen samples from serial passages in the marmoset, Abbott investigators used representational difference analysis (RDA) to compare pre- and post-inoculation marmoset sera [18]. Following selective amplification and subtractive cloning, a unique nucleic acid sequence was found in the post-inoculation specimen and shown to be absent in serum obtained from the marmoset prior to receipt of the GB inoculum. The sequence was expanded until the full genome was identified. Subsequently, it became apparent that there was more than one GB agent, and these were designated GBV-A, GBV-B and GBV-C. The genomic structure identified these agents as flaviviridae, but they showed little homology to HCV or other members of that family. Extensive population studies, studies of patients with and without liver disease and studies of marmosets established that GBV-A was a primary marmoset agent, that GBV-C was a human virus, and that GBV-B might be able to infect both species.

In independent investigations conducted at Gene Labs, Inc. in collaboration with investigators at NIH and the CDC, an agent was identified using an amplification strategy that did not require foreknowledge of the viral sequence [9]. This method, sequence independent single primer amplification (SISPA), amplified a nucleic acid sequence that was novel to the Gene Bank, coded for a gene product that induced antibodies in humans, occurred in some patients with non-A, non-B hepatitis, and was recovered from the original patient serum as well as the amplified clonal derivative. This agent was originally thought to be a novel hepatitis virus and was designated the hepatitis G virus (HGV). By "walking the genome" the investigators identified HGV as a flavivirus distinct from HCV [9]. Subsequent sequence comparisons revealed that GBV-C and HGV were essentially the same agent, representing strain variants of a new member of the flaviviridae family. Disappointingly, clinical studies showed that although GBV-C/HGV was transmitted by blood transfusion and found in cases of community-acquired non-ABC hepatitis, there was no apparent causal relationship between the presence of the virus and the development of hepatitis. In studies of transfusion-associated hepatitis [1a], it was shown that the agent was found in two to four percent of blood donors, that it was readily transmitted by blood transfusion, and that it could lead to persistent infection in recipients. Nonetheless, the virus was found with equal frequency in patients who did and did not develop hepatitis, and no consistent relationship was shown between the level of viremia and the degree of liver damage. Further, the agent has not been proved to replicate in the liver. Rather, PCR identification of the agent in liver tissue appears to reflect contamination from serum and/or circulating blood cells [16]. Despite extensive worldwide investigations over the past decade, GBV-C/HGV has not been shown to cause hepatitis or other known liver or non-liver disease.

TT virus

In 1997, Nishizawa and coworkers (1997) in Japan employed RDA to compare pre- and post-hepatitis sera from five patients with transfusion-associated hepatitis (TAH). A viral clone, designated N22, yielded a 500-nucleotide sequence that showed little homology to published sequences and that was of nonhuman origin. This sequence was absent prior to the onset of hepatitis and was subsequently found in three of the five TAH cases studied. In addition, there was a correlation between the titer of the virus and the level of ALT. The novel sequence was originally isolated from the serum of a patient whose initials were TT, and the presumed virus was then designated the TT virus (TTV). Biophysical characterization by investigators in Dr. Makoto Mayumi's lab [15] revealed several important features of the agent: 1) the agent banded in sucrose gradients at 1.26 g/cm^3 and in cesium chloride at 1.31-1.32 g/cm^3, suggesting that it was particle associated; 2) the band density did not change after treatment with Tween 80, suggesting that it was non-enveloped; 3) the genome was shown to be sensitive to DNase I and Mung Bean Nuclease, suggesting that it represented single-stranded DNA; 4) the full sequence consisted of 3,739 bases, and it appeared to contain at least two open reading frames. These data, in composite, suggested that TTV was a novel, non-enveloped, single-stranded human DNA virus. The agent showed no significant homology to established human hepatitis viruses and initially was thought to be a new member of the parvovirus family. Further studies, however, showed that the DNA in TTV was circular and that the agent was most closely related to circoviridae, a family of animal and plant viruses, not previously associated with human disease (Mushahwar IK, 1999). A representative circovirus is the chicken anemia virus. Continued investigations into TTV showed considerable diversity among isolates. It was initially classified into two genetic groups that differed by 30% and were designated G1 and G2, and then into subgroups that differed in sequences by 11%-15%, resulting in the classifications of G1a and G1b as well as G2a and G2b. The genetic diversity has continued to expand as more and more isolates have been studied and in 1999, Okamoto [15] reported that TTV could be classified into at least 16 genotypes separated by an evolutionary distance of >0.30. Sequence divergence among the most separated members of the family exceeds 50%.

TTV has been claimed to replicate in the liver based on PCR detection of the genome in the liver at titers equal to or greater than that in the serum. While such data are suggestive of hepatotropism, more definitive evidence has recently been reported by in-situ hybridization. Rodriguez-Inigo, et al. (2000) in Spain analyzed the presence of TTV DNA by PCR and in-situ hybridization in liver biopsies from 30 patients with liver disease, among whom 15 were TTV-DNA positive and 15 TTV-DNA negative in serum. They also tested the livers from eight patients without liver disease. TTV DNA was detected in the liver of each of the 15 patients with liver disease in whom it was detected in serum, and the TTV DNA titers in the liver were generally 10 times higher than in serum. TTV DNA was also detected in two of eight normal livers from TTV-positive patients. In-situ hybridization showed a positive signal in the 17 patients infected with TTV, but in none of the TTV-negative patients. The percentage of positive hepatocytes ranged from 2% to 30% and correlated with TTV DNA titers in the liver. There were no morphologic changes in the liver cells that showed hybridization signals, and there was no correlation between the percentage of TTV-infected hepatocytes and the histologic activity index or its composite scores. Thus, although this study indicates that TTV can infect liver cells, it does not establish this agent's role in the causation of hepatitis. Proof that TTV replicates in the liver is still lacking and will require the demonstration of replicative intermediates within hepatocytes.

Epidemiologic studies have confirmed that TTV is a parenterally transmitted agent, as demonstrated by donor-recipient linkage in transfused patients and by a high prevalence among hemophiliacs and intravenous drug abusers. In addition, TTV has been shown to be enterically transmitted and has been recovered from both bile and stool. Although other agents, such as hepatitis A virus, can be transmitted by both enteral and parenteral routes, usually there is a marked preference for one mode of transmission over the other; uniquely, TTV appears to be very efficiently spread by both these major routes of transmission. In the original studies of TTV in Japan [14], the agent was found in 34/290 (12%) healthy donors compared to 9/19 (47%) patients with fulminant non-A to G hepatitis, 41/90 (46%) with non-A-G chronic liver disease and 19/28 (68%) hemophiliacs. While these data suggested a relationship to acute and chronic liver disease, this has not been borne out in subsequent studies. Further, as investigators utilized more inclusive primers that targeted conserved sequences and encompassed a broader spectrum of the heterogeneous TTV family, the background prevalence increased dramatically, and in one study using conserved primers in the non-coding region, 93% of the Japanese population studied was infected [15]. With background rates this high, establishing disease causality becomes extremely difficult.

In follow-up to the initial report from Japan showing high TTV prevalence in non-A to G fulminant and chronic liver disease, Naoumov [12] studied 126 adults in England, among whom 72 had a range of liver diseases, predominantly hepatitis C (33 patients), hepatitis B (10 cases) and non A-G liver disease with and without transplant (29 cases). Also included were 24 who had recovered from hepatitis C and 30 healthy controls. TTV DNA was found in 25% of the 72 patients with chronic liver disease compared to 10% of controls. This difference was not significant ($p = 0.15$). The rate of TTV infection was similar among patients with various liver diseases and did not define the group with non-A to G hepatitis. The majority of TTV-infected patients had no biochemical or histologic evidence of liver damage. In Taiwan, Kao et al. [7] found TTV DNA in five of 12 (42%) patients with acute non-A to E hepatitis, and in five of 11 (45%) with fulminant non-A to E hepatitis compared to 10 of 100 (10%) healthy adults. While these differences were significant ($p < 0.01$), it was found that viremia was present substantially before the onset of hepatitis, and that TTV levels remained constant throughout the course of hepatitis and were not associated with fluctuations in ALT; this suggested that these patients were chronic TTV carriers, who had an unrelated, superimposed acute hepatitis. Further, the authors point out that the higher rates observed in those with acute or fulminant hepatitis may not imply causality, but rather that these patients had a higher rate of past parenteral exposures. Among patients in this study with Thalassemia, who had TTV infection in the absence of other hepatitis viruses, most had normal ALT and the others only minimal elevations.

Matsumoto [10] studied TTV infection in the transfusion setting using the more restrictive primers utilized in the original publications on TTV. The background prevalence in the volunteer donor population was 7.5%, statistically similar to the prevalence in patients prior to transfusion (11.0%). Prospective follow-up of transfusion recipients revealed that 26% developed new TTV infections following transfusion compared to 4.7% of those who were not transfused ($p < 0.0001$). There was a strong corrclation between the rate of infection and the number of units transfused. Although infection was clearly transfusion transmitted, near 5% of non-transfused patients developed nosocomial infections. The key to the NIH study was that the frequency of new TTV infections was identical in patients with non-A to G hepatitis (23%) and control patients who did not develop hepatitis (22%). Since the vast majority of patients in the study did not develop hepatitis, and since the rate of TTV infection was equal in those with and without hepatitis, less than 4% of TTV infections were associated with hepatitis. Even in the cases where an association was found, there was poor correlation between TTV DNA levels and ALT levels. Hence, as had occurred in investigations with HGV, the NIH prospective series did not support a causal association between TTV infection and post-transfusion hepatitis. However, there are caveats to the interpretation that TTV lacks pathogenicity in that the agent may cause disease in only a minority of infected individuals who have particular host susceptibility factors, or there may be particular TTV variants that are pathogenic, while the wild type virus is not. In addition, the NIH study focused only on the original TTV agent and not the wide array of variants that subsequently emerged.

SANBAN, YONBAN and TLMV

The laboratory of Dr. Shunji Mishiro has worked extensively on TTV variants and has reported a new isolate designated SANBAN that was TTV-negative by the prototype PCR assay, but positive by a new PCR assay using more conserved primers that detect a broader range of TTV variants [6]. SANBAN is quite distant from the prototype TTV agent, showing only 57% sequence homology and 34% amino acid homology. Within ORF-1 sequences, SANBAN was only very distantly related to the six major TTV genotypes. It was concluded that SANBAN might represent a new TTV-like viral species and not merely a genotype of TTV. Little is known at this writing regarding the clinical significance of the SANBAN agent.

In performing further phylogentic analyses, Mishiro's laboratory has uncovered still another distant variant of the TTV family that they have designated YONBAN. Little is known of YONBAN at this writing, but its discovery further emphasizes the diversity of this family. As opposed to HCV, where variants primarily represent strain differences of one to two percent (quasispecies), or genotypes diverging by about 15%, in the TTV family, sequence differences between variants frequently exceed 30% and sometimes exceed 50%. These differences are so great that the agents, though linked by common biophysical characteristics, may have totally different clinical spectrums and disease associations.

In additional studies from this laboratory, Takahashi [19] reported a new human virus resembling TTV and the chicken anemia virus (CAV) that has been designated the TTV-like mini virus (TLMV). Like TTV, this agent is non-enveloped and has single-stranded, circular DNA, placing it in the circoviridae family. This agent, however, is smaller than TTV, having a genome of 2860 nucleotides compared to the 3852 nucleotides in the prototype TTV isolate (TA278). Despite its smaller genome, TLMV has a similar density in cesium chloride and, like TTV, appears to be negative-stranded. In contrast, TLMV is larger than CAV (2319 nucleotides). Since CAV differs considerably from other animal circoviruses, it has been proposed that it might be classified with TTV and TLMV under a new family designated Paracircoviridae.

SEN virus

A viral discovery program conducted by Diasorin Corp. uncovered what was at the time a novel agent, designated SEN for the initials of the patient in whom it was found. The investigators reasoned that any new parenterally transmitted agent was most likely to be found in the serum of an HIV-infected intravenous drug abuser. This approach enhanced the possibility of exposure and the likelihood that viral titers would be high due to the immunosuppression. Daniele Primi, who headed these investigations, then performed PCR on this patient's serum using highly degenerate primers from the prototype TTV agent. A viral sequence was discovered that was sufficiently distinct from TTV and other sequences deposited in the Gene Bank that the agent was considered novel. Sequence homology with the prototype TTV strain was only 50% and amino acid homology only 30%. Hence, investigations proceeded to determine the nature of SEN-V and its clinical relevance. Like TTV, SEN-V proved to be a small, non-enveloped, single-stranded DNA virus, but initially it appeared to be linear rather than circular. SEN-V was not only widely divergent from TTV, but represented a subfamily of very heterogeneous agents wherein variants were designated sequentially from SENV-A to SENV- I. These variants, grouped within the SEN-V family, differed by 15%-50% from each other in nucleotide sequences and differed from TTV by 40%-60%. However, these comparisons were made with the prototype TTV agent (TA278), and as the TTV family expanded to include SANBAN, YONBAN and TLMV, it has become apparent that SEN-V is most closely related to SANBAN. In particular the SEN-V variant designated "I" shows 90% homology with SANBAN, whereas other SEN-V variants diverge widely from SANBAN (50% sequence homology). Despite its independent discovery, it is best to consider SEN-V another member of the enlarging TTV family of circoviridae.

Whatever name is ultimately applied to the SEN agent, the key question is whether any of the SEN variants or other members of the TTV family have clinical relevance. At NIH, we studied two SEN virus agents designated SENV-D and SENV-C/H. It was originally thought that SENV-C and H were distinct agents, but it was subsequently shown that they were minor variants of each other, and primers were developed that would detect both variants simultaneously. We concentrated on SENV-D and SENV-C/H out of the eight SENV variants, because screening assays suggested that they occurred in relatively low frequency in the normal control population and because, on initial screening, they appeared to have the strongest association with transfusion-associated non-A to E hepatitis. We thus screened our prospectively-followed population of transfusion recipients and controls for new SEN-V infections. SENV-D and/or C/H were found in 1.8% of 436 current donors and 1.1% of 175 donors, prior to the implementation of HCV donor screening (1990). SEN-V was unequivocally transfusion-transmitted occurring in 40% of 155 transfused subjects compared to 3% of 97 non-transfused controls ($p < 0.0001$) [21]. In addition, there was a significant relationship to transfusion volume, and donor-recipient linkage was established by sequencing. It is noteworthy that new SENV infections occurred in 3% of patients who were not transfused, suggesting nosocomial transmission or reactivation of latent virus.

In the NIH prospective study of transfusion-associated hepatitis [21], 13 cases of non- A to E hepatitis were observed. Of these, one was infected with SEN-V prior to transfusion. Remarkably, among the remaining 12 susceptible recipients, 11 (92%) became SENV-D and or C/H positive following transfusion, and there was a good, though imperfect, temporal association between the level of virus and the level of ALT elevation. In contrast, acute SEN-V infection was observed in 24% of transfused patients who did not develop hepatitis ($p < 0.0001$). Despite the strong statistical link to cases of transfusion-associated non-A to E hepatitis, it was projected that no more than 6% of SEN-V infections were accompanied by biochemical evidence of hepatitis. Thus, if SEN-V is a hepatitis agent, it causes disease in only a small minority of infected individuals, the difference perhaps depending upon host susceptibility, viral load or immune responsiveness. A parallel might be drawn to viruses such as CMV or EBV that also cause disease in only a minority of infected individuals.

Long-term follow-up of a subset of 31 patients with either SEN-V infection alone or SEN-V/HCV coinfection demonstrated that the virus was cleared within one year in 61% and within five years in 87%; the infection persisted greater than 10 years in 6%. Two of the 11 patients (18%) with acute SEN-V-associated hepatitis had persistent infection with biochemical evidence of chronic hepatitis. However, liver biopsies were not obtained to histologically confirm the chronic hepatitis. There was no apparent clinical effect of SEN-V infection on coexistent hepatitis C, either in the severity of the acute disease or the probability of developing chronic hepatitis C. In separate studies involving patients in the U.S., Japan and Germany, we were unable to show an association between SEN-V infection and acute liver failure or cryptogenic cases of chronic hepatitis, cirrhosis or HCC. Thus, the only clinical correlation that we have thus far observed is the strong statistical association with acute, transfusion-associated hepatitis.

Summary and conclusions

Despite confusing nomenclature and uncertain clinical relevance, it now seems firmly established that there is a newly discovered complex family of viruses capable of infecting humans. Indeed, this appears to be a "super-family" of relatively small (3500-4000 nt), non-enveloped, single-stranded, circular DNA viruses akin to previously described animal viruses designated circoviridae. These agents have been found in high prevalence in healthy populations, particularly in Japan, and the prevalence is highly dependent on the inclusivity of the primer sets utilized. Each member of this family exhibits considerable heterogeneity within its local cluster, and the "super-family" encompasses viruses that are widely divergent, sometimes exhibiting less than 50% sequence homology and only 30% amino acid homology. The major components of this family are the originally described TT virus, SANBAN, SEN virus, YONBAN and perhaps TLMV. These viruses are readily transmitted by blood transfusion and other parenteral routes, but also appear to be transmitted by enteric routes, and TTV has been found in bile and feces. The agents have not been proved to replicate in the liver, but several studies using PCR suggest that the virus is concentrated in the liver, and one study has shown the virus within hepatocytes by in-situ hybridization. An additional study suggests that replicative intermediates can be found in the liver. However, the association of these agents with liver disease is uncertain. The vast majority of infected patients have no evidence of liver disease, and hepatocytes harboring the agent by in-situ hybridization did not show morphologic evidence of hepatitis. Although early data on TTV showed an association with fulminant liver disease and cryptogenic hepatitis, this has not been confirmed. In the NIH prospective transfusion study [21], there is a very strong association between two strains of SEN-V and the development of acute, transfusion-associated non-A to E hepatitis. However, because the majority of SEN-V infected patients do not develop hepatitis, causality is difficult to establish.

Because the circoviruses are so diverse, the agents within this family may have very different disease manifestations. This will make clinical investigations difficult, because each agent will have to be assessed independently for its pathogenic potential. That potential may not be restricted to liver disease. In terms of proving causation in liver disease, it will be necessary to confirm intrahepatic localization by in-situ hybridization and to prove intrahepatic replication through the demonstration of replicative intermediates within hepatocytes. Once the optimal primers are defined, there is need for large-scale testing of liver disease populations and appropriate controls. There is also a need to develop antibody assays to define total exposure and to reassess transmission rates in relationship to immune susceptibility status. Finally, there is a need to reclassify and rename the agents based on careful phylogenetic analysis and established taxonomic principles.

The power and sophistication of molecular technology virtually insures that novel genetic sequences and new viral agents will continue to be discovered. Some of these agents may be pathogenic, some benign and others perhaps beneficial as commensal organisms. Finding a new virus in a patient with liver disease does not establish causality, and the more prevalent the agent, the more difficult the proof. How, then, does one prove causality in this age of molecular discovery? Since most such discoveries involve agents that have not been visualized and cannot be grown in tissue culture or reliably transmitted to small animals, the classic tenets of causality epitomized in Koch's postulates rarely apply. There is a need to develop a new paradigm of causation, and this issue is nicely addressed in a treatise by Fredericks and Relman (Fredericks

DN and Relman DA, 1996). In a simplistic adaptation of their proposed guidelines for causality, it would seem that establishing a causal relationship between a new agent and a given disease would require the following set of rules: 1) the sequence of the putative pathogen should be present in most cases of the disease; 2) the sequences should be found preferentially in the target (pathologic) organ; 3) fewer or no copies of the putative agent should be found in hosts or tissues without the disease; 4) the sequences should be found in areas of pathology by in-situ hybridization and/or visualized in these tissues by EM; 5) sequenced-based evidence should be reproducible both within the lab and among independent laboratories; 6) with resolution of the disease, the copy number should decrease or become undetectable; 7) temporality should be demonstrated, wherein sequence detection should predate the disease, and/or the copy number should correlate with disease severity.

Using these guidelines, the TTV-related circoviridae have not yet been established to have a causal role in liver disease. Nonetheless, some of these elements have been fulfilled for individual members of the family, and it is worthwhile to continue to pursue causal associations, once the interrelationships of the agents are established and the most relevant primers are defined.

References

1. Alter HJ, Purcell RH, Shih JW, Melpolder JC, Houghton M, Choo Q-L, Kuo G. Detection of antibody to hepatitis C virus in prospectively followed transfusion recipients with acute and chronic non-A, non-B hepatitis. *N Engl J Med* 1989;321:1494-1500.

1a. Alter HJ, Nakatsuji Y, Melpolder J, Wages J, Wesley R, Shih JW, Kim JP. (1997) The Incidence of transfusion-associated hepatitis G Virus Infection and its relation to Liver Disease. *The New England Journal of Medicine;* 336:747-754.

2. Alter HJ, Bradley DW. Non-A, Non-B Hepatitis unrelated to the hepatitis C virus (non-ABC). *Sem Liv Dis* 1995;15:110-120.

3. Alter MJ, Margolis HS, Krawczynski K, Judson FN, Mares A, Alexander WJ, Hu PY, Miller JK, Gerber MA, Sampliner RE, Meeks EL, Beach MJ. The natural history of community-acquired hepatitis C in the United States. *N Engl J Med* 1992;327:1899-1905.

4. Fredricks DN, Relman DA. Sequence-based identification of microbial pathogens: a reconsideration of Koch's postulates. *Clin Microbiol Rev* 1996;9:18-33.

5. Hibbs JR, Frickhofen N, Rosenfeld SJ, Feinstone SM, Kojima S, Bacigalupo A, Locasciulli A, Tzakis AG, Alter HJ, Young NS. Aplastic anemia and viral hepatitis. Non-A, Non-B, Non-C? *JAMA* 1992;267:2051-2054.

6. Hijikata M, Takahashi K, Mishiro S. Complete circular DNA genome of a TT virus variant (Isolate name SANBAN) and 44 partial ORF2 sequences implicating a great degree of diversity beyond genotypes. *Virology* 1999;260:17-22.

7. Kao JH, Chen W, Hsiang SC, Chen PJ, Lai MY, Chen DS. Prevalence and implication of TT virus infection: minimal role in patients with non-A-E hepatitis in Taiwan. *J Med Virol* 1999;59:307-312.

8. Kuo G, Choo Q-L, Alter HJ, Gitnick GL, Redeker AG, Purcell RH, Miyamura T, Dienstag JL, Alter MJ, Stevens CE, Tegtmeier GE, Bonino M, Colombo M, Lee W-S, Kuo C, Berger K, Shuster JR, Overby LR, Bradley DW, Houghton M. An assay for circulating antibodies to a major

etiologic virus of human non-A, non-B hepatitis. *Science* 1989;244:362-364.

9. Linnen J, Wages J Jr, Zhang-Keck ZY, Fry KE, Krawczynski KZ, Alter H, Koonin E, Gallagher M, Alter M, Hadziyannis S, Karayiannis P, Fung K, Nakatsuji Y, Shih JW-K, Young L, Piatak M Jr, Hoover C, Fernandez J, Chen S, Zou JC, Morris T, Hyams KC, Ismay S, Lifson JD, Hess G, Fong SKH, Thomas H, Bradley D, Margolis H, Kim JP. Molecular cloning and disease association of Hepatitis G virus: A transfusion-transmissible agent. *Science* 1996;271:505-508.
10. Matsumoto A, Yeo AE, Shih JW, Tanaka E, Kiyosawa K, Alter HJ. Transfusion-associated TT Virus infection and its relationship to liver disease. *Hepatology* 1999;30:283-288.
11. Mushahwar IK, Erker JC, Muerhoff AS, Leary TP, Simons JN, Birkenmeyer LG, Chalmers ML, Pilot-Matias TJ, Dexai SM. Molecular and biophysical characterization of TT virus: evidence for a new virus family infecting humans. *Proc Natl Acad Sci USA* 1999;96:3177-3182.
12. Naoumov NV, Petrova EP, Thomas MG, Williams R. Presence of a newly described human DNA virus (TTV) in patients with liver disease. *Lancet* 1998;352:195-197.
13. Nishizawa T, Okamoto H, Konisi K, Yoshizawa H, Miyakawa Y, Mayumi M. A novel DNA virus (TTV) associated with elevated transaminase levels in posttransfusion hepatitis of unknown etiology. *Biochem Biophys Res Commun* 1997;241:92-97.
14. Okamoto H, Nishizawa T, Kato N, Ukita M, Ikeda H, Iizuka H, Miyakawa Y, Mayumi M. Molecular cloning and characterization of a novel DNA virus (TTV) associated with posttransfusion hepatitis of unknown etiology. *Hepatol Research* 1998;10:1-16.
15. Okamoto H, Takahashi M, Nishizawa T, Ukita M, Fukuda M, Tsuda F, Miyakawa Y, Mayumi M. Marked genomic heterogeneity and frequent mixed infection of TT virus demonstrated by PCR with primers from coding and noncoding regions. *Virology* 1999;259:428-436.
16. Pessoa MG, Terrault NA, Detmer J, Kolberg J, Collins M, Hassoba HM, Wright TL. Quantitation of hepatitis G and C viruses in the liver: evidence that hepatitis G virus is not hepatotropic. *Hepatology* 1998;27:877-880.
17. Rodriguez-Iñigo E, Casqueiro M, Bartolomé J, Oritz-Movilla N, López-Alcorocho JM, Herrero M, Manzaebeitia F, Oliva H, Carreño V. Detection of TT virus DNA in liver biopsies by *in situ* hybridization. *Am J Pathol* 2000;156:1227-1234.
18. Simons JN, Leary TP, Dawson GJ, Pilot-Matias TJ, Muerhoff AS, Schlauder GG, Desai SM, Mushahwar IK. Isolation of novel virus-like sequences associated with human hepatitis. *Nat Med* 1995;1:564-569.
19. Takahashi K, Iwasa Y, Hijikata M, Mishiro S. Identification of a new human DNA virus (TTV-like mini virus, TLMV) intermediately related to TT virus and chicken anemia virus. *Arch Virol* 2000;145:979-993.
20. Tanaka Y, Primi D, Wang RY, Umemura T, Yeo AE, Mizokami M, Alter HJ, Shih JW. Genomic and molecular evolutionary analysis of a newly identified infectious agent (SEN virus) and its relationship to the TT virus family. *J Infect Dis* 2001;183:359-367.
21. Umemura T, Yeo AET, Sottini Á, Moratto D, Tanaka Y, Wang RYH, Shih JWK, Donahue P, Primi D, Alter HJ. SEN virus infection and its relationship to transfusion-associated hepatitis. *Hepatology* (2001, in press).

IMMUNOLOGY AND VACCINES

Virus-specific CD8+ cell immune responses in acute and chronic hepatitis B virus infection

GEORGE J.M. WEBSTER and GEOFFREY M. DUSHEIKO

Centre for Hepatology, Royal Free Campus, Royal Free and University College Medical School, Rowland Hill Street, London, UK, NW3 2PF

Abstract

Hepatitis B virus-specific cytotoxic T lymphocytes (CTL) have previously been thought to be the principle mediators of control of viral replication following HBV infection, through the direct lysis of infected hepatocytes. Models of HBV infection have led to the importance of non-cytolytic mechanisms being recognized. Recent longitudinal studies performed from the incubation phase of acute infection, in animal models and man, have led to a better definition of the interaction between viral replication and liver injury. The development of tetramer technology, which enables the direct quantification of antigen-specific CTL, has also improved our understanding of the role of HBV-specific CTL in the immunopathogenesis of acute and chronic hepatitis B.

Introduction

The interaction between host and virus following hepatitis B virus (HBV) infection may result in a range of clinical outcomes, and the balance of this interaction may have significant health implications. In more than 90% of immunocompetent adults, HBsAg is cleared from the circulation following acute infection, often in association with a clinical hepatitis, and there are no long-term sequelae. In 5% of adults, and more than 90% of infected infants, the virus is not adequately controlled, as demonstrated by detectable HBsAg, and subsequent chronic infection may lead to cirrhosis and hepatocellular carcinoma [1]. Control of HBV appears to depend on coordinated innate and adaptive, humoral and cellular immune responses [2], and as the virus is usually non-cytopathic, the host immune response is thought to mediate not only viral control, but also liver injury. The cellular immune response has been thought to be particularly important in these processes, with cytotoxic T lymphocytes (CTL) being final effectors of both viral control and liver injury. The application of new techniques for defining HBV-specific CTL responses are leading to improvements in our understanding of the interaction between virus, specific and nonspecific immune responses, and liver injury in acute and chronic hepatitis B, and will be the focus of this brief review. There is consensus that HBV-specific CD8+ T lymphocytes recognize infected hepatocytes

Frontiers in Viral Hepatitis Ed. by RF Schinazi, J-P Sommadossi and CM Rice. 49 — 58

through the presentation of viral epitopes by MHC class 1 molecules on the hepatocyte membrane [2]. Bound epitopes are derived from the processing of HBV genome within the cell into nine to 10 amino acid peptide sequences. CD8+ cells bearing a T-cell receptor corresponding to this peptide then bind the peptide-HLA class 1 molecule complex. For a range of infections, binding of virus-specific CD8+ cytotoxic T lymphocytes (CTL) has been shown to be associated with viral control. The relative importance of virus-specific CTL, and their mechanisms of action, in the immunopathogenesis of acute and chronic hepatitis B has been a focus of research over the last few years.

Studying the CD8+ cell response in hepatitis B

Our understanding of the role of host immune responses, and CTL mechanisms in particular, in HBV control and liver injury has advanced remarkably over the last few years, despite a range of factors which complicate their study:

1. HBV infects and replicates only in man, chimpanzees, and possibly gorillas, therefore limiting the availability of models of infection. Although duck hepatitis B virus, and woodchuck hepatitis virus are hepadnaviral homologues of HBV the immune systems within these hosts are less well defined, and extrapolation to human infection is difficult.
2. The virus cannot be easily grown in tissue culture.
3. Study of immune response at the major site of viral replication (i.e., the liver), particularly sequentially over time, may pose technical and ethical difficulties in man.
4. Patients with acute infection are usually identified only after the onset of jaundice, therefore precluding studies of immune and viral dynamics during the early period of infection.
5. Previous methods to define the HBV-specific CD8+ cell response, including limiting dilution assays, have depended upon repeated rounds of *in vitro* peptide stimulation, which precludes analysis of the true frequency of virus-specific cells within a cell population, and may bias the identification of cells with particular functional capacity.

The development, by Chisari and colleagues, of a transgenic mouse model of HBV infection [3, 4], which expresses HBV gene products and replicates the viral genome within the hepatocytes, led to significant advances in the understanding of the sequential recruitment of components of the cellular immune response, and the importance of cytolytic and non-cytolytic mechanisms. A limitation of this model, however, is that the mice are not infected by the virus, precluding the study of the dynamics of viral replication and propagation. The study of chimpanzees [5] and woodchucks [6] after inoculation with HBV, and humans during the incubation phase of clinical disease [7], has shed new light on the dynamics of viral control and liver injury, and is discussed below.

Until recently, the *ex vivo* demonstration of virus-specific CD8+ cells has depended upon their *in vitro* expansion, following specific peptide stimulation [8, 9, 10]. Limiting dilution precluded an accurate assessment of the true frequency of these cells within the blood or liver. The development of tetrameric HLA-peptide complexes [11] has therefore been an important advance [12], allowing the direct quantification of virus-specific CD8+ cells within the blood and tissue lymphocyte populations of a range of infections [13, 14], including hepatitis B [15]. Each tetramer consists of four biotinylated HLA class 1 molecules, each folded with a specific peptide, and multimerized by the addition of flurochrome-labelled streptavidin (Figure 1). Tetramers have been made to incorporate nine to 10 amino acid peptides corresponding with previously defined HLA-A2-associated HBV CTL epitopes (including core 18-27, polymerase 335-343, envelope 575-583). The multimeric HLA class 1-peptide complex has a high avidity for CD8+ cells displaying the T cell receptor (TCR) corresponding to the specific epitope used. Fluoresence labelling of the tetramer allows these specific cells to be identified using flow cytometry. It has been observed that the frequency of circulating virus-specific CD8+ cells in acute infection with HBV [15] or EBV, as shown using tetramer complexes, may be up to 40-fold higher than was demonstrated by limiting dilution techniques. It has been recognized that the potential of these cells to expand is significantly influenced by their activation status, in that highly activated, antigen-specific cells appear to have a lower expansion potential than those of a resting phenotype, and this phenomenon may explain the lower cell frequencies found using limiting dilution techniques. Previous work has defined a number of CTL epitopes in HBV-infected individuals with the HLA-A2 haplotype [16], and the most immunodominant of these epitopes have been incorporated into the tetramers presently used in the study of hepatitis B [15]. It may be that other, as yet unidentified, HBV epitopes also play a role in the CTL response to hepatitis B, and it needs to be

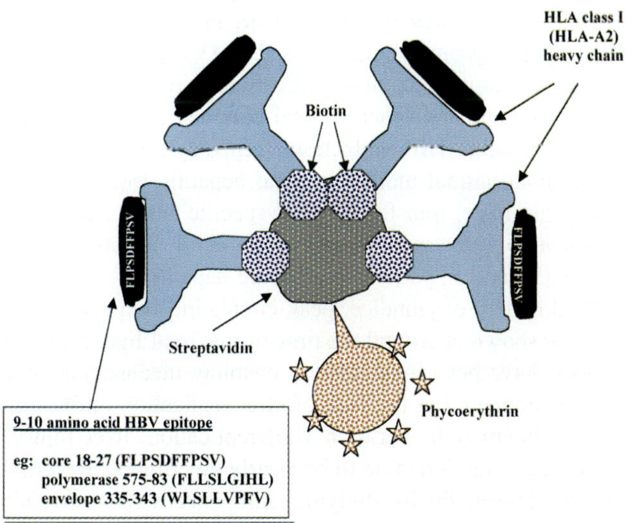

Figure 1. Schematic representation of HLA class 1 tetramer. The incorporation of the four HLA-A2-HBV peptide complexes into a tetrameric form, by multimerization with fluorochrome-labelled streptavidin, increases the stability of binding to the specific T-cell receptor of CD8+ cells, and allows these cells to be identified by flow cytometry.

borne in mind that CD8+ cells which are not found to be HBV-specific using present techniques are not necessarily 'antigen non-specific.' Notwithstanding these cautions, the development of tetramer technology, allowing direct quantification of HBV-specific CTL in man, in conjunction with data from transgenic mice and animal models of HBV infection, has led to recent improvements in our understanding of the immunopathogenesis of acute and chronic hepatitis B.

Acute hepatitis B

Acute icteric hepatitis is almost always associated with clearance of HBsAg. Following neonatal infection, however, icteric hepatitis and clearance of HBsAg are rare, and chronic hepatitis B occurs in 90% of neonates. Immunosuppression is associated with an absence of acute hepatitis after infection, and predisposes to chronicity. These clinical observations, and laboratory evidence accrued over the last 15 years, provided support for the argument that control of HBV replication and acute liver injury occur as a direct result of lysis of infected hepatocytes by HBV-specific CD8+ cells.

The presence of an inextricable link between the control of viral replication and liver injury has more recently been questioned. The finding that virtually 100% of hepatocytes are infected after woodchuck hepatitis virus infection [17] suggests that processes other than just cytolysis must be important, as massive hepatic necrosis leading to fulminant liver failure is a relatively rare clinical outcome. Studying HBV transgenic mice, Guidotti and colleagues have shown that HBV replication within hepatocytes may be abolished by cytokine-mediated mechanisms (involving IFNγ, TNFα), which do not require cell death [18]. Non-cytolytic control of infection has also been shown for other viruses that infect the liver, including murine cytomegalovirus (CMV) [19] and lymphochoriomeningitis virus (LCMV) [20]. Despite these findings in support of non-cytolytic control of viral replication, hepatocytes lysis, as inferred by the development of jaundice and other clinical parameters of hepatocytes injury, is a characteristic feature of acute HBV infection. Hepatocyte lysis has also been clearly demonstrated to occur in animal models of viral hepatitis [6], and to be mediated by CTL [21]. In transgenic mice, transfer of HBV-specific MHC class 1 restricted CD8+ cells has been shown to subsequently lead to an acute hepatitis and destruction of infected hepatocytes [3], and in patients with acute hepatitis B, studied at various time points after the development of jaundice, peak circulating frequencies of HBV-specific CD8+ cells have been shown at around the time of maximal liver injury [15].

Transgenic models have been invaluable in enabling mechanisms of viral clearance and liver injury to be defined, but the lack of viral replication in these models has not allowed the dynamic interactions between viral replication, liver injury, and immune responses during natural acute infection to be clearly determined. Recent data have shed light on this issue. By longitudinally studying chimpanzees soon after inoculation with HBV, Guidotti et al. [5] demonstrated that serum and intrahepatic levels of HBV DNA reduced markedly prior to liver injury, and that this reduction in viral replication also occurred before any significant influx of CD8+ cells into the liver could be detected. Reduction in viral replication has also been shown to occur prior to significant liver injury following woodchuck hepatitis virus infection, subsequent to the influx of CD4+ and CD8+ cells into the liver, and the production of IFNγ and TNFα [6].

We have recently had the opportunity to compare these findings with events during the early phase of human HBV infection, through the study of patients infected during a large, common-source outbreak of hepatitis B, arising from an acupuncture clinic in London [22]. As part of a lookback study involving 356 patients, 57 were shown to have been infected with HBV, and 30 of 33 HBsAg-positive individuals were actively infected with an identical variant of HBV, confirming the common source of infection. A number of these patients were identified in the preclinical phase of infection, thus offering a unique opportunity to study in man the interactions between viral control, liver injury, and HBV-specific cellular immune responses during both the incubation period and clinical phase of primary HBV infection. In four patients who subsequently developed acute icteric hepatitis, whilst serum ALT had begun to increase at the time of the initial fall in serum HBV DNA, maximal reduction in circulating virus occurred prior to peak liver injury, and more than 90% of circulating HBV DNA was cleared by the time of symptomatic hepatitis. Using tetramer complexes and proliferation assays to analyse the frequency of circulating HBV-specific CD8+ and CD4+ cells, respectively, we showed that core and polymerase-specific CD8+ cells (Figure 2), and core-specific CD4+ cells, are present in the circulation of patients in the incubation phase of disease, during the period of maximal reduction in HBV DNA. Natural killer (NK) cells, which are thought to play an early role in the response to acute viral infection, through cytolytic and cytokine-mediated mechanisms [23], were also seen to be at their highest circulating frequency during the earliest point of the incubation phase. In the single patient identified soon after infection who failed to clear HBsAg, no evidence of clinical hepatitis or HBV-specific cellular immune responses was seen.

Taken together, our data on acute hepatitis B suggest that the incubation phase of HBV infection is not simply the period when the virus establishes a reservoir of infected cells, and the presence of HBV-specific CD8+ and CD4+ cells during this phase suggests that these cells may play an important early role in the control of infection and in the initiation of events that lead to liver damage. The data do not allow a conclusion to be drawn as to whether the HBV-specific CD8+ cells present during the incubation phase are acting primarily through cytolytic or non-cytolytic mechanisms (during acute hepatitis B these cells have been shown to both lyse cells and produce IFNγ [15]), and both processes may be important.

What are the main cellular mediators of liver injury in acute hepatitis B? In animal models of acute hepatitis B, intrahepatic levels of unspecified CD8+ cells peak at the time of maximal liver injury [5]. Although peak levels of HBV-specific CD8+ cells were seen at the time of maximal liver injury in patients with acute hepatitis B (up to 1.4% of circulating CD8+ cells) (Figure 2), the marked increase in total activated CD8+ cells suggests that many cells may be nonspecifically activated. In transgenic mice, although transfer of HBV-specific MHC class 1 restricted CD8+ cells has been shown to subsequently lead to an acute hepatitis and destruction of infected hepatocytes [3], this lysis does not occur immediately following adoptive transfer of HBV-specific cells, but up to 12 hours later, in association with a large influx of non-antigen-specific inflammatory cells into the liver [24]. Recruitment of non-antigen-specific CD8+ cells

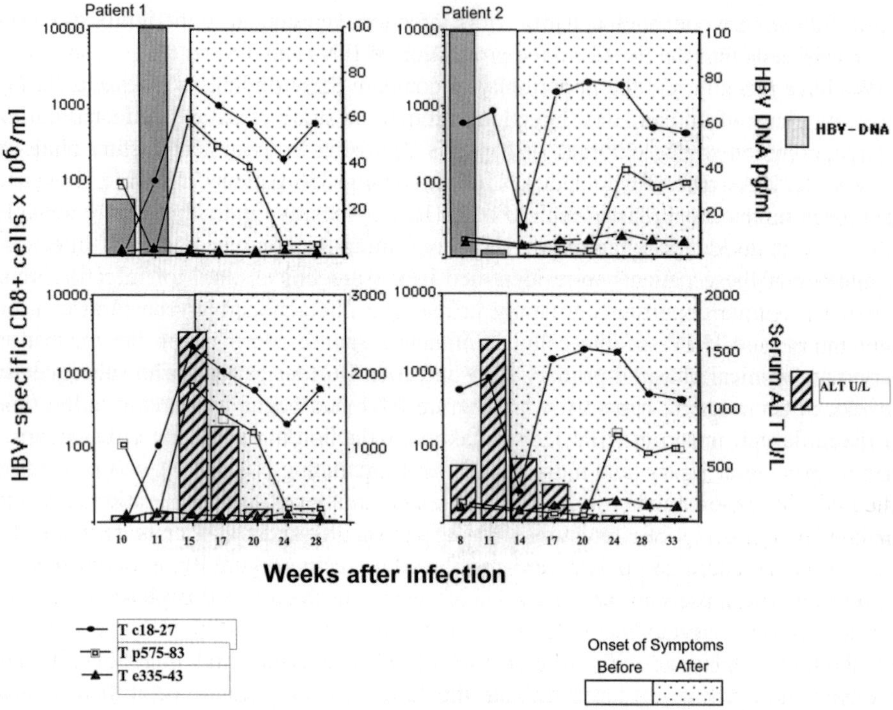

Figure 2. Longitudinal analysis of circulating HBV-specific CD8+ cells, serum HBV-DNA, and serum ALT concentrations, during incubation and clinical phase of acute hepatitis B. Data are shown for two patients who were identified during the incubation phase of acute hepatitis B. Circulating HBV-specific CD8 cells visualised by three HLA-A2/HBV tetramers (Tc18-27, Tp575-83 and Te335-43) were quantified at each time point. Numbers of core 18-27, pol 575-83, and env 335-43 specific CD8 cells per ml of blood (calculated as explained in methods) are represented in relation to time after infection (horizontal axis) and HBV-DNA level (expressed as a percentage of maximal HBV DNA concentration, upper panels), or serum ALT concentrations (lower panels).

is thought to mediate lung injury following high viral exposure in the mouse model of influenza [25]. The finding that HBV has been virtually cleared prior to significant liver injury also lends weight to the argument that liver injury is not only directly due to HBV-specific CD8+ cells, and implicates the importance of 'bystander' activation of non-antigen-specific cells in the pathognesis of liver injury in viral hepatitis [26].

Chronic hepatitis B

Acute and chronic hepatitis B are discussed separately here, but it is increasingly recognised that, clinically and pathogenetically, they represent a continuum of control of viral replication. The demonstration of HBV-specific CD8+ cell responses months or years after complete clinical resolution of acute hepatitis B, and the potential for reactivation of disease in HBsAg-negative individuals following immunosuppression, emphasizes that a persistent, lifelong interaction between virus and HBV-specific CD8+ cells may occur in most, if not all, patients who have been infected with HBV. Persistence of HBV in the liver [27] and blood [28, 29] of many patients who apparently previously 'cleared' the virus, and are HBsAg negative, with no evidence of liver injury, demonstrates that immunological control of virus, rather than eradication, is responsible. The clinical distinctions in chronic hepatitis B between 'replicating' (HBeAg+, high levels of HBV DNA) and 'non-replicating' (HBeAg-, low levels of HBV DNA) disease may also represent relative differences in the efficacy and specificity of the host cellular immune mechanisms.

It has previously been shown that, in contrast to the vigorous, multispecific HBV-specific CD8 response seen in acute disease, a response is barely detectable in the periphery of patients with chronic hepatitis B [30]. For the technical reasons outlined above, the role of HBV-specific CD8+ cells in mediating viral control and injury within the livers of patients with chronic hepatitis has been difficult to study, and hence has not been well defined. Using HBV-peptide tetramer complexes, circulating and intrahepatic HBV-specific CD8+ cells have recently been studied in two groups of chronically infected patients: one group with significant liver inflammation and high levels of HBV DNA (HBeAg+, HBV DNA >800pg/ml, raised ALT), the other with low levels of virus and minimal inflammation (anti-HBe+, HBV DNA <2pg/ml, normal ALT) [31]. In both groups, lower frequencies of HBV-specific CD8+ cells (approximately 0.1% of total circulating CD8+ cells) were found in the periphery than were seen in acute disease [15]. Within the liver, a similar absolute number of HBV-specific CD8+ cells were seen in both groups, but those in the group with liver inflammation were diluted within a large non-antigen-specific CD8+ cell infiltrate. These data suggest that in patients with inactive chronic hepatitis, HBV-specific CD8+ cells (which represent up to 9% of CD8+ cells within the liver) may adequately control virus in the absence of liver injury, and that intrahepatic HBV-specific CD8+ cells in chronic HBV infection may be associated with either protection or liver injury. Where virus is not controlled by virus-specific cells, recruitment of a large non-HBV-specific cellular infiltrate, including activated cells of the innate immune response [32], may contribute to the liver injury seen in chronic hepatitis.

In the transgenic model of influenza, the non-antigen-specific cellular infiltration that follows the adoptive transfer of virus-specific CD8+ cells, and which is associated with lung injury, appears to be IFNγ dependent, as it may be prevented with anti-IFNγ antibodies [25]. This finding also reiterates the fact that this cytokine may have both beneficial effects (non-cytolytic control of viral replication), and deleterious effects (initiation of T cell recruitment, TNF-mediated tissue injury) in the immune response to viral infection. The different clinical and pathological responses in the two groups of chronic hepatitis B patients discussed above, despite similar absolute numbers of virus-specific CD8+ cells within the liver, also suggests that these cells are behaving functionally different. The finding that HBV-specific CD8+ cells in the periphery of patients who are controlling the virus (but not those with high levels of virus) have a resting phenotype, and can be expanded on further stimulation [31], suggests that this is the case.

Future questions

The development of models of HBV infection, and new techniques to study virus-specific T cells, has enhanced our understanding of the pathogenesis of hepatitis B, and may offer the potential of improved therapies. Despite the advantages of tetrameric complexes in allowing the direct quantification of virus-specific CD8+ cells, detailed functional analysis of these cells, particularly of those within the liver, is awaited. Does the cytokine profile of these cells differ between chronically infected patients with high or low levels of viral replication, and minimal or significant liver injury? What influence do chemo-attractant factors, such as cellular chemokine receptor expression, have on the ability of virus-specific CD8+ cells to migrate to the site of viral replication within the liver? At present, tetramer staining of intrahepatic lymphocytes can only be performed after isolating the cells from the liver. The very recent description of in-situ staining of antigen-specific cells, using tetramer complexes and confocal microscopy [33], might allow the location of HBV-specific cells within the chronically infected liver to be more clearly defined. The role of non-HBV-specific inflammatory cells in the liver injury associated with acute and chronic hepatitis merits further study. Are these cells truly 'bystander' cells, as seems likely, or do they represent a large population of virus-specific cells, targeted against undefined epitopes, as suggested in acute EBV infection? [34]. If they are nonspecific bystander cells, why do they become activated during hepatitis B?

Recent data have shown that the peripheral HBV-specific CD8+ cell hyporesponsiveness characteristic of replicating chronic hepatitis B may be reversed following the lowering of viral replication with lamivudine, an antiviral nucleoside analogue [35]. In view of the fact that these cells are functionally active, and that, as discussed above, HBV-specific CD8+ cells may control virus without inducing significant liver injury, the potential for new immunotherapies in chronic hepatitis B exists. Considerable interest is now focused on the development of peptide vaccines, incorporating known CTL epitopes (such as core 18-27 [36]), which may act by augmenting host virus-specific CD8+ cell responses. Antiviral agents to directly lower viral replication, in conjunction with immunotherapeutic techniques to augment the host virus-specific CD8+ cell responses [37], may represent an important approach to achieving, and maintaining, HBeAg seroconversion in the future.

Acknowledgements

Special thanks to Antonio Bertoletti for his advice on the manuscript.

References

1. Lee WM. Hepatitis B virus infection. *N Engl J Med* 1997;337:1733-45.
2. Chisari FV, Ferrari C. Hepatitis B virus immunopathogenesis. *Annu Rev Immunol* 1995;13:29-60.
3. Moriyama T, Guilhot S, Klopchin K, Moss B, Pinkert CA, Palmiter RD, Brinster RL, Kanagawa O,

Chisari FV. Immunobiology and pathogenesis of hepatocellular injury in hepatitis B virus transgenic mice. *Science* 1990;248:361-4.
4. Chisari FV. Hepatitis B virus transgenic mice: insights into the virus and the disease. *Hepatology* 1995;22:1316-25.
5. Guidotti LG, Rochford R, Chung J, Shapiro M, Purcell R, Chisari FV. Viral clearance without destruction of infected cells during acute HBV infection. *Science* 1999;284:825-9.
6. Guo JT, Zhou H, Liu C, Aldrich C, Saputelli J, Whitaker T, Barrasa MI, Mason WS, Seeger C. Apoptosis and regeneration of hepatocytes during recovery from transient hepadnavirus infections. *J Virol* 2000;74:1495-505.
7. Webster GJM, Reignat S, Maini MK, Whalley S, Ogg GS, King AS, Vergani D, Williams R, Dusheiko GM, Bertoletti A. Incubation phase of acute hepatitis B in man: dynamic of cellular immune mechanisms. *Hepatology* 2000;32:1117-24.
8. Rehermann B, Lau D, Hoofnagle JH, Chisari FV. Cytotoxic T lymphocyte responsiveness after resolution of chronic hepatitis B virus infection. *J Clin Invest* 1996;97:1655-65.
9. Ferrari C, Penna A, Bertoletti A, Fiaccadori F. Cell mediated immune response to hepatitis B virus nucleocapsid antigen. *Arch Virol Suppl* 1993;8:91-101.
10. Rehermann B, Fowler P, Sidney J, Person J, Redeker A, Brown M, Moss B, Sette A, Chisari FV. The cytotoxic T lymphocyte response to multiple hepatitis B virus polymerase epitopes during and after acute viral hepatitis. *J Exp Med* 1995;181:1047-58.
11. Altman JD, Moss PAH, Goulder PJR, Barouch DH, McHeyzer-Williams MG, Bell JI, McMichael AJ, Davis MM. Phenotypic analysis of antigen-specific T lymphocytes. *Science* 1996;274:94-6.
12. Schwartz RS. Direct visualization of antigen-specific cytotoxic T cells-a new insight into immune defenses. *N Engl J Med* 1998;339:1076-8.
13. Gallimore A, Glithero A, Godkin A, Tissot AC, Pluckthun A, Elliott T, Hengartner H, Zinkernagel R. Induction and exhaustion of lymphocytic choriomeningitis virus-specific cytotoxic T lymphocytes visualized using soluble tetrameric major histocompatibility complex class I-peptide complexes. *J Exp Med* 1998;187:1383-93.
14. Ogg GS, King AS, Dunbar PR, McMichael AJ. Isolation of HIV-1-specific cytotoxic T lymphocytes using human leukocyte antigen-coated beads. *AIDS* 1999;13:1991-3.
15. Maini MK, Boni C, Ogg GS, King AS, Reignat S, Lee CK, Larrubia JR, Webster GJ, McMichael AJ, Ferrari C, Williams R, Vergani D, Bertoletti A. Direct ex vivo analysis of hepatitis B virus-specific CD8(+) T cells associated with the control of infection. *Gastroenterology* 1999;117:1386-96.
16. Ferrari C, Bertoletti A, Penna A, Cavalli A, Valli A, Missale G, Pilli M, Fowler P, Giuberti T, Chisari FV. Identification of immunodominant T cell epitopes of the hepatitis B virus nucleocapsid antigen. *J Clin Invest* 1991;88:214-22.
17. Kajino KA, Jilbert AR, Saputelli J, Aldrich E, Cullen J, Mason WS. Woodchuck hepatitis virus infections: very rapid recovery after a prolonged viraemia and infection of virtually every hepatocyte. *J Virol* 1994;68: 5792-803.
18. Guidotti LG, Chisari FV. To kill or to cure: options in host defense against viral infection. *Curr Opin Immunol* 1996;8:478-83.
19. Tay CH, Welsh RM. Distinct organ-dependent mechanisms for the control of murine cytomegalovirus infection by natural killer cells. *J Virol* 1997;71:267-75.
20. Guidotti LG, Borrow P, Brown A, McClary H, Koch R, Chisari FV. Noncytopathic clearance of lymphocytic choriomeningitis virus from the hepatocyte. *J Exp Med* 1999;189:1555-64.
21. Kondo T, Suda T, Fukuyama H, Adachi M, Nagata S. Essential roles of the Fas ligand in the development

of hepatitis. *Nat Med* 1997;3:409-13.

22. Webster GJ, Hallett R, Whalley SA, Meltzer M, Balogun K, Brown D, Farrington CP, Sharma S, Hamilton G, Farrow SC, Ramsay ME, Teo CG, Dusheiko GM. Molecular epidemiology of a large outbreak of hepatitis B linked to autohaemotherapy. *Lancet* 2000;356:379-84.
23. Biron CA. Initial and innate responses to viral infections--pattern setting in immunity or disease. *Curr Opin Microbiol* 1999;2:374-81.
24. Ando K, Moriyama T, Guidotti LG, Wirth S, Schreiber RD, Schlicht HJ, Huang SN, Chisari FV. Mechanisms of class I restricted immunopathology. A transgenic mouse model of fulminant hepatitis. *J Exp Med* 1993;178:1541-54.
25. Moskophidis D, Kioussis D. Contribution of virus-specific CD8+ cytotoxic T cells to virus clearance or pathologic manifestations of influenza virus infection in a T cell receptor transgenic mouse model. *J Exp Med* 1998;188:223-32.
26. Abrignani S. Bystander activation by cytokines of intrahepatic T cells in chronic viral hepatitis. *Semin Liver Dis* 1997;17:319-22.
27. Cacciola I, Pollicino T, Squadrito G, Cerenzia G, Orlando ME, Raimondo G. Occult hepatitis B virus infection in patients with chronic hepatitis C liver disease. *N Engl J Med* 1999;341:22-6.
28. Michalak TI, Pasquinelli C, Guilhot S, Chisari FV. Hepatitis B virus persistence after recovery from acute viral hepatitis. *J Clin Invest* 1994;93:230-9.
29. Rehermann B, Ferrari C, Pasquinelli C, Chisari FV. The hepatitis B virus persists for decades after patients' recovery from acute viral hepatitis despite active maintenance of a cytotoxic T- lymphocyte response. *Nat Med* 1996;2:1104-8.
30. Bertoletti A, Costanzo A, Chisari FV, Levrero M, Artini M, Sette A, Penna A, Giuberti T, Fiaccadori F, Ferrari C. Cytotoxic T lymphocyte response to a wild type hepatitis B virus epitope in patients chronically infected by variant viruses carrying substitutions within the epitope. *J Exp Med* 1994;180:933-43.
31. Maini MK, Boni C, Lee CK, Larrubia JR, Reignat S, Ogg GS, King AS, Herberg J, Gilson R, Alisa A, Williams R, Vergani D, Naoumov NV, Ferrari C, Bertoletti A. The role of virus-specific CD8(+) cells in liver damage and viral control during persistent hepatitis B virus infection. *J Exp Med* 2000;191:1269-80.
32. Nuti S, Rosa D, Valiante NM, Saletti G, Caratozzolo M, Dellabona P, Barnaba V, Abrignani S. Dynamics of intra-hepatic lymphocytes in chronic hepatitis C: enrichment for Valpha24+ T cells and rapid elimination of effector cells by apoptosis. *Eur J Immunol* 1998;28:3448-55.
33. Haanen JBAG, van Oijen MGCT, Tirion F, Oomen LCJM, Kruisbeek AM, Vyth-Dreese FA, Schumacher TNM. In situ detection of virus- and tumor-specific T-cell immunity. *Nat.Med.* 2000;6:1056-60.
34. Callan MF, Tan L, Annels N, Ogg GS, Wilson JD, O'Callaghan CA, Steven N, McMichael AJ, Rickinson AB. Direct visualization of antigen-specific CD8+ T cells during the primary immune response to Epstein-Barr virus In vivo. *J Exp Med* 1998;187:1395-402.
35. Boni C, Bertoletti A, Penna A, Cavalli A, Pilli M, Urbani S, Scognamiglio P, Boehme R, Panebianco R, Fiaccadori F, Ferrari C. Lamivudine treatment can restore T cell responsiveness in chronic hepatitis B. *J Clin Invest* 1998;102:968-75.
36. Heathcote J, McHutchison J, Lee S, Tong M, Benner K, Minuk G, Wright T, Fikes J, Livingston B, Sette A, Chestnut R. A pilot study of the CY-1899 T-cell vaccine in subjects chronically infected with hepatitis B virus. The CY1899 T Cell Vaccine Study Group. *Hepatology* 1999; 30:531-6.
37. Perrillo R. Short-term corticosteroid therapy in combination with lamivudine: A case of deja vu? *Hepatology* 2000;32:663-5.

Cell-mediated immunity and the outcome of HCV infection in chimpanzees

CHRISTOPHER M. WALKER

Department of Pediatrics, Division of Molecular Medicine,
The Children's Research Institute and The Ohio State University,
Columbus, OH, 43205, USA

Abstract

The common chimpanzee *Pan troglodytes* is the only animal model for human HCV infection, and emerging data suggest that mechanisms of protective immunity and viral persistence are identical in both species. The few individuals who spontaneously resolve infection have robust cell-mediated immune responses. CD4+ and CD8+ T helper cells targeting multiple class II and class I restricted epitopes, respectively, are found in the peripheral blood and liver of chimpanzees and humans coincident with termination of plasma viremia. In contrast persistent, lifelong infection in the majority of chimpanzees and humans is characterized by low-frequency T lymphocyte responses that appear to be largely compartmentalized to the liver. These data suggest that the same lesion in host immunity facilitates persistence of the virus in both species. Thus the chimpanzee model is likely to be important for the development of vaccines and other immunotherapies designed to terminate ongoing HCV replication.

Introduction

Chronic infection with the hepatitis C virus (HCV) is a global public health problem. Persistent virus replication over a period of years to decades causes deterioration of liver function through a process of inflammation and cirrhosis. Permanent termination of HCV replication is the ultimate goal of therapy, so replicase, helicase, or protease enzymes required for production of new virions are obvious targets for drug development. Vaccines that trigger or enhance host immune responses may be an important alternative or adjunct if drug therapies are limited by toxicity, emergence of resistant HCV strains, or high cost. An animal model of human HCV infection is important for defining protective immune mechanisms that might be elicited by vaccination. The only animal with known susceptibility to HCV infection is the common chimpanzee, Pan troglodytes. Their very close genetic relationship to humans could provide significant advantages for the study of HCV immunity and persistence. The value of the model depends entirely, however, on how closely key features of infection resemble those in humans. For instance, chimpanzees

Frontiers in Viral Hepatitis Ed. by RF Schinazi, J-P Sommadossi and CM Rice. 59 — 70

are the natural host for HIV-1, but they are not commonly used for studies of AIDS pathogenesis or vaccine development. HIV-1 replication is low or only sporadically detectable in many animals, and its interaction with the immune system of these two species is fundamentally different for reasons that aren't yet clear.

Chimpanzees were vital to the discovery of HCV [1]. Passage of infection from humans to animals proved that non-A, non-B hepatitis was an infectious disease probably caused by a small enveloped virus. Moreover, plasma from infected animals provided a pedigreed starting material for molecular cloning of the HCV genome. This article summarizes the key features of HCV infection and immunity in chimpanzees and why these rare, endangered animals continue to be an invaluable model for human infection and development of effective vaccines.

Advantages of an animal model for HCV infection

Understanding why some individuals spontaneously resolve acute hepatitis C would provide an important starting point for rational design of immunotherapies. Correlates of protective immunity are difficult to study in human subjects. Individuals with acute hepatitis C aren't easily identified because symptoms are often mild or indistinguishable from other acute viral syndromes. Experimental infection of chimpanzees therefore provides a unique opportunity to define the earliest events in the host-virus interaction. In addition, animals can be infected with genetically defined virus stocks, including infectious molecular clones that facilitate studies of HCV evolution and immune selection pressure [2, 3]. Reagents for detecting cellular immune responses, including recombinant viral proteins and vaccinia viruses that contain HCV sequences, are genetically matched with HCV-1 and HCV-H strains commonly used for experimental infections. Most antibodies directed against human lymphocyte surface antigens and cytokines also cross-react with chimpanzee homologues, so it is possible to dissect the immune responses with great precision. Indeed, newer approaches for quantification of virus-specific T cells in humans, including soluble tetrameric class I MHC molecules, intracellular cytokine staining and enzyme-linked immunospot (Elispot) assays [4], are readily adapted to chimpanzees.

Immunogenetics of the chimpanzee

Class I and II MHC loci govern the repertoire of viral peptides presented on the surface of infected cells to CD8+ and CD4+ T lymphocytes, respectively. The immunogenetic complex of humans (HLA) and chimpanzees (Patr) are remarkably conserved. Three orthologous class I loci designated A, B and C are present in both species [5]. Each encodes a 44 Kd heavy chain that forms a trimeric complex with β-2 microglobulin and a short antigenic peptide of about eight to 10 amino acids generated by proteasome-mediated digestion of viral proteins in the cytoplasm of infected cells. Both species also express heterodimeric DR, DP, and DQ class II molecules formed from α and β chains that bind antigenic peptides generated in endosomes [6].

Class I and II loci in humans and chimpanzees encompass several dozen polymorphic alleles. Discovery of new alleles has accelerated with the use of the common chimpanzee for studies of HCV immunity and pathogenesis. The number of known Patr class I alleles now exceeds 18 for the A locus, 33 for the B locus, and 13 for the C locus, and nucleotide sequence homology of human and chimpanzee class I molecules exceeds 95% and there are no species-defining polymorphisms. Nonetheless, identical class I A, B or C alleles have not been found in humans and chimpanzees, reflecting five million years of evolution since the two species diverged from a common ancestor [5]. Chimpanzees appear to lack an equivalent of the human HLA-A2/A11 family of alleles [5, 7, 8], and HLA-B lineage alleles are not conserved in chimpanzees. Moreover, the class I B and C loci have evolved at a faster rate in chimpanzees than humans [9]. A key question is whether some human and chimpanzee alleles are functionally equivalent, presenting the same repertoire of antigenic peptides to T lymphocytes. Some alleles from both species have highly conserved peptide binding grooves that might be predicted to present an identical or largely overlapping set of antigenic peptides. Consistent with this hypothesis, epitopes derived from HIV, HBV, and HCV that are presented by human class I molecules such as HLA-A2 and –B7 also bind to chimpanzee B cell lines [10]. Cross-binding of these peptides has been confirmed using recombinant class I MHC proteins derived from the chimpanzee B cell lines [11]. The most striking functional homology was between the human HLA-B*0702 and chimpanzee Patr-B*1301 class I molecules. Overlap in the peptide binding repertoire of these class I molecules was a remarkable 92%. Both bound peptides were nine amino acids in length with a strict requirement for proline at position 2 and either an aromatic or aliphatic residue at the C terminus.

In summary, the immunogenetic complex of the common chimpanzee closely resembles that of humans in overall organization and extent of allelic diversity. Thus the T cell response against HCV is unlikely to be restricted or fundamentally different in chimpanzees when compared with that of humans. Functional homology between some HLA and Patr class I allotypes might also facilitate the development and testing of human HCV vaccines in chimpanzees.

HCV infection in the chimpanzee

Key features of HCV replication are similar in both species. HCV RNA levels range from 10^4 to 10^6 genome equivalents per milliliter of plasma in most chronically infected humans and chimpanzees [12]. The kinetic of acute phase virus replication is not as well defined. Within a few days of experimental infection, HCV proteins and RNA can be visualized in chimpanzee hepatocytes using *in situ* techniques, and plasma viremia is detectable by PCR [12]. Whether this reaches a peak that then subsides to a "setpoint" as described for HIV remains unknown. The frequency of persistent infection and mutation rate of the quasispecies is also probably similar in both species [13, 14]. At least 70% of humans transfused with contaminated blood products become persistently viremic. While the number of chimpanzees infected to date is relatively small, at least half of them developed a lifelong viremia. Thus this animal model is important for comparing host immune responses in chronic and resolved hepatitis C as well as mechanisms of HCV persistence. The animal model may be of limited utility for the study of HCV pathogenesis. Chimpanzees infected at least 10 years ago have not yet developed the progressive liver disease observed in many humans. Inflammation and cirrhosis usually take their toll on the human liver over a period of decades, so it is conceivable that disease will eventually develop in chimpanzees. Many were infected as juveniles so age is a potentially important variable that cannot be excluded. Finally, the rate of disease progression in humans is probably regulated at least in part by genetic or environmental factors that may not be replicated in the chimpanzee model.

Cellular immune responses
T lymphocytes may have a dual function in HCV infection, controlling virus replication while at the same time causing hepatocellular injury. Although a detailed understanding of these mechanisms is not yet in hand, a consensus on involvement of virus-specific T cell responses in human and chimpanzee HCV infections is beginning to emerge. Key features of HCV persistence and cellular immune responses are probably the same in both species, thus the animal model may be very useful for exploring immunotherapies that will eventually be applicable to humans.

CD4+ T helper cell responses
Chimpanzees and humans who spontaneously resolve HCV infection have robust T helper cell activity in their peripheral blood. HCV-specific CD4+ T cells are detectable in blood coincident with termination of plasma viremia in human subjects [15-17]. Multiple class II MHC-restricted epitopes in structural and nonstructural HCV proteins are targeted. Some epitopes may be more dominant than others, including one located in nonstructural protein 3 (NS3) that is presented by multiple human class II allotypes. The kinetic and antigen specificity of acute phase CD4+ T helper cell responses has not been adequately described in chimpanzees that successfully resolve infection. However, strong HCV-specific T helper cells targeting multiple epitopes persist in both species for very long periods of time after clearance of plasma viremia. Most of these studies utilized γ-IFN elispot assays that allow for quantification of antigen-specific T cells. Briefly, peripheral blood mononuclear cells are stimulated with recombinant HCV antigens in microtiter wells; γ-IFN produced locally by responding cells is captured and detected using anti-γ-IFN antibodies. T cell frequencies are then calculated from the number of spots in each well. CD4+ T cells recognizing HCV proteins were detected in the peripheral blood of women approximately 20 years after they resolved an accidental HCV infection [18]. This finding is consistent with other studies, including one that demonstrated high frequencies of CD4+ T cells in peripheral blood several months after resolution of infection using the γ-IFN elispot assay [19]. Strong priming of T helper cell activity was also observed in four chimpanzees who resolved infection three to four months after experimental infection and were virus-free during several years of follow-up [20]. Blood collected at the four-year time point had high frequencies of HCV-specific T helper cells against the core and most nonstructural proteins as assessed in the γ-IFN elispot assay. Remarkably, CD4+ T cells responding to HCV antigens were also isolated from the liver of these animals. Intrahepatic CD4+ T cells were expanded by *in vitro* stimulation with anti-CD3 monoclonal antibodies rather than HCV antigens, suggesting that they are in that tissue at high frequency. One interpretation of this data is that HCV-specific T helper cells remain compartmentalized in the liver years after plasma viremia became undetectable. It is possible that the liver is a unique

repository of memory T cells or that HCV continues to replicate in the liver at levels too low to detect by PCR.

In contrast, a deficiency of functional class II restricted T cells targeting structural and nonstructural proteins has been documented in the blood of individuals with persistent viremia. Preliminary studies in chimpanzees failed to detect HCV-specific CD4+ T helper cell activity in peripheral blood, mirroring the situation in humans where proliferation of PBMC induced by recombinant HCV antigens is low in comparison with standard recall antigens. Moreover, most subjects recognized only a subset of the HCV proteins, suggesting a restriction in the number of epitopes that are targeted [12]. It is likely that CD4+ T cells are not routinely detected in blood because they are compartmentalized to the liver in at least some subjects. One recent survey demonstrated that HCV antigen-responsive CD4+ T cells are present in at least some chronically infected subjects, and multispecific CD4+ T cells are more frequently detected in liver than blood [19]. T helper cells from these two tissue compartments may also differ in function. Comparison of liver and blood–derived CD4+ T cell lines from a limited number of chronically infected subjects were compared and found to be distinct in T cell receptor usage, patterns of cytokine production, and their ability to provide help for immunoglobulin class switching [21]. Whether this reflects an influence of the liver microenvironment on T cell function or selective trafficking of some clonotypes to that organ is uncertain.

In summary, from a limited set of data it appears that key features of the HCV-specific CD4+ T cell response are similar in chimpanzees and humans. These include a strong association between resolution of infection and robust, durable CD4+ T cell responses, and a more limited response in chronically infected individuals. These similarities help establish the validity of the chimpanzee model for studies of human HCV infection and development of therapies to augment immunity.

CD8+ T cell responses

Chimpanzees are an ideal model for studying the evolution of HCV-specific CD8+ T cell responses during the acute and chronic phases of infection. Responses in two animals with self-limited hepatitis C merit special mention [22]. Intrahepatic CD8+ T cells were isolated from biopsy specimens collected at various times after experimental HCV infection and then expanded *in vitro* with anti-CD3 monoclonal antibodies and interleukin 2. These antibodies deliver a mitogenic signal through the T cell receptor that should allow for expansion of all T lymphocytes regardless of antigen specificity. After about two weeks of culture, the CD8+ T cells were then tested for lysis of autologous target cells that expressed individual HCV antigens. Strong cytolysis was observed against almost all structural and nonstructural antigens within three to five weeks of infection. Remarkably, plasma viremia was terminated shortly after HCV-specific CD8+ T cells were detected in the liver [22]. Cloning of these effector cells at limiting dilution revealed that at least eight to nine different epitopes in HCV structural and nonstructural proteins were targeted, and these were presented by Patr class I A, B, and C molecules. Similar findings were reported in two studies of human subjects with acute hepatitis C [23, 24]. Multispecific CTL were detected in the peripheral blood of individuals using an Elispot assay for γ-IFN production [23, 24]. The acute phase of infection in chimpanzees and humans who develop persistent viremia is characterized by weaker or more narrowly focused CD8+ T cell responses during the acute phase of infection [22-24]. This temporal relationship between a multispecific CD8+ T lymphocyte response and spontaneous resolution of infection strongly suggests a key role for cellular immune responses. We cannot rule out the possibility that this CD8+ T cell activity is a surrogate marker for other effector mechanisms, including CD4+ T helper activity, that could play a direct role in termination of virus replication.

Involvement of virus-specific T cells in the pathogenesis of chronic liver disease and perhaps partial containment of virus replication is uncertain. Treatment of humans with immune suppressive drugs clearly increases HCV replication, sometimes with a lessening of liver inflammation, and thus provides support for this concept [25]. HCV-specific CD8+ T cells are present in the peripheral blood and liver of some individuals after years of persistent HCV replication. Virus-specific CD8+ T cells can be expanded from the blood of some human subjects using synthetic HCV peptides that bind class I MHC molecules such as HLA-A*0201 [26-28]. Peptide stimulation must be repeated at least three to four times for detection of cytolytic cells, suggesting that they are present at a low frequency. Soluble tetrameric HLA-A*0201 complexed to HCV peptides have been used to visualize HCV-specific T cell populations by flow cytometry [29]. They have revealed that at least some T cell populations are indeed present in blood at low frequencies, and preliminary data suggest that they might be compartmentalized to the liver.

CD8+ T cell lines targeting HCV structural and nonstructural proteins have been established from the liver of chronically infected humans [30-34] and chimpanzees [35, 36]. The true scope of the intrahepatic CD8+ CTL response has been difficult to gauge, because access to tissue is restricted, and small numbers of lymphocytes are recovered from biopsy specimens. We have recently completed an analysis of four chimpanzees that were experimentally infected with the HCV-1/910 virus stock. Remarkably, all four animals had very robust intrahepatic CTL activity, even after five to seven years of chronic infection [20]. CD8+ T cells were cloned by limiting dilution in the presence of anti-CD3 antibodies immediately after isolation from the liver. Approximately 300 independently derived CD8+ T cell lines were then screened for lysis of target cells expressing HCV proteins. The frequency of virus-specific clones in this panel ranged from two to 10% for these four persistently viremic animals. Mapping of peptide epitopes and class I restriction elements revealed that the response was also multispecific; T cell lines targeted four to six different epitopes located in structural and nonstructural HCV proteins. This is probably a minimum estimate of the number of CTL populations in the liver of these animals given the relatively small number of CD8+ T cell lines (≅300) that were screened for antiviral activity. Data from humans with chronic hepatitis C suggest that these findings are not unique to chimpanzees. Virus-specific T cell lines were established from about 40% of persistently infected humans [33]. These were usually directed against only one or two viral proteins, with the exception of one individual who had multispecific CTL targeting at least five different HCV proteins. Unlike chimpanzees, most individuals are infected with highly variable (and largely uncharacterized) HCV quasispecies. Therefore it is difficult to rule out the possibility that dominant T cell populations in humans are missed, because screening is limited to available recombinant viruses or proteins based on the HCV-1 or HCV-H sequences.

In summary, the data indicate that HCV replicates efficiently for years in an organ infiltrated with virus-specific CD8+ T lymphocytes. The longevity or turnover rate of HCV-specific CD8+ T cells in the liver could influence their ability to control the rapidly replicating HCV quasispecies. Long-term follow-up of intrahepatic CD8+ T cell populations in one chronically infected chimpanzee provided a means to address this issue [20]. Panels of CTL lines generated from liver biopsies collected at seven and 84 months postinfection were compared for recognition of HCV epitopes presented by Patr-A and -B class I molecules. T cell populations established from the liver at 84 months postinfection targeted six epitopes located in C, E1, E2, NS3, NS4, and NS5. Remarkably, the identical E1, E2 and NS3 epitopes were recognized by T cell populations recovered from the liver at month 7 postinfection, almost seven years earlier. Results are summarized schematically in Figure 1. It is very likely that the NS4- and NS5-specific populations were also present at the earliest time point; recombinant vaccinia viruses expressing those nonstructural proteins had not been constructed when the first biopsy specimen was collected. These data suggest that the most dominant T cell populations are not deleted from the repertoire and indeed appear to be remarkably stable over time despite high levels of virus replication.

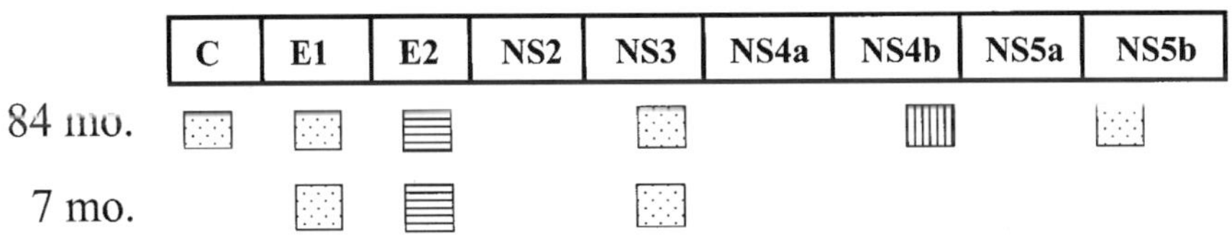

Figure 1. Stable repertoire of HCV-specific CD8+ T cells during seven years of chronic infection in a chimpanzee. CD8+ T cell lines generated from the liver of a chronically infected chimpanzee at seven and 84 months after experimental infection. The class I MHC restriction and HCV protein of origin are shown for each epitope. Epitopes presented by Patr-A*0401 ( ), B*1601 ( ), and B*1701 ( ) are indicated.

It is important to emphasize that these studies involved very few humans and chimpanzees with acute hepatitis C. Common findings in both species do, however, provide a model or framework for successful containment of virus replication where robust cell mediated immune responses directed against multiple class I (or class II) restricted epitopes facilitate complete control of virus replication. One critical area for future exploration is the relative contribution of CD4+ versus CD8+ T cells in this process. The outcome of these studies will undoubtedly influence the design of vaccines that prevent establishment of a persistent HCV infection.

Mechanisms of HCV persistence

One key unanswered question is why HCV-specific T cells with cytotoxic potential fail to terminate infection. Three general mechanisms can be envisioned, including deletion or anergy of these effector cells in the liver, interference with antigen processing or presentation pathways in infected hepatocytes, or mutation of the virus to evade immune recognition. The latter mechanism deserves special consideration because HCV is a rapidly replicating RNA virus with an error prone, RNA-dependent RNA replicase. Mutation in a class I MHC-restricted HCV epitope that facilitated escape from CTL activity was first demonstrated in a persistently infected chimpanzee [37], and changes in epitopes targeted by human CD8+ T cells have also been described [38-40]. A significant role for immune selection pressure in establishment or maintenance of persistence is complicated by the observation that at least some chimpanzees and humans have intrahepatic CTL directed against multiple class I epitopes. Mutations that break T cell recognition would have to occur in all or most of these epitopes. One model that accommodates mutation in several class I MHC epitopes is illustrated in Figure 2.

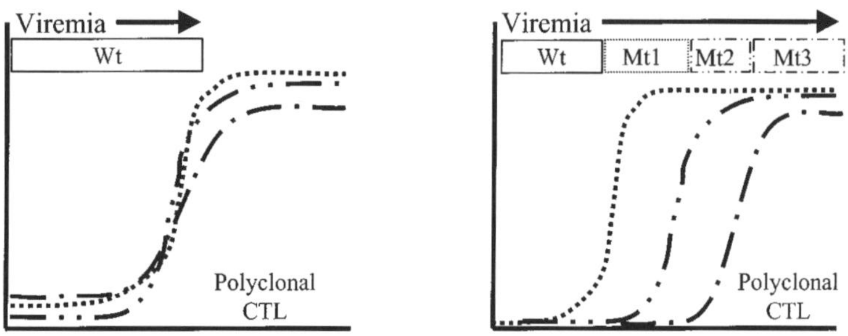

Figure 2. A model for generation of mutations in multiple class I MHC epitopes. Panel A shows termination of wild-type (Wt) HCV replication in the face of multispecific CTL that simultaneously infiltrate the liver. CTL populations targeting different epitopes are indicated by dashed lines. Panel B shows sequential selection of escape mutations in individual epitopes (Mt1, Mt2, and Mt3) when CTL populations develop in a staggered pattern over time.

Panel A summarizes observations in the two chimpanzees (ch-497 and ch-482) with self-limited infections [22]. Simultaneous appearance of several class I MHC-restricted T cell populations in the liver is disadvantageous for virus replication and leads to early termination of infection. Preliminary data indicate that chronically infected chimpanzees (and probably humans) target fewer epitopes during the earliest stages of infection. It is proposed that T cell populations targeting HCV epitopes develop in a staggered pattern over the first few weeks or months of infection (Panel B). In its simplest form this model predicts that immune selection pressure is focused on one epitope at a time. Thus, it is not necessary to postulate simultaneous mutation of all HCV epitopes, even though multiple intrahepatic CTL populations are sometimes found in chronically infected individuals. Evolution of virus and T lymphocyte populations is clearly a dynamic process, and the balance between persistence or resolution of infection is probably delicate. Some temporal overlap between developing T cell populations is likely, but they may not be uniformly distributed in a large solid organ like the liver, especially if frequencies are low. Viruses replicating in individual hepatocytes or lobules would be subject to selection pressure only by T cell clonotypes present in that microenvironment. Mutations in class II MHC restricted epitopes of HCV could facilitate persistence of HCV, and accumulating evidence supports this mechanism [41, 42].

Summary

HCV and HIV readily acquire resistance to host immune responses and drugs that inhibit rapid replication of their RNA genomes. This is probably the most significant scientific hurdle to development of effective therapies for these viruses. For instance, it is very likely that a combination of drugs targeting different HCV enzymes will be required for effective therapy. Complicated dosing regimens and hepatotoxicity could be significant barriers to successful treatment of patients who otherwise have few symptoms of chronic hepatitis C. Moreover, approximately 100 million infected individuals live in developing countries where combination drug therapies for HCV will not be widely available. An inexpensive and effective vaccine to treat chronic hepatitis C would be highly desirable.

Understanding how HCV is successfully controlled in individuals who spontaneously resolve infection will provide an important starting point for this effort. There is an emerging consensus that resolution of acute hepatitis C in humans and chimpanzees is associated with a vigorous cell-mediated immune response. In contrast, CD4+ T helper cell activity as measured by lymphoproliferation or γ-IFN production is lacking in chronically infected individuals. Moreover, the CD8+ T cell response may be locked on class I MHC-restricted epitopes that have mutated to avoid recognition. It is tempting to speculate that interventions to augment Th activity, broaden the CTL response to additional epitopes, or both, could lead to resolution of infection. Candidate HIV vaccines designed to elicit long-lasting CD4+ and CD8+ T cell responses are about to enter human clinical trials. Some of these will involve vaccination of chronically infected subjects taking antiviral drugs to lower HIV viral burden. Results of these trials could hold important clues for selection of HCV vaccine strategies.

Data reviewed here support the notion that the same lesion in cellular immunity facilitates persistence of HCV in humans and chimpanzees. Moreover, through the study of HCV infection, we have learned that the immunogenetic complex of chimpanzees and humans is remarkably similar. These observations establish the importance of the chimpanzee model for more detailed studies of the host response against HCV and for testing the safety and efficacy of candidate vaccines.

References

1. Choo QL, Kuo G, Weiner A, Wang KS, Overby L, Bradley D, Houghton M. Identification of the major, parenteral non-A, non-B hepatitis agent (hepatitis C virus) using a recombinant cDNA approach. *Semin Liver Dis* 1992;12:279-88.
2. Kolykhalov AA, Agapov EV, Blight KJ, Mihalik K, Feinstone SM, Rice CM. Transmission of hepatitis C by intrahepatic inoculation with transcribed RNA. *Science* 1997;277:570-4.
3. Yanagi M, Purcell RH, Emerson SU, Bukh J. Transcripts from a single full-length cDNA clone of hepatitis C virus are infectious when directly transfected into the liver of a chimpanzee. *Proc Natl Acad Sci U S A* 1997;94:8738-43.
4. McMichael AJ, O'Callaghan CA. A new look at T cells. *J Exp Med* 1998;187:1367-71.
5. Parham P, Lawlor DA, Lomen CE, Ennis PD. Diversity and diversification of HLA-A, B, C alleles. *J Immunol* 1989;142:3937-50.
6. de Groot NG, Bontrop RE. The major histocompatibility complex class II region of the chimpanzee: towards a molecular map. *Immunogenetics* 1999;50:160-7.
7. Watkins DI. The evolution of major histocompatibility class I genes in primates. *Crit Rev Immunol* 1995;15:1-29.
8. de Groot NG, Otting N, Arguello R, Watkins DI, Doxiadis GG, Madrigal JA, Bontrop RE. Major histocompatibility complex class I diversity in a West African chimpanzee population: implications for HIV research. *Immunogenetics* 2000;51:398-409.
9. Adams EJ, Cooper S, Thomson G, Parham P. Common chimpanzees have greater diversity than humans at two of the three highly polymorphic MHC class I genes. *Immunogenetics* 2000;51:410-24.
10. Bertoni R, Sette A, Sidney J, Guidotti LG, Shapiro M, Purcell R, Chisari FV. Human class I supertypes and CTL repertoires extend to chimpanzees. *J Immunol* 1998;161:4447-55.
11. McKinney DM, Erickson AL, Walker CM, Thimme R, Chisari FV, Purcell R, Sidney J, Sette A. Identification of five different Patr class I molecules which bind HLA supertype peptides and definition of their peptide binding motifs. *Journal of Immunology* 2000;in press.
12. Walker CM. Comparative features of hepatitis C virus infection in humans and chimpanzees. *Springer Semin Immunopathol* 1997;19:85-98.
13. Seeff LB. Natural history of hepatitis C. *Am J Med* 1999;107:10S-15S.
14. Bukh J, Miller RH, Purcell RH. Genetic heterogeneity of hepatitis C virus: quasispecies and genotypes. *Semin Liver Dis* 1995;15:41-63.
15. Missale G, Bertoni R, Lamonaca V, Valli A, Massari M, Mori C, Rumi MG, Houghton M, Fiaccadori F, Ferrari C. Different clinical behaviors of acute hepatitis C virus infection are associated with different vigor of the anti-viral cell-mediated immune response. *J Clin Invest* 1996;98:706-14.
16. Diepolder HM, Zachoval R, Hoffmann RM, Wierenga EA, Santantonio T, Jung MC, Eichenlaub D, Pape GR. Possible mechanism involving T-lymphocyte response to non-structural protein 3 in viral clearance in acute hepatitis C virus infection. *Lancet* 1995;346:1006-7.
17. Diepolder HM, Zachoval R, Hoffmann RM, Jung MC, Gerlach T, Pape GR. The role of hepatitis C virus specific CD4+ T lymphocytes in acute and chronic hepatitis C. *J Mol Med* 1996;74:583-8.
18. Takaki A, Wiese M, Maertens G, Depla E, Seifert U, Liebetrau A, Miller JL, Manns MP, Rehermann B. Cellular immune responses persist and humoral responses decrease two decades after recovery from a single-source outbreak of hepatitis C. *Nat Med* 2000;6:578-82.
19. Schirren CA, Jung M, Worzfeld T, Mamin M, Baretton GB, Gruener NH, Gerlach JT, Diepolder HM, Zachoval R, Pape GR. Cytokine profile of liver- and blood-derived nonspecific T cells after liver

transplantation: T helper cells type 1/0 lymphokines dominate in recurrent hepatitis C virus infection and rejection. *Liver Transpl* 2000;6:222-8.

20. Walker CM. Cell-mediated immunity and the outcome of infection in chimpanzees. Third International Conference on Therapies for Viral Hepatitis. Hawaii, USA, December 12-16, 1999.
21. Minutello MA, Pileri P, Unutmaz D, Censini S, Kuo G, Houghton M, Brunetto MR, Bonino F, Abrignani S. Compartmentalization of T lymphocytes to the site of disease: intrahepatic CD4+ T cells specific for the protein NS4 of hepatitis C virus in patients with chronic hepatitis C. *J Exp Med* 1993;178:17-25.
22. Cooper S, Erickson AL, Adams EJ, Kansopon J, Weiner AJ, Chien DY, Houghton M, Parham P, Walker CM. Analysis of a successful immune response against hepatitis C virus. *Immunity* 1999;10:439-49.
23. Lechner F, Wong DK, Dunbar PR, Chapman R, Chung RT, Dohrenwend P, Robbins G, Phillips R, Klenerman P, Walker BD. Analysis of successful immune responses in persons infected with hepatitis C virus. *J Exp Med* 2000;191:1499-512.
24. Gruner NH, Gerlach TJ, Jung MC, Diepolder HM, Schirren CA, Schraut WW, Hoffmann R, Zachoval R, Santantonio T, Cucchiarini M, Cerny A, Pape GR. Association of hepatitis C virus-specific CD8+ T cells with viral clearance in acute hepatitis C [In Process Citation]. *J Infect Dis* 2000;181:1528-36.
25. Rice CM, Walker CM. Hepatitis C virus-specific T lymphocyte responses. *Curr Opin Immunol* 1995;7:532-8.
26. Cerny A, McHutchison JG, Pasquinelli C, Brown ME, Brothers MA, Grabscheid B, Fowler P, Houghton M, Chisari FV. Cytotoxic T lymphocyte response to hepatitis C virus-derived peptides containing the HLA A2.1 binding motif. *J Clin Invest* 1995;95:521-30.
27. Battegay M, Fikes J, Di Bisceglie AM, Wentworth PA, Sette A, Celis E, Ching WM, Grakoui A, Rice CM, Kurokohchi K, et al. Patients with chronic hepatitis C have circulating cytotoxic T cells which recognize hepatitis C virus-encoded peptides binding to HLA-A2.1 molecules. *J Virol* 1995;69:2462-70.
28. Wentworth PA, Sette A, Celis E, Sidney J, Southwood S, Crimi C, Stitely S, Keogh E, Wong NC, Livingston B, Alazard D, Vitiello A, Grey HM, Chisari FV, Chesnut RW, Fikes J. Identification of A2-restricted hepatitis C virus-specific cytotoxic T lymphocyte epitopes from conserved regions of the viral genome. *Int Immunol* 1996;8:651-9.
29. He XS, Rehermann B, Lopez-Labrador FX, Boisvert J, Cheung R, Mumm J, Wedemeyer H, Berenguer M, Wright TL, Davis MM, Greenberg HB. Quantitative analysis of hepatitis C virus-specific CD8(+) T cells in peripheral blood and liver using peptide-MHC tetramers. *Proc Natl Acad Sci U S A* 1999;96:5692-7.
30. Koziel MJ, Dudley D, Wong JT, Dienstag J, Houghton M, Ralston R, Walker BD. Intrahepatic cytotoxic T lymphocytes specific for hepatitis C virus in persons with chronic hepatitis [published erratum appears in J Immunol 1993 Mar 15;150(6):2563]. *J Immunol* 1992;149:3339-44.
31. Koziel MJ, Dudley D, Afdhal N, Choo QL, Houghton M, Ralston R, Walker BD. Hepatitis C virus (HCV)-specific cytotoxic T lymphocytes recognize epitopes in the core and envelope proteins of HCV. *J Virol* 1993;67:7522-32.
32. Koziel MJ, Dudley D, Afdhal N, Grakoui A, Rice CM, Choo QL, Houghton M, Walker BD. HLA class I-restricted cytotoxic T lymphocytes specific for hepatitis C virus. Identification of multiple epitopes and characterization of patterns of cytokine release. *J Clin Invest* 1995;96:2311-21.
33. Wong DK, Dudley DD, Afdhal NH, Dienstag J, Rice CM, Wang L, Houghton M, Walker BD, Koziel MJ. Liver-derived CTL in hepatitis C virus infection: breadth and specificity of responses in a cohort of persons with chronic infection. *J Immunol* 1998;160:1479-88.

34. Nelson DR, Marousis CG, Davis GL, Rice CM, Wong J, Houghton M, Lau JY. The role of hepatitis C virus-specific cytotoxic T lymphocytes in chronic hepatitis C. *J Immunol* 1997;158:1473-81.
35. Erickson AL, Houghton M, Choo QL, Weiner AJ, Ralston R, Muchmore E, Walker CM. Hepatitis C virus-specific CTL responses in the liver of chimpanzees with acute and chronic hepatitis C. *J Immunol* 1993;151:4189-99.
36. Kowalski H, Erickson AL, Cooper S, Domena JD, Parham P, Walker CM. Patr-A and B, the orthologues of HLA-A and B, present hepatitis C virus epitopes to CD8+ cytotoxic T cells from two chronically infected chimpanzees. *J Exp Med* 1996;183:1761-75.
37. Weiner A, Erickson AL, Kansopon J, Crawford K, Muchmore E, Hughes AL, Houghton M, Walker CM. Persistent hepatitis C virus infection in a chimpanzee is associated with emergence of a cytotoxic T lymphocyte escape variant. *Proc Natl Acad Sci U S A* 1995;92:2755-9.
38. Giuggio VM, Bonkovsky HL, Smith J, Rothman AL. Inefficient recognition of autologous viral sequences by intrahepatic hepatitis C virus-specific cytotoxic T lymphocytes in chronically infected subjects. *Virology* 1998;251:132-40.
39. Tsai SL, Chen YM, Chen MH, Huang CY, Sheen IS, Yeh CT, Huang JH, Kuo GC, Liaw YF. Hepatitis C virus variants circumventing cytotoxic T lymphocyte activity as a mechanism of chronicity. *Gastroenterology* 1998;115:954-65.
40. Chang KM, Rehermann B, McHutchison JG, Pasquinelli C, Southwood S, Sette A, Chisari FV. Immunological significance of cytotoxic T lymphocyte epitope variants in patients chronically infected by the hepatitis C virus. *J Clin Invest* 1997;100:2376-85.
41. Frasca L, Del Porto P, Tuosto L, Marinari B, Scotta C, Carbonari M, Nicosia A, Piccolella E. Hypervariable region 1 variants act as TCR antagonists for hepatitis C virus-specific CD4+ T cells. *J Immunol* 1999;163:650-8.
42. Wang H, Eckels DD. Mutations in immunodominant T cell epitopes derived from the nonstructural 3 protein of hepatitis C virus have the potential for generating escape variants that may have important consequences for T cell recognition. *J Immunol* 1999;162:4177-83.

Adoptive immune transfer as a therapeutic approach for persistent hepatitis B virus infection

DANIEL SHOUVAL

Liver Unit, Division of Medicine, Hadassah University Hospital, P.O. Box 12000, Jerusalem, Israel

Complete resolution of persistent hepatitis B virus (HBV) infection using available licensed or experimental antiviral agents is still an unaccomplished goal in over 50% of treated patients. We have explored new means for improving the efficacy of antiviral therapy for hepatitis B. One avenue of research has examined the use of adoptive transfer of immunity to HBV as a means of overcoming immune tolerance to the virus in hepatitis B surface antigen (HBsAg) carriers. For this purpose we have recruited a population of bone marrow donors (BMDs) and bone marrow transplant recipients (BMTs). In these patients seroconversion, as manifested by detection of antibodies to HBsAg (anti-HBs), may be induced in BMT recipients who receive their BMT from HLA-matched BMDs immunized against HBV. Transfer of peripheral blood lymphocytes (PBL) from such BMDs to HBV-naïve BMT recipients has also induced anti-HBs seroconversion in the majority of patients tested. Adoptive transfer of HBV immune cells from HBV-immune BMDs has also been utilized for induction of hepatitis B clearance in BMT recipients persistently infected with HBV. These results have provided the justification for further evaluation of the role of vaccination in patients already infected with hepatitis B.

Introduction

Persistent hepatitis B virus (HBV) infection may develop in 10-90% of patients, depending on age at infection and adequacy of immune response. Resolution of HBV infection requires an intact cytolytic T cell response against nucleocapsid viral epitopes for clearance of intra-hepatocyte infection [1]. Acquired humoral response against the envelope protein(s) is essential for neutralizing circulating viruses and for future protection against HBV infection. Immune memory against HBV, whether acquired through resolution of infection or through vaccination, will usually remain for life. In contrast, a significant proportion of newborns and adults infected with HBV are unable to clear the infection and become HBsAg carriers. Currently, available antiviral therapy is only partially effective, and at best only one third of α-Interferon-treated patients may clear the virus from their circulation. New nucleoside analogues such as lamivudine may be effective in suppressing viral replication. However, with lamivudine

Frontiers in Viral Hepatitis Ed. by RF Schinazi, J-P Sommadossi and CM Rice. 71 — 75

there is evidence that treatment must be given indefinitely, since discontinuation may lead to re-emergence of HBV markers in the blood. On the other hand, prolonged administration of lamivudine will be associated with emergence of YMDD mutants. Thus, additional means are necessary to restore immune non- or hyporesponsiveness against HBV. In recent years several attempts have been made to induce cessation of HBV replication through active immunization against HBsAg using Pre-S/S HBV vaccines [2, 3]. Results of these preliminary clinical trials are not conclusive. We have chosen to study other means for inducing clearance of HBV infection through adoptive transfer of immunity. The hypothesis that the immune response against HBV can be transferred from immunocompetent donors to immune suppressed recipients was tested in mice and humans. Bone marrow obtained from human BMDs who recovered from HBV or were immunized against HBsAg was transplanted to HBV-naïve BMT recipients who required a marrow transplantation for their hematologic disease. The data obtained suggest that HBV-naïve individuals can acquire immunity against hepatitis B through adoptive transfer of immunity using the immunologic maneuver described above [4-8].

Transplantation of bone marrow or peripheral blood lymphocytes for human donors immunized against hepatitis B

In the early 1990s we made the first observation that 12/178 HBV-naïve recipients in our institution received their BM from healthy anti-HBc$^+$/anti-HBs$^+$ BMDs. All 12 BMT patients seroconverted to anti-HBc$^+$/anti-HBs$^+$ following transplantation [5]. Out of six patients followed for a mean of four years (range 1-6.2 years), three had evidence of humoral anti-HBs response, with serum anti-HBs levels ranging from 63-189 mIU/ml. Later, seroconversion to anti-HBs$^+$ was also documented in 22/35 (63%) BMT recipients whose BMDs were immunized at least once against HBV, using a second generation yeast-derived HBV vaccine (10-20 μg/dose) [5]. Seroconversion occurred between days 9-52 post-BMT. Although anti-HBs levels were low, some patients responded with a secondary rise in anti-HBs titers following one to several booster vaccinations given up to one year post-BMT. In seven out of nine patients followed for a longer period with a mean follow-up of 2.5 ± 4.3 months, anti-HBs levels remained above the lower threshold of protective levels (mean 102 ± 13 mIU/ml, range 22-183). Adoptive transfer of immunity to HBsAg was also accomplished in six out of eight BMT recipients following transplantation of PBLs from human donors immunized against HBsAg [7]. In four out of six patients in whom seroconversion was documented 27-45 days post-transplantation of PBL, a secondary rise in anti-HBs titer could be documented following immunization with a conventional HBV vaccine.

Resolution of persistent HBV infection following BMT from an HBV-immune donor

Clearance of HBV DNA and of HBsAg with seroconversion to anti-HBs$^+$ was documented for the first time in a child with chronic lymphocytic leukemia who received a BMT from his HLA-matched brother [9]. This brother, who was initially anti-HBc$^+$/anti-HBs$^+$, received a recombinant HBsAg vaccine booster injection prior to the harvesting of his bone marrow. Clearance of HBsAg and anti-HBs seroconversion in the BMT recipient was accompanied by a rise in aminotransferase levels, but with no adverse clinical symptoms. This first documentation of resolution of persistent HBV infection was later confirmed in a number of Chinese, $HBsAg^{+}$ patients in Hong Kong who received a BMT from HBV-immune donors [10, 11].

Evidence for long-term maintenance of immune memory in BMT recipients following adoptive transfer of immunity to HBV

Patients post-BMT have been contacted within one to two years of BMT for evaluation of residual PBL activity against rHBsAg *in vitro*. Briefly, PBLs obtained from healthy adults either non-immunized or immunized against HBV, or from BMT recipients receiving bone marrow from anti-HBs or $anti\text{-}HBc^{+}/anti\text{-}HBs^{+}$ donors, were stimulated *in vitro* with rHBsAg for seven days. After a pulse with ^{3}H-thymidin the specific stimulation index rose from 2.2 to 63 in BMT recipients from immunized donors following a booster injection one year or more post-BMT. This cell proliferation was also documented in healthy vaccinees; in BMT recipients from $anti\text{-}HBc^{+}/anti\text{-}HBs^{+}$ donors, but not in healthy controls [12].

Comment

Persistent HBV infection is one of the most common infections worldwide. The consequences of acute hepatitis B are serious not only in East Asia or Africa but also in the U.S. and Europe, where 32,000-90,000 new patients with chronic hepatitis B are added to the pool of patients with chronic liver disease each year. Such patients who are at risk for developing cirrhosis and hepatocellular carcinoma must be provided with an efficient means for suppressing or resolving active viral replication and slowing down the hepatic inflammatory and fibrotic processes. Unfortunately, so far currently available antiviral agents such as α-Interferon, lamivudine and other newer nucleoside analogues have not been shown to induce permanent resolution of the viral infection.

In recent years much attention has been given to a first attempt to augment the natural immune response against HBV in HBsAg carriers through active immunization with a Pre-S_2/s mammalian-derived hepatitis B vaccine. Coullin, Pol and coworkers have shown that repeated immunization of such carriers may reduce the viral load in about one third or more of patients [2]. Although the statistical significance of this treatment is not yet proven, this observation should lead to further attempts to test the effects of "*vaccinotherapy*" in patients with chronic hepatitis B. Recently Yap and coworkers conducted a placebo-controlled clinical trial in Indonesia where 108 patients were randomized to receive four doses of a mouse-cell-derived HBV vaccine containing Pre-S_1/Pre-S_2/S antigens, followed by a nine month interval and again several courses of immunization [3]. Although this study lacked power, a trend toward reducing viral replication and even seroconversion to anti-HBs was observed in those patients with elevated aminotransferase levels. Several similar clinical trials using preconditioning with antiviral agents followed by vaccination against HBV are now in progress. Two of these studies introduced new formulations of hepatitis B vaccines containing novel adjuvants intended to shift part of the cellular immune response toward T cell TH1 response.

Meanwhile, we are continuing our own efforts using adoptive transfer of immunity against HBV. In the clinical experiments described above, we take advantage of the intact immune response of healthy BMDs. Obviously, adoptive transfer of immunity through bone marrow transplantation is not a realistic option for the hundreds of millions of HBsAg carriers worldwide. Nevertheless, the concept of replacing or resuscitating a hyporesponsive immune system against HBV has been tested and shown effective under the conditions described above. Further confirmation of the initial observations was provided by the BMT group from Hong Kong who have been able to induce resolution of HBV infection in several BMT recipients with persistent HBV infection using the method of adoptive transfer of immunity [10, 11]. These investigators have elegantly documented the recovery of the anti-HBV immune response in $HBsAg^+$ BMT recipients transplanted with bone marrow from $anti\text{-}HBc^+$/$anti\text{-}HBs^+$ donors. Thus, recovery and seroconversion was accompanied by a fortunately mild hepatitis manifested by ALT elevation. It is evident that such a maneuver may be associated with a risk for induction of an immune attack against the infected hepatocytes, once immune response against HBV has been recovered [13]. The extent of such a response can only partially be controlled when BMT is used. However, we have shown that similar effects can be controlled through transplantation of HBV immune lymphocytes or stem cells instead of bone marrow [7]. Thus, better control of flare-ups may be possible, especially at a point where stem cell transplantation has replaced the conventional bone marrow transfer.

In summary, adoptive transfer of immunity to HBV was evaluated as a possible tool for inducing resolution of HBV infection in individuals who were unable to develop an adequate immune response against HBV. Further clinical trials should be designed to test the protective role of such an immunological maneuver as adjuvant therapy to conventional antiviral agents.

References

1. Chisari FV, and Ferrari C. Hepatitis B virus immunopathogenesis. *Annual Review of Immunology* 1995;13:29-34.
2. Coullin J, Pol S, Mancini M, Driss F, Brechot C, Trollais P and Michel ML. Specific vaccine therapy in chronic hepatitis B: Induction of T cell proliferative responses specific for envelope antigens. *Journal of Infectious Diseases* 1999;180:15-26.
3. Yap SP, Sulaiman A, Lesmana L, Dickson B, Vanhoutte F, Hadiyanto Y, Williams A and Young M. Immunotherapy of chronic hepatitis B in Asian patients using a novel triple antigen hepatitis B vaccine (Hepacare). *Antiviral Therapy* 2000;5(Suppl. 1):B.68.
4. Shouval D, Adler R and Ilan Y. Adoptive transfer of immunity to hepatitis B virus in mice by bone marrow transplantation from HBV immune donors. *Hepatology* 1993;17:955–959.
5. Ilan Y, Nagler, A, Adler, R., Naparstek E, Or R, Slavin S and Shouval D. Adoptive transfer of immunity to hepatitis B in humans following T-depleted bone marrow transplantation from HBV immune donors. *Hepatology* 1993;18:246-252.

6. Ilan Y, Nagler A, Ackerstein A, Or R, Kapelushnik J, Adler R, Slavin S and Shouval D. Development of antibodies to hepatitis B virus surface antigen in bone marrow transplant recipient following treatment with peripheral blood lymphocytes from immunized donors. *Journal of Clinical Experimental Immunology* 1994;97:299-302.
7. Shouval D and Ilan Y. Transplantation of hepatitis B immune lymphocytes as means for adoptive transfer of immunity to HBV. *Journal of Hepatology* 1995;23:98-101.
8. Shouval D and Ilan Y. Adoptive transfer of immunity to hepatitis B: development of the concept and evolution of the research project for targeted immunotherapy against hepatic cells which express a viral antigen. *Advances in Drug Delivery Reviews* 1995;17:317–320.
9. Ilan Y, Nagler A, Adler R, Tur Kaspa R, Slavin S and Shouval D. Ablation of persistent hepatitis B by allogeneic bone marrow transplantation from an HBV immune donor. *Gastroenterology* 1993;104:1818-1821.
10. Lau GK, Lok AS, Liang RH, Lai CL, Chiu EK, Lau YL and Lam SK. Clearance of Hepatitis B surface antigen after bone marrow transplantation: Role of adoptive immunity transfer. *Hepatology* 1997;25:1497-501.
11. Lau GK, Liang R, Lee CK, Yuen ST, Hou J, Lim WL and Williams R. Clearance of persistent hepatitis B virus infection in Chinese bone marrow transplant recipients whose donors were anti-hepatitis B core and anti-hepatitis B surface antibody-positive. *Journal of Infectious Diseases* 1998;176:1585-91.
12. Ilan Y, Nagler A, Zeira E, Adler R, Slavin S and Shouval D. Maintenance of immune memory to the hepatitis B envelope protein following adoptive transfer of immunity in bone marrow transplant recipients. *Bone Marrow Transplantation* 2000;26:633-638.
13. Strasser SI and McDonald GB. Hepatitis viruses and hematopoietic cell transplantation: A guide to patient and donor management. *Blood* 1999; 93:1127-1131.

Perspectives in HCV vaccine development

ERIK DEPLA

Innogenetics, N.V., Industriepark Zwijnaarde 7, Box 4, Ghent B-9052, Belgium

Introduction

The discovery of HCV in 1989 was followed by a decade of growing awareness about the full impact of this slowly progressing disease. The recent and dramatic increases in end-stage liver diseases, including hepatocellular carcinoma as reported for the US [1] and Japan [2], have been attributed to the boom of HCV infections during the 70s and 80s. For several years, HCV has become the leading cause of liver transplantation, and recent figures show that the hospitalization and indirect costs caused by HCV in the US increased to 1.5 billion US$ already in 1995 [3]. Moreover, there still remains a huge number of people who are unaware of their infections but will present to their physicians within the next decades with signs of progressive liver disease.

The only therapy approved today is (pegylated) interferon-α monotherapy or a combination of interferon with ribavirin. Although effective in achieving sustained response in up to 80% of some patient groups (e.g., genotype 2- or 3-infected), efficacy is only about 40% for the predominant genotype 1 infections [4, 5]. Moreover, many patients need to stop therapy because of adverse events, or they are excluded because of markers predicting side effects. Consequently, the demand for alternative therapies remains high. So is the need for prophylaxis due to the intrinsicly high cost of this disease and its therapy. Vaccines are currently being developed, and some have entered the phase of clinical testing, for prophylaxis and therapy.

Preclinical studies in chimpanzees have shown that infection can be prevented by active vaccination with E1E2 complexes [6], but this protection seems to be limited to low dose and homologous challenges. Therapeutic vaccination of chimpanzees with E1 resulted in strong and not previously noted immune responses which were capable of altering disease status by reducing signs of liver damage. However, this type of vaccination was not able to clear the infection [7].

The development of HCV vaccines is hampered by 1) the lack of knowledge concerning correlates of immune protection, 2) the technical difficulties encountered in the production of good quality envelope antigens, and 3) the lack of information on the structural restraints for these envelope proteins, which need to be taken into account for optimal antigen presentation within a vaccine context. In turn, many of these problems relate to the lack of an efficient *in vitro* cultivation system for this virus.

Frontiers in Viral Hepatitis Ed. by RF Schinazi, J-P Sommadossi and CM Rice. 77 — 85

In addition, the existence of genotypes and subtypes with a high genetic diversity is not favorable for vaccine development.

On the other hand, some recent studies (discussed below) provide new insights on how viral infections that may lead to persistence can be controlled by the host immune surveillance, or how the virus is able to avoid this control. Growing experience with therapy in HCV and other persistent viral infections is opening new possibilities that also apply to the field of vaccination. Finally, the ongoing clinical trials involving both prophylactic and therapeutic vaccines for HCV, as well as other viral infections including HIV and HBV, will in the near future shed even more light on the desired immune responses to combat HCV, even if such trials are only partially successful.

Persistent viral infection and the host immune system

As reviewed by Biron [8], the initial responses to viral infection lead to activation of NK cells either by potentiating their cytolytic function or by increasing their interferon-γ-mediated antiviral activity. The type of cytokines released during the early stages of infection may determine the activity of the NK cells. Induction of the type I interferon-α and-β promotes the cytolytic pathway, while induction of tumor necrosis factor-α, interleukin-6, and interleukin-12 activates the non-cytolytic but antiviral interferon-γ pathway.

The importance of this non-cytolytic clearance of an hepatocytic infection was recently demonstrated in two studies. HBV infection may lead to persistent infection, but the majority of individuals clear the infection spontaneously. A recent study [9] of HBV infection in chimpanzees gave some insight into the mechanisms involved in this viral resolution. Within eight to 12 weeks after infection, almost every hepatocyte was infected by HBV. However, this massive infection could be cleared mainly by a non-cytolytic pathway in which the cytokines interferon-γ and tumor necrosis factor-α were the major players. These cytokines are not released by CD8 cells, as they appear only later in the liver, probably to clear the remaining infectious sites, thereby resulting in an ALT peak. Finally, anti-HBsAg antibodies appear, and the animals recover completely from infection. In a second study, the same authors demonstrated that lymphocytic choriomeningitis virus infection is also cleared from mouse livers based on the same principle, but clearance of this virus from other tissues probably requires efficient killing [10].

The role of CD8 responses in clearing viral infections is well accepted, while that for neutralizing antibody is somewhat debated and may depend both on the infecting agent and the host. Nevertheless, several studies show that both CTL and humoral responses are required to achieve sustained elimination of viral infections that may lead to persistence. One of the best studied models is probably lymphocytic choriomeningitis virus, which infects mice and thus provides an easy and well-known animal model. This virus can initially be well controlled by neutralizing antibody, but in the absence of CD8 cells, escape mutants will appear [11]. Inversely, adoptive transfer experiments [12] and infection in B-cell-deficient mice [13] revealed that in the absence of B cells, the initial control of the virus by CD8 cells appears to be in vain. Studies with SIV in

CD8-depleted animals have shown that the CD8 response may even be a prerequisite to allow for the emergence of the neutralizing antibodies [14]. Although the neutralizing antibodies do not clear disease in the case of SIV, they are thought to slow down disease progression, as also shown for HIV [15].

Whether or not the immune response is successful may depend on many factors influencing a critical balance. Many viruses have developed mechanisms which result in a shift of the balance to persistence. Viral interference with cytokine function and antigen presentation are common, and include infection of antigen-presenting cells and alteration of MHC class I expression [for review see 16-18]. In addition, hiding or mutation of neutralizing epitopes (both humoral and cellular) is frequently observed [19, 20] in combination with the aforementioned escape strategies.

Persistence or resolution in HCV

Whether similar mechanisms lead to resolution of HCV remains to be evaluated. The lack of correlates of immune protection is remarkable, since spontaneous resolution of HCV is not such a unique event [around 20% of infections; 21]. One of the problems related to the acute phase of HCV is, however, the lack of clear-cut and severe symptoms. Consequently, not many people with acute HCV report to the clinic, and this important period goes by unattended. Most studies trying to unravel the mechanism of resolution have focused on chimpanzee experiments or unique cohorts of patients either those treated many years after the infection itself or patients on interferon-based therapies.

For HCV, there is evidence that resolution may occur without the help of antibodies. This resolution should then be governed by a strong and multispecific Th1 response [22] combined with high and also multispecific CTL activation, as observed in the chimpanzee [23]. Also for humans, resolution in the acute phase has been seen going hand in hand with high CD4 reactivity against NS3 [24]. In patients resolving infection, specific CTL responses can still be observed many years after resolution, and this in the absence of detectable antibody [25]. These studies are tempting many to conclude that a decent Th1 response combined with CTL activation and, preferably, with a high multispecificity, will clear HCV infection. Nevertheless, there is evidence that the virus can escape both CD4 [26] and CTL [27] responses by mutation. Furthermore, the studies of Takaki et al. [25] have not been able to provide further insight into the immune mechanisms involved in resolving the infection during the acute phase itself.

Also in HCV, there is ample evidence for the existence of neutralizing antibody and its role in resolving infections. A study by Zibert and coworkers [28] indicates that in acute resolving infections, antibodies to the hypervariable region 1 (HVR1) of E2 appear earlier than in patients who will evolve to chronic infection. Ishii and coworkers [29] reported that 'NOB' (neutralization of binding) titers against E2 were significantly higher in chimpanzees clearing infection after vaccination and in patients spontaneously resolving HCV. These NOB titers were later related to antibodies inhibiting binding of E2 to CD81, a putative HCV receptor [30]. Specific reports on the use of HBIG administered in the liver transplant setting indicate that the incidence of HCV recurrence or newly acquired infection was significantly lower prior to screening of blood donations for HCV antibodies and removal of anti-HCV-positive blood units prior to the preparation of HBIG [31]. Although sexual transmission may be an uncommon route of transmission, it can also be prevented by passive administration of an anti-HCV-positive immunoglobulin preparation [32]. Similarly, passive administration of human immunoglobulin preparations was able to delay the onset of the disease in chimpanzees [33].

Unfortunately, no epitopes within the envelope regions have been identified which give rise to neutralizing antibodies, except for the hypervariable region at the N-terminus of E2. For the latter, both *in vitro* [34, 35] and *in vivo* chimpanzee experiments [36, 37] showed that infection can be inhibited solely by antibodies against this region. As the hypervariability of this region gives the virus the possibility to escape, the options to use this region for prophylactic vaccine development are thereby limited.

Remarkably, once the chronic HCV infection is established, a vigorous CD4 and CD8 response to many HCV proteins remains detectable both in the circulation and in the liver [38-41], and this combined with antibodies against the envelope regions and, more specifically, the hypervariable region [38, 42]. There may be a diversity of reasons why this immune response is not able to clear infection, including viral escape mechanisms, as indicated by the lack of recognition of autologous HCV sequences by the intrahepatic CD8 cells [43].

Of greater potential significance is the fact that the persistent viral infection may have altered the functional capacity of the immune system to respond in an effective way. The failure of a CTL vaccine for treatment of HBV infection was attributed to the fact that the T helper cells of HBV carriers have a reduced interleukin-12/interferon-γ secretion in response to the vaccine, as compared to healthy volunteers [44]. Also, HCV may be interfering with many defense mechanisms, as suggested by the interactions of NS5A [45, 46] and E2 [47] with the interferon pathways and the interaction of core with cytokine receptors [48, 49]. In addition, HCV is infecting dendritic cells which may lead to reduced antigen presentation [50]. A recent study revealed that a lowered immune response to an HBV vaccine occurs in HCV chronic carriers, which further supports the concept of a weakened immune response, which is in this case not even restricted to HCV [51]. A failure of interleukin-2 secretion upon specific T cell stimulation by HCV protein further emphasizes that the interference with the immune response may be complex [52].

Nevertheless, once HCV viral titers can be reduced by interferon therapy in chronic HCV carriers, the preexisting immunity both on the cellular [39] and humoral levels [53, 54] may determine the outcome of treatment. During successful treatment newly arising CD4 and CD8 responses are observed [55, 56]. Even without suppression of the viral load, the induction of neo-antibodies to the envelope region of HCV by therapeutic vaccination resulted in amelioration of chronic active disease. Remarkably, this was achieved by immunization with E1, indicating that this antigen may not be devoid of neutralizing epitopes [7].

Conclusion

There is sufficient evidence supporting the notion that a CD8 response or a humoral response may lead to resolution of HCV infection. However, there is also ample proof that both may fail to do so. Studies in other models have revealed that the combined action of both is the best guarantee for clearance of viral infection. Protection against disease solely by CTL responses, as shown for HIV [57] and also suggested for HCV by the presence of unique Th1 responses in some apparently protected cohorts [58], may be limited to a minority of the infection events. Detailed analysis of both B- and T-cell responses in the same cohort of preferentially acutely infected patients, is still required to elucidate the role of both compartments of the immune system in HCV resolution. Based on currently available knowledge, a prophylactic vaccine should aim at arming both the CD8 and B-cell arm of the immune system, at least in a way sufficient to prevent persistent infection, which is the major clinical problem with HCV. The careful selection of an antigen capable of raising neutralizing antibodies is one of the major tasks still lying ahead. As these neutralizing epitopes will be located within the envelope regions, the production of qualitatively good antigens and the means to determine this quality need to be established as well. On the other hand, HCV seems to be gifted with several antigens containing conserved T-cell epitopes for both CD4 and CD8 cells, and which are mainly located in the nonstructural genes and core. Nevertheless, it is still essential to determine which epitopes are involved in the generation of protective responses. However, the separation of antigens for humoral and cellular responses may allow the combination of each with an adjuvant, maximizing the desired response.

For therapeutic vaccination, the host may be given a second chance to mount an adequate immune response leading to resolution, by taking over the role of the innate immune system through antiviral therapy using compounds directly affecting the life cycle of HCV. The interference of the virus with the host immune responses can be alleviated in this way and the massive infection reduced to a level which can again be controlled by a specific immune response. Inversely, antiviral therapy with small compounds interfering with the viral life cycle may not only provide a window for therapeutic vaccination, but the vaccination may be required to achieve success in a therapeutic approach for HCV which will most likely be plagued by resistance. The finding that Th1 responses in HBV carriers are restored under lamivudine therapy [59] already gives some support for antiviral-vaccine combination therapy and, at the same time, confirms that the virus is indeed directly influencing the host immune system.

Antivirals for HCV are slowly appearing on the horizon, and the insight into natural HCV resolution is growing. This can be combined with an increasing knowledge of how to produce HCV envelope proteins [60-63] or how to generate broadly cross-reacting mimotopes of the hypervariable region [64]. An interesting and promising decade for HCV vaccine development lies ahead.

References

1. El-Serag HB, Mason AC. Rising incidence of hepatocellular carcinoma in the United States. N Engl J Med 1999;340:745-750.
2. Tsuji K, Yatsuhashi H, Ohata K, Matsumoto T, Inoue O, Kog M, Yano M. Natural history of chronic hepatitis B and C: risk of hepatocellular carcinoma in 25 year follow-up study. Third International Conference on Therapies for Viral Hepatitis Maui, Hawaii, 1999). Antiviral therapy 1999;4 Supplement 4): abstract 63.
3. Kim WR, Gross JB, Poterucha JJ, Locke GR, Dickson ER, Outcome of hospital care of liver disease associated with hepatitis C in the United States. Hepatology. 2001;33:201-206.
4. Manns MP, McHutchison JG, Gordon SC, Rustgi VK, Shiffman M, Reindollar R, Goodman ZD, Koury K, Ling MH, Albrecht JK. Pegintron alfa-2b plus ribavirin compared with interferon alpha-2b plus ribavirin for initial treatment of chronic hepatitis C: a randomised trial. The Lancet. 2001;358:958-965.
5. Poynard T, Marcellin P, Lee SS, Niederau C, Minuk GS, Ideo G, Bain V, Heathcote J, Zeuzem S, Trepo C, Albrecht J. Randomised trial of interferon alpha2b plus ribavirin for 48 weeks or for 24 weeks versus interferon alpha2b plus placebo for 48 weeks for treatment of chronic infection with hepatitis C virus. Lancet. 1998;352:1426-1432.
6. Choo QL, Kuo G, Ralston R, Weiner A, Chien D, Van Nest G, Han J, Berger K, Thudium K, Kuo C, Kansopon J, McFarland J, Tabrizi A, Ching K, Moss B, Cummins LB, Houghton M, Muchmore E. Vaccination of chimpanzees against infection by the hepatitis C virus. Proc Natl Acad Sci U S A. 1994;91:1294-1298.
7. Depla E, Priem S, Verschoor E, Roskams T, Desmet V, Van Doorn LJ, Fuller S, Vandeponseele P, Bosman F, Heeney J, Kos A Maertens G. Therapeutic vaccination of chronically infected chimpanzees with the HCV E1 protein. Third International Conference on Therapies for Viral Hepatitis Maui, Hawaii, 1999). Antiviral therapy 1999;4 Supplement 4):abstract 39.
8. Biron CA. Initial and innate responses to viral infections--pattern setting in immunity or disease. Curr Opin Microbiol. 1999;2:374-381.
9. Guidotti LG, Rochford R, Chung J, Shapiro M, Purcell R, Chisari FV. Viral clearance without destruction of infected cells during acute HBV infection. Science. 1999;284:825-829.
10. Guidotti LG, Borrow P, Brown A, McClary H, Koch R, Chisari FV. Noncytopathic clearance of lymphocytic choriomeningitis virus from the hepatocyte. J Exp Med. 1999;189:1555-1564.
11. Ciurea A, Klenerman P, Hunziker L, Horvath E, Senn BM, Ochsenbein AF, Hengartner H, Zinkernagel RM. Viral persistence in vivo through selection of neutralizing antibody-escape variants. Proc Natl Acad Sci U S A. 2000;97:2749-2754.
12. Planz O, Ehl S, Furrer E, Horvath E, Brundler MA, Hengartner H, Zinkernagel RM. A critical role for neutralizing-antibody-producing B cells, CD4+. T cells, and interferons in persistent and acute infections of mice with lymphocytic choriomeningitis virus: implications for adoptive immunotherapy of virus carriers. Proc Natl Acad Sci U S A. 1997;94:6874-6879.
13. Thomsen AR, Johansen J, Marker O, Christensen JP. Exhaustion of CTL memory and recrudescence of viremia in lymphocytic choriomeningitis virus-infected MHC class II-deficient mice and B-cell-deficient mice. J Immunol. 1996;157:3074-3080.
14. Schmitz JE, Kuroda MJ, Santra S, Sasseville VG, Simon MA, Lifton MA, Racz P, Tenner-Racz K, Dalesandro M, Scallon BJ, Ghrayeb J, Forman MA, Montefiori DC, Rieber EP, Letvin NL, Reimann KA. Hepatitis C virus core protein interacts with a human DEAD box protein DDX3. Virology. 1999;257:330-340.

15. Cao Y, Qin L, Zhang L, Safrit J, Ho DD. Virologic and immunologic characterization of long-term survivors of human immunodeficiency virus type 1 infection. N Engl J Med. 1995;332:201-208.
16. Estcourt MJ, Ramshaw lA, Ramsay AJ. Cytokine responses in virus infections: effects on pathogenesis, recovery and persistence. Curr Opin Microbiol. 1998;1:411-418.
17. Oldstone MB. Viral persistence: mechanisms and consequences. Curr Opin Microbiol. 1998;1:436-441.
18. Ploegh HL. Viral strategies of immune evasion. Science. 1998;280:248-253.
19. Arendrup M, Akerblom L, Heegaard PM, Nielsen JO, Hansen JE. The HIV-1 V3 domain on field isolates: participation in generation of escape virus in vivo and accessibility to neutralizing antibodies. Arch Virol. 1995;140:655-670.
20. Salzwedel K, Smith ED, Dey B, Berger EA. Sequential CD4-coreceptor interactions in human immunodeficiency virus type 1 Env function: soluble CD4 activates Env for coreceptor-dependent fusion and reveals blocking activities of antibodies against cryptic conserved epitopes on gp120. J Virol. 2000;74:326-333.
21. Boyer N, Marcellin P. Pathogenesis, diagnosis and management of hepatitis C. J. Hepatol. 2000; 32:98-112.
22. Lamonaca V, Missale G, Urbani S, Pilli M, Boni C, Mori C, Sette A, Massari M, Southwood S, Bertoni R, Valli A, Fiaccadori F, Ferrari C. Conserved hepatitis C virus sequences are highly immunogenic for CD4+. T cells: implications for vaccine development. Hepatology. 1999;30:1088-1098.
23. Cooper S, Erickson AL, Adams EJ, Kansopon J, Weiner AJ, Chien DY, Houghton M, Parham P, Walker CM. Analysis of a successful immune response against hepatitis C virus. Immunity. 1999;10:439-449.
24. Diepolder HM, Zachoval R, Hoffmann RM, Wierenga EA, Santantonio T, Jung MC, Eichenlaub D, Pape GR. Possible mechanism involving T-lymphocyte response to non-structural protein 3 in viral clearance in acute hepatitis C virus infection. Lancet. 1995;346:1006-1007.
25. Takaki A, Wiese M, Maertens G, Depla E, Seifert U, Liebetrau A, Miller JL, Manns MP, Rehermann B. Cellular immune responses persist and humoral responses decrease two decades after recovery from a single-source outbreak of hepatitis C. Nat Med. 2000;6:578-582.
26. Wang H, Eckels DD. Mutations in immunodominant T cell epitopes derived from the nonstructural 3 protein of hepatitis C virus have the potential for generating escape variants that may have important consequences for T cell recognition. J Immunol. 1999;162:4177-4183.
27. Weiner A, Erickson AL, Kansopon J, Crawford K, Muchmore E, Hughes AL, Houghton M, Walker CM. Persistent hepatitis C virus infection in a chimpanzee is associated with emergence of a cytotoxic T lymphocyte escape variant. Proc Natl Acad Sci U S A. 1995;92:2755-2759.
28. Zibert A, Meisel H, Kraas W, Schulz A, Jung G, Roggendorf M. Early antibody response against hypervariable region 1 is associated with acute self-limiting infections of hepatitis C virus. Hepatology. 1997;25:1245-1249.
29. Ishii K, Rosa D, Watanabe Y, Katayama T, Harada H, Wyatt C, Kiyosawa K, Aizaki H, Matsuura Y, Houghton M, Abrignani S, Miyamura T. High titers of antibodies inhibiting the binding of envelope to human cells correlate with natural resolution of chronic hepatitis C. Hepatology. 1998;28:1117-1120.
30. Pileri P, Uematsu Y, Campagnoli S, Galli G, Falugi F, Petracca R, Weiner AJ, Houghton M, Rosa D, Grandi G, Abrignani S. Binding of hepatitis C virus to CD81. Science. 1998;282:938-941.
31. Feray C, Gigou M, Samuel D, Ducot B, Maisonneuve P, Reynes M, Bismuth A, Bismuth H. Incidence of hepatitis C in patients receiving different preparations of hepatitis B immunoglobulins after liver transplantation. Ann Intern Med. 1998;128:810-816.
32. Piazza M, Sagliocca L, Tosone G, Guadagnino V, Stazi MA, Orlando R, Borgia G, Rosa D, Abrignani S, Palumbo F, Manzin A, Clementi M. Sexual transmission of the hepatitis C virus and

efficacy of prophylaxis with intramuscular immune serum globulin. A randomized controlled trial. Arch Intern Med. 1997;157:1537-1544.

33. Krawczynski K, Fattom A, Spelbring J, Kamili S, Basham L, Purdy M, Sapan C, Naso R and Darson D. Immune treatment of HCV infection: passive transfer of anti-HCV in acutely infected chimpanzees. 6th International symposium on HCV and related viruses 1999, Washington, abstract 9.4.
34. Zibert A, Schreier E, Roggendorf M. Antibodies in human sera specific to hypervariable region 1 of hepatitis C virus can block viral attachment. Virology. 1995;208:653-661.
35. Zhou YH, Shimizu YK, Esumi M. Monoclonal antibodies to the hypervariable region 1 of hepatitis C virus capture virus and inhibit virus adsorption to susceptible cells in vitro. Virology. 2000;269:276-283.
36. Farci P, Shimoda A, Wong D, Cabezon T, De Gioannis D, Strazzera A, Shimizu Y, Shapiro M, Alter HJ, Purcell RH. Prevention of hepatitis C virus infection in chimpanzees by hyperimmune serum against the hypervariable region 1 of the envelope 2 protein. Proc Natl Acad Sci U S A. 1996;93:15394-15399.
37. Esumi M, Rikihisa T, Nishimura S, Goto J, Mizuno K, Zhou YH, Shikata T. Experimental vaccine activities of recombinant E1 and E2 glycoproteins and hypervariable region 1 peptides of hepatitis C virus in chimpanzees. Arch Virol. 1999;144:973-980.
38. Mondelli MU. Is there a role for immune responses in the pathogenesis of hepatitis C? J Hepatol. 1996;25:232-238.
39. Nelson DR, Marousis CG, Ohno T, Davis GL, Lau JY. Intrahepatic hepatitis C virus-specific cytotoxic T lymphocyte activity and response to interferon alfa therapy in chronic hepatitis C. Hepatology. 1998;28:225-230.
40. Chang KM, Gruener NH, Southwood S, Sidney J, Pape GR, Chisari FV, Sette A. Identification of HLA-A3 and -B7-restricted CTL response to hepatitis C virus in patients with acute and chronic hepatitis C. J Immunol. 1999;162:1156-1164.
41. Jackson M, Smith B, Bevitt DJ, Steward M, Toms GL, Bassendine MF, Diamond AG. Comparison of cytotoxic T-lymphocyte responses to hepatitis C virus core protein in uninfected and infected individuals. J Med Virol. 1999;58:239-246.
42. Depraetere S and Leroux Roels G. Hepatitis C virus envelope proteins: immunogenicity in humans and their role in diagnosis and vaccine development. J Viral Hepatitis;5:113-146.
43. Giuggio VM, Bonkovsky HL, Smith J, Rothman AL. Inefficient recognition of autologous viral sequences by intrahepatic hepatitis C virus-specific cytotoxic T lymphocytes in chronically infected subjects.Virology. 1998:10;251:132-140.
44. Livingston BD, Alexander J, Crimi C, Oseroff C, Celis E, Daly K, Guidotti LG, Chisari FV, Fikes J, Chesnut RW, Sette A. Altered helper T lymphocyte function associated with chronic hepatitis B virus infection and its role in response to therapeutic vaccination in humans. J Immunol. 1999;162:3088-3095.
45. Gale MJ Jr, Korth MJ, Tang NM, Tan SL, Hopkins DA, Dever TE, Polyak SJ, Gretch DR, Katze MG. Evidence that hepatitis C virus resistance to interferon is mediated through repression of the PKR protein kinase by the nonstructural 5A protein. Virology. 1997;230:217-227.
46. Francois C, Duverlie G, Rebouillat D, Khorsi H, Castelain S, Blum HE, Gatignol A, Wychowski C, Moradpour D, Meurs EF. Expression of hepatitis C virus proteins interferes with the antiviral action of interferon independently of PKR-mediated control of protein synthesis. J Virol. 2000;74:5587-5596.
47. Taylor DR, Shi ST, Romano PR, Barber GN, Lai MM. Inhibition of the interferon-inducible protein kinase PKR by HCV E2 protein. Science. 1999;285:107-110.
48. Owsianka AM, Patel AH. Hepatitis C virus core protein interacts with a human DEAD box protein DDX3. Virology. 1999;257:330-340.
49. Matsumoto M, Hsieh TY, Zhu N, VanArsdale T, Hwang SB, Jeng KS, Gorbalenya AE, Lo SY, Ou JH,

Ware CF, Lai MM. Hepatitis C virus core protein interacts with the cytoplasmic tail of lymphotoxin-beta receptor. J Virol. 1997;71:1301-1309.
50. Bain C, Fatmi A, Zoulim F, Zarski JP, Trépo C, Inchauspé G. Impaired allostimulatory function of dendritic cells in chronic hepatitis C infection. Gastroenterology. 2001;201:512-524.
51. Wiedmann M, Liebert UG, Oesen U, Porst H, Wiese M, Schroeder S, Halm U, Mossner J, Berr F. Decreased immunogenicity of recombinant hepatitis B vaccine in chronic hepatitis C. Hepatology. 2000;31:230-234.
52. Eckels DD, Tabatabail N, Bian TH, Wang H, Muheisen SS, Rice CM, Yoshizawa K, Gill J. In vitro human Th-cell responses to a recombinant hepatitis C virus antigen: failure in IL-2 production despite proliferation. Hum Immunol. 1999;60:187-199.
53. Hattori M, Yoshioka K, Aiyama T, Iwata K, Terazawa Y, Ishigami M, Yano M, Kakumu S. Broadly reactive antibodies to hypervariable region 1 in hepatitis C virus-infected patient sera: relation to viral loads and response to interferon. Hepatology. 1998;27:1703-1710.
54. Depraetere S, Van Kerschaever E, Van Vlierberghe H, Elewaut A, Brouwer JT, Niesters HG, Schalm SW, Maertens G, Leroux-Roels G. Long term response to interferon treatment in chronic hepatitis C patients is associated with a significant reduction in anti-E1 envelope antibody titers. J Med Virol. 2000;60:126-132.
55. Lohr HF, Gerken G, Roth M, Weyer S, Schlaak JF, Meyer zum Buschenfelde KH. The cellular immune responses induced in the follow-up of interferon-alpha treated patients with chronic hepatitis C may determine the therapy outcome. J Hepatol. 1998;29:524-532.
56. Lohr HF, Schmitz D, Arenz M, Weyer S, Gerken G, Meyer zum Buschenfelde KH. The viral clearance in interferon-treated chronic hepatitis C is associated with increased cytotoxic T cell frequencies. J Hepatol. 1999;31:407-415.
57. Rowland Jones SL, Dong T, Dorrell L, Ogg G, Hansasuta P, Krausa P, Kimani J, Sabally S, Ariyoshi K, Oyugi J, MacDonald KS, Bwayo J, Whittle H, Plummer FA, McMichael AJ. Broadly cross-reactive HIV-specific cytotoxic T-lymphocytes in highly-exposed persistently seronegative donors. Immunol Lett. 1999;66:9-14.
58. Cramp ME, Rossol S. HCV-specific T helper cell responses in HCV exposed but uninfected cases. AASLD meeting Chicago, 1998). Hepatology 1998;28:200A.
59. Boni C, Bertoletti A, Penna A, Cavalli A, Pilli M, Urbani S, Scognamiglio P, Boehme R, Panebianco R, Fiaccadori F, Ferrari C. Lamivudine treatment can restore T cell responsiveness in chronic hepatitis B. J Clin Invest. 1998;102:968-975.
60. de Martynoff G, Venneman A, Maertens G. Analysis of post-translational modifications of HCV structural proteins by using the vaccinia virus expression system. Proceedings of IX Triennial International Symposium on viral hepatitis and liver disease, Rome, Italy 1996. pp 219-224.
61. Baumert TF, Vergalla J, Satoi J, Thomson M, Lechmann M, Herion D, Greenberg HB, Ito S, Liang TJ. Hepatitis C virus-like particles synthesized in insect cells as a potential vaccine candidate. Gastroenterology. 1999;117:1397-1407.
62. Mustilli AC, Izzo E, Houghton M, Galeotti CL. Comparison of secretion of a hepatitis C virus glycoprotein in Saccharomyces cerevisiae and Kluyveromyces lactis.Res Microbiol. 1999;150:179-187.
63. Dubuisson J. Folding, assembly and subcellular localization of hepatitis C virus glycoproteins. Curr Top Microbiol Immunol. 2000;242:135-148.
64. Puntoriero G, Meola A, Lahm A, Zucchelli S, Ercole BB, Tafi R, Pezzanera M, Mondelli MU, Cortese R, Tramontano A, Galfre G, Nicosia A. Towards a solution for hepatitis C virus hypervariability: mimotopes of the hypervariable region 1 can induce antibodies cross-reacting with a large number of viral variants. EMBO J. 1998;17:3521-3533.

VIRAL HEPATITIS B AND C INFECTIONS IN CHILDREN

Maternal/fetal/pediatric HBV and HCV infections

RICHARD A. SCHREIBER

Associate Professor of Pediatrics, University of British Columbia, Division of Pediatric Gastroenterology, BC Children's Hospital, Vancouver BC Canada

Introduction

On a worldwide basis most cases of viral hepatitis occur in children. Although acute hepatitis in the pediatric age group is often self limited and chronic hepatitis is usually mild, the long-term outcome may not be so benign. Indeed, the major burden of morbidity and mortality of childhood viral hepatitis occurs in adulthood. The following article will provide an update of viral hepatitis B and C as it pertains to the pediatric population. Issues particularly relevant to infants and children, such as vertical transmission rates, natural history of disease, strategies for prevention and current treatment options will be discussed. Some of the important differences of viral hepatitis B and C infections in children compared to adults will be highlighted.

Hepatitis B

Hepatitis B virus (HBV) is a partially double stranded DNA virus, which causes acute and chronic hepatitis. It is the most common bloodborne infection in the world. Over two billion people have been infected with HBV, and 350 million have become chronic hepatitis B surface antigen (HBsAg) carriers with the attendant risk for developing chronic active hepatitis, cirrhosis and hepatocellular carcinoma. Worldwide, approximately one million people die each year from HBV infection. In the United States it is estimated that there are 300,000 new cases of hepatitis B annually and one million chronic carriers. Each year 4,000 deaths in the United States are attributed to hepatitis B. Children account for a small proportion of the new cases of hepatitis B reported in the USA. Only eight percent of newly reported cases occur in those under ten years old and 10% in those 11-19 years of age [1]. Although the vast majority of pediatric HBV infections are asymptomatic, cases of fulminant hepatitis B, hepatitis B-related liver cirrhosis and hepatocellular carcinoma do occur in children.

Frontiers in Viral Hepatitis Ed. by RF Schinazi, J-P Sommadossi and CM Rice. 89 — 96

Epidemiology

The highest prevalence rates (>8%) for hepatitis B are found in Asia, the African basin, the Amazon basin of South America, Alaska and Northern Canada. In the remainder of North America, the prevalence rates are low (<2%). Data collected from the US national surveys NHANES II and III between 1976 and 1994 show that the overall age-adjusted prevalence rate for hepatitis B is about 5% [2, 3]. In the US, hepatitis B prevalence rates are low in infants and young children up until the age of 12, and thereafter rates increase in all racial groups, with the highest rates (over 20%) in the non-Hispanic, African-American population compared to rates of 4% in non-Hispanic Caucasians. Thus, children have a low but appreciable risk for acquiring hepatitis B infection — a risk that increases significantly through adolescence, presumably at the onset of first sexual activity or other high risk behaviors. Similar data have been reported in Canada, with annual rates of acute hepatitis B increasing dramatically in the 15 to 19-year-old age group [4].

The principle mode for HBV transmission in a child is by the perinatal route from HBsAg-carrier pregnant mothers to their newborns. In many hyperendemic areas this transmission route accounts for 40-50% of all HBsAg carriers. Another means of HBV infection is by horizontal transmission through either intrafamilial spread from infected family members, sexual activity, the parenteral route or in institutionalized children. Of these, the two most important routes of horizontal transmission are highly infectious family members or improperly sterilized syringes [5]. With regard to sexual activity in the pediatric population, young adolescents practice high risk sexual behaviour. Recent data from the CDC have found that 50% of males and 32% of females by the age of 16 have had first heterosexual intercourse [6]. By the age of 19 the rates increase to 86% and 75%, respectively. Yet 57% of males and only 32% of females were found to have used condoms at their last sexual intercourse. Moreover, many teenagers have multiple sex partners. An understanding and appreciation of these risk factors for both perinatal and horizontal HBV transmission in the pediatric population has formed the basis for current disease prevention strategies.

Natural history

One of the most striking aspects of HBV infection is the age dependence of the chronicity rate. The outcome of HBV infection is very different for neonates and young infants compared to older children and adults. The risk for developing chronic HBV infection is inversely proportional to the age at acquisition. Whereas only 5% of adults go on to develop chronic hepatitis B after an acute infection, over 90% of newborns and infants less than one year of age who acquire HBV will have persistent infection. Children infected between the ages of four to six have an intermediate chance of becoming chronic carriers, estimated at ten to forty percent.

Chronic hepatitis B infection is defined by the presence of HBsAg in the serum for more than six months. Most children who are chronic HBsAg carriers are asymptomatic. The presence of jaundice and hepatic dysfunction or growth failure in chronically HBV-infected pediatric patients is very unusual. Extrahepatic manifestations may occur.

Membranous nephropathy has been strongly associated with chronic carriers, particularly in those children who were infected horizontally. Polyarteritis nodosa and essential mixed cryoglobulinemia are very rare in pediatric HBV infection.

HBeAg is a marker of active HBV replication. For reasons that are poorly understood, HBV replication may be reduced as the child ages, and the HBeAg can gradually clear. For children, HBeAg clearance is usually an insidious event. In a study of 420 Taiwanese HBsAg-positive children aged one month to 17 years who were followed for one to 12 years, 331 children HAD acquired their HBV infection through vertical transmission and 89% of them (375 children) were initially HBeAg positive [7]. During the follow-up period, 90 of the 375 children (24%) became HBeAg negative. Only 10 children became HBsAg negative. The annual HBsAg clearance in this study was 0.6% per year. In another study of 185 Italian and Spanish children aged one to 16 years, vertical transmission was the mode of infection in only 14% of patients, and 90% of cases were initially HBeAg positive [8]. During a mean follow-up of 13 years, 86% of children lost HBeAg, and 7% had clearance of HBsAg. The spontaneous HBsAg clearance rate in this cohort was 0.5%/yr. These differences in eAg clearance rates between Western and Asian populations probably reflect the age of acquisition and longer duration of infection in the Asian population, the effects of early eAg presentation on the development of immune tolerance and host genetic factors.

In another study of 39 children who cleared HBeAg, 87% and 58% of cases had detectable HBV DNA by PCR within five and 10 years after seroconversion, respectively [9]. Acute exacerbation of hepatitis with reactivation of HBV replication is unusual in children once anti-HBe appears. Moreover, the progression of liver disease and the development of liver cirrhosis is rare in those children who are HBe seroconverters. A recent study by Ruiz-Moreno reported that most children who had seroconverted demonstrated improvement in their liver histology [10]. Yet despite the disappearance of HBeAg or improved histology, integration of the HBV genome may occur, although the development of hepatocellular carcinoma is rare during childhood. Only 51 cases of hepatocellular carcinoma were reported over a 13-year study period in Taiwanese children aged three to 16 years [11]. Approximately 80% of these children were anti-HBe positive, but all of them were HBsAg positive.

Treatment

The first step to the treatment of hepatitis B is prevention. Immunoprophylaxis against hepatitis B infection is key. One of the first universal infant vaccine programs was introduced in Taiwan in 1984, achieving an 85-94% immunization rate [12]. The HBsAg carrier rate decreased from 10% in 1982 to less than 1% in 1994. Moreover, the rate of childhood hepatocellular carcinoma in this population declined from 0.7/100,000 in 1981-1986 to 0.36/100,000 by 1990-1994. In the United States, screening of all pregnant women for hepatitis B surface antigen and universal vaccination of all newborns at zero, one and six months is now standard practice. Hepatitis B immune globulin is also administered at birth to all neonates of HBsAg-positive mothers. Catch up vaccination is now recommended in the United States for older children, so that by adolescence all children should be vaccinated. As predicted, the introduction of this vaccination strategy in the United States has led to a marked reduction in the incidence of HBV infection [13]. The effect of hepatitis B vaccine on disease prevalence has been one of the great achievements of the latter half of the 20th century. Unfortunately, only 109 of the world's 211 countries have instituted universal infant vaccine programs, and many do not even achieve a 50% vaccination rate. The major obstacles for implementation of global vaccine programs continue to lie with difficulties in vaccine administration and vaccine cost.

Limited treatment options exist for children already infected with HBV. In a large multinational, multicentered, randomized controlled trial of interferon therapy for hepatitis B that included 144 patients aged one to 17 years who were HBsAg positive (for more than six months), eAg and HBV DNA positive and had serum ALT greater than 1.5 times normal, 26% of the treatment group had eAg seroconversion and loss of HBV DNA compared with 11% of the controls [14]. Although this was a statistically significant response, an even more important finding was that 10% of the treated patients also lost HBsAg. Predictors of response were female sex, low HBV DNA levels (<50pg/ml) and younger age.

More recently, a five-year follow-up study from Italy found that the proportion of interferon-treated children who eventually lost HBeAg did not differ significantly from that observed in the untreated controls. However, the interferon-treated group did have a higher rate of HBsAg loss [15]. Thus the true benefit of interferon therapy for children with hepatitis B may be that it simply accelerates the process of seroconversion and loss of HbsAg.

There are a number of unresolved issues unique to pediatric HBV infection. The vast majority of children are asymptomatic carriers with normal ALT levels, yet treatment strategies for this patient population have not been developed. The natural history of disease progression in non-Asian children who are chronic carriers or who have spontaneously seroconverted is not well defined. For those patients who have responded to interferon, the long-term risks for hepatocellular carcinoma or other complications are unknown. Trials of lamuvidine in the treatment of HBV in children are currently underway, and results should be available within a year.

In summary, pediatric HBV is often a benign condition during childhood that portends a significant long-term morbidity and mortality. Although interferon therapy is the sole treatment agent currently approved for use in children with chronic HBV, the role and safety of other antiviral agents alone or in combination remain unclear. While treatment recommendations for young patients chronically infected with HBV are constantly evolving, prevention remains a key strategy. Universal infant and childhood vaccination programs have a proven track record. We should all advocate strongly for efficient worldwide vaccination programs.

Hepatitis C

Hepatitis C virus (HCV) is a small, single stranded RNA virus roughly 9600 nucleosides in length, belonging to the flavivirus family. Infection with HCV causes both acute and chronic hepatitis. However unlike adults acutely infected with hepatitis B where the risk for chronicity is only 5%, the chronicity rate for adults with hepatitis C is very high, upwards of 75-80%. It is estimated that 170 million people are infected with hepatitis C worldwide, but probably most of these cases are not the result of childhood infection. Indeed, hepatitis C is uncommon in children.

Epidemiology

Data from studies of infants and children with hepatitis C are just beginning to emerge. The recently published US National Health and Nutrition Epidemiologic Survey shows the prevalence of anti-HCV in children aged six to 11 years old is only 0.2% and rises to only 0.4% in those aged 12 to 19 [16]. In this report only 30% of the anti-HCV-positive children had HCV RNA, suggesting that the chronicity rate of HCV in the pediatric population is less than half that of adults. This is the opposite of what occurs in hepatitis B, where the chronicity rates in children are much higher than in adults.

Historically, the major risk for acquisition of hepatitis C in children was the parenteral route. Thus, hepatitis C has been common in children with hemophilia or thalassemia, those on renal dialysis or cancer chemotherapy for leukemia, those who received contaminated immune globulin, or with a history of blood transfusions while in the neonatal intensive care, those on ECMO or who have had congenital heart or other surgery. These cases represent mostly children who received contaminated blood or blood products prior to 1992 (or contaminated IVIG 4/93-2/94), so they would be at least eight years of age now. With the introduction of more advanced approaches to the screening and processing of blood and blood products, the parenteral route for transmission of hepatitis C is rare, now at an estimated risk of 1 in 100,000 units transfused. At present, the major risk factor for acquisition of hepatitis C in the pediatric population is maternal infant transmission, occurring in about 5% of cases. With maternal coinfection of HCV and HIV, the transmission rates are much higher, upwards of 15%. The maternal viral load is an important determinant. The risk for having one newborn infected through maternal transmission does not appear to influence the risk for the second pregnancy, although there is one report of all three children in one family infected through maternal transmission [17, 18]. Other risk factors that might influence the transmission rate, such as the mode of delivery or type of obstetrical intervention, have not yet been clarified. However, in a recent study from the CDC of 323 infants born to anti-HCV-positive mothers, among the 252 infants who were followed for at least one year, only 2.8% (seven patients) were infected based on detection of HCV RNA on at least two follow-up visits [19]. No child born to an HCV RNA negative mother was infected. A multivariate analysis found that a maternal HCV-RNA-titre greater than 10^6 genome eq/ml, fetal monitoring and early rupture of membranes were additional risk factors. Results of numerous studies suggest breast-feeding does not appear to be a risk factor for transmission, although HCV RNA has been detected in breast milk. There is little or no risk for the intrafamilial spread of hepatitis C among household members.

Natural history

The natural history of hepatitis C infection in children has not been well characterized, however the mode of transmission and age of acquisition of hepatitis C are likely to be important determinants of outcome. Losasciulli et al. reported data on 114 childhood patients with leukemia, of whom 56 (49%) were HCV RNA positive at the end of chemotherapy [20]. After a 17-year follow-up of the HCV-RNA-positive group, all were asymptomatic, the ALT values were normal in 71%, and 16 of the 56 (29%) had spontaneously cleared their viremia and had become HCV RNA negative. In one of the most comprehensive outcome studies, Vogt et al. followed 458 children who were transfused at cardiac surgery, at a time before blood donor screening for hepatitis C existed [21]. The patients at operation had a mean age of 2.8 years and were followed for a mean of 19 years. None had received prior or subsequent transfusions, and none had mothers who were HCV RNA positive. At follow-up, anti-HCV was detected in 67 (14.6%) patients compared with three (0.7%) in an age- and sex-matched control group. Of these, 55% (37/67) were HCV RNA positive and 45% seem to have spontaneously cleared their infection. Only one patient had an abnormal ALT. Of the seven patients who underwent liver biopsy, all but three had minimal inflammation and no fibrosis. Of the three patients with significant histological change, two with portal fibrosis had ongoing congestive heart failure, and the third with micronodular cirrhosis was coinfected with hepatitis B. The authors concluded that chronic hepatitis C in childhood is more benign or more slowly progressive than in adults.

There are few studies of the natural history of hepatitis C in children who acquired their infection through vertical transmission. A summary of 14 reports published between 1995 and 1999 would include only 120 infants who were identified as being HCV RNA positive after birth. Of these 31 patients, 25.8% appeared to have spontaneously cleared the infection. A small study by Garcia-Monzon compared the outcome of liver histology in 24 HCV-positive children with 22 HCV-infected adults [22]. After a mean follow-up of 11 years with both age groups having similar viral loads and genotype, the histologic grade and stage was 0.6 ± 0.7 and 0.5 ± 0.5, respectively, in the pediatric group compared with 3.2 ± 1.1 and 2.6 ± 1.2 in adults. Thus, over an 11 year period, both the intensity of hepatic inflammation and degree of fibrosis were markedly less in children than in adults. The available data from these studies, although still sparse, consistently show a milder outcome of hepatitis C infection in the first two decades of life with a high rate of spontaneous recovery as evidenced by the loss of HCV RNA.

Treatment

There have been few published trials of treatment with interferon for children with chronic HCV (Table 1). Many of these are of small sample size, and few are randomized or controlled. Moreover, the study design and treatment doses varied widely, making it difficult to judiciously pool the data. The sustained response rates varied from 0-50%. It is still unclear whether interferon is an effective therapy for children with chronic hepatitis C. At the last NIH consensus conference, no firm treatment recommendations were made for patients under the age of 18. It was recommended that treatment decisions be taken individually by the patient and their physician, and that wherever possible, treatment should be introduced in the context of a clinical trial. To date, there have been no published trials of combination ribavirin and interferon for the treatment of hepatitis C in children. The efficacy of pegylated interferon, where weekly rather than daily injections would be a welcomed advantage for children, has unfortunately not yet been studied.

In summary, hepatitis C infection may differ in the pediatric population compared with adults. Although historically the burden of disease has been in those young patients who were infected by contaminated blood and blood products, with improvements in blood bank screening and blood product processing, vertical transmission has become the most important source of infection for children. We need to focus our research to better identify risk factors for maternal infant transmission and to more fully characterize the natural history of HCV disease in this cohort. Although the treatment strategies for HCV infection continue to evolve, novel agents need to be specifically evaluated in children in a timely manner to properly assess their efficacy and safety in this age group. The limited data garnered so far suggest important epidemiological and outcome differences of chronic HCV in children compared to adults. Whether in regards to the natural history of disease or its treatment, it is now quite clear that the adult HCV experience should not be applied de facto to the pediatric population.

Table 1. Hepatitis C in children. Summary of published α interferon treatment trials.

Study Author	Pub yr	Number of patients: Treatment	Number of patients: Control	Mean Age (yr)	Mean Disease Duration (yr)	αIFN Dose (mu/m^2)	Follow Up (mo)	Sustained Response (%)
Clemente	94	21	14	14	??	3 x 15	36	37
Bortolotti	95	14	13	8	3.5	5 x 12	24	43
Iorio	96	11	10	7.5	4.9	3 x 12	30	45
Ruiz Moreno	92	12	0	8.4	-	3 x 6	18	45
Dimarco	97	70	0	14.1	8.1	5 x 2, 3 x 10	36	40
Jonas	98	23	0	10.6	5.3	3 x 12	12	33
Sawada	98	24	0	10.6	4.1	0.1 mu/kg x 6	48	50

References

1. Alter MJ, Mast EE: The epidemiology of viral hepatitis in the United States. In Martin P, Freidman L eds. Gastroenterol Clin N Amer: Viral Hepatitis Philadelphia WB Saunders 1994: 437-455
2. Coleman PJ, McQuillan GM, Moyer LA, Lambert SB, Margolis HS: Incidence of hepatitis B virus infection in the United States 1976-1994:estimates from the National Health and Nutrition Examination Surveys *J Inf Dis* 1998 178: 954-9
3. McQuillan GM, coleman PJ, Kruszn-Moran D, Moyer LA, Lambert SB, Margolis HS: Prevalence of hepatitis B virus infection in the United States: the National Health and Nutrition examination Surveys 1976-1994 *Am J Pub Health* 1999 898:145-18
4. Bulletin, Minister of Public Works and Government Services, Canada 1998

5. Hsu SC, Chang MH, Ni YH et al: Horizontal transmission of hepatitis B virus in children *J Ped Gi Nutr* 1993 105:1173-8
6. Youth Risk Behaviour Surveillance: National College Health risk behaviour survey-United States MMWR 46(SS-6);1-54
7. Hsu HY, Chang MH, Lee Cy et al: Spontaneous loss of HbsAg in children with chronic hepatitis B virus infection. *Hepatology* 1992 15:380-386
8. Bortolotti F, Jara P, crivellaro C, Hieroo L, Cadrobbi P, Frauca E et al: Outcome of hepatitis B in Caucasian children during a 20 year observation period. *J Hepatol* 1998 29:184-190
9. Bortolotti F, Wirth S, Crivellaro C et al: Long term persistence of hepatitis B virus DNA in the serum of children with chronic hepatitis B after hepatitis e antigen to antibody seroconversion *J Ped Gastr Nutr* 1996 22:270-274
10. Ruiz Moreno M, Otero M, Millan A, Castillo I et al: clinical and histological outcome after hepatitis B e antigen to antibody seroconversion in children with chronic hepatitis B *Hepatology* 1999 29:572-575
11. Chang MW, Chen DS, Hsu HC et al: Maternal transmission of hepatitis B virus in childhood hepatocellular carcinoma. *Cancer* 1989; 64: 2377-80
12. Chang MW, Chen CJ, Lai MS et al: Universal hepatitis B vaccination in Taiwan and the incidence of hepatocellular carcinoma in children. *NEJM* 1997 336:1855-1859
13. Margolis H: Prevention of acute and chronic liver disease through immunization: hepatitis B and beyond *J Inf Disease* 1993 168:9-14
14. Sokal EM, Conjeevaram HS, Roberts EA, Alvarez F, Bern EM et al: Interferon alfa therapy for chronic hepatitis B in children: a multinational randomized controlled trial *Gastroenterology* 1998 14:988-995
15. Bortolotti F., Jara P, Barbera C, Gregorio GV et al: Long term effect of alpha interferon in children with chronic hepatitis B. *Gut* 2000 46:715-718
16. Alter MJ, Kruszon-Moran D, Nainan OV, McQuillan GM et al: The prevalence of hepatitis C virus infection in the United States 1988 through 1994. *NEJM* 1999 341:556-562
17. Resti M, Bortolotti F, Azzari C, Giacchino R et al: Transmission of hepatitis C virus form infected mother to offspring during subsequent pregnancies *J Ped GI Nutr* 2000 30:491-3
18. Schreiber RA, Krajden M, Chaudhary R, Dobson R, Israel DM: Vertical transmission of hepatitis C: all three children in one family *J Ped GI Nutr* 2000 31:S55
19. Mast EE, Hwang LY, Nolte FS, Kelly MG, Alter MJ: Perinatal hepatitis C virus transmission: Maternal risk factors and optimal timing of diagnosis. *Hepatology* 1999 30: 499A
20. Loscasciulli A, Testa M, Pontisso P et al: Prevalence and natural history of hepatitis C infection in patients cured of childhood leukemia. *Blood* 1997 11:4628-33
21. Vogt M, Lang T, Frosner G et al: Prevalence and clinical outcome of hepatitis C infection in children who underwent cardiac surgery before the implementation of blood-donor screening *NEJM* 1999 341:866-870
22. Garcia-Monzon C, Jara P, Fernandez-Bermejo M et al:Chronic hepatitis C in children: a clinical and immunohistochemical comparative study with adults. *Hepatology* 1998 28:1696-1701

Effects of interferon treatment in children with post-transfusional chronic hepatitis B

MARIA POP, M. SERBAN, L. CIONCA,
R. COSTA and C. JINCA

University of Medicine Timisoara, III-rd Pediatric Clinic Timisoara, Romania

Introduction

Infection with hepatitis B virus (HBV) is considered as a major health problem worldwide, with 5% of the global population, that is over 350,000,000 people, being chronic carriers of HBV [1]. However, its geographic distribution is uneven; while chronic carriers represent less than 1% of the population in industrialized countries, in underdeveloped or developing countries the percentage amounts to 5-15%. In Romania too, the prevalence of HBV infection is on average 7-10% [2], which entails also a high rate of post-transfusional hepatitis infection.

At present the only therapy with benefits that have been confirmed in the treatment of chronic viral hepatitis is alpha interferon (IFN-α), lamivudine, and hepsera (adefovir dipivoxil). Further antiviral nucleoside analogues (famciclovir, lobucavir, ganciclovir, etc.) remain under evaluation.

The purpose of this treatment is a long-term eradication of HBV/DNA viremia, remission of the inflammatory process, and prevention of the progression to cirrhosis and development of hepatocellular carcinoma.

This study is intended to evaluate the efficiency of IFN-α alone or combined with lamivudine in the treatment of children with chronic hepatitis B, especially those with post-transfusional chronic hepatitis.

Patients and method

The present study is a retrospective analysis of 20 consecutive patients with chronic hepatitis B divided in two groups: A — post-transfusional hepatitis and B — non-transfusional hepatitis (Table 1). There have been included all patients with infection and replication markers (HBsAg, HBeAg, ± HBV-DNA), with high levels of alanine aminotransferase (ALT) for at least six months and with histologic evidence of liver inflammation have been included.

Frontiers in Viral Hepatitis Ed. by RF Schinazi, J-P Sommadossi and CM Rice. 97 — 105

Table 1. Study group distribution

Sex distribution:	13 male and 7 female	
Age range:	8-17 years; mean 13.4 years	
Group A: With previous transfusions		
• Idiopathic thrombocytopenic purpura (ITP)		- 4 cases
• Acute lymphoblastic leukemia (ALL)		- 2 cases
• Gaucher disease (with splenectomy)		- 1 case
• Haemophilia		- 2 cases
• Non-Hodgkin's lymphoma (NHL)		- 2 cases
Group B: Without previous transfusions		
• Chronic hepatitis B without associated pathology		- 7 cases
• Compensated cirrhosis — Child stage A		- 1 case
• Chronic hepatitis B associated with secondary nephrotic syndrome		- 1 case

The histological diagnosis was carried out according to international criteria [3], and the histological activity index (HAI) [4] was used to evaluate histological activity. As exclusion criteria we considered HIV and HDV positivity; none of the patients presented biological markers of autoimmune hepatitis. Biochemical and hematological parameters were assessed using the standard methods (Table 2).

Table 2. Clinical and biochemical evaluation of patients

Clinical examination;

Laboratory tests:

- complete BCC;
- serum biochemical tests- ALT, AST, LDH, bilirubin, alkaline phosphatase, prothrombine time, albumin;
- immunological tests- serum immunoglobulin levels (IgM, IgG, IgA);
- virological markers-HBsAg, anti-HBs, HBeAg, anti-HBe, anti-HBc, anti-HCV, anti-HDV.

Histopathological examination by means of liver biopsy, evaluating the necrotic and inflammatory activity by the "Histological Activity Index" (HAI) developed by Knodell.

Viral markers were determined by Elisa immunoassays of IInd and IIIrd generation. All patients were clinically and biologically monitored according to parameters indicated in (Table 3).

The long-term evolution has been evaluated using clinical, biochemical and virological markers (Table 4). The regimen of interferon therapy was: 3MU/day, three times/week for six to 12 months (17 cases) and 5MU/day, three times/week with lamivudine 100 mg/day, for six months (3 cases). The follow-up observation period ranged from six to 12 months.

Table 3. Follow-up parameters for evaluation of the response to treatment

Clinical examination:
- three times/week in the first week
- weekly in the first month
- monthly the next five (11) months

Biological parameters:
- complete BCC weekly
- ALT, AST monthly
- virological markers
  - before start of therapy
  - at three months after start of therapy
  - at six and 12 months after end of therapy

Table 4. Types of response to IFN treatment in HBV chronic hepatitis

Criteria	Complete	Incomplete	Transitory	Absent
Clinical improvement	+	+	+	+
Normalization of serum ALT	+	+	+	-
Seroconversion from HBeAg to anti-HBe	+	+	+/-	-
Seroconversion from HBsAg to anti-HBs	+	-	-	-
Clearance of HBV DNA	+	+	+	-

Results

The results are presented in tables 5a and 5b. Seroconversion from HBeAg to anti-HBe occurred in three cases (27.27%) from group A, and in four cases (44.44%) from group B (Tables 5c and 5d). Complete seroconversion (HBeAg to anti-HBe, HBsAg to anti-HBs) occurred only in two cases from group A. HBV DNA level, determined because of the prohibitive costs only in three patients of group B, dropped to normal values in one, remaining at high values in the other two patients. In all cases serum ALT levels dropped to normal values at the end of treatment. In the groups studied, HAI scores ranged between six to 12 whereas the fibrosis scores ranged between 0 and 3. No liver biopsy was performed after the end of treatment. The therapy was well tolerated

Table 5a. Personal and biological data of the patients who underwent previous transfusions

Ctrl. No.	Name	Age Years	Sex	Concomitant Diseases	Virologic markers before treatment					Serum amino-transferase levels	Inflammatory syndrome	Duration of infection (years)
					HBsAg	Anti-HBs	HBeAg	Anti- HBe	Anti-HCV			
1	BD	9	M	ITP	+	-	+	-	-	2N	+	1.5
2	MC	10	M	ITP	+	-	+	-	-	2N	-	4.5
3	RV	12	M	ITP	+	-	+	-	-	N	-	2.5
4	RC	10	F	ITP	+	-	+	-	-	1.5N	+	3
5	BA	11	F	ALL	+	-	+	-	-	10N	+	2
6	BC	17	M	ALL	+	-	+	-	-	10N	+	8
7	CA	11	M	Gaucher	+	-	+	-	-	8N	+	4
8	RB	9	M	NHL	+	-	+	-	-	1.5N	+	1.5
9	RB	12	M	Haemophilia	+	-	+	-	-	2N	+	5
10	GL	11	M	Haemophilia	+	-	+	-	+	8N	+	1
11	AI	12	M	NHL	+	-	+	-	+	10N	+	1.5

Table 5b. Response to IFN ± lamivudine therapy in patients with post-transfusional chronic hepatitis

Patients			1	2	3	4	5	6	7	8	9	10	11
Treatment	IFN	Dose (MU/week)	3 x 3										
		Duration (months)	12	12	6	6	12	12	12	2	6	6	12
	LMV	Dose (100 mg/day)	-	-	-	-	-	-	-	-	-	-	-
Results of treatment	ALT		N	N	N	N	N	N	N	N	N	N	N
	HBsAg		+	+	+	+	+	+	+	+	+	-	-
	HBeAg		+	-	-	+	+	+	-/+	+	+	-	-
	Anti-HBs		-	-	-	-	-	-	-	-	-	+	+
	Anti-HBe		-	+	-	-	-	-	+/-	-	-	+	+
	Anti-HCV		-	-	-	-	-	-	-	-	-	+	+
Types of response	Complete											+	+
	Incomplete			+	+								
	Transitory								+				
	Absent		+			+	+	+		+	+		

Table 5c. Personal and biological data of the patients without history of previous transfusions

Patients		1	2	3	4	5	6	7	8	9
Name		TM	UP	SP	IC	NI	TC	EL	AG	BP
Age		12	10	8	11	17	13	9	9	14
Gender		M	M	M	F	M	F	F	F	F
Concomitant diseases		-	NS	-	-	-	-	-	-	-
Virological markers before treatment	HBsAg	+	+	+	+	+	+	+	+	+
	Anti-HBs	-	-	-	-	-	-	-	-	-
	HBeAg	+	+	+	+	+	+	+	+	+
	Anti-HBe	-	-	-	-	-	-	-	-	-
Serum aminotransferase levels		1.5N	N	1.5N	2N	N	1.5N	2N	2.5N	N
Inflammatory syndrome		+	+	+	+	+	+	+	+	+
Duration of infection (years)		4	1	4	5	3	4	6	2	4.5

Table 5d. Response to IFN ± lamivudine therapy in patients with non-transfusional chronic hepatitis B

Patients			1	2	3	4	5	6	7	8	9
Treatment	IFN	Dose	3x3	3x3	3x3	3x3	3x3	6x3	3x3	3x3	3x3
		(MU/week)	5x3		5x3	5x3					
		Duration	6	12	9	6	6	6	6	12	6
		(months)	6		3	6					
	LMV	Dose	+	-	+	+	-	-	-	-	-
		(100 mg/day)									
		Duration	6	-	6	6	-	-	-	-	-
Results of treatment		ALT	N	N	N	N	N	N	N	N	N
		HBsAg	+	+	+	+	+	+	+	+	+
		HBeAg	-	-	+	+	-	+	-	+	+
		Anti-HBs	-	-	-	-	-	-	-	-	-
		Anti-HBe	+	+	-	-	+	-	+	-	-
Types of response		Complete									
		Incomplete	+	+			+		+		
		Transitory									
		Absent			+	+		+		+	+

in all children. The adverse reactions were similar to those reported in adults. During the first injection, most of the children suffered a flu-like syndrome with fever (>38°C), headache, asthenia and anorexia. These symptoms tended to ameliorate or disappear after two weeks of treatment. One case developed transitory depression and one case, vitiligo. None of them required cessation of treatment.

Discussions

Unlike in developed countries, where the incidence of HBV is entirely circumstantial (adopted children and adult immigrants from countries with high endemicity) [5] numerous factors of a socioeconomic and medical nature are responsible for the still high rate of infection in developing countries, such as ours.

The high endemicity (AgHBs positivity among the general population is 7.3%, and 32% for the children living in orphanages) [6] is partly responsible for the high prevalence of bloodborne infection with HBV; in our cohort of haemophilic patients its percentage amounts to 35.4 [7].

The belated introduction of hepatitis B immunization in the general population only five years ago, lack of vaccination and revaccination in high risk population groups (multiple transfused patients, patients undergoing haemodialysis, transplanted patients, etc.) as well as the usage, on a large scale, of blood products not properly virus-inactivated (fresh frozen plasma, cryoprecipitate), represent additional responsible factors.

Post-transfusional hepatitis stands out among other types of hepatitis due to its characteristic feature of secondary disease; it is a concomitant disease, being in fact always associated with a main disease, requiring haemotherapy: congenital coagulopathies, talassemia, malignant diseases, etc. The disease requiring transfusional therapy confers certain peculiarities on the patient: haemochromatosis, numerous viral co-infections and a disimmune status (autoimmunity or immunodeficiency) in order to interfere with viral clearance.

Therapeutic experience with chronic HBV infection (carrier, chronic hepatitis) is relatively poorly reflected in literature, due to the loss of interest in developed countries for HBV infection, especially at this stage, when treatment with IFN and antiviral medication has become part of the therapeutic regimen for hepatitis infections. As for therapeutic efficacy, factors such as immunologic reactivity, especially multiple infection with hepatitis viruses (HDV, HCV) or non-hepatitis viruses (HTLV, TTV, HIV), would suggest resistance of post-transfusional hepatitis to IFN therapy. Surprisingly enough, contrary to what was expected, the transfusion has not been referred to as an unfavorable prediction factor for chronic hepatitis B in IFN therapy [8].

However, in our study the percentage of good responses (complete and incomplete) was only 27.27% in patients with transfusional history, as compared to 44.44% in patients without transfusional history. The small number of patients does not allow a statistical evaluation, however it suggests an unfavorable prediction factor in previously transfused patients with actual chronic B hepatitis. Interestingly the two cases of complete favorable response were those with HBV+HCV co-infection. These results would run counter to the literature data, according to which the response to interferon is poor in the simultaneous presence of two viruses that would have an increased cytopathic effect. However, molecular biology studies have shown the existence of interconnection between the two viruses, with HCV inhibiting HBV activity.

The interpretation must be handled cautiously, considering the reciprocal effect on the replication status of each virus. Therefore, even in the absence of simultaneous replication parameters, the frequency of severe evolution to cirrhosis is significantly higher in dual and triple hepatitis infection [9].

At present we evaluate the efficacy of lamivudine associated with IFN therapy in resistant forms of disease.

The preliminary conclusions are pessimistic as far as the performed therapeutic regimen is concerned. These results indicate an urgent need for developing and promoting new therapeutic schedules, more efficient for these types of diseases, especially when we consider that there are over 350,000,000 people infected with HBV in the world, of whom a significant number are condemned to an evolution towards cirrhosis or even neoplasms.

References

1. Ying C, De Clercq E, Neyts J. Lamivudine, adefovir and tenofovir exhibit long-lasting anti-hepatitis B virus activity in cell culture. *J Viral Hepat* 2000; 1:79
2. Moraru E. Chronic hepatitis in children, *Editura Medicala* 1999: 129
3. International Group. Acute and chronic hepatitis revised. *Lancet* 1977;914-919
4. Knodell RG, AndoY, Sonnerborg A et al. Formulation and application of a numerical scoring system for assessing histological activity in asymptomatic chronic active hepatitis. *Hepatology* 1981;1:431-435
5. Sangfelt P, Norder H, Magnius LO, Alaeus A, Carlsson T and Reichard O. Interferon α 2b treatment in hepatitis B carriers. Effect on hepatitis B virus DNA levels in children infected with different genotypes. *Acta pediatr.* 1997; 86:135-137
6. Rosiu N, Brehar Cioflec D., Vaida A.M., et al. Studies regarding viral hepatitis in south-western Romania. *Romanian communication session - Herculane, Romania: Infections with hepatitis viruses – a present health problem 1996.*
7. Serban M., Pop M., Cucuruz M., et al. Infectious complications of the therapy with blood and blood products. *Congress of onco-pediatrics – June 1996 - Bucharest, Romania.*
8. Neudorf-Grauss R, Bujanover Y, Dinari G, Broide E, Neveh Y, Zahavi I, Reif S. Chronic hepatitis B virus infection in children in Israel: clinical and epidemiological characteristics and response to interferon therapy. *Isr.Med Assoc J* 2000;2(2):164-168
9. Mathurin P., Thibault V., Kadidja K., Ganne-Carrié N. et al. Replication status and histological features of patients with triple (B, C, D) and dual (B, C) hepatic infections. *Journal of Viral Hepatitis* 2000; 7: 15 – 22.

GENETICS, PATHOLOGY AND VIRAL DIAGNOSIS

Effects of genotypic variations on hepatitis C virus nonstructural protein 5B structure and activity

ZHI HONG*, ERIC B. FERRARI, ANGELA SKELTON, JACQUELYN WRIGHT-MINOGUE, WEIDONG ZHONG and CHARLES A. LESBURG[†] *

Department of Antiviral Therapy and [†]Department of Structural Chemistry, Schering-Plough Research Institute, 2015 Galloping Hill Road, Kenilworth, NJ 07033-0539

Abstract

Nonstructural protein 5B (NS5B) of hepatitis C virus (HCV) possesses an RNA-dependent RNA polymerase (RdRp) activity responsible for viral genome replication. It presents an excellent target for antiviral development. Recent studies revealed that removal of the C-terminal hydrophobic domain improved the solubility of NS5B to a level suitable for enzymatic characterization and structural determination. This hydrophobic C-terminal tail is highly conserved among all six genotypes of HCV, indicating an important functional and structural role, presumably as a membrane anchor for the assembly of a replication complex. Similar hydrophobic domains were also identified in related viruses such as pestiviruses and GB viruses. Removal of these hydrophobic domains had a universal impact on enzyme solubility and resulted in production of soluble polymerases from all six HCV genotypes, as well as from pestiviruses and GB viruses. Biochemical characterization demonstrated that the activity of RdRps from different HCV genotypes/subtypes varied and lacked a clear correlation either to the response to combination therapy or to the plasma viremia levels. Structure-based surface variability analysis further identified highly conserved regions in the active site and predicted asymmetric distribution of important functionality and critical structural elements essential for replication.

Introduction

HCV is the causative agent for most cases of non-A and non-B hepatitis [1], with an estimated prevalence of 170 million cases (i.e., 2-3%) globally [2]. Close to four million individuals

* To whom correspondence should be addressed: Department of Structural Chemistry, K-15-1800, Schering-Plough Research Institute, 2015 Galloping Hill Road, Kenilworth, New Jersey 07033-0539. Phone: 908-740-3515; Fax: 908-740-7664; E-mail: Charles.Lesburg@spcorp.com.

Frontiers in Viral Hepatitis Ed. by RF Schinazi, J-P Sommadossi and CM Rice. 109 — 121

are infected in the United States alone [3]. In most instances, the virus establishes chronic and insidious infection that persists for decades. This usually results in recurrent and progressively worsening liver inflammation, which often leads to more severe disease states such as cirrhosis and hepatocellular carcinoma [4, 5]. Currently, there are no broadly effective treatments for the debilitating progression of chronic HCV infection.

HCV, a member of the *Flaviviridae* family, is a positive-stranded RNA virus. Its life cycle consists of several interrelated processes that occur primarily in the cytoplasm of the host cells [6]. RNA replication is the centerpiece of the viral proliferation cycle. Despite many years of research, RNA-dependent RNA replication is poorly characterized. The virally encoded polymerase, a product of NS5B in HCV, is the key enzyme that dictates the entire replication process. The interplay between viral polymerase and its substrates (template, primer and incoming nucleotide) defines the basic framework for viral replication. Although the RNA-dependent RNA polymerase (RdRp) presents an excellent target for antiviral development, no therapeutic inhibitors have been brought to the market thus far. This is, in part, due to the lack of understanding about RdRps at the molecular level until recently. As a distinct class of polymerases, HCV NS5B RdRp utilizes RNA template exclusively and catalyzes RNA synthesis via either copy-back [7, 8] or *de novo* [9, 10] mechanisms. Unlike many related RdRps, such as that of poliovirus ($3D^{pol}$), HCV NS5B has acquired a hydrophobic domain at the C-terminus, believed to anchor the viral polymerase to the endoplasmic reticulum (ER) membrane. Many earlier studies using the full-length NS5B have been complicated by the poor solubility of this viral enzyme [11, 12]. Removal of this hydrophobic domain improves the solubility of NS5B [11-13] and allows the determination of the crystal structure of the NS5B apoenzyme [14-16]. These structural studies have revealed unique features of RdRps and have provided useful information for the comparative analysis of RdRps in relation to other classes of polymerases. This knowledge will in turn help to advance our understanding of viral replication at the molecular level for positive-stranded RNA viruses.

Although the mechanism of HCV replication initiation remains unclear, the "copy-back" RNA synthesis shown *in vitro* [7, 8] is unlikely to be the mode of replication in the infected cells due to the lack of repetitive terminal sequence motifs in the HCV genome. *De novo* initiation is likely to play a critical role in HCV replication *in vivo* [9, 10, 17, 18]. Further delineation of the molecular processes at the initiation step requires detailed mechanistic analysis of the reaction pathway of HCV NS5B-catalyzed nucleotide incorporation. Recent studies in our laboratories have begun to address the stoichiometric assembly of the polymerase with its RNA/NTP substrates, which permits efficient nucleotide incorporation for subsequent kinetic analyses. These studies have demonstrated that HCV NS5B has developed a novel structural mechanism to ensure strict terminal initiation from the 3' end of the viral genome. An RNA template with a single-stranded 3' terminus docks precisely in the polymerase active site, which allows the initiating nucleotide(s) to base pair with the terminal template base(s) [19, 20].

In this chapter, we further explore the biological importance of the functional and structural elements in HCV NS5B from a genetic aspect. Phylogenetic relatedness and divergence are analyzed, by comparing all six major genotypes of HCV NS5B. In addition, ribavirin 5'-triphosphate (RTP) is shown to be a weak inhibitor against HCV polymerases from all six major genotypes. A map of conserved functional domains as well as structural surfaces accessible to protein-protein, protein-RNA and protein-NTP interactions will impact our understanding of HCV replication, and more importantly, the inhibitor development, which most likely targets these conserved regions important for viral replication.

The C-terminal hydrophobic domain

Several earlier studies revealed that the full-length HCV NS5B had poor solubility and required high concentrations of salts, glycerol and detergent to remain in solution [11, 12]. Even so, the full-length protein formed high molecular weight aggregates and was unstable in solution [12]. Removal of this 21-amino-acid C-terminal domain resulted in a truncated NS5B which displayed an excellent solubility profile (i.e., monodisperse in solution and free of aggregates) [11, 12]. Furthermore, the truncated NS5B exhibited higher RdRp activity than the full-length protein, which might have a higher proportion of inactive enzyme [12]. Nevertheless, the excellent solubility observed after the C-terminal truncation allowed the determination of the NS5B crystal structure which we would be unlikely to attain from the full length NS5B [14-16].

Despite the lack of detrimental effect on NS5B RdRp activity by the removal of the C-terminal domain, this hydrophobic tail has been hypothesized to play a role in anchoring the NS5B protein to the ER membrane where the replication is believed to take place [6]. This hypothesis is consistent with the subcellular localization of NS5B [21, 22]. To further assess the biological function of this hydrophobic domain, the C-terminal 21 amino acids from 11 subtypes representing all six major genotypes of HCV NS5B were compared. The sequence alignments (Figure 1A) show that all HCV NS5B polymerases contain this highly hydrophobic domain. Surprisingly, this domain is also highly conserved. Several hydrophobic amino acid clusters, such as "LLLL", "GVG" and "LLP", are strictly conserved, suggesting that the hydrophobic C-terminal tail plays an important structural and/or functional role during replication.

Similar hydrophobic C-terminal tails were also present in NS5B of pestiviruses (bovine viral diarrhea virus, BVDV) and the newly identified GB viruses (GB virus B, GBV-B) as illustrated by the hydropathy profiles of these related NS5Bs (Figure 1B). Interestingly, NS5 of flaviviruses (yellow fever virus, YFV) lacks the apparent hydrophobic tail at the C-terminus. There appears to be a correlation between the cleavage of NS5 into NS5A/NS5B and the presence of the hydrophobic C-terminal domain in the hepaciviruses and pestiviruses. It is conceivable that NS5B alone associates with the ER membrane via an instrinsic structural element at the C-terminus, whereas NS5 (equivalent to covalently attached NS5A and NS5B) associates with the ER membrane using a different mechanism. Nevertheless, the effect of the C-terminal hydrophobic domain on NS5B solubility was similar for BVDV and GBV-B, in that removal of the hydrophobic domains resulted in production of soluble and active viral polymerases [23, 24]. Furthermore, soluble NS5 of YFV can be over-expressed in bacterial cells without the requirement of any terminal truncations (data not shown), consistent with the hydropathy analysis of NS5.

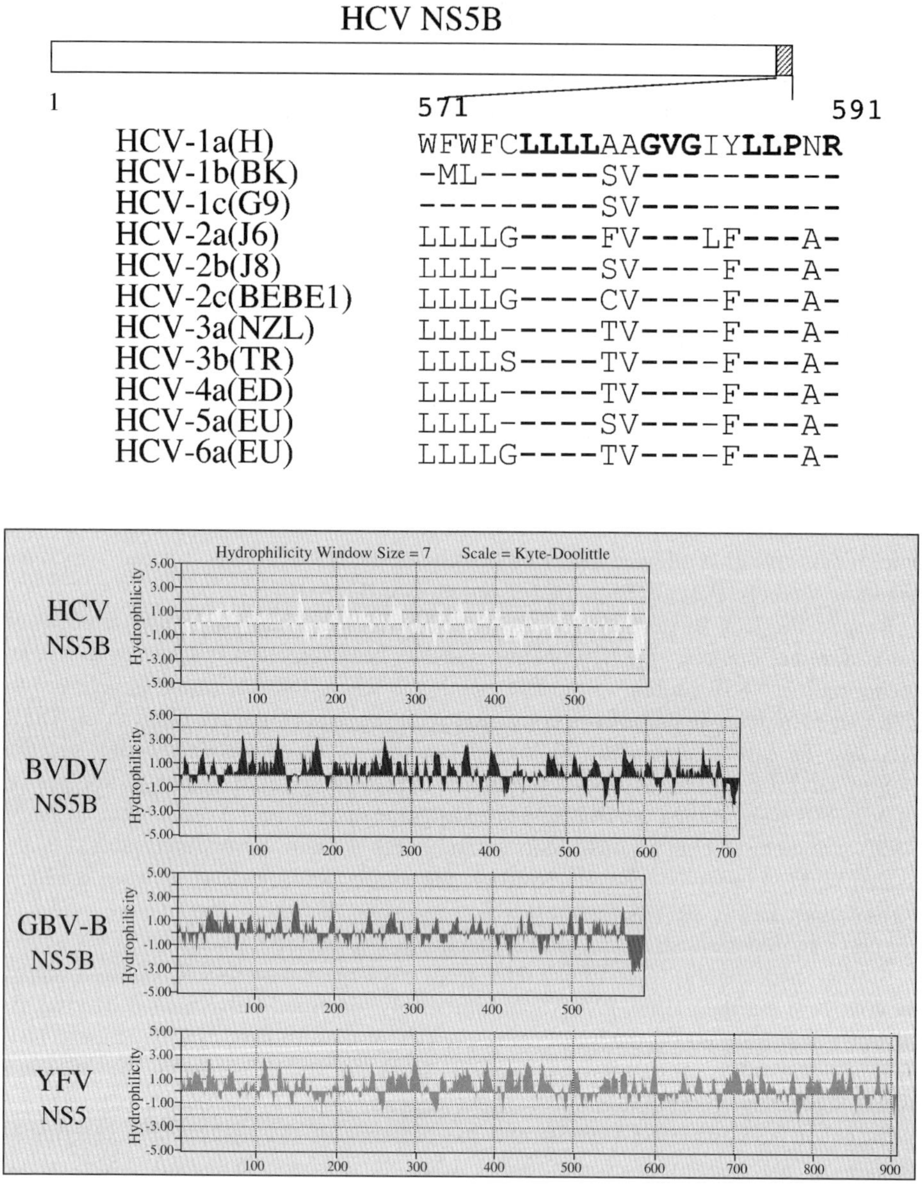

Figure 1. The C-terminal hydrophobic domain is highly conserved in HCV and related viruses. A) Representative amino acid sequences at the C-termini of NS5Bs from 11 different subtypes representing all six major genotypes of HCV were compared. All of the sequences were obtained from the Genbank database using an advanced BLAST search. Clusters of hydrophobic amino acids which are absolutely conserved are in boldface type. Short dashes ("–") represent identical amino acids compared to the lead sequence in (H77 isolate; HCV-1a). B) Hydropathy profiles of the prototype viruses from each genus in the *Flaviviridae* family were compared.

Activity comparison of HCV polymerases from all six major genotypes

NS5B genes from nine different subtypes representing all six major genotypes of HCV were isolated from patient sera, and soluble proteins were produced from each subtype after the removal of the C-terminal 21 amino acids. Consensus NS5B genes were obtained by sequencing multiple cDNA clones from each subtype. The activities of these C-terminally truncated NS5B RdRps were compared. The results in Figure 2A demonstrate that the *in vitro* enzymatic activities vary within one order of magnitude. The difference in activity does not correlate with the viremia levels in patient sera (data not shown). We further isolated NS5Bs from 10 isolates in subtype 1b that respond differentially to the interferon alpha-2b and ribavirin combination therapy (Rebetron^{TM}, Schering-Plough Corporation). Five isolates were from patients who failed to respond to the treatment (designated as NR), and five additional isolates were from patients who had achieved sustained response (SR). All of the proteins were produced as C-terminally truncated soluble proteins, and the RdRp activities were analyzed and compared (Figure 2B). There was no apparent correlation between the RdRp activity and the response to Rebetron. Also, the viremia levels did not parallel the RdRp activity (data not shown).

Inhibition by ribavirin 5'-triphosphate

Ribavirin is a purine analogue with broad-spectrum antiviral activity against many RNA and DNA viruses. However, its molecular mechanism(s) of action have not been fully understood. The clinical efficacy of ribavirin in combination with interferon alpha-2b (Rebetron^{TM}) against HCV infection has led to many hypotheses, none of which alone can convincingly account for all of the observed antiviral effects. One theory proposes that ribavirin enhances the T-helper cells' Type 1 cytokine-mediated immune response while suppressing the Type 2 cytokine response, thus exerting its antiviral activity as an immune modulator [25, 26]. Another theory is based on the inhibitory activity of ribavirin 5'-monophosphate on host cellular inosine monophosphate dehydrogenase, which is responsible for converting inosine 5'-monophosphate to guanosine 5'-monophosphate, an important and rate-limiting step in the biosynthesis of guanosine 5'-triphosphate (GTP). Since GTP is one of the nucleotide substrates for RNA synthesis, depletion of the cellular GTP pool could lead to reduced levels of viral RNA replication [27]. A third theory suggests that ribavirin 5'-triphosphate (RTP), an intracellular metabolite of ribavirin, has a direct antiviral effect against viral polymerases [28-33]. This direct effect is also supported by the estimation that ribavirin exists principally as the triphosphate form, with a ratio of tri- to di- to mono-phosphate close to 25:5:1 [34].

Using our optimized HCV RNA-dependent RNA polymerase (RdRp) assay [11], RTP was shown to inhibit all six genotypes of HCV RdRps (measured by [^{3}H]-GMP incorporation), with IC_{50} values ranging from 50-150 μM (12-37 μg ribavirin equivalent/mL; Figure 3), suggesting that RTP is a weak inhibitor of HCV polymerase. To estimate the intrahepatic concentration of ribavirin in patients during therapy, tissue distribution studies in animal species (rat, mouse and dog) were carried out, showing that the local

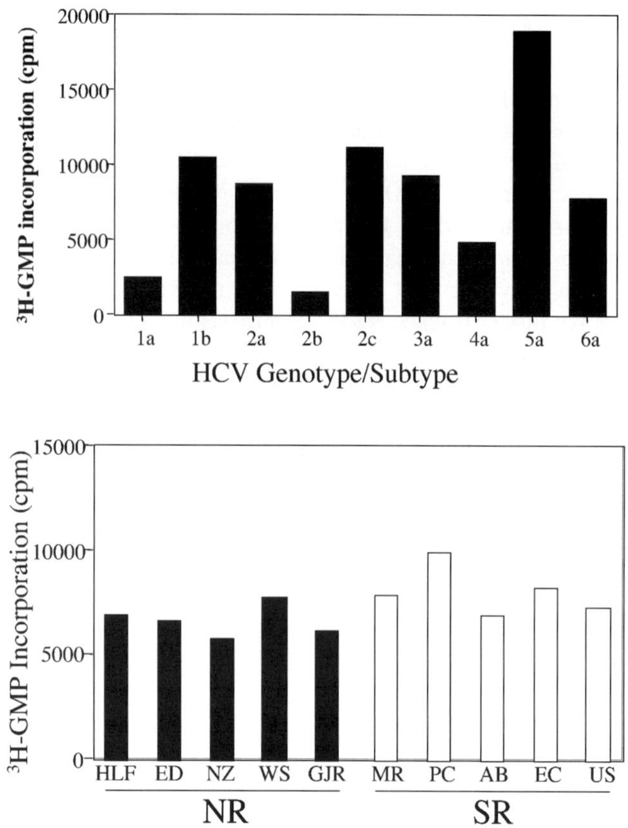

Figure 2. RdRp activity comparison among NS5Bs of various genotypes/subtypes. A) RdRp activity from 9 different subtypes of HCV. NS5B genes were isolated either by PCR from a molecular clone (isolate H77, provided by Dr. Charles Rice, Washington University at St. Louis) or by RT-PCR directly from patient sera. Multiple cDNA clones (from 3 to 6) were sequenced and compared. Consensus sequences were derived, and the clones with the consensus sequences were identified and subject to further characterization. All NS5B cDNAs were subcloned into either pET-21a or pET-28a for expression in bacterial cells as described previously [11]. For production of soluble protein, the C-terminal 21 amino acids were deleted from all of the NS5Bs. The production and purification of each NS5B protein were similarly described [11]. A scintillation proximity assay (SPA) was developed to analyze the RdRp activity for each NS5B polymerase [11]. Briefly, the reaction components are as follow: 20 mM HEPES pH7.3, 5 mM dithiotreitol (DTT), 50 mM NaCl, 7.5 mM $MnCl_2$, 1 unit of RNasin, 0.25 μg poly(C), 0.025 μg biotinylated oligo$(G)_{12}$, 0.05 μCi/5 μM [^{3}H]-GTP and 50 nM NS5B. The reactions were carried out at room temperature (~22°C) for 3 h and quenched by adding 50 mM EDTA in phosphate-buffered saline (PBS). 0.5 mg of streptavidin-coated SPA beads were added to each reaction to capture the RNA products (incubation at room temperature for 15 minutes). The beads were harvested onto a filter plate (GF/B filter, Packard, Meriden, CT) using a TOMTEC Mach 3U Harvester (Hamden, CT). The radioactivity was counted using a TopCount Scintillation/Luminescence Counter (Packard). B) RdRp activity from 10 isolates of HCV-1b with differential response to Rebetron therapy. Ten patients were identified according to their response to Rebetron™ therapy. Five patients had sustained response (SR) to the therapy and the remaining five were nonresponders (NR). Consensus NS5Bs were isolated from each patient and produced in bacterial cells. The RdRp activity was analyzed as described above.

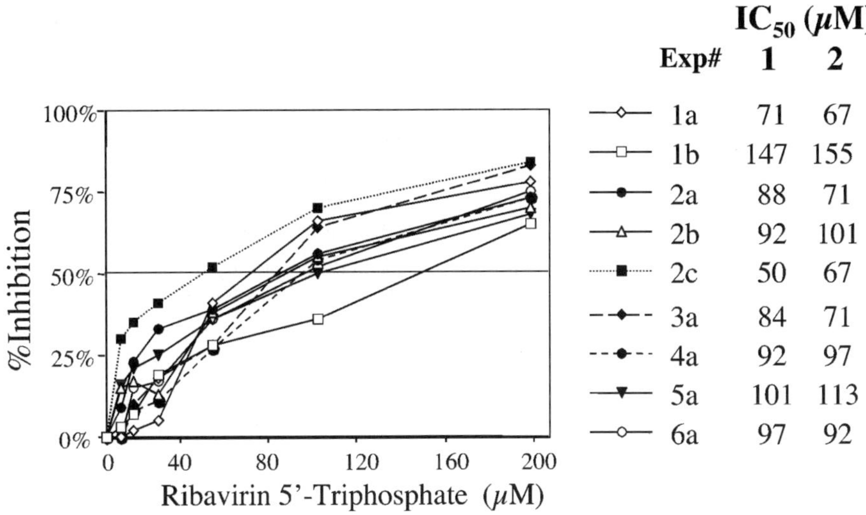

Figure 3. RTP is a weak inhibitor of HCV polymerase. RTP with more than 97% purity was obtained from Moravek Biochemicals, Inc (Brea, CA). RTP (1.5–200 μM) was added to each reaction together with the nucleotide substrate (5 μM GTP). The RdRp activity in the presence of RTP was normalized to that without RTP (100% activity and 0% inhibition). The percentage of inhibition was calculated and plotted. Each reaction was repeated at least twice, and the half maximum inhibitory concentrations (IC_{50}) are listed.

concentrations of ribavirin in liver tissue were 10- to 25-fold higher than the plasma level or in other tissues (data not shown). The average steady-state plasma concentration of ribavirin in patients treated with 1,000-1,200 mg of ribavirin daily is about 10 μM (2.4 μg/mL). Based on this information, we calculate that the intrahepatic concentration of ribavirin in humans is expected to be approximately 100-250 μM, which is similar to or higher than the IC_{50} values of RTP against HCV RdRp. This proposed ribavirin action is further supported by the positive correlation between the steady-state plasma ribavirin level and the proportion of patients showing a complete and sustained virological response (for both HCV genotypes 1 and non-1 infection) based on a large clinical database (data not shown).

Structural variability of HCV polymerases from different genotypes

Viral polymerases are validated targets for antiviral development. Two classes of inhibitors have been developed against HIV reverse transcriptase (RT): nucleoside analog inhibitors (NRTIs) and non-nucleoside analog inhibitors (NNRTIs) [35, 36]. One of the major differences between these two classes of inhibitors is the viral specificity. While NNRTIs are highly specific and only active against HIV-1 [37],

NRTIs have a much broader spectrum against HIV and related viruses, such as hepatitis B virus [38]. It is now known that the viral specificity profile correlates with the modes of action of these inhibitors in that NRTIs compete with the nucleotide substrates (NTPs) for binding at the active site, while NNRTIs bind to a lipophilic pocket near the active site [39, 40]. While the NTP binding site is highly conserved among various related viruses, the NNRTI binding pocket is only present in HIV-1, conferring the high specificity of this type of inhibitor [36]. Clearly, the determination of the crystal structure of HIV RT has contributed tremendously towards our understanding of the mechanistic aspects of these potent polymerase inhibitors and enhanced our knowledge in predicting the viral specificity and drug resistance profiles of new inhibitors [39].

Traditional analysis of amino acid sequence conservation is quite useful in identifying motifs which are important for function and structural integrity. Such conservation analysis may be extended to three dimensions with the availability of the crystal structure of HCV NS5B polymerase [14, 15, 16]. The relative variation entropy (RVE), a measure of sequence variation [41], is plotted on the surface of the enzyme (Figure 4) and ranges from strictly conserved (colored white) to hypervariable (colored purple). This surface variability analysis (SVA) allows for identification of regions on the protein surface which are conserved, even though the neighboring residues which contribute to such a surface may not be sequentially located in the primary amino acid sequence. The surface variability of HCV NS5B indicates strong conservation along the putative trajectory of the RNA template strand as well as the direction of the incoming NTP (Figure 4). It is clear that the NTP binding site which defines the active site, located at the center of the structure, is highly conserved. This conserved NTP binding surface is likely to define the binding pocket of a nucleoside analog inhibitor. Surface variation begins to increase along the direction of the extruded RNA product, away from the active site.

Further examination of the overall structure showed that one side of the NS5B polymerase from which the nascent RNA product exits (Figure 5B, back view) is more variable than the other side (Figure 5A, front view). Comparison of the average RVE values for the two faces of the NS5B molecule revealed that the side with the visible β-hairpin (Figure 5B) is approximately 50% less conserved than the other face (Figure 5A). This difference suggests that most of the HCV polymerase activities occur primarily on the more conserved side of the enzyme, where the incoming NTP enters the polymerase. The assembly of the replication complex is also likely to occur on the more conserved face where protein-protein interactions with other viral/host factors may take place. The more variable face of the enzyme, away from the replication center, appears to have little pressure for conservation and may thus be the consequence of host immune response.

Summary

A highly conserved hydrophobic domain at the C-terminus of NS5B in HCV and related viruses predicts an important replication strategy employed by these viruses. This C-terminal domain is proposed to serve as an anchor for association with the ER

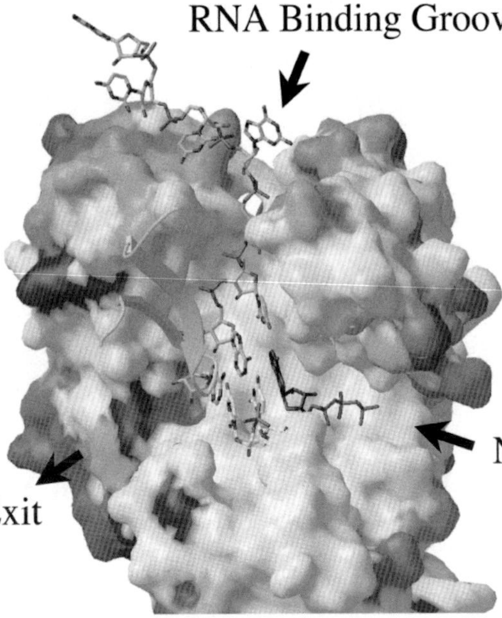

Figure 4. Active site variability of HCV NS5B polymerases from different genotypes. Representative sequences from each of six HCV genotypes (isolates H77, RP, TSS, 266676, SA13 and RJ) were chosen for calculation of surface variability or relative variation entropy (RVE) [41] calculation. The most conserved positions have a value of 0.0 while the most variable positions have a value of 1.0. A value of 1.0 indicates that each amino acid has an equal probability of existing at a particular position. Since only six sequences are being considered, the maximal RVE value in this analysis is 0.6. The RVE calculation does not consider the degree of similarity among multiple amino acids found at a particular position. A molecular surface has been constructed about the atoms of HCV NS5B [14] and colored according to the RVE of the underlying residue which contributes to that surface point. This construction gives a representation of the amino acid variability presented on the surface of the HCV NS5B structure. Only side-chain atoms contribute to the coloring as the backbone atoms are always conserved. The surface is colored smoothly from white (RVE = 0.0) via orange to purple (RVE = 0.6). This Figure was produced using the programs GRASP [42], Molscript [43] and Raster3D [44].

membrane at the site of viral replication [11]. Enzymatic characterization demonstrated that the C-terminal domain is dispensable for RdRp activity, suggesting that membrane association is not required for activity [8, 11, 12]. In the crystal structure of HCV NS5B with the C-terminal 21 amino acids deleted, the newly generated C-terminal tail packs against the active site via interactions with the β-hairpin and blocks the passage of the nascent RNA product [14]. We believe that, in the presence of the hydrophobic domain, the C-terminal tail is unlikely to fold back towards the active site. Indeed, 55 or 62

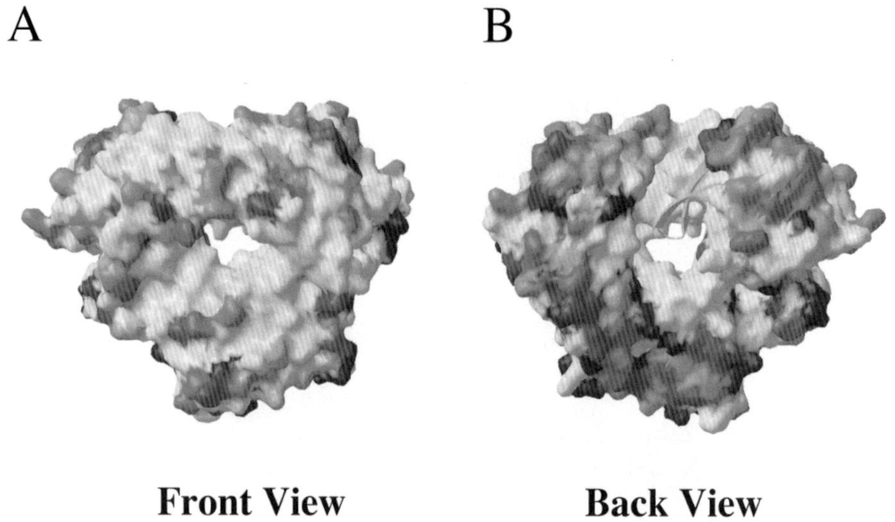

Figure 5. Overall surface variation among polymerases from different genotypes. The surface of NS5B molecule was sliced down the middle (in the plane of the paper), with equal numbers of surface modules on each side (a total of more than 35,000 modules). On the front face of the polymerase (panel A), 60% of the surface (colored white) is strictly conserved, i.e., the RVE value is 0.0. On the back face where the β-hairpin is visible (panel B), only 40% of the surface is strictly conserved. The degree of variability on the back face is also higher, with more clusters of hypervariable regions (colored purple).

amino acids can be removed from the C-terminus without any adverse effects on the RdRp activity. Rather, higher activity was associated with these larger truncations at the C-terminus [8, 11]. This is consistent with our hypothesis that the C-terminal domain is involved in membrane association and, during infection, is located away from the catalytic site of the polymerase.

Surface variability analysis allows for the identification of pockets with high degrees of inter-genotypic homology and thus provides candidates of potential inhibitor binding sites for antiviral development. Highly conserved regions such as those shown in the active site of NS5B (Figure 4) are suitable local targets for inhibitor binding. Detailed analysis of the molecular architectures of these conserved surface pockets accessible by small molecules will shed light on inhibitor design and have predictive value in evaluating HCV NS5B inhibitors for broad-spectrum activity as well as potential resistance profiles.

Acknowledgment

We thank Gregory R. Reyes and Bahige M. Baroudy for support.

References

1. Choo QL, et al. Isolation of a cDNA clone derived from a blood-borne non-A, non-B viral hepatitis genome. *Science* 1989;244, 359-62.
2. World Health Organization. Hepatitis C. Seroprevalence of hepatitis C virus (HCV) in a population sample. *Wkly Epidemiol Rec* 1996;71, 346-9.
3. Alter MJ, et al. The prevalence of hepatitis C virus infection in the United States, 1988 through 1994. *N Engl J Med* 1999;341, 556-62.
4. Saito I, et al. Hepatitis C virus infection is associated with the development of hepatocellular carcinoma. *Proc Natl Acad Sci U S A* 1990;87, 6547-9.
5. Shimotohno K. Hepatitis C virus as a causative agent of hepatocellular carcinoma. *Intervirology* 1995;38, 162-9.
6. Rice CM. Flaviviridae: The Viruses and Their Replication. in *Fields Virology* (eds. Fields BN, Knipe DN and Howley PM) 931-959 (Lippincott - Raven Publishers, Phladelphia, 1996).
7. Behrens SE, Tomei L and De Francesco R. Identification and properties of the RNA-dependent RNA polymerase of hepatitis C virus. *EMBO J* 1996;15, 12-22.
8. Lohmann V, Korner F, Herian U and Bartenschlager R. Biochemical properties of hepatitis C virus NS5B RNA-dependent RNA polymerase and identification of amino acid sequence motifs essential for enzymatic activity. *J Virol* 1997;71, 8416-28.
9. Zhong W, Uss AS, Ferrari E, Lau JY and Hong Z. De novo initiation of RNA synthesis by hepatitis C virus nonstructural protein 5B polymerase. *J Virol* 72000;4, 2017-22.
10. Luo G, et al. De novo initiation of RNA synthesis by the RNA-dependent RNA polymerase (NS5B) of hepatitis C virus. *J Virol* 2000;74, 851-63.
11. Ferrari E, et al. Characterization of soluble hepatitis C virus RNA dependent RNA polymerase expressed in Escherichia coli. *J Virol* 1999;73, 1649-54.
12. Tomei L, et al. Biochemical characterization of a hepatitis C virus RNA-dependent RNA polymerase mutant lacking the C-terminal hydrophobic sequence. *J Gen Virol* 2000;81 Pt 3, 759-67.
13. Yamashita T, et al. RNA-dependent RNA polymerase activity of the soluble recombinant hepatitis C virus NS5B protein truncated at the C-terminal region. *J Biol Chem* 1998;273, 15479-86.
14. Lesburg CA, et al. Crystal structure of the RNA-dependent RNA polymerase from hepatitis C virus reveals a fully encircled active site. *Nat Struct Biol* 1999;6, 937-43.
15. Ago H, et al. Crystal structure of the RNA-dependent RNA polymerase of hepatitis C virus. *Structure Fold Des* 1999;7, 1417-26.
16. Bressanelli S, et al. Crystal structure of the RNA-dependent RNA polymerase of hepatitis C virus. *Proc Natl Acad Sci U S A* 1999;96, 13034-9.
17. Oh JW, Ito T and Lai MM. A recombinant hepatitis C virus RNA-dependent RNA polymerase capable of copying the full-length viral RNA. J Virol 1999;73, 7694-702.
18. Sun XL, Johnson RB, Hockman MA and Wang QM. De novo RNA synthesis catalyzed by HCV RNA-dependent RNA polymerase. *Biochem Biophys Res Commun* 2000;268, 798-803.
19. Zhong W, et al. Template/primer requirements and single nucleotide incorporation by hepatitis C virus nonstructural protein 5B polymerase. *J Virol* 2000;73, 9134-9143.
20. Hong Z, et al. Hepatitis C virus NS5B employs a novel mechanism to ensure terminal initiation during replication. *Virology* 2000;285, 6-11.
21. Hwang SB, Park KJ, Kim YS, Sung YC and Lai MM. Hepatitis C virus NS5B protein is a membrane-associated phosphoprotein with a predominantly perinuclear localization. *Virology* 1997;227, 439-46.

22. Tu H, et al. Hepatitis C virus RNA polymerase and NS5A complex with a SNARE-like protein. *Virology* 1999;263, 30-41.
23. Lai VC, et al. Mutational analysis of bovine viral diarrhea virus RNA-dependent RNA polymerase. *J Virol* 1999;73, 10129-36.
24. Zhong W, et al. RNA-dependent RNA polymerase activity encoded by GB virus nonstructural protein 5B. *J. Viral Hepat* 2000;7, 335-342.
25. Hultgren C, Milich DR, Weiland O and Sallberg M. The antiviral compound ribavirin modulates the T helper (Th) 1/Th2 subset balance in hepatitis B and C virus-specific immune responses. *J Gen Virol* 1998;79, 2381-91.
26. Tam RC, et al. Ribavirin polarizes human T cell responses towards a Type 1 cytokine profile. *J Hepatol* 1999;30, 376-82.
27. Markland W, McQuaid TJ, Jain J and Kwong AD. Broad-spectrum antiviral activity of the IMP dehydrogenase inhibitor VX-497: a comparison with ribavirin and demonstration of antiviral additivity with alpha interferon. *Antimicrob Agents Chemother* 2000;44, 859-66.
28. Toltzis P, O'Connell K and Patterson JL. Effect of phosphorylated ribavirin on vesicular stomatitis virus transcription. *Antimicrob Agents Chemother* 1988;32, 492-7.
29. Wray SK, Gilbert BE. and Knight V. Effect of ribavirin triphosphate on primer generation and elongation during influenza virus transcription in vitro. *Antiviral Res* 1985;5, 39-48.
30. Wray SK, Gilbert BE, Noall MW and Knight V. Mode of action of ribavirin: effect of nucleotide pool alterations on influenza virus ribonucleoprotein synthesis. *Antiviral Res* 1985;5, 29-37.
31. Fernandez-Larsson R and Patterson JL. Ribavirin is an inhibitor of human immunodeficiency virus reverse transcriptase. *Mol Pharmacol* 1990;38, 766-70.
32. Fernandez-Larsson R, O'Connell K, Koumans E and Patterson JL. Molecular analysis of the inhibitory effect of phosphorylated ribavirin on the vesicular stomatitis virus in vitro polymerase reaction. *Antimicrob Agents Chemother* 33, 1668-73 (1989).
33. Fernandez-Larsson R and Patterson JL. Altered ATP function of a vesicular stomatitis virus mutant detected by kinetic analysis of the transcriptase using phosphorylated ribavirin. *J Gen Virol* 1989;70, 2791-7.
34. Smith RA. Mechanisms of action of ribavirin. in *Ribavirin: a broad spectrum antiviral agent* (eds. Smith RA and Kirkpatrick W) 99-118 (Academic Press, New York, 1980).
35. De Clerq E. Antiviral therapy for human immunodeficiency virus infections. *Clin Microbiol Rev* 1995;8, 200-239.
36. De Clerq E. What can be expected from non-nucleoside reverse transcriptase inhibitors (NNRTIs) in the treatment of human immunodeficiency virus 1 (HIV-1) infections? *Rev Med Virol* 1998;6, 97-117.
37. Pauwels R, et al. Potent and selective inhibition of HIV-1 replication in vitro by a novel series of TIBO derivatives. *Nature* 1990;343, 470-474.
38. Balzarini J, et al. Anti-HIV and anti-HBV activity and resistance profile of 2', 3'-dideoxy-3'-thiacytidine (3TC) and its arylphosphoramidate derivative CF 1109. *Biochem Biophys Res Commun* 1996;225, 363-9.
39. Kohlstaedt LA, Wang J, Friedman JM, Rice PA and Steitz TA. Crystal structure at 3.5 Å resolution of HIV-1 reverse transcriptase complexed with an inhibitor. *Science* 1992;256, 1783-90.
40. Spence RA, Kati WM, Anderson KS and Johnson KA. Mechanism of inhibition of HIV-1 reverse transcriptase by nonnucleoside inhibitors. *Science* 1995;267, 988-93.
41. Sander C and Schneider R. Database of homology-derived protein structures and the structural meaning of sequence alignment. *Proteins* 1991;9, 56-68.

42. Nicholls A, Sharp KA and Honig B. Protein folding and association: insights from the interfacial and thermodynamic properties of hydrocarbons. *Proteins* 1991;11, 281-96.
43. Kraulis PJ. MOLSCRIPT: a program to produce both detailed and schematic plots of protein structure. *J Appl Crystallogr* 1991;24, 946-950.
44. Merritt E and Bacon DJ. Raster3D: photorealistic molecular graphics. *Meth Enzymol* 1997;276, 505-524.

Compartmentalization of hepatitis C viral quasispecies

XIAOFENG FAN, ANDRE CASTRO LYRA and
ADRIAN M. DI BISCEGLIE

*From the Department of Internal Medicine,
Saint Louis University School of Medicine, Saint Louis, Mo*

Introduction

The hepatitis C virus (HCV) has a single-stranded RNA genome approximately 9, 000 nucleotides in length [4]. This RNA genome is subject to considerable variability. At least six different genotypes have been identified, each nucleotide sequence differing by 30 to 35% [23]. Within these genotypes are subtypes and isolates. Isolates derived from individual patients at specific time points are also subject to variability, and their nucleotide sequences may differ from each other by 1% to 2%. These minor variants make up the quasispecies diversity of HCV, and HCV is said to circulate as a quasispecies swarm [13]. Minor variants may be generated by nucleotide substitutions occurring due to lack of fidelity of the HCV RNA-dependent RNA polymerase or perhaps by selection of variants, either by immune pressure or functional efficiency.

Identification of quasispecies

HCV variants making up the quasispecies have been identified by variation in nucleotide sequence within certain specific regions of the HCV genome. Regions of the genome which are subject to variability and have been useful in identifying variants include the envelope (particularly E2) and NS5A regions of the genome [2].

These regions of the genome have been studied using various techniques [9, 10, 14, 19, 26]. Of these techniques, the most thorough and complete is the direct determination of the nucleotide sequence of an isolate. To demonstrate variability, it is necessary to sequence multiple clones from a particular isolate. Thus, for HCV it is not sufficient to sequence simply the product of amplification by reverse transcription PCR. Multiple clones of PCR product must first be obtained for sequencing. Furthermore, it is necessary to sequence large numbers of clones to obtain sequences representative of the major variants present in an isolate. Because cloning and sequencing are very tedious and cumbersome, other methods to screen for the presence of variants have been evaluated. These techniques include PCR followed by single-stranded conformational polymorphism (PCR-SSCP) and heteroduplex mobility assays (HMA). While PCR-SSCP has proved to be an unreliable method for studying HCV quasispecies, HMA has

Frontiers in Viral Hepatitis Ed. by RF Schinazi, J-P Sommadossi and CM Rice. 123 — 130

been found to be useful as a way of identifying the number of variants present and the degree of variability between them [9, 19, 26].

HVR1

Two hypervariable regions have been identified within the E2 glycoprotein of HCV. The larger of these two is found at the 5' end of the E2 region of the genome and is about 81 base pairs in length, coding for approximately 27 amino acids and referred to as HVR1 [24]. This region has been the subject of considerable attention, as it has been thought to play an important role in the host immune response to HCV infection [25]. Thus it is predicted to be the site of both B cell and T cell epitopes, and because of its considerable variability, it is thought to play a role in escape from immune surveillance. Patients with acute self-limiting hepatitis have an earlier and stronger antibody reactivity to HVR1 and also have a rapidly diminishing number of HCV variants. A recently published study which clearly implicated humoral immunity in persistence of HCV followed a plan very similar to our proposed studies. Zibert and coworkers studied serum samples from a group of women infected with the same strain of HCV from contaminated lots of anti-D serum used in management of Rh incompatibility. Using synthetic peptides derived from the HVR1 region of the infecting HCV, they tested for antibodies in serum of infected patients. Interestingly, those patients who developed acute, self-limited HCV infection developed higher titers more rapidly to HVR1 peptide than those who went on to chronicity [28]. These findings are compatible with the notion that high titers of anti-HVR1 were able to neutralize and eliminate infecting HCV, whereas lower titers permitted development of escape mutants and thus led to chronicity. Developmental vaccines against HCV which make use of recombinant E2/NS1 have been shown to be at least partly protective in chimpanzees [3], another observation suggesting that envelope proteins of HCV may contain important neutralizing epitopes.

Interestingly, other flaviviruses do not have regions analogous to HVR1, and they cause only acute infection. Finally, exacerbations and remission of liver injury due to HCV, as indicated by fluctuations in serum aminotransferase values, are associated with appearance and clearance, respectively, of new HVR1 variants [25]. Against this is the recent finding that little change was found in HVR1 consensus sequence over time in two chimpanzees inoculated with an infectious clone of HCV. Both animals became chronically infected and, although amino acid substitutions occurred over the first year of infection, these were few and were largely confined to E1, E2, p7, NS3 and NS5 [12].

Significance of HCV quasispecies

Several investigators have tried to understand the biological and clinical significance of HCV quasispecies variants by correlating their presence with clinical manifestations of HCV infection, such as development of liver disease, response to interferon therapy and viral load in serum [8, 9, 10, 14, 15, 19, 22]. It has been suggested that increasing complexity of quasispecies variants is associated with a relative lack of interferon responsiveness and that some quasispecies variants are more resistant to interferon than others, although these findings may not have been adequately corrected for viral titer and genotype. Recently, Farci and coworkers studied the significance of quasispecies variants evolution among patients with acute HCV infection. She found that patients with acute resolving infection had a rapidly diminishing number of quasispecies variants in serum, while those who went on to develop chronic HCV infection had a progressive increase in the number of quasispecies variants [6]. However, the clinical significance of quasispecies variants still remains to be elucidated, particularly with regard to liver disease severity. Most studies have focused on HCV quasispecies variants in serum rather than within the liver (the major site of HCV replication), and it is possible that hepatic viral genotypes, subtypes and quasispecies variants may correlate better with clinical disease caused by HCV than those found in serum.

Genetic diversity and response to interferon

Alpha interferon is commonly used in the therapy of chronic hepatitis C, but no more than about 40% of patients achieve a sustained virologic response with long-term clearance of HCV RNA from serum. Some viral factors that play an important role in determining response to interferon include HCV genotype and the level of HCV RNA in serum [11]. However, it has also been suggested that HCV genetic diversity may affect the outcome of therapy. Polyak and coworkers found a greater degree of genetic diversity and HCV complexity among nonresponders to interferon compared to responders [19]. Hassoba and coworkers also pointed out that interferon therapy may induce the formation of HCV quasispecies. Patients who were treated with interferon but did not respond to therapy often had new HVR1 variants appear following therapy [9].

Tissue compartmentalization of HCV

Most studies of HCV quasispecies have been based on isolates from serum of infected individuals. However, the liver appears to be the major site of HCV replication. Liver tissue contains much higher titers of HCV RNA than serum, and the negative-strand replicative intermediate of HCV is more readily detectable within the liver [7]. Furthermore, HCV antigens and RNA can be observed within the liver by immunostaining and *in situ* hybridization [17, 27]. It is reasonable to question whether there are differences in HCV diversity within the liver where HCV is replicating, compared to the circulation. In addition, there are some suggestions that HCV may replicate within other cells and tissues, such as lymphocytes [1]. Certainly HCV RNA can be identified within lymphocytes, although it is not clear that they represent a major site of viral replication.

Few studies have been done of HCV quasispecies in compartments other than serum, probably because of the lack of suitable liver tissue. Navas and colleagues compared HVR1 sequences from isolates within peripheral blood mononuclear cells (PBMC), liver tissue and serum. They found that genetic variability appeared to be greater in serum than liver or PBMC. Furthermore, phylogenetic analysis showed segregation of sequences by tissue compartment. Finally, sequences from liver and PBMC were more closely related to each other than to sequences from serum [16]. Okuda and coworkers studied PBMC, liver and serum from 13 patients with chronic HCV infection. Figure 1 shows that although common HVR1 amino acid sequences could be identified within all three compartments, some sequences were found only within liver, serum or PBMC [18].

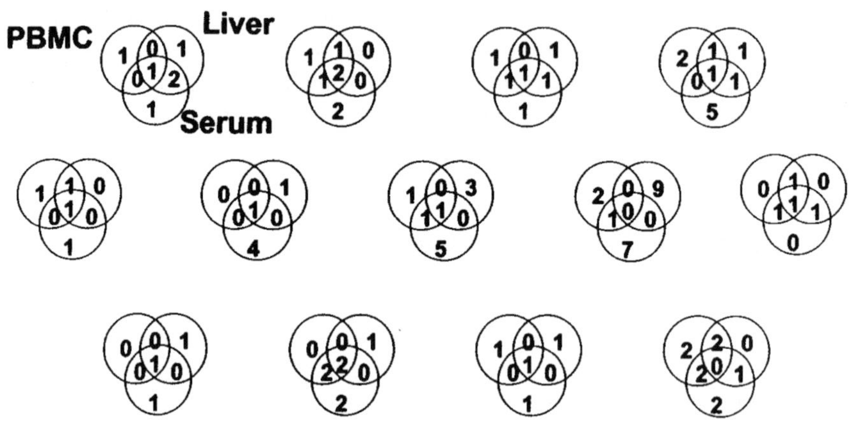

Figure 1. Compartmentalization of HVR1 quasispecies: Common amino acid sequences found in liver, serum and PBMC in 13 patients with chronic hepatitis C (adapted from reference 18, with permission).

One of the more detailed published comparisons of HCV nucleotide diversity in serum and liver was recently published by Sakai et al. [20]. They studied eight patients with chronic HCV infection and found significantly different degrees of diversity between these two compartments in seven of eight cases (Table 1). Interestingly, greater diversity was not consistently found in either serum or liver - this appeared to vary from patient to patient [20]. These investigators also studied liver tissue derived from three different regions of the liver and found significantly greater diversity within some portions of the liver than others (Table 2). Only the study of Sakamoto and colleagues showed no differences in HCV variants by consensus sequencing of PCR products and by single strand conformational polymorphism [21].

We have conducted similar studies of HCV diversity by evaluating matched serum and liver samples tested by reverse transcription polymerase chain reaction amplification and single-stranded conformation polymorphism analysis of the hypervariable portion of the E2/NS1 region of the HCV genome [5]. The number of quasispecies found was compared to the amount of HCV RNA and HCV genotype. Sixteen of 40 patients studied had HCV RNA detectable in serum and liver. The HCV genotype was identical in serum and liver in all but one case. HCV RNA levels were approximately tenfold higher in liver than serum. The number of HCV quasispecies detectable in serum by

Table 1. Nucleotide diversity in serum and liver (adapted from reference 20 with permission)

	Nucleotide Diversity (%)		
Pt.	Serum	Liver	p Value
1	1.87	2.47	<0.01
2	1.05	0.81	<0.01
3	1.61	0.46	<0.01
4	3.82	3.33	n.s.
5	2.91	2.48	<0.05
6	0.74	1.02	<0.05
7	4.10	2.73	<0.01
8	2.57	1.74	<0.01

n.s.: not significant

Table 2. Nucleotide diversity within the liver (adapted from reference 20 with permission)

	Nucleotide Diversity (%)			
Pt.	Sample 1	Sample 2	Sample 3	p Value
1	2.60	2.66	2.14	n.s.
2	0.99	0.63	0.81	n.s.
3	0.47	0.54	0.37	n.s.
4	3.62	3.63	2.75	<0.05
5	2.40	2.54	2.52	n.s.
6	1.02	1.48	0.57	<0.01
7	3.08	2.38	2.74	<0.05
8	1.80	1.99	1.43	<0.05

n.s.: not significant

SSCP ranged between two and six (median 3.0) and in the liver between two and 19 (median 3.5, mean liver/serum ratio 1 to 6.3, median 1.8). The number of quasispecies in the liver was equal to or greater than that in serum in all cases. We concluded that the number of hepatic HCV quasispecies usually exceeds that in serum, independent of the amount of HCV RNA and HCV genotype, and we surmised that this finding was compatible with clearance of some quasispecies from serum, but not the liver, by putative neutralizing antibodies.

We were not able to confirm these results when we studied some of the same samples using the more specific method of cloning and sequencing of HCV variants. The hypervariable region of the genome and adjacent flanking sequences of the E2/NS1 envelope region of the hepatitis C virus serum and liver samples of two patients was amplified by PCR and cloned into M13. Approximately 50 clones from each sample were sequenced, and the nucleotide sequences analyzed to determine their relationship to each other. Amino acid variations and antibody reactivity to these variations were compared between liver and serum. We found 27 quasispecies (defined as having a single nucleotide variation) in sample 1, with an equal number in both liver and serum, and 28 variants in sample 2. One sample had the same single dominant quasispecies with multiple minor variants in both liver and serum, while the other had one dominant and one subdominant variant with multiple minor variants. Based on this more refined methodology, we concluded that the same dominant viral quasispecies variants are found within liver and serum of chronically infected patients. We have also analyzed HCV variability within different regions of the liver by testing three separate areas of an HCV-infected liver obtained at the time of liver transplantation and found that, although minor variability occurred both in serum and liver isolates, phylogenetic analysis did not confirm segregation of variants by location within the liver.

Summary and conclusions

HCV quasispecies remain an interesting biologic phenomenon which may have important clinical implications. Studies of HCV variability within different compartments have yielded conflicting results. Some have found significant differences in variants within liver, serum and PBMC, while others have not. Our own studies have had the advantage of studying large amounts of liver tissue obtained at the time of transplantation. We have also sequenced large numbers of HCV clones from each isolate. Based on these detailed studies, we do not find significant differences in HCV quasispecies within liver and serum. An important implication of this finding is that it is acceptable for future studies of HCV quasispecies diversity to be done using serum from infected individuals, rather than having to rely on the more difficult to obtain liver tissue compartment.

References

1. Artini M, Natoli G, Avantaggiati ML, Balsano C, Chirillo P, Costanzo A, Bonavita MS, Levrero M. Detection of replicative intermediates of viral RNA in peripheral blood mononuclear cells from chronic hepatitis C virus carriers. Arch Virol 1993; 8:23-29.
2. Bukh J, Miller RH, Purcell RH. Genetic heterogeneity of hepatitis C virus: quasispecies and genotypes. Semin Liver Dis 1995; 15: 41-63.
3. Choo QL, Kuo G, Ralston R, Weiner A, Chien D, Van Nest G, Han J, Berger K, Thudium K, Kuo C,

Kansopon J, McFarland J, Tabrizi A, Ching K, Moss B, Cummins LB, Houghton M, Muchmore E. Vaccination of chimpanzees against infection by the hepatitis C virus. Proc. Natl. Acad. Sci. USA 1994; 91:1294-1298.

4. Choo QL, Richman KH, Han JH, Berger K, Lee C, Dong C, Gallegos C, Coit D, Medina Selby R, Barr PJ, Weiner AJ, Bradley DW, Kuo G, Houghton M. Genetic organization and diversity of the hepatitis C virusProc Natl Acad Sci U S A 1991; 88:2451-2455.
5. Fan X, Solomon H, Poulos JE, Neuschwander Tetri BA, Di Bisceglie AM. Comparison of genetic heterogeneity of hepatitis C viral RNA in liver tissue and serum. Am J Gastroenterol 1999; 94:1347-1354.
6. Farci P, Shimoda A, Coiana A, Diaz G, Peddis G, Melpolder JC, Strazzera A, Chien DY, Munoz SJ, Balestrieri A, Purcell RH, Alter HJ. The outcome of acute hepatitis C predicted by the evolution of the viral quasispecies. Science 2000; 288:339-344.
7. Fong TL, Shindo M, Feinstone SM, Hoofnagle JH, Di Bisceglie AM. Detection of replicative intermediates of hepatitis C viral RNA in liver and serum of patients with chronic hepatitis C. J Clin Invest 1991; 88:1058-1060.
8. Gonzalez-Peralta RP, Qian K, She JY, Davis GL, Tomoyoshi O, Mizokami M, Lau JYN. Clinical implications of viral quasispecies heterogeneity in chronic hepatitis C. J Med Virol 1996; 49: 242-247.
9. Hassoba HM, Bzowej N, Berenguer M, Kim M, Zhou S, Phung Y, Grant R, Pessoa MG, Wright TL. Evolution of viral quasispecies in interferon-treated patients with chronic hepatitis C virus infection. J Hepatol 1999; 31: 618-627.
10. Honda M, Kaneko S, Sakai A, Unoura M, Murakami S, Kobayashi K. Degree of diversity of hepatitis C virus quasispecies and progression of liver diseases. Hepatology 1994; 20:1144-1151.
11. Hoofnagle JH, Di Bisceglie AM. The treatment of chronic viral hepatitis. N Engl J Med 1997; 336:347-356.
12. Major ME, Mihalik K, Fernandez J, Seidman J, Kleiner D, Kolykhalov AA, Rice CM, Feinstone SM. Long-term follow-up of chimpanzees inoculated with the first infectious clone for hepatitis C virus. J Virol 1999; 73: 3317 3325.
13. Martell M, Esteban JI, Quer J, Genesca J, Weiner A, Esteban R, Guardia J et al. Hepatitis C virus (HCV) circulates as a population of different but closely related genomes: quasispecies nature of HCV genome distribution. J Virology 1992; 66:3225-3229.
14. Moribe T, Hayashi N, Kanazawa Y, Mita E, Fusamoto H, Negi M, Kaneshige T, Hirotsune I, Takaenobu K, Uchida K. Hepatitis C viral complexity detected by single-strand conformation polymorphism and response to interferon therapy. Gastroenterology 1995; 108:789-795.
15. Naito M, Hayashi N, Moribe T, Hagiwara H, Mita E, Kanazawa Y, Kasahara A, Fusamoto H, Kamada T. Hepatitis C viral quasispecies in hepatitis C virus carriers with normal liver enzymes and patients with type C chronic liver diseases. Hepatology 1995; 22:407-412.
16. Navas S, Martín J, Quiroga JA, Castillo I, Carreño V. Genetic diversity and tissue compartmentalization of the hepatitis C virus genome in blood mononuclear cells, liver, and serum from chronic hepatitis C patients. J Virol, 1998; 72: 1640-1646.
17. Nouri-Aria KT, Sallie R, Mizokami M, Portmann BC and Williams R. Intrahepatic expression of hepatitis C virus antigens in chronic liver disease. J Pathol 1995; 175:77-83.
18. Okuda M, Hino K, Korenaga M, Yamaguchi Y, Katoh Y, Okita K. Differences in hypervariable region 1 quasispecies of hepatitis C virus in human serum, peripheral blood mononuclear cells, and liver. Hepatology 1999; 29: 217-222.
19. Polyak SJ, Faulkner G, Carithers RL, Corey L, Gretch DR. Assessment of hepatitis C virus quasispecies

heterogeneity by gel shift analysis: correlation with response to interferon therapy. J Infect Dis 1997; 175:1101-1107.

20. Sakai A, Kaneko S, Honda M, Matsushita E, Kobayashi K. Quasispecies of hepatitis C virus in serum and in three different parts of the liver of patients with chronic hepatitis. Hepatology 1999; 30: 556-561.
21. Sakamoto N, Enomoto N, Kurosaki M, Asahina Y, Maekawa S, Koizumi K, Sakuma I, Murakami F, Marumo T, Sato C. Comparison of the hypervariable region of hepatitis C virus genomes in plasma and liver. J Med Virol 1995; 46:7-11.
22. Shindo M, Arai K, Sokawa Y and Okuno T. The virological and histological states of anti-hepatitis C virus-positive subjects with normal liver biochemical values. Hepatology 1995; 22: 418-425.
23. Simmonds P, Alberti A, Alter HJ, Bonino F, Bradley DW, Brechot C, Brouwer JT, Chan SW, Chayama K, Chen DS (and 36 additional authors). A proposed system for the nomenclature of hepatitis C viral genotypes [letter] Hepatology 1994; 19: 1321-1324.
24. Weiner AJ, Brauer MJ, Rosenblatt J, Richman KH, Tung J, Crawford K, Bonino F, Saracco G, Choo QL, Houghton M, and Han JH. Variable and hypervariable domains are found in the regions of HCV corresponding to the flavivirus envelope and NS1 proteins and the pestivirus envelope glycoproteins. Virology 1991;180:842-848.
25. Weiner AJ, Geysen HM, Christopherson C, Hall JE, Mason TJ, Saracco G, Bonino F, Crawford K, Marion CD, Crawford KA, Brunetto M, Barr PJ, Miyamura T, McHutchinson J and Houghton M. Evidence for immune selection of hepatitis C virus (HCV) putative envelope glycoprotein variants: Potential role in chronic HCV infections. Proc Natl Acad Sci USA 1992; 89:3468-3472.
26. Wilson JJ, Polyak SJ, Day TD, Gretch DR. Characterization of simple and complex hepatitis C virus quasispecies by heteroduplex gel shift analysis: correlation with nucleotide sequencing. J Gen Virol 1995; 76: 1763-1771.
27. Yamada G, Nishimoto H, Endou H, Doi T, Takahashi M, Tsuji T, Yoshizawa H, Nozawa M, Koji T and Nakane PK. Localization of hepatitis C viral RNA and capsid protein in human liver. Dig Dis Sci 1993; 38: 882-887.
28. Zibert A, Meisel H, Kraas W, Schulz A, Jung G and Roggendorf M. Early antibody response against hypervariable region 1 is associated with acute self-limiting infections of hepatitis C virus. Hepatology 1997; 25:1245-1249.

In situ localization of PCR-amplified hepatitis C virus RNA on human erythrocytes

SUSAN SIMON[1], GABOR LOTZ[1], FRITZ KURY[2],
BIRGIT REIPERT[3], ALEXANDER STEINKASSERER[4,5],
MARTHA M. EIBL[4] and ZSUZSA SCHAFF[1]

[1] *2nd Department of Pathology, Semmelweis University, Budapest, Hungary*
[2] *ViennaLab Labordiagnostika GmbH, Vienna, Austria*
[3] *Baxter Hyland Immuno AG, Vienna, Austria*
[4] *Immunology Outpatient Clinic, Vienna, Austria*
[5] *Present address: Department of Dermatology, University of Erlangen - Nürnberg, Erlangen, Germany*

Summary

Erythrocytes from 43 patients chronically infected with hepatitis C virus (HCV) were analysed by reverse transcriptase *in situ* polymerase chain reaction (RT-*in situ* PCR). The positive strand of the viral RNA genome was associated with the erythrocyte cell membrane as demonstrated by fluorescence microscopy in 40 out of the 43 patients. None of the red blood cells from 10 healthy individuals and seven of the patients with diseases unrelated to HCV showed positive signals for HCV RNA. These data suggest that HCV RNA can attach to the RBC surfaces by immunoadherence and can possibly play an important role in the pathogenesis or transmission of hepatitis C virus.

Introduction

Hepatitis C virus (HCV) is the most common cause of posttransfusion hepatitis [1]. It is well known that hepatocytes are the main source for HCV replication, however, several groups have proved that HCV can also be carried by and replicated in lymphoid cells [2, 3, 4, 5].

It has been documented that whole blood contains more HCV RNA copies than plasma [6], however, it is unclear which compartment of the whole blood is the primary source for HCV [7]. The high risk of transfusion-transmitted HCV infections via fresh packed red blood cells from anti-HCV antibody-negative donors has been frequently reported [8, 9, 10].

Direct cellular localization of HCV RNA is best accomplished by RT *in situ* PCR analyses [11, 12]. Using this method, even the relatively low copy number of the virus

Frontiers in Viral Hepatitis Ed. by RF Schinazi, J-P Sommadossi and CM Rice. 131 — 138

can be detected in a given productive infection [13]. In the present study we prepared erythrocyte smears from chronically infected HCV patients and analysed them for the presence of HCV RNA using reverse transcriptase *in situ* polymerase chain reaction (RT-*in situ* PCR) [14, 15].

Patients and methods

Patients

Blood was taken from 43 patients with known histories of HCV infection. Thirty-five patients had chronic hepatitis with varying histology activity index [16]. Chronic HCV infection was proven six to 12 months before enrollment into the study by (i) consistent detection of anti-HCV antibodies using commercially available, second generation, enzyme-linked immunosorbent assay kits (Ortho Diagnostic System, Raritan, NJ), (ii) elevation of serum alanine transaminase (ALT), (iii) liver needle biopsy, and (iiii) detection of HCV RNA in the serum. Control blood samples were taken from seven patients with liver disease unrelated to HCV infection, and from 10 healthy individuals. The protocol was in accordance with the ethical guidelines of the 1975 Declaration of Helsinki and was approved by the ethical committee of the Semmelweis University, Budapest.

Cell preparation

Four ml of EDTA blood (Vacutainer EDTA (K3), Becton Dickinson Vacutainer Venous Blood Collection System; Franklin Lakes, NJ, USA) was obtained from each HCV-infected patient and from control individuals.

The coded blood samples taken from the HCV-infected patients and controls were analysed for solution phase and RT-*in situ* PCR to detect HCV RNA. Cells ($1x10^7$) from whole blood were fixed at room temperature for 20 minutes in 4% (w/v) paraformaldehyde (pH: 7.4) in a total volume of 1 ml. The fixed cells were washed twice with phosphate-buffered saline (PBS) and their cell number adjusted to $1x10^5$ cells/ml. Then 200 μl of this solution were transfered onto silane-coated sildes and allowed to adhere at room temperature for two hours as described by Wilkinson [17]. Non-adherent cells were washed away with PBS. The slides were then air dried and sequentially treated with 0.1% Triton X-100/PBS (pH:7.4) and 0.2M HCl for 10 minutes each, and then with 3 μg/ml proteinase K (Boehringer Mannheim, Mannheim, Germany) in buffer (10 mM Tris, pH:8, 0, 2 mM CaCl2, 50 mM EDTA) at 37°C for 6 min to permeabilize the cell membranes. This reaction was stopped by rinsing the slides with ice-cold 0.1M glycine/PBS (pH:7.2) for 10 min. DNase treatment was then performed overnight in a humidified chamber at 37°C in a total volume of 10 μl using 10 U DNase (RNase-free; Boehringer Mannheim) in buffer (10^5 mM Sodium Acetate, 5 mM MgSO4). Standard precautions were used to prevent RNase contamination.

RT *in situ* PCR

Amplification of the 5' non-coding region from the HCV genome was chosen in order to detect the positive HCV RNA strand [4, 18, 19, 20] (Table 1). Slides with blood smears were placed on the flat heating block of the thermal cycler (BIOMED Thermocycler 60, Biotrade, Vienna, Austria) and kept for 1 hour at 42°C.

Table 1. Positive strand HCV RNA oligonucleotides used for RT-*in situ* PCR and solution phase RT-PCR

Primer	Nucleotides
HCV 11	5' CCATAGATCACTCCCCTGTG 3'
HCV 8	5' GCACGGTCTACGAGACCT 3'
HCV 3	5' CTGTGAGGAACTACTGTCTTCACGCAG 3'
HCV 4	5' CGGTTCCGCAGACCACTATG 3'

A mixture of 20 µl RT buffer (50 mM TRIS-HCI, 75 mM KCI, 3 mM MgCI2 containing 10 mM dithiothreitol), 200 U cloned Moloney murine leukemia virus reverse transcriptase (RT) (GIBCO), 40 Units RNase inhibitor (Boehringer Mannheim) and 1 mM of each dNTP were added to the blood smears. Primer HCV8 (Genset, Paris, France) (50 pmol/ml) was used for reverse transcription. The RT reaction was stopped by heating the thermal block for five minutes at 94°C.

For amplification the HCV RNA slides were preheated (70°C) using a thermal cycler. The PCR amplification solution, containing primers HCV 11, HCV 3 and HCV 4 (Genset, Paris, France) was kept at 95°C for 15 minutes to eliminate primer oligomerization and to activate the AmpliTaq Gold enzyme (Perkin Elmer, Vienna, Austria). Twenty µl of the PCR amplification solution containing 2.5 µl 10x PCR buffer, 2.25 mM MgCl2, 250 µM dNTP's + 1,0 nm dig-11-UTP + digoxigenin-11 dUTP (Mannheim, Boehringen) + 5U AmpliTaq Gold polymerase and 10 pmol/ml of each primer were laid on top of the smears. After an initial denaturation step at 94°C for three minutes, 20 PCR cycles were performed using the following cycle steps: denaturing (94°C), annealing (55°C), extension (72°C), each for one minute.

Posthybridization treatment and detection

To reduce the nonspecific primer hybridization in the RT-*in situ* PCR reaction, a high stringency wash was included using 1 x SSC, 0.15 mM NaCl, 0.015 mM sodium citrate containing 0.1% BSA (Sigma Cat. No. 4628) at 56°C for 10 minutes. The PCR-amplified HCV cDNA was detected by immunohistochemistry using high affinity anti-digoxigenin (anti-DIG) antibody (1:4 dilution in PBS) conjugated to fluorescein (fluorescein 5 (6)-carboxy-fluorescein-N-hydroxysuccinimide ester, Enzo, Boehringer Mannheim).

To eliminate unspecific background signals, blocking solution (No: 1096176 Boehringer Mannheim) was used as recommended by the manufacturer. Fluorescein-conjugated digoxigenin -11 dUTP signals were detected by fluorescence microscopy (NIKON Alphaphot 2-H microscope; Nikon Corporation, Tokyo, Japan) using triple band filter (DAPI; FITC; TEXAS RED) at 500-fold magnification. Numbers of positive erythrocytes were semiquantitatively evaluated, counting 10 fields on each smear.

Detection of HCV RNA by solution phase RT-PCR

All patients and controls enrolled in this study were also evaluated by solution phase RT-PCR using samples of the same blood drawings as for RT-*in situ* PCR. HCV RNA was detected from the serum using the Roche Diagnostic System (Amplicor^{TM} test for hepatitis C virus detection, Vienna, Austria). After evaluating the results, the samples found positive by RT-*in situ* PCR and negative by solution phase PCR were reprobed by both methods up to three times within one year.

Results

Analyses of erythrocyte smears by fluorescence microscopy

Out of 60 blood smears (43 HCV-infected and 17 controls) analysed by RT-*in situ* PCR, the PCR-amplified viral RNA was clearly localized to the erythrocyte cell membrane in 40 HCV-infected cases (Figure 1A). Samples from three HCV-infected patients gave inconclusive results because of high background, and were finally considered as negative. None of the ten healthy individuals and seven patients with liver disease unrelated to HCV gave positive signals (Fig.1B). Morphologically, the RT-*in situ* PCR-amplified viral RNA detected on the erythrocyte membrane by fluorescence microscopy showed a high signal variety. The fluorescence signals appeared as bright or dim green lines, semicircles or dots localized to the erythrocyte membrane (Figure 1A). Ten to 80 percent of erythrocytes showed positive fluorescence signals in the smears derived from HCV-infected individuals.

Solution phase PCR

Solution phase PCR analyses of the sera taken from HCV-infected patients were carried out parallel with *in situ* RT PCR analyses. In 30 cases a positive signal was obtained with solution phase PCR, whereas in 13 patients we could not detect viral RNA in their sera. In comparison, using RT-*in situ* PCR only three out of 43 patients gave negative results. All the controls were HCV negative when checked by solution phase PCR and by *in situ* PCR.

Subsequently, 12 out of the 13 cases found to be positive by RT-*in situ* PCR and negative by solution phase PCR were repeatedly analysed for up to three times by both methods within one year. One solution phase PCR-negative patient, who was

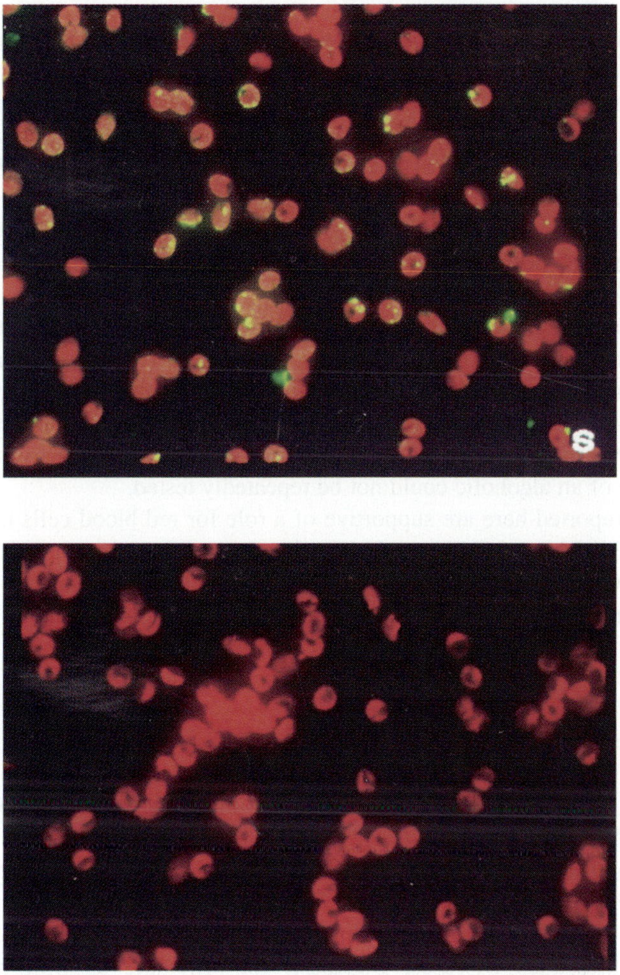

Figure 1. Bright HCV-specific signals attached to the erythrocyte membrane were detected by fluorescence microscopy (A). Negative control (B) (A, B: 400 x).

an alcoholic, could be checked only once. All 12 samples were positive by RT-*in situ* PCR by the repeated testing. Nine samples were repeatedly positive by solution phase PCR, while three samples were repeatedly negative. These three patients found to be negative had undergone a combined interferon plus ribavirin treatment during the testing period.

Discussion

In our study the PCR-amplified HCV RNA signal identified by RT-*in situ* PCR was observed localized on the erythrocyte membrane. Fluorescence microscopy confirmed these data, showing that the signals were localized to the cell membrane and demonstrating that RBCs can carry membrane-bound HCV RNA.

Transmission of HCV likely relates to cell free and cell bound virus in the blood [21]. Cell free mature virion is predominantly associated with circulating immune complexes (IC) [22]. It has been suggested that HCV might also be concentrated on the RBC surfaces by immunoadherence [20]. Adherence of circulating immune complexes to erythrocytes has been studied widely [23, 24]. Complement receptor 1 (CR1, CD35), present at the surface of the erythrocytes, is responsible for immune adherence reactions as described by Nelson [25].

All but three cases with proven HCV infection were positive by RT-*in situ* PCR. Interestingly, 13 out of the 43 cases were negative with solution phase PCR. Nevertheless, nine of these 13 became positive within one year by repeated testing, indicating that they carried HCV. Three out of the four remaining negative cases underwent Interferon + Ribavirin therapy, and remained negative by solution phase PCR. One case of an alcoholic could not be repeatedly tested.

The results reported here are supportive of a role for red blood cells in the transport of HCV. The RBC-bound HCV might be missed if only the sera are analysed for the detection of HCV by PCR. It remains to be proven whether or not the association of RBC to HCV is the result of adherence of HCV RNA-carrying complexes (cryoglobulin complex), or whether it may be attributed to a different mechanism.

Acknowledgements

This work has been supported by grants AKP 98-78 3, 2; OTKA T 023579; T 029266 and FKFP 0305/1999.

We wish to thank Drs. F. Szalay and M. Abonyi from the 1st Dept. of Internal Medicine, as well as Dr. G. Lengyel from the 2nd Dept. of Internal Medicine (Semmelweis University, Budapest), furthermore, Drs. E. Ibranyi and L. Telegdy (Hospital for Infectious Diseases, Budapest) for providing us with blood samples from HCV-infected patients, Dr. R. Zeillinger (University of Vienna) for his helpful advice, and K. Olas (Baxter Hyland Immuno AG, Vienna) for the technical assistance. Dr. S. Simon gratefully acknowledges fruitful discussions with and technical advice given by Dr. G. J. Nuovo (MGN Medical Research Laboratories, New York).

References

1. Seeff LB, Buskell-Bales Z, Right EC, Durako SJ, Alter HJ, Iber FL, Hollinger FB, et al. Long-term mortality after transfusion-associated non-A, non-B hepatitis. *N Engl J Med* 1992; 327:1906-1911.
2. Müller HM, Pfaff E, Goeser T, Kallinowski B, Solbach C, Theilmann L. Peripheral blood leucocytes serve as a possible extrahepatic site for hepatitis C virus replication. *J Gen Virol* 1993; 74:669-676.
3. Chang TT, Young KC, Yang YJ, Lei HY, Wu HL. Hepatitis C virus RNA in peripheral blood mononuclear cells: Comparing acute and chronic hepatitis C virus infection. *Hepatology* 1996; 23:977-981.

4. Muratori L, Gibellini D, Lenzi M, Cataleta M, Muratori P, Morelli MC, Bianchi FB. Quantification of hepatitis C virus-infected peripheral blood mononuclear cells by in situ reverse transcriptase-polymerase chain reaction. *Blood* 1996; 88:2768-2774.
5. Moldvay J, Deny P, Pol S, Brechot C, Lamas E. Detection of hepatitis C virus RNA in peripheral blood mononuclear cells of infected patients by in situ hybridization. *Blood* 1994; 83:269-273.
6. Schmidt WN, WU P, Cederna J, Mitros FA, LaBrecque DR, Stapleton JT. Surreptitious hepatitis C virus (HCV) infection detected in the majority of patients with cryptogenic chronic hepatitis and negative HCV antibody test. *J Infect Dis* 1997; 176:27-33.
7. Schmidt WN, Wu P, Han JQ, Perino MJ, LaBrecque DR, Stapleton JT. Distribution of hepatitis C virus (HCV) RNA in whole blood and blood cell fraction: Plasma HCV RNA analysis underestimate circulating virus load. *J Infect Dis* 1997; 176:20-26.
8. Taliani G, DeBac S, Maioz S, Vania A, Aron MC. HCV transmission by fresh packed red cells from anti-HCV-negative donors. *Lancet* 1991;338:62.
9. Tabor E, Hewlett I, Yu M-Y.W, Farshid M, Epstein JS. Summary of a Food and Drug Administration workshop on nucleic acid testing to screen donations of blood and plasma for the hepatitis C virus. *Transfusion* 1999; 39:912-913.
10. Conry-Cantilena C, VanRades M, Gibble J, Melpolder J, Shakh AO, Viladomiu L, Cheung L, et al. Routes of infection, viremia, and liver disease in blood donors found to have hepatitis C virus infection. *N Engl Med* 1996; 334:1691-1696.
11. Nuovo GJ, Lidonnici K, MacConnell P, Lane B. Intracellular localization of polymerase chain reaction (PCR) - amplified hepatitis C cDNA. *Am J Surg Pathol* 1993; 17:683-690.
12. Nouri Aria KT, Sallie R, Sangar D, Alexander GJM, Smith H, Byrne J, Potmann B, et al. Detection of genomic and intermediate replicative strands of hepatitis C virus in liver tissue by in situ hybridization. *J Clin Invest* 1993, 91:2226-2234.
13. Negro F, Pacchioni D, Shimizu Y, Miller RH, Bussolati G, Purcell RH, Bonino F. Detection of intrahepatic replication of hepatitis C virus RNA by in situ hybridization and comparison with histopathology. *Proc Natl Acad Sci* 1992; 89:2247-2251.
14. Nuovo GJ. PCR in situ hybridization. Protocols and applications. 3th edition, Philadelphia, New York, Lippincott-Raven 1997.
15. Simon S, Reipert B, Eibl MM, Steinkasserer A. Detection of phosphatidylinositol glycan class A gene transcripts by RT in situ PCR hybridization: A comparative study using fluorescein, Texas red, and digoxigenin-11 dUTP for color detection. *J Histochem Cytochem* 1997; 45:1659-1664.
16. Desmet VJ, Gerber M, Hoofnagle JH, Manns M, Scheuer PJ. Classification of chronic hepatitis: diagnosis, grading and staging. *Hepatology* 1994; 19:1513-1520.
17. Wilkinson DG. In situ Hybridization A Practical Approach. IRL Press 1992; pp.86-92.
18. Choo QL, Richman KH, Han JH, Berger K, Lee C, Dong C, Gallegos C, et al. Genetic organization and diversity of the hepatitis C virus. *Proc Natl Acad Sci* 1991; 88:2451-2455.
19. Lanford RL, Sureau C, Jacob JR, White R, Fuerst TR. Demonstration of in vitro infection of chimpanzee hepatocytes with hepatitis C virus using strand-specific RT/PCR. *Virology* 1994; 202:606-614.
20. Garson JA, Tedder RS, Briggs M, Tuke P, Glazebrook JA, Trute A, Parker D, et al. Detection of hepatitis C viral sequences in blood donation by "nested" polymerase chain reaction and prediction of infectivity. *Lancet* 1990; 335:1419-1422.
21. Pivetti S, Novarino A, Calvo L, Massaro AL, Brunetto MR, Caligaris CF, Bonino F. Hepatitis C virus infection in patients with haematological diseases: evidence for the association with erythrocytes transfusion and liver disease. *Int Hepatol Commun* 1995; 4:9-15

22. Rocatello D, Morsica G, Picciotto G, Cesano G, Ropolo R, Bernardi MT, Cacace G, et al. Impaired hepatosplenic elimination of circulating cryoglobulins in patients with essential mixed cryoglobulinaemia and hepatitis C virus (HCV) infection. *Clin Exp Immunol* 1997; 110:9-14.
23. Pascual M, Schifferli JA. Another function of Erythrocytes: Transport of circulating immune complexes. *Infusionstherapie* 1995, 22:310-315.
24. Madi N, Paccaud JP, Steiger G, Schifferli JA. Immune complex binding efficiency of erythrocyte complement receptor 1 (CR1). *Clin Exp Immunol* 1991; 84:9 -14.
25. Nelson RA. The immune adherence phenomenon: an immunologically specific reaction between micro-organisms and erythrocytes leading to enhanced phagocytosis. *Science* 1953;118:733

Nucleic acid-based antiviral approaches to HBV

H.C. SPANGENBERG and J.R. WANDS

Liver Research Center, Rhode Island Hospital and Brown University School of Medicine, 55 Claverick Street, 4th floor, Providence, RI 02903

Introduction

The hepatitis B virus (HBV), discovered in 1966, belongs to a family of closely related, small enveloped DNA viruses [1]. This family, called hepadnaviruses, includes the woodchuck (WHBV), ground squirrel (GSHV), duck (DHBV) and heron (HHV) hepatitis B viruses. Such infectious agents are characterized by hepatotropism and cause acute and chronic hepatitis. Despite the availability of a vaccine and passive immunization against HBV, more than 350 million people worldwide are chronically infected [2]. Furthermore, approximately one million deaths occur annually due to HBV-induced liver disease, which ranges from acute to chronic infection and from cirrhosis to hepatocellular carcinoma [3, 4]. Vaccination is the only effective approach to prevent chronic infection. Once individuals are chronically infected with the virus, only a few therapeutic options are available. Treatment possibilities involve the administration of interferon-α as well as the use of viral polymerase inhibitors such as nucleoside analogues either alone or in combination. Thus far, clinical success with these drugs is unsatisfactory, due to transient effects on HBV replication and emergence of drug-resistant strains [5]. The need for alternative therapeutic approaches has provided the impetus to develop novel reagents.

Extensive developments in molecular biology and recombinant DNA technology have led to more accurate diagnosis, therapy and prevention of human diseases. Molecular methods have facilitated the detection of the hepatitis B viral genome and have provided detailed information on the viral life cycle. Attachment of the virus to the cell membrane, internalization, uncoating, viral replication, gene expression, virus assembly and virion export offer possible targets for antiviral therapy (Figure 1). To influence gene expression, Paterson et al. demonstrated that single-stranded DNA was able to inhibit translation of a complementary HBV-specific RNA [6]. Thus, various different nucleic acid-based approaches including ribozymes, antisense oligodeoxynucleotides and RNA, dominant negative mutants, intracellular antibodies, and DNA-based immunization have been developed to potentially complement existing antiviral therapies [7-9]. To take advantage of these strategies against HBV, it is important to note that there is only modest nucleic acid sequence heterogeneity among HBV DNA strains compared to other viral agents, such as hepatitis C virus (HCV) and human immunodeficiency virus (HIV). Thus, HBV may be a good candidate for nucleic

Frontiers in Viral Hepatitis Ed. by RF Schinazi, J-P Sommadossi and CM Rice. 139 — 156

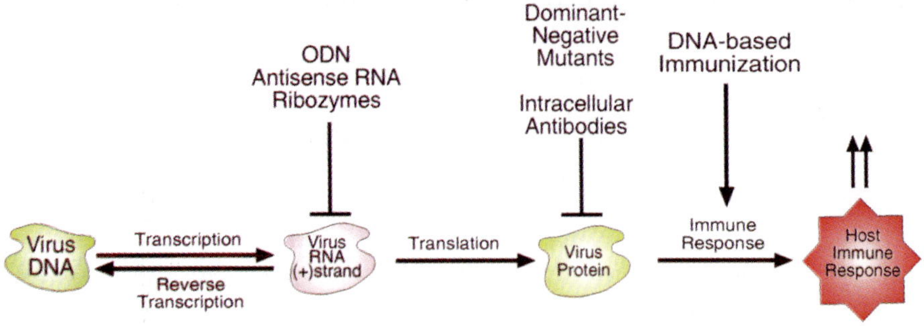

Figure 1. Steps in the viral life cycle of HBV and potential targets of nucleic acid-based approaches to HBV. HBV viral DNA is transcribed in several viral RNAs, and serves as the template for translation into viral proteins. HBV pregenomic RNA is reverse transcribed into viral DNA. Ribozymes, ODN and antisense RNA may bind to and interfere with viral RNA. Dominant negative mutants and intracellular antibodies may interfere with viral proteins. The host immune response against viral proteins may be augmented by DNA-based immunization.

acid-based antiviral approaches; however, efficient gene delivery and transfer systems to all HBV-infected cells will need to be developed. Before general application to HBV prevention and therapy, additional considerations for successful use of these agents must include assessments of the stability of the nucleic-acid based construct of interest to allow interaction with the viral target, as well as toxicity/safety issues [10].

We review, herein, the current molecular strategies designed for HBV infection, with emphasis on ribozymes, antisense molecules, dominant negative mutants of viral proteins, intracellular antibodies and DNA-based immunization, and examine their potential as antiviral agents for acute and chronic hepatitis B.

Ribozymes

Ribozymes are catalytic, active RNA whose structures are based on naturally occurring site-specific, self-cleaving RNA molecules [12-14]. Such molecules are potentially very efficient, because one ribozyme is able to cleave many target mRNAs. Four major classes of naturally occurring ribozymes have been discovered, and they serve as the basis for many artificially engineered ribozymes. Hammerhead and haipirin ribozymes (Figure 2A) have been extensively studied as experimental tools for suppression of gene expression and have possible therapeutic applications [14, 15]. The catalytic moiety of ribozymes recognize the specific nucleotide sequences GUX, or, for the hammerhead ribozymes, NUX (X = C, U or A: N = any nucleotide) [16, 17]. Because this nucleic acid sequence occurs frequently in RNA, the sequence complementary to the RNA target and flanking the catalytic sequence mediates the specific cleavage of the substrate [18]. *In vitro* experiments have shown cleavage of viral mRNA derived from HIV, arenavirus or lymphocytic choriomeningitis virus (LCMV) by engineered ribozymes [19-21]. Possible *in vivo* applications have been tested in Drosophila and murine models [22, 23]. Recently, the *in vivo* application of an allosterically controllable ribozyme that cleaves Bcr-Abl mRNA in chronic myelogenous leukemia cells was tested and revealed oncogene inactivation and enhanced survival of mice [24].

With respect to HBV, several studies using hammerhead or haipirin ribozymes have shown specific cleavage of HBV RNA. These investigations demonstrated that hammerhead ribozymes cleave HBV RNA in a cell free system [25] and in cell extracts [26], whereas no activity was apparent *in vivo*. Lack of an *in vivo* effect may be due, in part, to intracellular protein-RNA interactions as well as to low Mg2+ concentration. More recent experiments have shown activity of hammerhead ribozymes on other regions of HBV RNA. In these studies, the ribozyme attack was targeted to the hepatitis Bx-RNA sequence [26-29]. Regarding haipirin ribozymes, two studies have shown inhibitory effects on the HBV life cycle. One investigation demonstrated a decrease in virus particle production of 83%, as measured by an endogenous polymerase assay following the introduction of ribozymes into hepatoma cell lines by retroviral vectors [30]. Another study used a combinatorial screening method to select haipirin ribozymes that were subsequently shown to cleave HBV RNA. These ribozymes were cloned into eukaryotic expression vectors and then cotransfected with a replication-competent HBV genome. Under these experimental conditions, HBV replication was inhibited up to 80% and HBsAg secretion was decreased by 50% [31]. Thus, there is ample evidence that ribozymes have antiviral activity against HBV *in vitro*.

Antisense Strategies

Antisense approaches rely on the formation of reverse complementary Watson-Crick base pairs, which impair the utilization of messenger RNA (mRNA) and thereby inhibit translation (Figure 2B/C). The reverse nucleic acid complement may be DNA or RNA. For antisense oligodeoxynucleotides (ODN), short synthetic (15-40 nucleotide (nt)) sequences are designed. Modifications of the chemical backbone by phosphorothioates (PS), which prevent ODN-carrying phosphodiester bonds from degradation by nucleases, have improved the stability of ODNs both *in vitro* and *in vivo*. However, toxic side effects dependent on the route of administration and dosage schedule have been observed *in vivo*.

It is also possible to promote antisense regulation of gene expression [32] or splicing [33] by complementary RNAs. In this context, artificially designed antisense RNAs are usually longer than 50 nucleotides. The major advantage of using antisense RNAs compared to ODNs is delivery to the cell, since antisense RNA may be engineered as antisense genes and subsequently expressed in target cells using nonviral or viral vectors such as retroviruses [34] or adenoviruses [35]. If hybridization between the exogenous nucleotide sequence and the viral or cellular mRNA occurs, then RNA replication, reverse transcription or mRNA translation may be terminated. RNA-RNA and RNA-DNA duplexes can be unwound by a variety of repair/editing enzymes [36], which would abolish antisense activity in the cell. However, RNases such as

RNase H are ubiquitous nuclear enzymes that bind to the RNA-DNA duplexes and specifically cleave the RNA due to endonuclease activity [37] and, thus, produce the observed antisense effects.

The DNA ODN may be designed to be as short as 10 nucleotides [38] and is unaffected by RNase H activity. This small molecule may also hybridize with many other target mRNAs with the appropriate complementary sequence. In addition, such a short ODN sequence may initiate undesirable cellular damage by interfering with other cellular RNAs due to cross hybridization [39]. ODNs bearing a centrally located CpG motif have been shown to exhibit antiviral effects by inducing murine B-lymphocyte proliferation and immunoglobulin secretion *in vitro* and *in vivo* [40, 41]. For RNA-RNA duplexes, double-stranded (ds) RNA serves as a substrate for editing enzymes such as double-stranded adenosine deaminase [42, 43]. Deamination of adenosine leads to ionosine, which may target the mRNA for destruction. Furthermore, dsRNA is a potent substrate for rapid degradation by double-strand-specific RNases. It is also an activator of the interferon pathway [44], resulting in the activation of protein kinase PKR [45] and 2′5′ oligoadenylate synthetase [46], whose product in turn can activate a latent endonuclease (RNase L). Thus, unexpected cellular effects mediated by antisense molecules may or may not be beneficial with respect to antiviral activity and need to be carefully monitored.

Antisense ODN research has progressed rapidly and is being transferred to clinical trials involving treatment of malignant diseases, tissue inflammation and viral infections. Cellular targets of antisense molecules include protein kinase C isotype alpha [47-49], c-raf (a serine-threonine-specific protein kinase) [50, 51], BCR/ABL [52, 53] and Bcl2 [54] which are overexpressed in several tumors, as well as c-myc [55, 56], an immediate early growth response gene. Infectious disease targets have been identified as well and include HIV, human papilloma virus (HPV), cytomegalovirus (CMV), HCV and tuberculosis. Indeed, Vitravene, an ODN directed against CMV [57], is now approved for local treatment of retinitis and represents the first class of novel therapeutic agents based on antisense strategy that has been approved by the Federal Drug Administration in the United States. With respect to HBV, antisense ODNs have been successfully used *in vitro* and *in vivo* and promote antiviral effects. Antiviral activities were exhibited following cotransfection of antisense ODNs with a replication-competent HBV clone into hepatoma cells. The ODNs were directed against different viral target nucleotide sequences located in the viral polymerase, encapsidation signal, polyadenylation site and preS/S region [58-60]. Inhibitory effects of the ODN on viral replication/viral protein synthesis were apparent. For example, a 40-mer antisense ODN derived from the HBV polymerase gene was found to inhibit viral replication compared to a sense control ODN [61]. The first *in vivo* application of antisense ODNs was performed in Pekin ducks, where inhibition of DHBV replication was observed following infusion of a PS-modified antisense ODN directed against the 5′ region of the preS gene [62]. Additional *in vivo* studies in ducks, woodchucks and nude mice demonstrated antiviral effects by ODNs against other HBV RNA target sequences [63-65].

In addition, antisense RNA constructs prepared against HBV target nucleic acid sequences exhibited significant inhibition of HBV replication under different experimental conditions. For example, antisense RNA directed against the surface and core antigen encoding regions and delivered by retroviral vectors to HCC cells that constitutively produce HBV, effectively decreased HBsAg production and secretion of HBV DNA into the culture medium [66]. In another study, several regions of the HBV genome were examined for susceptibility to antisense RNA effects. Two constructs, when cotransfected into hepatoma cells with a replication-competent HBV genome, were found to inhibit viral replication by 75%. This study illustrates that antisense RNA may specifically target HBV sequences in the cell before the encapsidation of pregenomic (pg) RNA into the core particle [67]. It will be interesting to determine if these antisense molecules demonstrate antiviral effects *in vivo* using relevant animal model systems.

Dominant negative mutants and intracellular antibodies

Dominant negative (DN) molecules are generally mutated proteins that suppress the activity of their native counterparts. This approach, when used as an antiviral strategy, has been successful and found to inhibit virus replication of herpes simplex, HIV and hepadnaviruses [7, 68, 69]. A perfect HBV target for this strategy is to disrupt virus assembly (Figure 2D), in which HBV pgRNA and viral polymerase are packaged into an icosahedral nucleocapsid structure. This shell is self-assembled within the cell following dimerization of viral core proteins [70]. The core protein consists of 183 amino acids; the amino-terminal region is essential for virus assembly [71], whereas the carboxy-terminal domain contributes to the pgRNA packaging and DNA maturation [72-74]. Therefore, the introduction of mutated core proteins that retain the ability to assemble with their natural counterparts may disrupt viral replication through one or more blocking effects at this critical step of the life cycle (Figure 2E).

For avian and mammalian hepadnaviruses, various constructs including N-terminal extended, C-terminal truncated and polypeptides fused to the C-terminal part of the viral nucleocapsid protein were investigated. The DN mutants were cotransfected with replication-competent wild type virus or delivered by recombinant retroviral or adenoviral vectors. The results demonstrated that DN mutants disrupt nucleocapsid core protein assembly and specifically inhibit viral replication by up to 95%. These antiviral effects may be due, in part, to the disintegration of the viral nucleocapsids, which promotes loss of pgRNA packaging capability and/or defects in DNA maturation [75-81]. Interestingly, the overexpression of native precore protein has been shown to also exert a dominant negative effect both *in vitro* and *in vivo* [82, 83], as measured by inhibition of viral replication.

Another protein-based antiviral approach is the use of intracellular antibodies [84]. These antibodies are generally produced from cDNAs derived from monoclonal antibody variable regions that are directed against viral proteins. These cDNAs are isolated by PCR-based cloning techniques and subsequently used to generate expression constructs. Constructs encoding for Fab or single-chain antibody fragments (scFv) are capable of assuming a functional intracellular molecule under certain experimental conditions and may bind with high affinity to their viral targets (Figure 2F). Antibody modifications leading to or contributing to increased stability and steric inhibitory

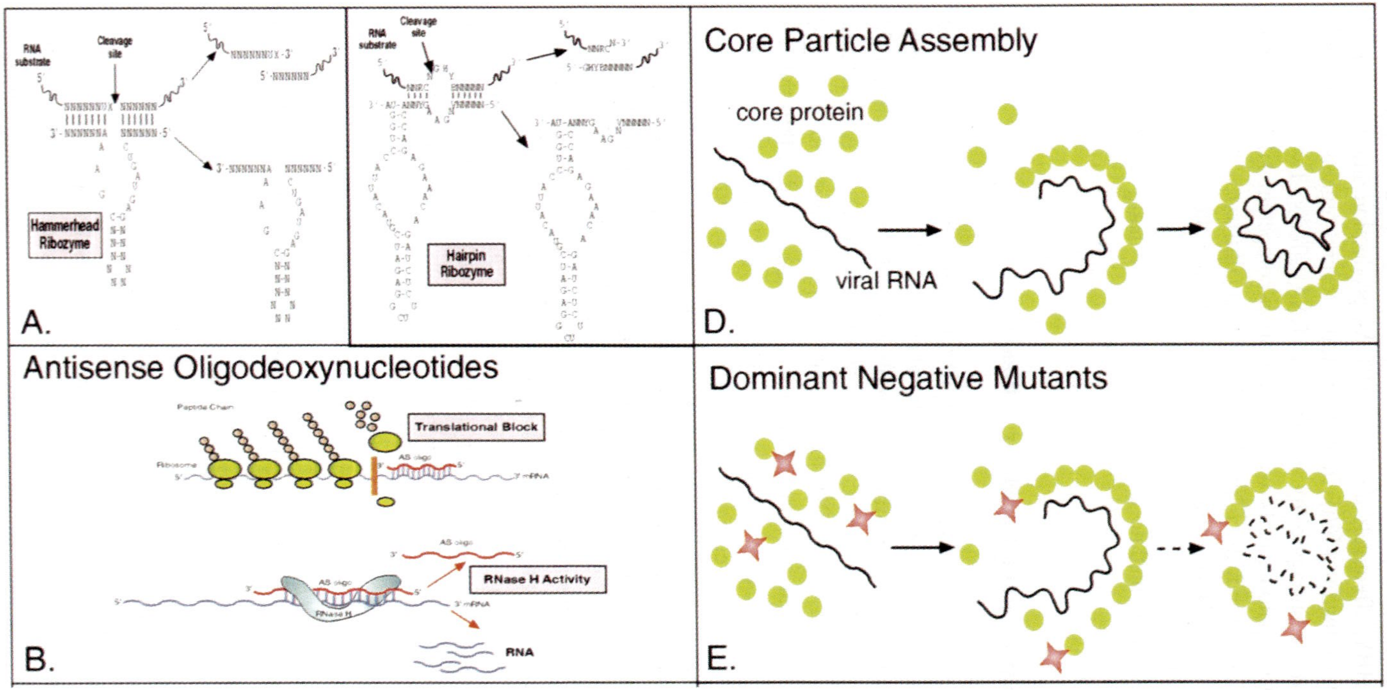

Figure 2. Cellular mechanisms of antiviral activity exhibited by nucleic acid-based approaches. **A.** Ribozymes: Illustration of the hammerhead and haipirin ribozymes. The hammerhead ribozyme cleaves its RNA substrate 3′ to nucleotide triplet NUX (N = any nucleotide; X = any base except G); the haipirin ribozyme cleaves its substrate RNA 5′ to a G in the sequence RCN/GHYB (R = G; N = any base; H = A, C or U; B = C, G or U;V = A, C or G) **B.** Antisense oligodeoxynucleotides: sequence - specific hybridization of antisense ODN to viral target RNA leads to block of translation and premature termination of peptide chain synthesis. DNA-RNA duplexes are recognized and degraded by endogenous RNases H. **C.** Antisense RNA: Sequence-specific hybridization of antisense RNA to viral target RNA generates an RNA-RNA duplex, which may be recognized and degraded by double-strand-specific RNase. RNA duplexes also serve as substrate for a deaminase and can activate components of the interferon pathway. **D.** Illustration of viral capsid assembly. Multiple subunits of the viral core protein form the viral capsid. **E.** Incorporation of dominant negative mutants of the core protein block the assembly process.

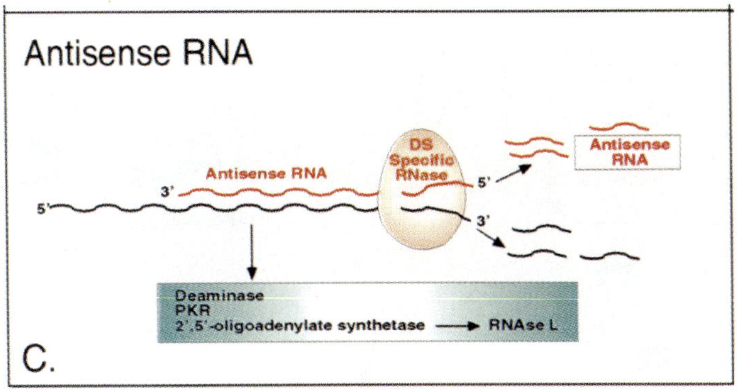

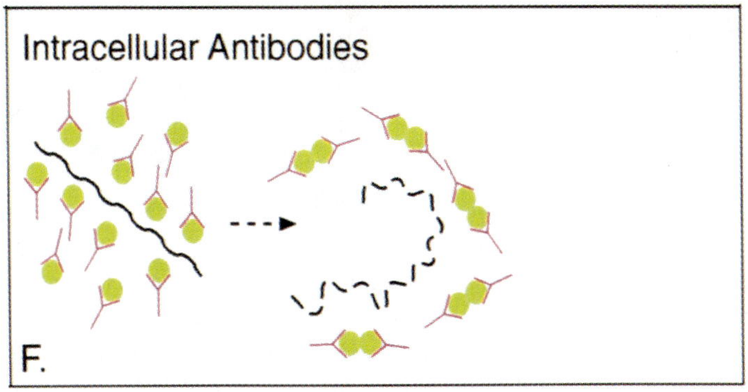

Figure 2. (Continued) **F.** Intracellular antibodies bind tightly to nucleocapsid or other viral proteins and interfere with nucleocapsid assembly.

activity have been observed when polypeptide sequences were added to the C-terminal region of these molecules. *In vitro* and *in vivo* studies have demonstrated the effectiveness of intracellular antibodies or "intrabodies", as illustrated by inhibition of HIV replication and altering the growth of tumors [85-87]. Intracellular single-chain antibody fragments directed against various antigens of HBV have now been generated [88-90]. For example, scFV expressing cDNAs and directed against the nucleocapsid protein have been stably cotransfected into an HBV-producing hepatoblastoma cell line. There was downregulation of HBV replication due to inhibition of reverse transcription from pgRNA to single-stranded DNA [91]. It is of interest that substantially reduced HBsAg secretion has been observed in a cell line transfected with a monoclonal antibody derived from a cDNA construct expressing a scFv fragment directed against HBsAg [92]. In conclusion, this new approach has potential as an antiviral strategy, but efficacy has yet to be demonstrated *in vivo*.

DNA-based immunization

The DNA-based immunization approach [93, 94] (also called genetic vaccination) shows

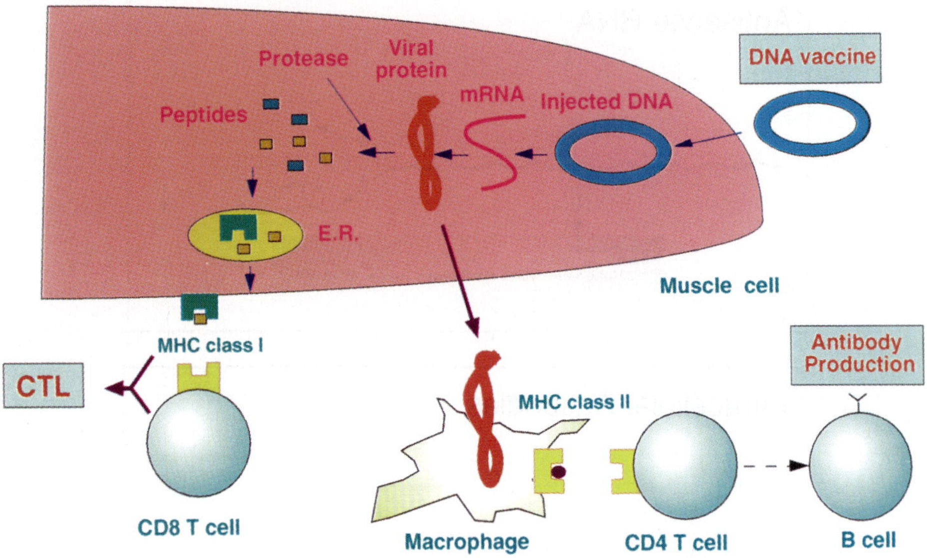

Figure 3. Illustration of the DNA-based immunization approach. A plasmid vector expressing the protein of interest under the control of an appropriate promoter is injected into the skin or muscle of the host. After uptake of the plasmid, the protein is produced endogenously and intracellularly processed into small peptides by proteases. These peptides are presented on the cell surface by MHC class I and, subsequently, CD8+ cytotoxic T cells are stimulated and evoke cell-mediated immunity. The foreign protein can also be presented by the MHC class II pathway by professional APCs, which may elicit CD4+ T cell responses. Humoral immune responses are also augmented by this technique.

great promise for potential therapy of chronic viral infections as well as human tumors. Naked plasmid DNA may be injected via several routes (intradermal, intravenous or intramuscular) [95]. The plasmid vector expressing the gene of interest under an appropriate promoter is taken up by muscle and antigen presenting cells and the gene product is endogenously produced and subsequently degraded by proteasomes into short peptides (Figure 3). These peptides (about 8-10 amino acids) enter the endoplasmatic reticulum through membrane-associated transporter, become bound to MHC class I and are eventually exported from the ER. The MHC-peptide complex is presented on the cell surface where circulating CD8+ T cells (CTLs) are stimulated and evoke cell-mediated immune responses. Such CTLs recognize virus infected cells and mediate virus clearance through cytolytic and non-cytolytic pathways that involve cytokines such as interferon γ (IFN-γ) and tumor necrosis factor-α (TNF-α).

Humoral immune responses may also be augmented by DNA-based immunization. This process is initiated following endocytosis of antigens by professional antigen-presenting cells (APC), subsequent degradation, and peptide loading onto MHC class II molecules and presenting on the cell surface to activate helper T (CD4+) cells. Depending on the subtype response of CD4+ cells, B cells are then stimulated to proliferate and produce antibodies of predefined specificity [96, 97].

Several advantages of this method, as compared to other nucleic acid-based approaches, or to other vaccine strategies, are notable. Plasmid vectors with the desired gene coding sequence can easily be manipulated [98, 99] and produced in cost-effective large amounts. In addition, several plasmids encoding for proteins with different biologic properties may be administered in combination [100-104]. Finally, the thermal stability of plasmid DNA offers an additional advantage where the need for uninterrupted refrigeration during storage has precluded the use of conventional protein- or peptide-derived vaccines in underdeveloped regions of the world.

Cellular and humoral immune responses against HBV antigens are believed to play a major role in elimination of the virus from the host. While cellular immune responses in acutely infected patients are strong, multispecific and polyclonal, chronically infected individuals have only weak or barely detectable and narrowly focused immune responses [105]. Following acute HBV infection, cytokines such as IFN-γ are released and subsequently down-regulate viral replication. Such cytokines, including TNF-α participate in viral clearance without causing hepatic injury and are active prior to the generation of cellular immune responses in the liver [106]. The immunological basis for viral persistence after infection is not well characterized. Possible explanations are T cell exhaustion, early localization of virus to immune privileged sites and the development of viral mutations which evade the immune response [107, 108]. However, chronically infected individuals may spontaneously clear the virus from the blood and liver. This phenomenon is usually accompanied by an increased proliferative CD4+ T cell activity to viral peptides and a transient increase of hepatic alanine aminotransferase levels, presumably reflecting liver injury due to elimination of viral infected cells.

Strategies to alter or to enhance the immune responses to HBV may influence clearance of the virus from the liver in chronically infected persons. Extensive studies using DNA-based immunization techniques against HBV viral structural proteins have been performed in animal models [96, 98, 104-110]. The immunogenicity of the nucleocapsid protein and the envelope proteins (middle and large) has been analyzed after genetic vaccination in mice [102, 112, 114-117]. Immunized animals developed high-titer antibodies against such proteins within seven to 10 days after intramuscular immunization [109]. Furthermore, generation of a strong antigen-specific, MHC class II-restricted CD4+ T lymphocyte response against HBV envelope and nucleocapsid proteins occurred.

Characterization of T-cell activation responses revealed a predominant release of TH-1-type cytokines, as determined by high levels of interleukin-2 (IL-2) and IFN-γ, but low levels of interleukin-4 (IL-4). In response to DNA immunization, it is remarkable that all HBV structural proteins induced strong MHC class I-restricted CD8+ CTL responses. For HBcAg, CTLs were evident as early as 16-21 days after immunization [114, 117-119] and maintained their activity for several months. Enhanced immunological effects have been observed by co-administration of cytokine-expressing plasmids, which enhances antigen presentation to APCs at the site of immunization. Additional potentially beneficial immunomodulatory effects of constructs containing CpG motifs (naturally occurring bacterial sequences with immunostimulatory properties) have been described [121-123].

The therapeutic potential of DNA-based immunization is illustrated by studies performed with transgenic animals. Transgenic mice expressing HBV envelope proteins have been immunized with a single administration of a plasmid encoding the MHBs (preS2 and S containing middle envelope protein) and HBsAg (small or S envelope protein) [124]. This approach induced anti-HBsAg antibodies in tolerant HBsA-expressing transgenic mice and led to clearance of HBsAg from the blood, and thus broke immunologic tolerance in these animals. The disappearance of HBsAg lasted for 20 weeks, which was principally due to the induction of specific anti-HBs antibodies. More importantly, HBV mRNA within the liver became undetectable without any signs of hepatic injury. It was postulated that DNA-based immunization led to downregulation of the transgene, due to the generation of HBsAg-specific T-cells and subsequent release of cytokines. Another study observed only humoral responses in two of five different HBV transgenic mice lineages [125]. These findings were partially confirmed by another recent report [126] where no humoral and cellular immune responses were generated after DNA-based immunization in transgenic mice expressing HBsAg. Therefore, the ability of DNA vaccination to break immunologic tolerance under these experiments remains controversial.

There are other experimental models that support the concept that generation of humoral and cellular immune responses to HBV enhances viral clearance from the liver, during persistent infection. Adoptive transfer of HBsAg immune spleen cells has been found to suppress HBsAg antigenemia in congenic transgenic mice, suggesting the presence of HBsAg-specific antibodies [126]. In this study, donor CD4+ T cells were required to support a long-lasting anti-HBsAg antibody response. In contrast to experiments described above, downregulation of the HBV mRNA derived from the transgene was not observed and hepatic injury did not occur. Adoptive transferred CTLs rapidly disappeared in their recipients, whereas CD4+ T cells were engrafted and were detectable for months. Generation of similar immune responses by DNA vaccines may also have therapeutic potential. For example, DNA-based immunization using the genes encoding for the envelope proteins protected ducks and woodchucks from natural infection following inoculation with wild type DHBV and WHV, respectively [127-129]. Indeed, DNA-based immunization of chronically infected ducks resulted in a significant decrease in viremia, and this effect was sustained for 42 weeks [128]. Immunization with a DHBV large envelope protein (preS and S containing protein) expression plasmid in breeding ducks led to maternal transmission of antibodies to the ducklings; such antibodies were protective to wild type virus challenge [130, 131]. Despite the controversial findings under different experimental settings, DNA vaccination shows promise as an antiviral approach not only in terms of preventing HBV infection, but also with respect to possible therapy for chronic viral carriers. The results of ongoing human clinical trials are eagerly awaited.

Current issues and future perspectives

Nucleic acid-based approaches are actively being pursued as antiviral therapy for chronic HBV infection. The therapeutic potential of ribozymes, antisense molecules, dominant negative mutant proteins, intracellular antibodies and DNA-based vaccination, has been clearly demonstrated in experimental systems both *in vitro* and *in vivo*. Future studies will need to evaluate these antiviral strategies in established or new animal systems involving ducks, woodchucks, and nude or transgenic mice. More effective methods of targeted gene delivery systems to all infected hepatocytes will have to be developed. It may also be necessary to pursue regulated gene expression systems for optimal therapeutic results. Due to genetic mutations, escape of HBV from nucleic acid-based strategies is anticipated and viral resistance may occur. Preclinical trials of pharmacokinetic, pharmacodynamic and toxic profiles of these new molecular agents will be required to ensure a safe translation to human subjects. Under these conditions, nucleic acid-based antiviral strategies may eventually contribute to existing therapies and augment the treatment and prevention of chronic HBV infection.

Acknowledgements

This work was supported by Grants CA-35711, AA-02666 and AA-08169 from the National Institutes of Health. H.C. Spangenberg is recipient of a grant by the Ernst Jung Stiftung fuer Wissenschaft und Forschung, Hamburg, Germany.

References

1. Purcell RH. The discovery of the hepatitis viruses. *Gastroenterology* 1993; 104:955-963.
2. Lee WM. Hepatitis B virus infection. *New Engl J Med* 1997; 337:1733-1745.
3. Lau JYN, Wright TL. Molecular Virology and pathogenesis of hepatitis B. *Lancet* 1993; 343:1335-1344.
4. Wands JR, Blum HE. Primary hepatocellular carcinoma. *New Engl J Med* 1991; 325:729-731.
5. Hoofnagle JH, Di Bisceglie AM. The treatment of chronic viral hepatitis. *New Engl J Med* 1997; 336:347-56.
6. Paterson BM, Roberts BE, Kuff EL. Structural gene identification and mapping by DNA-mRNA hybrid-arrested cell-free translation. *Proc Natl Acad Sci USA* 1977; 74:4370-4374.
7. Wands JR, Geissler M, zu Putlitz J, Blum HE, von Weizsaecker F, Mohr L, Yoon SK, Melegari M, Scaglioni PP. Nucleic acid-based antiviral and gene therapy of chronic hepatitis B infection. *J Gastroenterol Hepatol* 1997; 12:S354-369.
8. von Weizsaecker F, Wieland S, Koeck J, Offensperger WB, Offensperger S, Moradpour D, Blum HE. Gene therapy for chronic viral hepatitis: ribozymes, antisense oligonucleotides, and dominant-negative mutants. *Hepatology* 1997; 26;251-255.
9. Offensperger WB, Blum HE, Gerok W. Molecular therapeutic strategies in hepatitis B virus infection. *Clin Investig* 1994; 72: 737-741.
10. Verma IM, Somia N. Gene therapy - promises, problems and prospects. *Nature* 1997; 389:239-242.
11. Cech TR. The efficiency and versatility of catalytic RNA: implications of an RNA world. *Gene* 1993; 135:33-36.
12. Cech TR. Catalytic RNA: structure and mechanism. *Biochem Soc Trans* 1993; 21:221-22.7
13. Pyle AM. Ribozymes: a distinct class of metalloenzymes. *Science* 1993; 261:709-714.
14. Bartolome J, Madejon A, Carreno V. Ribozymes: structure, characteristics and use as potential antiviral agents. *J Hepatol* 1995; 22:57-64.

15. Fedor MJ. Structure and function of the haipirin ribozyme. *J Mol Biol* 2000; 297:269-291
16. Ruffner D, Dahm S, Uhlenbeck OC. Studies on the hammerhead RNA self-cleaving domain. *Gene* 1989; 82:31-41.
17. Symmons RH. Small catalytic RNAs. *Annu Rev Biochem* 1992; 61:641-671.
18. Haseloff J, Gerlach WL. Simple RNA enzymes with new and highly specific endoribonuclease activities. *Nature* 1988; 334:585-591.
19. Sarver N, Cantin EM, Chang PS, Zaia JA, Ladne PA, Stephens DA, Rossi JJ. Ribozymes as potential anti-HIV-1 therapeutic agents. *Science* 1990; 247:1222-1225.
20. Xing Z, Whitton JL. An anti-lymphocytic choriomeningitis virus ribozyme expressed in tissue culture cells diminishes viral RNA levels and leads to a reduction in infectious virus yield. *J Virol* 1993; 67:1840-1847.
21. Xing Z, Whitton JL. Ribozymes which cleave arenavirus RNAs: identification of susceptible target sites and inhibition by target site secondary structure. *J Virol* 1992; 66:1361-1369.
22. Zao JJ, Pick L. Generating loss-of-function phenotypes of the fushi tarazugene with a targeted ribozyme in drosophila. *Nature* 1993; 365:448-451.
23. Larsson S, Hotchkiss G, Andang M, Nyholm T, Inzuna J, Jansson I, Ahrlund-Richter L. Reduced beta–microglobulin mRNA levels in transgenic mice expressing a designed hammerhead ribozyme. *Nucleic Acids Res* 1994; 22:2242-2248.
24. Tanabe T, Kuwabara T, Warashina M, Tani K, Taira K, Asanao S. Oncogene inactivation in a mouse model. *Nature* 2000; 406:473-474.
25. von Weizsaecker F, Blum HE, Wands JR. Cleavage of hepatitis B virus RNA by three ribozymes transcribed from a single DNA template. *Biochem Biophys Res Commun* 1992; 189:743-748.
26. Beck J, Nassal M. Efficient hammerhead ribozyme-mediated cleavage of the structured hepatitis B virus encapsidation signal *in vitro* and in cell extracts, but not in intact cells. *Nucleic Acid Res* 1995; 23:4954-4962.
27. Kim YK, Junn E, Park I, Lee Y, Kang C, Ahn JK. Repression of hepatitis B virus X gene expression by hammerhead ribozymes. *Biochem Biophys Res Commun* 1999; 257:759-765.
28. Passmann M, Weinberg M, Kew M, Arbuthnot P. In situ demonstration of hammerhead ribozymes that are targeted to the hepatitis Bx sequence in cultured cells. *Biochem Biophys Res Commun* 2000; 268:728-733.
29. Weinberg M, Passmann M, Kew M, Arbuthnot P. Hammerhead ribozyme-mediated inhibition of hepatitis B virus X gene expression in cultured cells. *J Hepatol* 2000; 33:142-151.
30. Welch PJ, Tritz R, Yei S, Barber J, Yu M. Intracellular application of haipirin ribozyme genes against hepatitis B virus. *Gene Ther* 1997;4:736-743.
31. zu Putlitz J, Yu Q, Burke JM, Wands JR. Combinatorial screening and intracellular antiviral activity of haipirin ribozymes directed against hepatitis B virus. *J Virol* 1999; 73:5381-5387.
32. Eguchi Y, Itoh T, Tomizawa J. Antisense RNA. *Annu Rev Biochem* 1991; 60:631-652.
33. Madhani HD, Guthrie C. Dynamic RNA-RNA interactions in the spliceosome. *Annu Rev Genet* 1994; 28:1-26.
34. Arteaga CL, Holt JT. Tissue-targeted antisense c-fos retroviral vector inhibits established breast cancer xenografts in nude mice. *Cancer Res* 1996; 56:1098-1103
35. Fox JC, Shanley JR. Antisense inhibition of basic fibroblasts growth factor induces apoptosis in vascular smooth muscle cells. *J Biol Chem* 1996; 271:12578-12584.
36. Nellen W, Lichtenstein C. What makes an mRNA anti-sense-itive? *Trends Biochem Sci* 1993; 18:419-429.
37. Hogrefe HH, Hogrefe RI, Walder RY, Walder JA. Kinetic analysis of Escherichia coli Rnase H using

DNA-RNA-DNA/DNA substrates. *J Biol Chem* 1990; 265:5561-5566.

38. Woolf TM, Melton DA, Jennings CG. Specificity of antisense oligonucleotides *in vivo*. *Proc Natl Acad Sci USA* 1992; 89:7305-7309.
39. Branch AD. A hitchhiker's guide to antisense and nonantisense biochemical pathways. *Hepatology* 1996; 24:1517-1529.
40. Krieg AM, Yi AK, Matson S, Waldschmidt TJ, Bishop GA, Taesdale R, Karetzky GA, Klinman DM. CpG motifs in bacterial DNA trigger direct B-cell activation. *Nature* 1995; 374:546-549.
41. Monteith DK, Henry SP, Howard RB, Flournoy S, Levin AA, Bennett CF, Crooke ST. Immune stimulation – a class of effect of phosphorothioate oligodeoxy-nucleotides in rodents. *Anticancer Drug Des* 1997; 12:421-432.
42. Kim U, Nishikura K. Double-stranded RNA adenosine deaminase as a potential mammalian RNA editing factor. *Sem Cell Biol* 1993; 4:285-293.
43. Kim U, Wang Y, Sanford T, Zeng Y, Nishikura K. Molecular cloning of cDNA for double-stranded RNA adenosine deaminase, a candidate enzyme for nuclear RNA editing. *Proc Natl Acad Sci USA* 1994; 91:11457-11461.
44. Baglioni C, Nilsen TW. The activation of interferon at the molecular level. *Am Sci* 1981; 69:392-399.
45. Proud CG. PKR: a new name and new roles. *Trends Biochem Sci 1995*; 20:241-246.
46. Desai SY, Patel RC, Sen GC, Malhorta P, Ghadge GD, Thimmapaya B. Activation of interferon-inducible 2'-5' oligoadenylate synthetase by adenoviral VAI RNA. *J Biol Chem* 1995; 270:3454-3461.
47. Dean N, MacKay R, Miraglia L, Howard R, Cooper S, Giddings J, Nicklin P, Meister L, Ziel R, Geiger T, Muller M, Fabbro D. inhibition of growth of human tumor cell lines in nude mice by an antisense oligonucleotide inhibitor of protein kinase C-alpha expression. *Cancer Res* 1996; 56:3499-3507.
48. Zhang X, Wen J, Aletta JM, Rubin RP. Inhibition of expression of PKC-alpha by antisense mRNA is associated with diminished cell growth and inhibition of amylase secretion by AR4-2J cells. *Exp Cell Res* 1997; 233:225-231.
49. McGraw K, McKay R, Miraglia L, Boggs RT, Pribble JP, Muller M, Geiger T, Fabbro D, Dean NM. Antisense oligonucleotide inhibitors of isozymes of protein kinase: *in vitro* and *in vivo* activity, and clinical development as anti-cancer therapeutics. *Anticancer Drug Des* 1997; 12:315-327.
50. Monia BP. First- and second-generation antisense inhibitors targeted to human c-raf kinase: *in vitro* and *in vivo* studies. *Anticancer Drug Des* 1997; 12:327-341.
51. Monteith DK, Geary RS, Leeds JM, Johnston J, Monia BP, Levin AA. Preclinical evaluation of the effects of a novel antisense compound targeting C-raf kinase mice and monkeys. *Toxicol Sci* 1998; 46:365-375.
52. Vaerman JL, Lammineur C, Moureau P, Lewalle P, Deldime F, Blumenfeld M, Martiat P. BCR-ABL antisense oligodeoxyribonucleotides suppress the growth of leukemic and normal hematopoetic cells by a sequence specific but not an antisense mechanism. *Blood* 1995; 86:3891-3896.
53. Kronenwett R, Haas R. Specific bcr-abl-directed antisense nucleic acids and ribozymes: a tool for the treatment of chronic myelogenous leukemia? Recent Results *Cancer Res* 1998; 144:127-138.8
54. Kronenwett R, Haas R. Antisense strategies for the treatment of hematological malignancies and solid tumors. *Ann Hematol* 1998; 77:1-12.
55. Shi Y, Fard A, Galeo A, Hutchinson HG, Vermani P, Dodge GR, Hall DJ, Shaheen F, Zalewski A. Transcatheter delivery of c-myc antisense oligomers reduces neointimal formation in a porcine model of coronary artery balloon injury. *Circulation* 1994; 90:944-951.
56. Mannion JD, Ormont ML, Shi Y, O'Brien JE Jr, Chung W, Roque F, Zalewski A. Saphenous vein graft protection: effects of c-myc antisense. *J Thorac Cardiovasc Surg* 1998; 115:152-161.

57. Bochot A, Couvreur P, Fattal E. Intraviteal administration of antisense oligonucleotides: potential of liposome delivery. *Prog Retin Eye Res* 2000; 19:131-147.
58. Goodarzi G, Gross SC, Tewari A, Watabe K. Antisense oligoribonucleoides inhibit the expression of the gene for hepatitis B birus surface antigen. *J Gen Virol* 1990; 71:3021-3025.
59. Korba BE, Gerin JL. Antisense oligonucleotides are effective inhibitors of hepatitis B virus replication *in vitro*. *Antiviral Res* 1995; 28:225-242.
60. Wu GY, Wu CH. Specific inhibition of hepatitis B viral gene expression *in vitro* by targeted antisense oligonucleotides. *J Biol Chem* 1992; 267:12436-12439.
61. Blum HE, Galun E, von Weizsaecker F, Wands JR. Inhibition of hepatitis B virus by antisense oligodeoxynucleotides. *Lancet* 1991; 337;1230.
62. Offensperger WB, Offensperger S, Walter E, Teubner K, Igloi GM Blum HE, Gerok W. *In vivo* inhibition of duck hepatitis B virus replication and gene expression by phosphorthioate modified antisense oligodeoxynucleotides. *Embo J* 1993; 12:1257-1262.
63. Soni PN, Brown D, Saffie R, Savage K, Moore D, gregoriadis G, Dusheiko GM. Biodistribution, stability, and antiviral efficacy of liposome-entrapped phosphoro-thioate antisense oligodoxynucleotides in ducks for the treatment of chronic duck hepatitis B virus infection. *Hepatology* 1998; 28:1402-1410.
64. Bartholomew RM, Carmichael EP, Findeis MA, Wu CH, Wu GY. Targeted delivery of antisense DNA in woodchuck hepatitis virus-infected woodchucks. *J Viral Hepat* 1995; 2;273-278.
65. Yao Z, Zhou Y, Feng X, Chen C, Guo J. *In vivo* inhibition of hepatitis B viral gene expression by antisense phosphorothioate oligodeoxynucleotides in athymic mice. *J Viral Hepat* 1996; 3:19-22.
66. Ji W, Si CW. Inhibition of hepatitis B virus by retroviral vectors expressing antisense RNA. *J Viral Hepat* 1997; 4:167-173.
67. zu Putlitz J, Wieland S, Blum HE, Wands JR. Antisense RNA complementary to hepatitis B virus specifically inhibits viral replication. *Gastroenterology* 1998; 115:702-713.
68. Friedman AD, Triezenberg SJ, McKnight SL. Expression of a truncated trans-activator selectively impedes lytic infection by its cognate virus. *Nature* 1988; 335:352-354.
69. Trono D, Feinberg MB, Baltimore D. HIV-1 Gag mutants can dominantly interfere with the replication of the wild-type virus. *Cell* 1989; 59:113-120.
70. Zhou S, Standring DN. Hepatitis B virus capsid particles are assembled from core-protein dimer precursor. *Proc Natl Acad Sci USA* 1992; 89:100046-10050.
71. Khudyakov YE, Kalinina TI, Neplyueva VS, Gazina EV, Kadoshnikov YP, Bogdanova SL, Smirnov D. The effect of the structure of the terminal regions of the hepatitis B virus gene C polypeptide on the formation of core antigen (HBcAg) particles. *Biomed Sci* 1991; 2:257-265.
72. Beames B, Lanford RE. Carboxy-terminal truncations of the HBV core protein affect capsid formation and the apparent size of encapsidated HBV RNA. *Virology* 1993; 194:597-607.
73. Nassal M. The arginine rich domain of the hepatitis B virus core protein is recquired for pregenome encapsiation and productive viral positive-strand DNA synthesis but not for virus assembly. *J Virol* 1992; 66;4107-4116.
74. Schlicht HJ, Bartenschlager R, Schaller H. The duck hepatitis B virus core protein contains a highly phosphorylated C terminus that is essential for replication but not for RNA packaging. *J Virol* 1989; 63:2995-3000.
75. Delaney MA, Goyal S, Seeger C. Design of modified core genes that inhibit replication of woodchuck hepatitis virus. In: Hollinger FB, Lemon SM, Margoils H, eds. *Viral Hepatitis and Liver Disease.* Baltimore: William & Wilkins, 1991:667-668.
76. Scaglioni PP, Melegari M, Wands JR. Characterization of hepatitis B virus core mutants that inhibit

viral replication. *Virology* 1994; 205;112-120.

77. von Weizsaecker F, Wieland S, Blum HE. Inhibition of viral replication by genetically engineered mutants of the duck hepatitis B virus core protein. *Hepatology* 1996; 24:294-299.
78. Scaglioni P, Melegari M, Takahashi M, Chowdhury J, Wands JR. Use of dominant-negative mutants of the hepadnaviral core protein as antiviral agents. *Hepatology* 1996; 24:1010-1017.
79. Scaglioni P, Melegari M, Wands JR. Posttranssriptional regulation of hepatitis B virus replication by the precore protein. *J Virol* 1997; 71:345-353.
80. Koeck J, Wieland S, Blum HE, von Weizsaecker F. Duck hepatitis B virus nucleocapsids formed by N-terminally extended and C-terminally truncated core proteins disintegrate during viral DNA maturation. *J Virol* 1998; 72:9116-9120.
81. von Weizsaecker F, Koeck J, Wieland S, Offensperger WB, Blum HE. Dominant negative mutants of the duck hepatitis B virus core protein interfere with RNA pregenome packaging and viral DNA synthesis. *Hepatology* 1999; 30:308-315.
82. Lambert C, Nassal M, Velhagen I, Zentgraf H, Schroeder CH. Precore-mediated inhibition of hepatitis B virus progeny DNA synthesis. *J Virol* 1992; 67:3756-3762.
83. Guidotti LG, Matzke B, Pasquinelli C, Shoenberger JM, Rogler CE, Chisari FV. The hepatitis B virus precore protein inhibits HBV replication in transgenic mice. *J Virol* 1996; 70:7056-7061.
84. Rondon IJ, Marasco WA. Intracellular antibodies (intrabodies) for gene therapy of infectious diseases. *Annu Rev Microbiol* 1997; 51:257-283.
85. Richardson JH, Marasco WA. Intracellular antibodies: development and therapeutic potential. *Trends Biotechnol* 1995; 13:306-310.
86. Marasco WA, Haseltine WA, Chen SY. Design, intracellular expression, and activity of a human anti-humanimmunodeficiency virus type 1 gp120 single-chain antibody. *Proc Natl Acad Sci USA* 1993; 90:7889-7893.
87. Transductional efficacy and safety of an intraperitoneally delivered adenovirus encoding an anti-erbB-2 intracellular single-chain antibody for ovarian cancer genetherapy. *Gynecol Oncol* 1997; 64:378-385.
88. Canaan-Haden l, Ayala M, Fernandez-de-cossio ME, Pedroso I, Rodes L, Gavilondo JV. Purification and application of a single-chain Fv antibody fragment specific to hepatitis B virus surface antigen. *Biotechniques* 1995; 19:6060-608.
89. zu Putlitz J, Skerra A, Schroeder CH, Zentgraf H, Wands JR. Cloning, bacterial synthesis, and characterization of immunoglobulin variable regions of a monoclonal antibody specific for the hepatitis B virus X protein. *Gene* 1998; 221:143-149.
90. Sanchez L, Ayala M, Freyre F, Pedroso I, Bell H, Falcon V, Gavilondo JV. High cytoplasmic expression in E. coli, purification, and in viro refolding of a single chain Fv antibody fragment against the hepatitis B surface antigen. *J Biotechnol* 1999; 72:13-20.
91. Yamamoto M, Hayashi N, Takehara T, Ueda K, Mita E, Tatsumi T, Sasaki Y, Kashahara A, hori M. Intracellular single-chain antibody against hepatitis B virus core protein inhibits the replication of hepatitis B virus in cultured cells. *Hepatology* 1999; 30:300-307.
92. zu Putlitz J, Wands JR. Cloning, bacterial expression and chararcterization of immunoglobulin variable regions from a murine monoclonal antibody directed against hepatitis B virus surface antigen. (Abstract) *Hepatology* 1997;26;426A
93. Wolff JA, Malone RW, Williams P, Chong W, Acsadi G, Jani A, Felgner PL. direct gene transfer into mouse muscle *in vivo*. *Science* 1990; 247:1465-1468.
94. Ulmer JB, Donnelly JJ, Parker SE, Rhodes GH, Felgner PL, Dwarki VJ, Gromkowski SH, Deck RR, DeWitt CM, Friedman A, et al. Heterologous protection against influenza by injection of DNA encoding

a viral protein. *Science* 1993; 259:1745-1749.

95. Bohm W, Mertens T, Schirmbeck R, Reimann J. Routes of plasmid DNA vaccination that prime murine humoral and cellular immune responses. *Vaccine* 1998; 16;949-954.
96. Davis HL, Brazalot Milan CL. DNA-based immunization against hepatitis B virus. *Springer Semin Immunopathol* 1997; 19:195-209.
97. Corr M, Tigh H. Plasmid DNA vaccination: Mechanism of antigen presentation. *Springer Semin Immunopathol* 1997; 19:139-145.
98. Bohm W, Kuhrober A, Paier T, Mertens T, Reimann J, Schirmbeck R. DNA vector constructs that prime hepatitis B surface antigen-specific cytotoxic T lymphocyte and antibody responses in mice after intramuscular injection. *J Immunol Methods* 1996; 193:29-40.
99. Mancini M, Davis H, Tiollais P, Michel ML. DNA-based immunization against the envelope proteins of the hepatitis B virus. *J Biotechnol* 1996; 44:47-57.
100. Geissler M, Gesien A, Tokushige K, Wands JR. Enhancement of cellular and humoral immune responses to hepatitis C core protein using DNA-based vaccines augmented with cytokine expressing plasmids. *J Immunol* 1997; 158:1231-1237.
101. Geissler M, Schirmbeck R, Reimann J, Blum HE, Wands JR. Cytokine and hepatitis B virus DNA coimmunizations enhance cellular and humoral immune responses to the middle but not to the large hepatitis B virus surface antigen in mice. *Hepatology* 1998; 28:202-210.
102. Chow YH, Huang WL, Chi WK, Chu YD, Tao MH. Improvement of hepatitis B virus DNA vaccines by plasmids coexpressing hepatitis B virus suface antigen and interleukin-2. *J Virol* 1997; 71:169-178.
103. Chow YH, Chiang BL, Lee YL, Chi WK, Lin WC, Chen YT, Tao MH. Development of Th1 and Th2 populations and the nature of immune responses to hepatitis B virus DNA vaccines can be modulated by codelivery of various cytokine genes. J Immunol 1998; 160:1320-1329.
104. Xiang Z, Ertl HC. Manipulation of the immune response to a plasmid-encoded viral antigen by coinoculation with plasmids expressing cytokines. *Immunity* 1995; 2:129-35.
105. Chisari FV. Cytotoxic T cells and viral hepatitis. *J Clin Invest* 1997; 99:1472-1477.
106. Guidotti LG, Rochford R, Chung J, Shapiro M, Purcell R, Chisari FV. Viral clearance without destruction of infected cells during acute HBV infection. *Science* 1999; 284:825-829.
107. Franco A, Ferrari C, Sette A, Chisari FV. Viral mutations, T cell receptor antagonism and escape from the immune response. In: *Current Opinion in Immunology*. A. Sher and R. Ahmed, eds. Current Biology Ltd., London. 524-531.
108. Ando K, Guidotti LG, Wirth S, Ishikawa T, Missale G, Moriyama T, Schreiber RD, Schlicht HJ, Huang S, Chisari FV. Class I restricted cytotoxic T lymphocytes are directly cytopathic for their targets *in vivo*. *J Immunol* 1994; 152:3245-3253.
109. Michel ML, Davis HL, Schleef M, Mancini M, Tiollais P, Whalen RG. DNA mediated immunization to the hepatitis B surface antigen in mice: aspects of the humoral response mimic hepatitis B viral infections in humans. *Proc Natl Acad Sci USA* 1995; 92:5307-5311.
110. Davis HL, Michel ML, Mancini M, Schleef M, Whalen RG. Plasmid DNA-based immunization against the hepatitis B virus surface antigen. *Vaccine* 1994; 12:1503-1509.
111. Davis HL, Schirmbeck R, Reimann J, Whalen RG. DNA-mediated immunization in mice induces a potent MHC class I-restricted cytotoxic T lymphocyte response to the hepatitis B envelope protein. *Human Gene Ther* 1995; 6:1447-1456.
112. Davis Hl, Mancini M, Michel ML, Whalen RG. DNA-mediated immunization to hepatitis B surface antigen: Longevity of primary response and effect of boost. *Vaccine* 1996; 14:910-915.
113. Whalen RG, Leclerc C, Deriaud E, Schirmbeck R, Reimann J, Davis HL. DNA-mediated immunization

to the hepatitis B surface antigen. Activation and entrainment of the immune response. *Ann NY Acad Sci* 1995; 772:64-76.

114. Geissler M, Tokushige K, Chante CC, Zurawski VR, Wands JR. Cellular and humoral immune response to hepatitis virus structural proteins in mice after DNA-based immunization. *Gastroenterology* 1997; 112:1307-1320.
115. Sallberg M, Townsend K, Chen M, O'Dea J, Banks T, Jolly DJ, Chang SM, Lee WT, Milich DR. Characterization of humoral and CD4+ cellular responses after genetic immunization with retroviral vectors expressing different forms of the hepatitis B virus core and e antigens. *J Virol* 1997; 71:5295-5303.
116. Major ME, Vitvitski L, Mink MA, Schleef M, Whalen RG, Trepo C, Inchauspe G. DNA-based immunization with chimeric vectors for the induction of immune responses against the hepatitis C virus nucleocapsid. *J Virol* 1995; 69:5798-5805.
117. Schirmbeck R, Bohm W, Ando K, Chisari FV, Reimann J. Nucleic acid vaccination primes hepatitis B surface antigen specific cytotoxic T lymphocytes in nonresponder mice. *J Virol* 1995; 69:5929-5934.
118. Kuhrober A, Wild J, Pudollek HP, Chisari FV, Reimann J. DNA vaccination with plasmids encoding the intracellular (HBcAg) or secreted (HBeAg) from the core protein of the hepatitis B virus primes T cell responses to two overlapping Kb- and Kd-restricted epitopes. *Int Immunol* 1997; 9:1203-1212.
119. Kuhrober A, Pudollek HP, Reifenberg K, Chisari FV, Schlicht HJ, Reimann J, Schirmbeck R. DNA immunization induces antibody and cytotoxic T cell responses to hepatitis B core antigen in H-2b mice. *J Immunol* 1996; 156:3687-3695.
120. Davis HL, Michel ML, Whalen RG. DNA-based immunization induces continuous secretion of hepatitis B surface antigen and high levels of circulating antibody. *Hum Mol Genet* 1993; 2:1847-1851.
121. Davis HL, Weeranta R, Waldschmidt TJ, Tygrett L, Schorr J, Krieg AM. CpG DNA is potent enhancer of specific immunity in mice immunized with recombinat hepatitis B surface antigen. *J Immunol* 1998; 160:870-876.
122. Leclerc C, Deriaud E, Rojas M, Whalen RG. The preferential induction of Th1 immune response by DNA-based immunization is mediated by the immunostimulatory effect of plasmid DNA. *Cell Immunol* 1997; 179:97-106.
123. McCluskie MJ, Davis HL. CpG DNA is a potent enhancer of systemic and mucosal immune response against hepatitis B surface antigen with intranasal administration to mice. *J Immunol* 1998; 161:4463-4466.
124. Mancini M, Hadchouel M, Davis HL, Whalen RG, Tiollais P, Michel ML. DNA-mediated immunization in a transgenic mouse model of the hepatitis B surface antigen chronic carrier state. *Proc Natl Acad Sci USA* 1996; 93:12496-12501.
125. Shimuzi Y, Guidotti LG, Fowler P, Chisari FV. Dendritic cell immunization breaks cytotoxic T lymphocyte tolerance in hepatitis B virus transgenic mice. *J Immunol* 1998; 161:4520-4529.
126. Schirmbeck R, Wild J, Stober D, Blum HE, Chisari FV, Geissler M, Reimann J. Ongoing murine T1 or T2 immune responses to the hepatitis B surface antigen are excluded from the liver that express transgene-encoded hepatitis B surface antigen. *J Immunol* 2000; 164:4235-4234.
127. Triyatni M, Jilbert AR, Qiao M, Miller DS, Burrell CJ. Protective efficacy of DNA vaccines against duck hepatitis B virus infection. *J Virol* 1998; 72:84-94.
128. Rollier C, Sunyach C, Barraud L, Madani N, Jamard C, Trepo C, Cova L. Protective and therapeutic effect of DNA-based immunization against hepadnavirus large envelope protein. *Gastroenterology* 1999; 116:658-665.
129. Lu M, Hilken G, Kruppenbacher J, Kemper T, Schirmbeck R, Reimann J, Roggendorf M. Immunization of woodchucks with plasmids expressing woodchuck hepatitis virus (WHV) core antigen and suface

antigen suppresss WHV infection. *J Virol* 1999; 73:281-289.

130. Rollier C, Charollois C, Jamard C, Trepo C, Cova L. Maternally transferred antibodies from DNA-immunized avians protect offspring against hepadnavirus infection. *J Virol* 2000; 74:4908-4911.
131. Rollier C, Charllois C, Jamard C, Trepo C, Cova L. Early life humoral response of ducks to DNA immunization against hepadnavirus large envelope protein. *Vaccine* 2000; 18:3091-3096.

In vitro phenotype of HBV variants in patients with fulminant hepatitis B

MARTINA STERNECK[1,2] and T. KALININA[2]

[1] *Department of Liver Transplant Surgery, University Hospital, Hamburg, Eppendorf*
[2] *Heinrich Pette Institute, Martinistr. 52, 20246 Hamburg, Germany*

Summary

Several outbreaks of fulminant hepatitis B infections suggest that viral variants play an important role in the pathogenesis of this aggressive course of the infection. Here, the phenotypes of the viral mutants isolated from patients with fulminant hepatitis B (FHB) were investigated by transfection studies in human hepatoma cells. One of eight patients with FHB was infected with high-replicating viral variants. Furthermore, HBV mutants with a severe secretion defect were found in a mixed population in two patients investigated. These data show that a high-replicating or secretion-defective phenotype of the viral variants is not a general characteristic for patients with FHB, but may in some cases contribute to the disease pathogenesis.

Introduction

The pathogenesis of fulminant hepatitis B (FHB) is not well understood. Viral factors as well as the host's immune response may both play an important role. However, several outbreaks of FHB cases that could be traced back to one chronically infected transmitter suggest that specific viral variants with increased pathogenicity are responsible for the fulminant clinical course of the infection [1-5]. Based on two case reports, it was proposed that such HBV strains are characterised by a particularly high replication ability [6, 7]. Alternatively, a strong cytopathogenicity and/or a high immunogenicity of certain HBV variants may favour a fulminant disease course.

Analysis of the complete nucleotide sequences of the HBV populations from patients with FHB revealed that no specific mutation is associated with a fulminant clinical course of the infection [8]. However, it is conceivable that different mutations in the HBV genome could result in a similar viral phenotype.

Therefore, the aim of the current study was to functionally characterise the HBV strains isolated from patients with FHB. Complete HBV genomes, amplified by full-length polymerase chain reaction from the serum of patients with FHB, were cloned and subsequently transfected into human hepatoma cells [9]. Then transcription, replication

Frontiers in Viral Hepatitis Ed. by RF Schinazi, J-P Sommadossi and CM Rice. 157 — 164

competence and protein expression were studied by Northern blot, Southern blot, immunoblot and ELISA. In addition, PCR products were directly transfected to investigate the phenotype of the dominant viral population of the respective patient. Subsequent construction and functional analysis of viral hybrid genomes, in which parts of the mutant viruses were introduced into wildtype virus, allowed determination of the sequence changes responsible for the specific viral phenotype.

HBV variants with a high replicating phenotype

The replication competence of the HBV strains infecting eight patients with FHB was analysed. Two cloned HBV genomes of each patient and wildtype virus were transfected in Huh 7 cells [10]. Southern blot analysis of the HBV DNA in the cell cytoplasms revealed, only for the two cloned HBV genomes of patient 8, a markedly increased amount of intracellular HBV DNA compared to wildtype virus (Figure 1), indicating a high replication ability of these two variants [10]. In contrast, the HBV genomes of the other seven patients with FHB showed a replication competence comparable to wildtype virus (Figure 1). Direct transfection of the PCR-amplified HBV DNA from the serum of patient 8 also revealed an increased replication ability. This confirms that the two investigated cloned HBV genomes are representative of the heterogeneous viral population and that the dominant viral population present *in vivo* also shows a high-replicating phenotype. Interestingly, patient 8 was the only patient who suffered from fulminant HBV reinfection of his liver graft after transplantation. In summary, these data suggest that HBV variants with a high replication competence are not in general found in patients with FHB, but in some cases may contribute to the disease pathogenesis.

Mutations in the core promoter region are responsible for the high-replicating phenotype

In order to determine the sequence changes leading to the increased replication competence of the variants from patient 8, viral hybrid genomes were constructed. In the latter, the variant core promoter regions were introduced into wildtype virus. Functional analysis of such viral constructs also revealed a markedly increased level of intracellular HBV DNA compared to wildtype virus (data not shown), indicating that the high-replicating phenotype of the variants results from mutations in the core promoter region. By sequence analysis, two mutations (G1764T and C1766G) were identified in both cloned variant genomes, which create a putative binding site for the transcription factor HNF 3 [8]. Since it had been previously shown that mutations creating an HNF 1 or HNF 3 binding site in the core promoter region result in a high replicating phenotype [7, 11], we assume that in the case described here the G1764T and C1766G substitutions were responsible for the observed high replication competence. Further experiments will be performed to confirm this hypothesis. However, a sequence alignment with the DNA sequences of more than 40 HBV genomes from patients with FHB and 36 HBV genomes from patients without FHB revealed that the above identified mutations are rare in both patient groups.

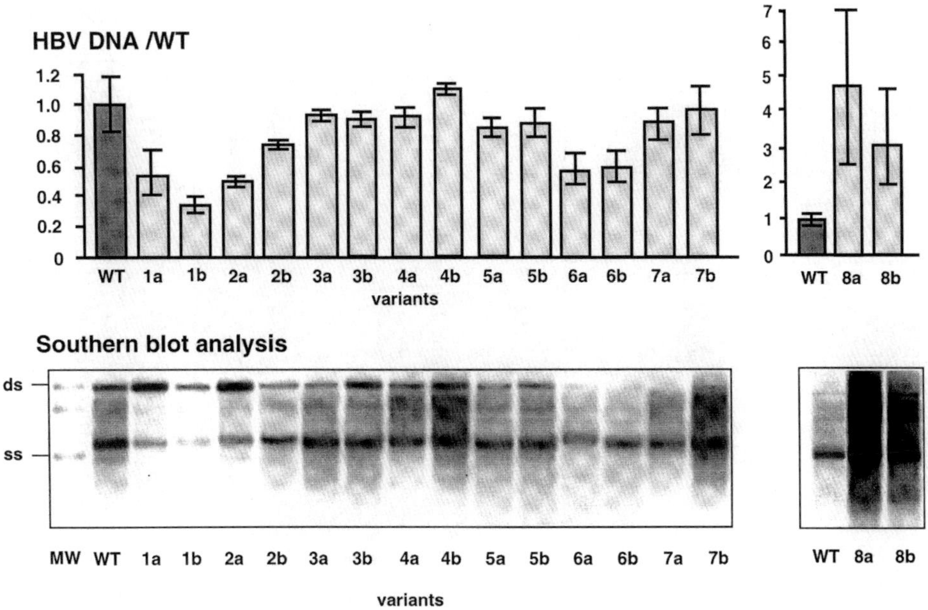

Figure 1. Transfection studies were performed with two (a and b) cloned HBV genomes of eight patients with FHB (1-8) and wildtype virus (WT). Core particles were purified from the cell cytoplasm, and HBV DNA was quantitatively assessed by Southern blot analysis. The amount of HBV DNA in cells transfected with the variants relative to the amount of HBV DNA in cells transfected with WT is given. Both variants of patient 8 showed increased levels of HBV DNA compared to WT, indicating a high replication efficiency, whereas the HBV genomes of the other seven patients showed a replication competence similar to WT.

HBV variants with a secretion defect

In order to study the secretion ability of the viral variants from the eight patients with FHB, the amount of HBsAg in the medium of the transfected cells was determined by ELISA. With both cloned HBV genomes of patient 4 and patient 8, the levels of extracellular HBsAg were very low compared to wildtype virus. To prove that this was due to a secretion defect of the variants and not due to an impaired recognition of the mutant HBsAg by the ELISA, S- and L-protein were in addition quantitatively assessed by immunoblot analysis using the monoclonal antibodies Mab 18/07 and Mab H166. Prior sequence analysis had confirmed that the mutant envelope proteins carried no mutations within the binding regions of these antibodies. Transfection studies with HBV variants from patient 4 (variant 4a and 4b) and patient 8 (variant 8a, 8b and 8d) revealed an intracellullar amount of mutant S- and L-protein similar or increased compared to wildtype virus (Figure 2, 3). In contrast, in the medium of cells transfected with these

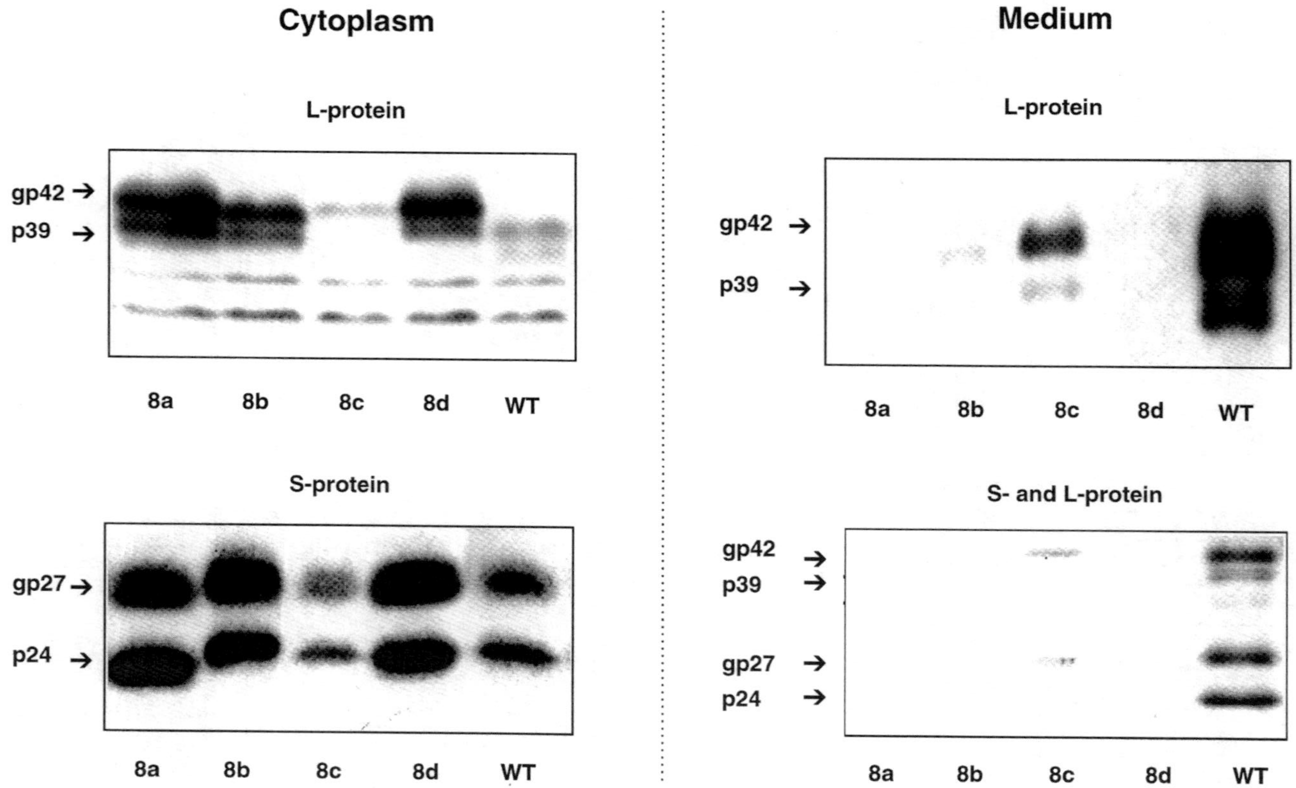

Figure 2. Four cloned HBV genomes isolated from patient 8 (8a-8d) and wildtype virus (WT) were transfected into Huh7 cells. After purification of viral particles from the medium of cells, S- and L-protein were detected by immunoblot using the monoclonal antibodies Mab H166 and Mab 18/07, respectively. With the HBV genomes 8a, 8b and 8d, S- and L-protein were detectable in the cell cytoplasm, but not in the cell culture medium, indicating an almost complete secretion defect of these HBV variants. In contrast, in the medium of cells transfected with variant 8c, L- and S-protein were present at a low level, indicating that viral particles were still secreted, although at a very low level compared to WT.

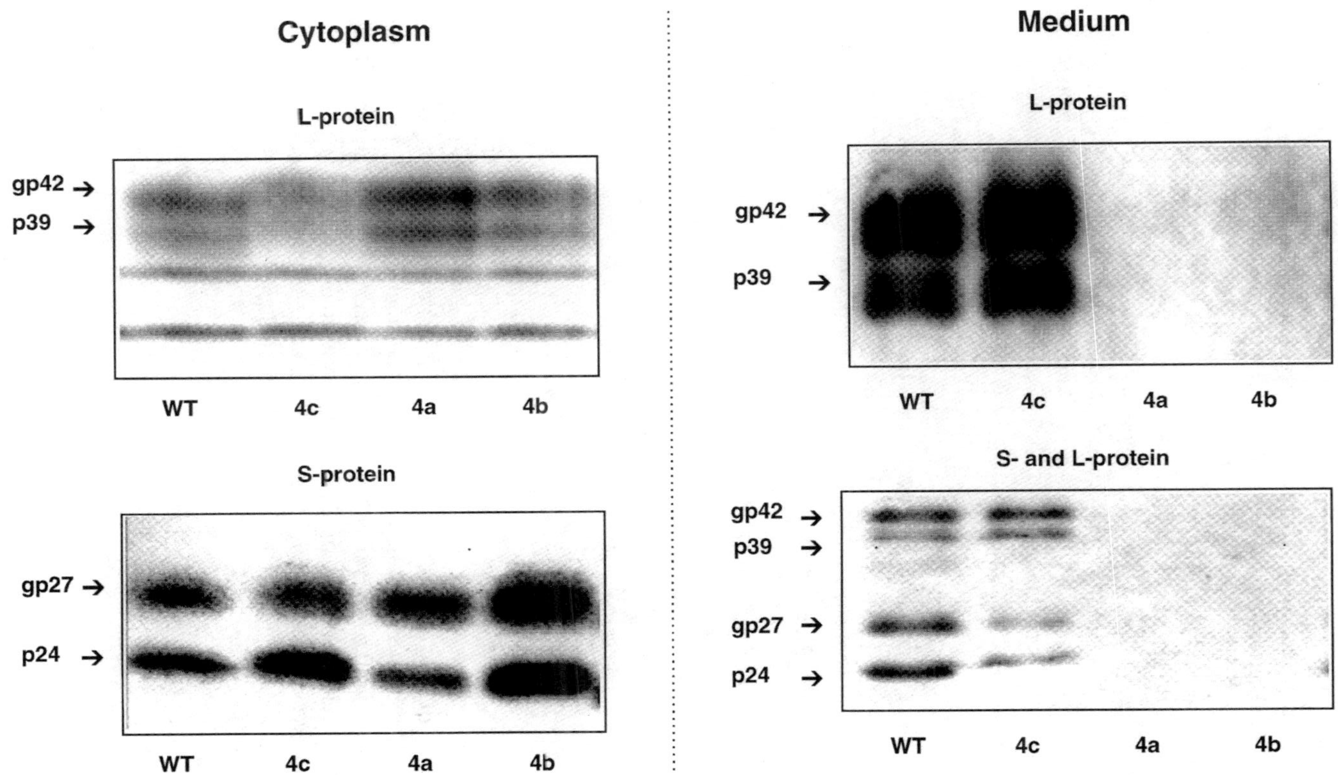

Figure 3. Transfection studies were performed with three cloned HBV genomes isolated from patient 4 (4a-4c) and wildtype virus (WT). S- and L- protein were quantitatively assessed by immunoblot using the same monoclonal antibodies as given above. In cells transfected with the variants 4a and 4b, S- and L-protein were both present in an amount comparable to WT, but in the cell culture medium both envelope proteins were absent-indicating a severe secretion defect. In contrast, in the supernatant of cells transfected with mutant 4c, levels of L- and S-protein were comparable to those found with WT. This indicates that secretion-defective HBV strains coexisted with secretion-competent viruses *in vivo*.

mutants, S- and L-proteins were hardly detectable (Figure 2, 3). This indicates that these HBV variants had an almost complete defect in the secretion of both subviral particles and virions. Further investigations showed that in both patients, HBV genomes with such a secretion defective phenotype represented a large fraction of the viral population. In addition, HBV genomes without a secretion defect were present (variants 4c and 8c, Figure 2 and 3).

In order to determine the dominant phenotype of the heterogeneous viral populations present in the serum of patients 4 and 8, HBV populations amplified by PCR were directly transfected into Huh7 cells. These experiments also revealed hardly detectable amounts of envelope proteins in the cell culture media, confirming that the dominant viral populations of patient 4 and patient 8 exhibited severe secretion defects. The presence of mixed viral populations with the possibility of complementation may explain why viral variants with a secretion defect can survive *in vivo*.

Mutations in the small S-gene determine the secretion defect of the variants

In order to determine the sequence changes responsible for the observed secretion defect in the HBV mutants, viral hybrid genomes were constructed in which the mutant pre-S regions, or alternatively the mutant S-regions, were introduced into wildtype virus. In both cases the constructs with the mutant S-regions, but not the constructs with the mutant pre-S regions, showed a secretion defect *in vitro* (Figure 4). This indicates that mutations in the S-gene are responsible for the almost complete secretion block. To our knowledge the occurrence of such mutants *in vivo* has not been described.

Pathogenesis of FHB

Our data indicate that some patients with FHB are infected with viral variants with a specific phenotype, i.e., one with a high replication ability and/or a secretion-defective phenotype. In one of the cases described, the combination of both the increased replication ability and the secretion defect may have contributed to the fulminant HBV reinfection of the liver graft. However, in the majority of cases neither a high replication competence nor a secretion defect of the variants was found to be associated with the aggressive disease course. Whether these viral variants play an important role for the clinical manifestation of infection, for example by inducing an enhanced immune response, is still unknown.

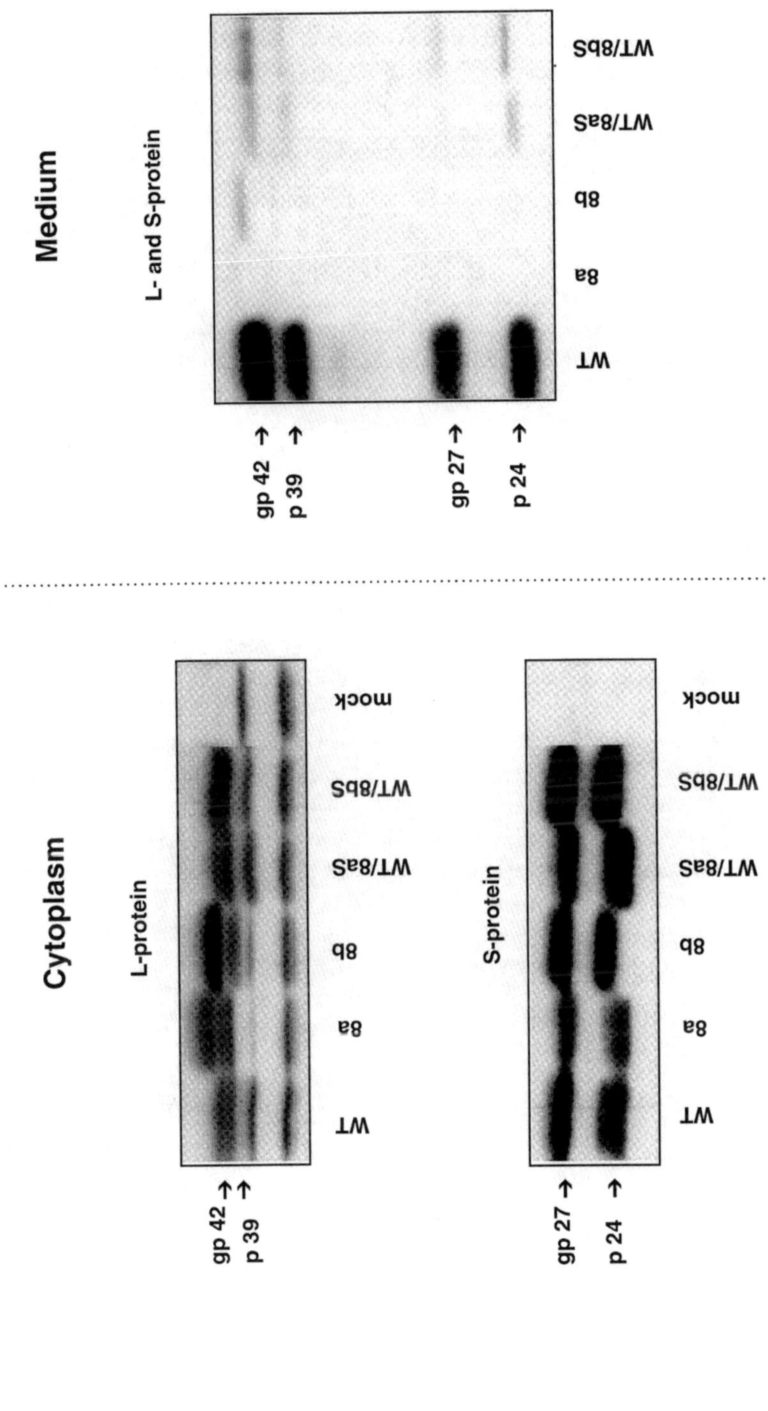

Figure 4. Transfection studies were performed with two cloned HBV genomes from patient 8 (variant 8a and 8b), WT and two hybrid genomes in which the S-regions of the variants 9a or 9b were introduced into WT (constructs WT/8aS and WT/8bS). In the medium of cells transfected with variants 8a and 8b, as well as in the medium of cells transfected with the constructs WT/8aS and WT/8bS, almost no S- and L-protein was found. This indicates that the secretion-defective phenotype of the variants 8a and 8b results from mutations in the S-region.

References

1. Zuckerman MA, Hawkins AE, Briggs M, Waite J, Balfe P, Thom B, Gilson RJ, Tedder RS. Investigation of hepatitis B virus transmission in a health care setting: application of direct sequence analysis. *Journal Of Infectious Diseases* 1995; 172(4): 1080-3.
2. Tanaka S, Yoshiba M, Iino S, Fukuda M, Nakao H, Tsuda F, Okamoto H, Miyakawa Y, Mayumi M. A common-source outbreak of fulminant hepatitis B in hemodialysis patients induced by a precore mutant. *Kidney International* 1995; 48(6): 1972-8.
3. Ogata N, Miller R, Ishak K, Purcell R. The complete nucleotide sequence of a precore mutant of hepatitis B virus implicated in fulminant hepatitis and its biological characterization in chimpanzees. *Virology* 1993; 194: 263-76.
4. Liang TJ, Hasegawa K, Rimon N, Wands J, Ben-Porath E. A hepatitis B virus mutant associated with an epidemic of fulminant hepatitis. *New England Journal of Medicine* 1991; 324: 1705-9.
5. Asahina Y, Enomoto N, Ogura Y, Sakuma I, Kurosaki M, Izumi M, Marumo F, Sato C. Complete nucleotide sequences of hepatitis B virus genomes associated with epidemic fulminant hepatitis. *Journal of Medical Virology* 1996; 48: 171-8.
6. Hasegawa K, Huang J, Rogers SA, Blum HE, Liang TJ. Enhanced replication of a hepatitis B virus mutant associated with an epidemic of fulminant hepatitis. *Journal of Virology* 1994; 68: 1651-9.
7. Pult I, Chouard T, Wieland S, Klemenz R, Yaniv m, Blum H. A hepatitis B virus mutant with a new hepatocyte nuclear factor binding site emerging in transplant-transmitted fulminant hepatitis. *Hepatology* 1997; 25: 1507-15.
8. Sterneck M, Guenther S, Santantonio T, Fischer L, Broelsch CE, Greten H, Will H. Hepatitis B virus genomes of patients with fulminant hepatitis do not share a specific mutation. *Hepatology* 1996; 24(2): 300-6.
9. Günther S, Li B, Miska S, Krüger D, Meisel H, Will H. A novel method for efficient amplification of whole hepatitis B virus genomes permits rapid functional analysis and reveals deletion mutants in immunosuppressed patients. *Journal of Virology* 1995; 69: 5437-44.
10. Sterneck M, Kalinina T, Guenther S, Fischer L, Santantonio T, Greten H, Will H. Functional analysis of HBV genomes from patients with fulminant hepatitis. *Hepatology* 1998; 28(5): 1390-7.
11. Günther S, Piwon N, Iwanska A, Schilling R, Meisel H, Will H. Type, prevalence and significance of core promoter/enhancer II mutations in hepatitis B viruses from immunosuppressed patients with severe liver disease. *Journal of Virology* 1996; 70: 8318-31.

Evaluation of three commercially available HBV viral load assays: Dynamic range, precision and clinical utility

ANDREA SNOW[1], FLORENCE MYRICK[1],
CHARLES WAKEFORD[1] and BRUCE MCCREEDY[2]

[1] *Triangle Pharmaceuticals, Inc., 4611 University Drive P.O. Box 50530, Durham, North Carolina 27717-0530, USA*
[2] *Intelligent Therapeutic Solutions, Inc., 2505 Meridian Parkway, Suite 200, Durham, North Carolina 27713, USA*

There is a need for a standardized assay to monitor viral load in patients chronically infected with hepatitis B virus (HBV) receiving antiviral therapy. We have performed a comparative analysis of three commercially available HBV viral load assays: the Quantiplex™ HBV DNA Assay (Chiron) from Chiron Corporation, the Digene® HBV Test Hybrid Capture® II (Digene) from Digene Corporation and the Amplicor HBV Monitor™ Test (Roche) from Roche Molecular Systems to determine the dynamic range, precision and clinical utility of each assay. Serum samples from HBV-infected patients enrolled in a clinical trial were collected and analyzed using each assay. Viral load results were compared, and a statistical analysis evaluating the correlation and the concordance of the three assays was performed. Overall the results generated using Digene correlated more closely with results obtained using Chiron than with Roche. The version of the Chiron method used was less sensitive than the other two methods. Digene showed an acceptable dynamic range but failed to quantify HBV DNA levels in patients with very low (<5, 000 copies/ml) viral loads. Roche was the most sensitive assay, to detecting as few as 400 copies/ml.

Introduction

Advances have been made with regard to the development of antiviral therapies against the hepatitis B virus (HBV). Nucleoside analogues such as (-)-β-L-2', 3'-Dideoxy-3'-thiacytidine (3TC), *cis*-5-fluoro-1-[2-(hydroxymethyl)-1, 3-oxathiolan-5-yl]-cytosine (FTC), (-)-β-D-2, 6-Diaminopurine dioxolane (DAPD) and 1-(2-fluoro-5-methyl-β-L-arabinofuranosyl)-uracil (L-FMAU) have been shown to have potent anti-HBV activity and are currently undergoing pre-clinical and clinical evaluation [1]. To assess the antiviral efficacy of these drugs in patients enrolled in clinical trials, an assay is needed that can quantitate viral load with precision over a broad dynamic range.

Several assays are available that measure different markers of HBV replication. Conventionally, the status of the e antigen (HBeAg) has been an indicator of active viral replication [8, 11]. However, precore mutations have been described that inhibit the

Frontiers in Viral Hepatitis Ed. by RF Schinazi, J-P Sommadossi and CM Rice. 165 — 172

production of the HBeAg regardless of the viral replication rate [4, 6, 8, 10]. In contrast to HIV, where reduction in viral load is an accepted surrogate marker of therapeutic efficacy [2], no consensus has been reached to date as to which marker is most appropriate for monitoring patients chronically infected with HBV [4, 9]. Nevertheless, the ability to quantify HBV viral load is emerging as an essential tool in the management of chronically infected patients. In addition to providing information about progression of the disease and drug efficacy, HBV viral load can also be an early predictor of treatment failure and drug resistance [5].

Unlike HIV, where viral loads can vary by 5-6 logs, HBV DNA in chronically infected patients can vary by 10 logs or more. Knowing that the HBV viral load can vary so dramatically poses some concern, since no single commercially available assay has the capability to quantify HBV viral loads over the entire range. Therefore, it may be necessary to use more than one assay to evaluate the HBV viral load in a patient throughout treatment. Again, this poses a problem since many of the commercially available assays use different technologies (i.e. bDNA, hybrid capture and PCR) and standards to detect and quantify HBV DNA. Because of these differences, the results obtained for a single sample using different assays can be very different.

We evaluated three assays: Quantiplex™ HBV DNA Assay (Chiron), Digene® HBV Test Hybrid Capture® II (Digene) and Amplicor HBV Monitor™ Test (Roche) and determined the dynamic range, precision and clinical utility of each assay. The HBV DNA samples used in these evaluations were from chronically infected patients enrolled in a dose-escalation study of Coviracil® (emtricitabine, FTC), a nucleoside analogue with potent anti-HBV activity [3]. The HBV DNA samples were collected prior to treatment to determine a baseline viral load and weekly throughout an 8-week dosing period. Samples were assayed for HBV viral load using each assay.

Our main objective was to identify a method with the appropriate sensitivity to accurately measure HBV DNA over a broad dynamic range. The utility of all three methods was evaluated and a correlation was established between the assays.

Description of the assays

Each of the three HBV viral load assays utilizes a different method of detection to measure HBV DNA in serum. The Chiron assay is a sandwich nucleic-acid hybridization assay in which HBV DNA from a specimen is captured on a plate via a set of specific synthetic oligonucleotide target probes. A second set of target probes then hybridizes to the viral DNA and branched DNA amplifiers. The two sets of target probes bind to specific sequences on the minus-sense strand of the viral DNA. Multiple copies of an alkaline-phosphatase-conjugated probe are then hybridized to this immobilized complex to amplify the signal. Detection is achieved by incubating the complex with a chemiluminescent substrate and measuring the light emitted. Light emission is directly proportional to the amount of HBV DNA present in each specimen, and results are recorded as luminescent counts by a plate luminometer. A standard curve is defined by light emission from standards with known concentrations of HBV DNA. The concentration of HBV DNA in specimens is determined from this standard curve.

The Digene assay is a signal amplification-hybridization antibody capture microplate test that uses chemiluminescent detection. Specimens containing the target DNA hybridize with an RNA probe, and the resultant RNA:DNA hybrids are captured onto the surface of microplate wells coated with antibodies specific for the RNA:DNA hybrids. Immobilized hybrids are then treated with alkaline-phosphatase-conjugated antibodies specific for the RNA:DNA hybrids. Several alkaline-phosphatase molecules are conjugated to each antibody, and multiple conjugated antibodies bind to each captured hybrid resulting in substantial signal amplification. The bound alkaline-phosphatase then cleaves a chemiluminescent substrate. The emitted light is measured as relative light units (RLUs) on a luminometer. A calibration curve of calibrators is plotted, and the RLU value of each specimen is compared to that of the curve to determine the concentration of HBV DNA in the specimen. If very low levels of HBV DNA are to be quantified, an ultrasensitive (US) test can be performed where the virions are concentrated through centrifugation prior to performing the test.

The Roche assay is based on four major processes: specimen preparation, PCR amplification of target DNA using HBV-specific complimentary primers, hybridization of the amplified products to oligonucleotide probes specific to the target, and detection of the amplified products by colorimetric determination. The quantification of HBV DNA is performed using an external standard curve generated with every run. A quality-control reagent (internal standard, IS) is incorporated into every standard and specimen at a known copy number and is carried through the amplification and detection steps. The ratio of HBV to IS signal is calculated for all standards and specimens to compensate for any differences in amplification or detection between samples. Six HBV standards are included in each run. The copy number of each standard is plotted against the HBV:IS ratio for each standard to generate a standard curve. HBV DNA levels in the unknown specimens are determined by comparing the individual HBV:IS ratios to the standard curve generated with each run. All three assays differ in dynamic range, as shown in Table 1.

Table 1. Overview of three commercially-available assays, including individual dynamic ranges

Assay Name	Technology	Sensitivity (LOQ)	Stated Dynamic Range
Quantiplex™ HBV DNA Assay	Branched DNA	7.0×10^5 Eq/ml	> 7.0×10^5 Eq/ml
Digene® HBV Test Hybrid Capture® II	Hybrid Capture	(US) 4.7×10^3 c/ml 1.42×10^5 c/ml	(US) $4.7 \times 10^3 - 5.6 \times 10^7$ c/ml $1.42 \times 10^5 - 1.7 \times 10^9$ c/ml
Amplicor HBV Monitor™ Test	PCR	4.0×10^2 c/ml	$4.0 \times 10^2 - 4.0 \times 10^7$ c/ml

Standardization issues and dynamic range

Currently, the ability to determine a pre-treatment viral load as well as to monitor a patient to maximum viral suppression requires that different assays be used in combination. Unfortunately, this does not give a true measure of viral load, since there is no standardization among the assays, nor is there a conversion factor that allows for the inter-assay comparison of results. Figure 1 shows an example of where the individual assays are limited in their ability to accurately report viral load as well as the lack of standardization between assays. Chiron is shown to be limited at the low end of viral load, while both Digene and Roche underestimate the viral load at the high end. The lack of standardization can be seen in the disparity between results generated for the same sample, despite the overlap in the dynamic ranges between 7.0 x 10^5 and 4.0 x 10^7 copies/ml.

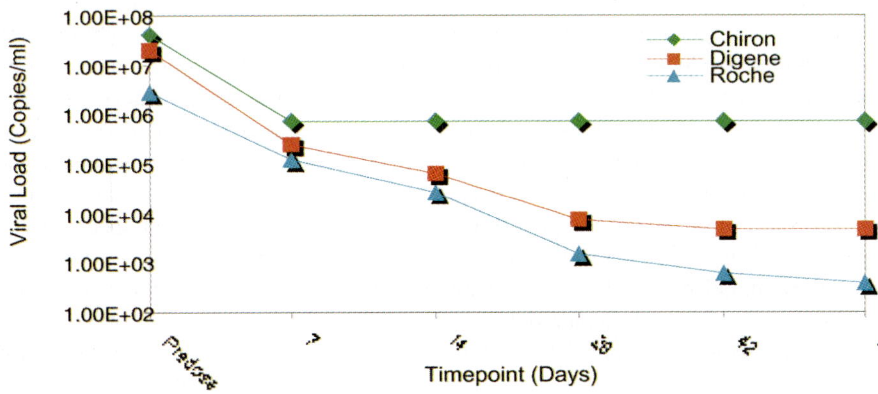

Figure 1. Viral load determination from one patient using three commercially-available assays.

In an attempt to expand the upper-end dynamic range of Digene and Roche, high-viral-load samples were diluted and re-tested. Statistical analyses indicate that we were successful at expanding the upper-end dynamic range of Digene to 4.35 x 10^{10} copies/ml and the dynamic range of Roche to 1.25 x10^9 copies/ml.

Statistical analysis

The concordance, which is a measure of how well pairs of results agree, was determined using the following statistical methodology. HBV DNA values were analyzed on a log 10 scale. Concordance was calculated as the percentage of Chiron (or Roche) data points that were within a specified tolerance value of the corresponding Digene data points. Concordance is stronger as its value approaches 100%. A tolerance value of 10% was chosen for the purposes of calculating concordance. Assuming a within-sample standard deviation (SD) of 0.2 log for Digene, this 10% tolerance corresponds to approximately three SD for assay values near six logs. Also determined was a linear correlation coefficient, which is a measure of the strength of linear association between two variables. A strong, positive linear relationship exists when the linear correlation coefficient (r) approaches one.

Two hundred and twenty-nine specimens were evaluated using both the Digene and Chiron assays, according to the individual manufacturer's instructions. The concordance was calculated to be 88.6%, and the correlation coefficient was 0.92. Included in this analysis are values where the dynamic ranges of the assays do not overlap (Panel 4, Table 2). Samples above Digene's dynamic range were diluted and re-tested. When these values were included in the analysis, the concordance strengthened slightly to 89.4%, increasing our confidence in the diluted-Digene results (Panel 3, Table 2). There were 201 matching data points where Digene and Chiron overlap, starting at Chiron's limit of sensitivity and stopping at Digene's upper end. Using a 10% tolerance, the concordance was 96.5%, and the correlation coefficient was 0.95 (Panel 2, Table 2). Lastly, when matching data points, including diluted values for Digene, were analyzed starting at Chiron's lower limit, the concordance strengthened slightly to 96.8%, and the correlation coefficient increased slightly (0.96) (Panel 4, Table 2). The range of concordance values (88.6% to 96.8%) and linear correlation coefficient values (0.92 to 0.96) indicate an overall strong agreement between Digene and Chiron.

Table 2. Statistical analysis results: Chiron versus Digene

Panel	Range (copies/ml)	n	Concordance (10% Tolerance)	Correlation Coefficient
1	Chiron > 7.0×10^5			
	Digene > 7.0×10^5	218	96.8%	0.96
2	Chiron > 7.0×10^5			
	7.0×10^5 < Digene < 1.7×10^9	201	96.5%	0.95
3	Chiron > 7.0×10^5			
	Digene > 4.7×10^3	246	89.4%	0.94
4	Chiron > 7.0×10^5			
	4.7×10^3 < Digene < 1.7×10^9	229	88.6%	0.92

Similar analyses were performed to compare Digene and Roche. Three hundred and seven specimens were tested using both Digene and Roche, according to the manufacturer's instructions. The concordance was 67.4%, and the correlation coefficient was 0.91. Included in this analysis are values where the dynamic ranges of the assays do not overlap (Panel 4, Table 3). The concordance strengthens slightly to 69.9% when diluted values are included for both Digene and Roche (Panel 3, Table 3).

Also determined was the concordance between the assays where the lower-end gap in the dynamic ranges of the assays is censored from the analysis. For the set of data which represents where Digene and Roche overlap, starting with Digene's lower limit and stopping at Roche's upper limit, the concordance is 72.8% (Panel 2, Table 3). Lastly, when values were analyzed starting at Digene's lower limit and included diluted values for both assays, the concordance strengthens to 75.7% (Panel 1, Table 3). The range of concordance values (67.4% to 75.7%) and linear correlation coefficient values (0.91 to 0.94) indicate a fairly strong agreement between Digene and Roche.

Table 3. Statistical analysis: Roche versus Digene

Panel	Range (copies/ml)	n	Concordance (10% Tolerance)	Correlation Coefficient
1	Roche > 4.7×10^3 4.7×10^3 < Digene < 1.7×10^9	304	75.7%	0.94
2	4.7×10^3 < Roche < 4.0×10^7 4.7×10^3 < Digene < 4.0×10^7	265	72.8%	0.90
3	Roche > 4.0×10^2 Digene > 4.7×10^3	342	69.9%	0.94
4	4.0×10^2 < Roche < 4.0×10^7 4.7×10^3 < Digene < 1.7×10^9	307	67.4%	0.91

A visual representation of the linear relationship and concordance between two methods can be seen in scatter plot graphs (Figure 2). Both plots represent how well the assays correlate over the best possible dynamic range, which is where the assays overlap according to the manufacturer's stated lower limit, and includes diluted values for both Digene and Roche. Consistent with the numerical findings, the relationship between Digene and Chiron appears to be slightly stronger than between Digene and Roche

Conclusions

The three commercially available assays evaluated in this study utilize different technologies to detect and quantify HBV DNA. In addition, there are significant differences in the dynamic ranges of all three assays. Upon initial evaluation each assay proved to be useful within certain ranges. Chiron proved to be useful for determining HBV viral loads > 7.0×10^5 Eq/ml. Roche was determined to be the most sensitive and was useful for determining low HBV viral loads, while Digene demonstrated the broadest dynamic range. The upper-end dynamic range of both Roche and Digene were successfully expanded through dilution and re-testing of high-viral-load samples. However, for Roche this became time consuming and expensive due to the large number

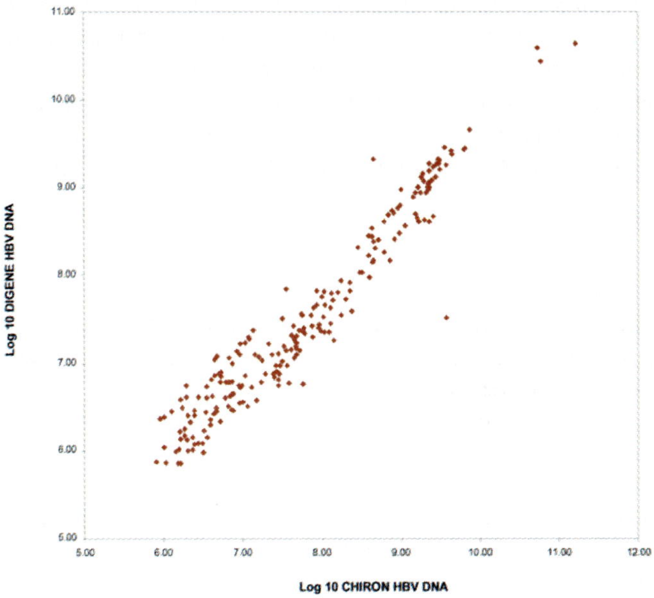

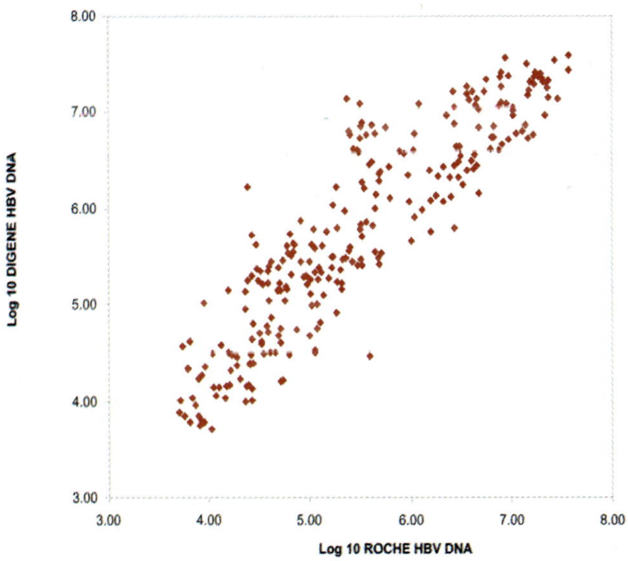

Figure 2. Assay comparison: Scatterplots

of samples that required dilutions. Based on the statistical findings, the concordance between Digene and Chiron was determined to be stronger than that between Digene and Roche, even though a strong, positive linear relationship exists between both sets of comparisons. Based on all of these observations, Digene was identified as a reliable, cost-efficient method that could be used for the determination of pre-treatment viral loads as well as to monitor patients while on therapy to as low as 4,700 copies/ml.

References

1. Chu Chung K, Boudinot F. Douglas, Peek Simon F., Hong Joon H., Choi Yongseok, Korba Brent E., Gerin John L., Cote Paul J., Tennant Bud C. and Cheng Yung-Chi. Preclinical investigation of l-FMAU as an anti-hepatitis B virus agent. Antiviral Therapy 3: Supplement 3 1998; 113-121.
2. Gerken G., Gomes J., Lampertico P., Colombo M., Rothaar T., Trippler M., Colucci G. Clinical evaluation and applications of the Roche Monitor test, a quantitative HBV DNA PCR assay. Journal of Virological Methods 1998; 4:2, 155-165.
3. Gish R.G., Leung N.W.Y., Wright T., et al. Anti-Hepatitis B Virus (HBV) Activity and Pharmacokinetics of FTC in a 2-Month Trial in HBV-Infected Patients. Abstract 2216. Digestive Disease Week, May 16-19, 1999, Orlando, FL.
4. Ho Stephen K. N., Chan Tak Mao, Cheng Ignatius K. P. and Lai Kar Neng. Comparison of the Second-Generation Digene Hybrid Capture Assay with the Branched-DNA Assay for Measurement of Hepatitis B Virus DNA in Serum. Journal of Clinical Microbiology 1999; 37:8 2461-2465.
5. Hodinka R.L. The clinical utility of viral quantitation using molecular methods. Clinical and Diagnostic Virology 1998; 10:1, 25-47.
6. Hunt Christine M., McGill James M., Allen Marchelle I., Condreay Lynn D. Clinical Relevance of Hepatitis B Viral Mutations. Hepatology 2000; 31:5, 1037-1044.
7. Krajden M., Minor J., Cork L., Comanor L. Multi-measurement method comparison of three commercial hepatitis B virus DNA quantification assays. J Viral Hepat 1998; 5:6, 415-422.
8. Niitsuma Hirofumi, M.D., Ishii Motoyasu, M.D., Miura Masahito, M.D., Kobayashi Koju, M.D. and Toyota Takayoshi, M.D. Low Level Hepatitis B Viremia Detected by Polymerase Chain Reaction Accompanies the Absence of HBe Antigenemia and Hepatitis in Hepatitis B Virus Carriers. The American Journal of Gastroenterology 1997; 92:1 119-123.
9. Pawlotsky Jean-Michel, Bastie Anne, Lonjon Isabelle, Remire Jocelyne, Darthuy Francoise, Soussy Claude-James and Dhumeaux Daniel. What technique should be used for routine detection and quantification of HBV DNA in clinical samples? Journal of Virological Methods 1997; 65 245-253.
10. Thomas H. C. and Carman W. F. The Host Immune Response May Be Responsible for Selection of Envelope and Precore/Core Variants of HBV. Progress In Liver Diseases 1998, Chapter 11 239-251.
11. Zaaijer H. L, Borg F. Ter, Cuypers H. T. M., Hermus M. C. A. H. and Lelie P. N. Comparison of Methods for Detection of Hepatitis B Virus DNA. Journal of Clinical Microbiology 1994; 32:9 2008-2091.

CELL SYSTEMS AND ANIMAL MODELS

Cell lines that allow regulated expression of HCV proteins: principles and applications

DARIUS MORADPOUR[1*], MARKUS H. HEIM[2], ANDREAS CERNY[3], CHARLES M. RICE[4] and HUBERT E. BLUM[1]

[1] *Department of Medicine II, University of Freiburg, D-79106 Freiburg, Germany*
[2] *Department of Research, University Hospital Basel, CH-4031 Basel, Switzerland*
[3] *Clinica Medica, Ospedale Civico, CH-6903 Lugano, Switzerland*
[4] *Center for the Study of Hepatitis C, Rockefeller University, New York, NY 10021*

Abstract

Investigation of hepatitis C virus (HCV) replication and pathogenesis is limited by the lack of an efficient cell culture system. Using a tetracycline-regulated gene expression system, we have established and characterized a comprehensive panel of continuous human cell lines inducibly expressing HCV structural and nonstructural proteins. The cellular and viral proteolytic machineries and posttranslational modification pathways were fully functional in these cell lines. Steady-state expression levels could be regulated over a broad range by the concentration of tetracycline present in the culture medium. As shown by a number of recent applications, these inducible cell lines represent a unique model system to analyze structural and functional properties of HCV proteins and their interactions with cellular proteins and pathways. In addition, these cell lines should prove useful for the evaluation of novel antiviral strategies in a well-defined and highly reproducible cellular context.

Introduction

The lack of an efficient cell culture system permissive for hepatitis C virus (HCV) infection and replication has limited the systematic study of the viral life cycle and pathogenesis as well as the development and evaluation of novel antiviral strategies. Infection of primary hepatocytes and established cell lines *in vitro* [1-3] and transient expression of presumed full-length HCV RNA [4, 5] yielded only low-level and often poorly reproducible viral replication. The recent establishment of selectable subgenomic HCV replicons represents a major breakthrough in this direction [6]. The current generation of HCV replicons, however, does not include the structural

Frontiers in Viral Hepatitis Ed. by RF Schinazi, J-P Sommadossi and CM Rice. 175 — 186

proteins. An alternative approach involves the generation of cell lines stably expressing viral sequences from chromosomally integrated cDNA (Figure 1). This strategy has proven useful, e.g., for the study of hepatitis B virus where the HepG2-2.2.15 [7] and, more recently, the HepG2-4A5 [8] cell lines have significantly contributed to the understanding of the viral life cycle and the evaluation of antiviral agents. However, for unknown reasons that may include transcriptional *trans*-suppression of certain promoters [9, 10], hypermethylation of the transgene [11], or toxicity of viral gene products, it has been difficult to date to establish cell lines constitutively expressing HCV cDNAs at high levels.

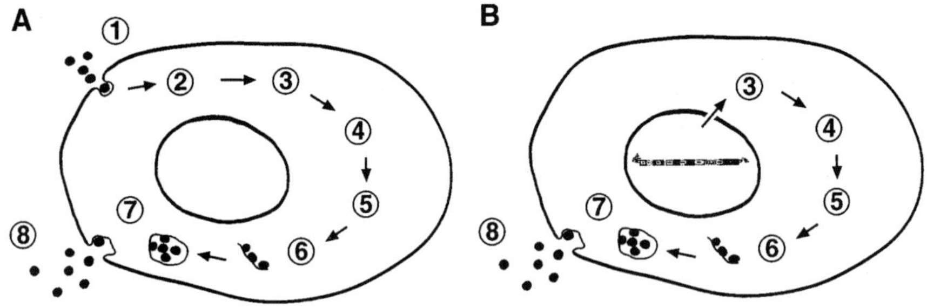

Figure 1. Hypothetical HCV replication cycle and principle of stably transfected cell lines. **(A)** The presumed HCV life cycle includes (1) binding to a cell surface receptor and internalization into the host cell, (2) cytoplasmic release and uncoating of the viral RNA genome, (3) internal ribosome entry site (IRES)-mediated translation, (4) polyprotein processing by cellular and viral proteases, (5) RNA replication, (6) packaging and assembly, (7) virion maturation, and (8) release from the host cell. **(B)** In stably transfected cell lines viral sequences are expressed from chromosomally integrated cDNA.

Cell lines that allow regulated expression of HCV proteins

By the use of a gene expression system that is based on regulatory elements of the tetracycline-resistance operon of *Escherichia coli*, we have over the past years established a comprehensive panel of continuous human cell lines that allow the inducible expression of HCV structural and nonstructural proteins [12-15]. Since the initial description by Gossen and Bujard [16] the tetracycline-regulated gene expression system, schematically illustrated in Figure 2, has been successfully applied to the study of gene function and regulation both *in vitro* and *in vivo* [17, 18]. Inducible cell lines were generated by two successive transfection and selection steps. A founder cell line constitutively expressing the tetracycline-controlled transactivator (tTA) was established first, followed by stable transfection of the cDNA constructs, shown in Figure 3, under the transcriptional control of a tTA-dependent promotor. The U-2 OS human osteosarcoma-derived founder cell line UTA-6 [19] was our preferred cellular background, because these cells display a relatively well-preserved architecture and

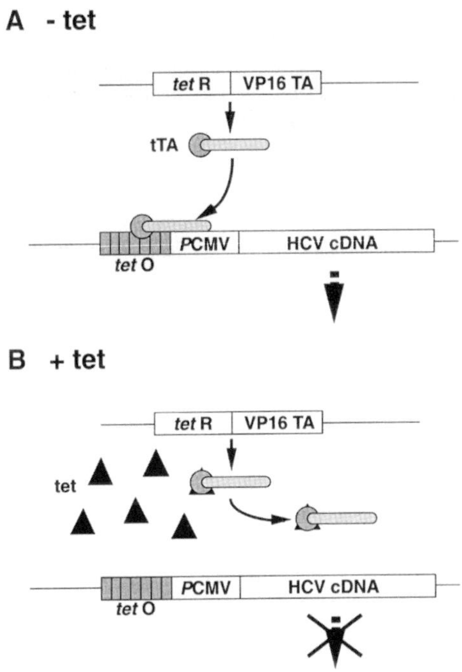

Figure 2. Tetracycline-regulated gene expression system. The system consists of a tetracycline-controlled transactivator (tTA), which is composed of the tetracycline repressor (*tet* R) fused to the activating domain of VP16 of herpex simplex virus, and of a tTA-dependent promoter, which is composed of a minimal sequence derived from the cytomegalovirus intermediate early promoter (CMV P) combined with heptameric tetracycline operator (*tet* O) sequences. **(A)** The tTA-dependent promoter is virtually silent in many cell types in the presence of low concentrations of tetracycline (tet), which prevents the tTA from binding to *tet* O sequences. **(B)** In the absence of tetracycline, the tTA binds to the *tet* O sequences to activate transcription from the minimal promoter.

fine morphology which facilitates studies on the subcellular localization of viral gene products. In addition, important signaling pathways, including interferon-α (IFN-α)-induced activation of the Jak-STAT pathway [20], tumor suppressor (wild-type *p53* and *Rb* genes) and apoptotic functions [19] as well as major histocompatibility complex (MHC) class I antigen processing and presentation pathways [21] were found to be functional in U-2 OS cells. Inducible cell lines were characterized in detail and maintained in continuous culture for at least 12 (in some cases >36) months and after more than 50 passages with stable characteristics and without loss of tightly regulated gene expression. Individual clones of a given cell line contained different numbers of HCV transgenes chromosomally integrated in a head-to-tail fashion. HCV-specific transcripts of the expected length were inducibly expressed upon tetracycline withdrawal. The size and characteristics of HCV structural and nonstructural proteins produced in this expression system were consistent with data from cell-free and transient cellular

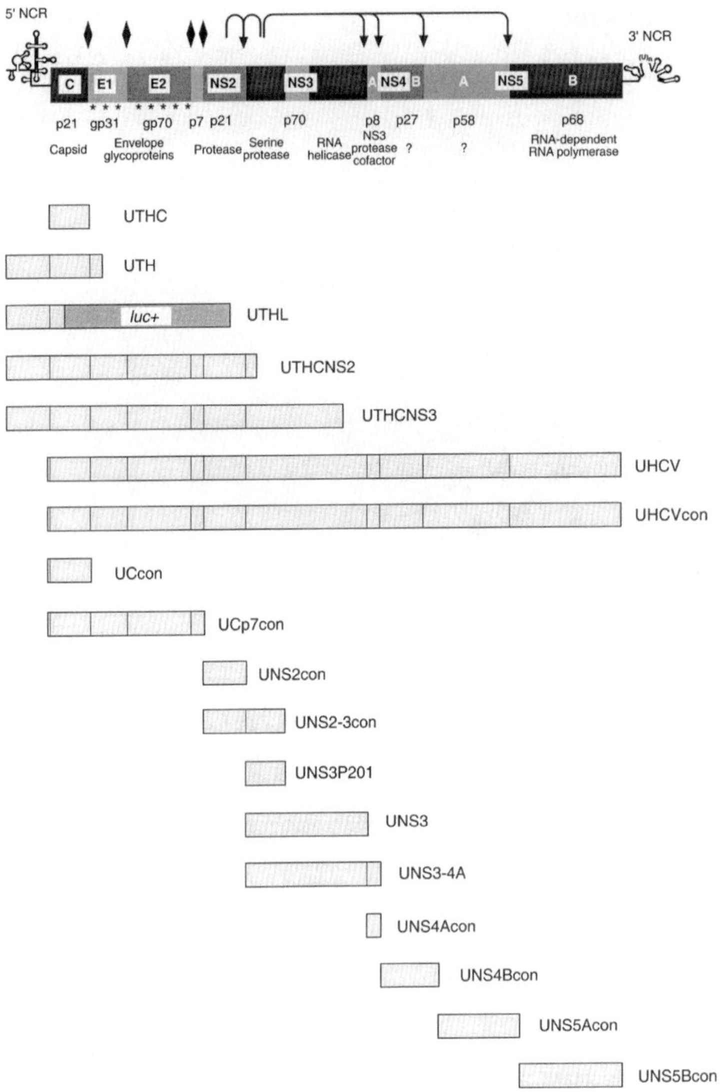

Figure 3. Cell lines that allow the regulated expression of HCV proteins. The genetic organization and polyprotein processing of HCV are depicted at the top. Postulated RNA secondary structures in the 5' and 3' NCRs are schematically illustrated based on published studies (35-37). Asterisks in the E1 and E2 region indicate glycosylation of the envelope proteins. Diamonds denote cleavages of the HCV polyprotein precursor by the endoplasmic reticulum signal peptidase and arrows indicate cleavages by HCV NS2-3 and NS3 proteases. The cell lines UTHC (D.M. and H.E.B., unpublished data), UTH (12), UTHL (12), UTHNCS2 (D.M. and H.E.B., unpublished data), and UTHCNS3 (13) were derived from a genotype 1b cDNA, termed TH (13). UHCV (14), UNS3P201, UNS3, and UNS3-4A (15) cell lines were derived from a prototype HCV H cDNA (genotype 1a) (22). The second-generation UHCVcon cell line and the cell lines UCcon, UCp7con, UNS2con, UNS2-3con, UNS4Acon, UNS4Bcon, UNS5Acon, and UNS5Bcon (D.M., C.M.R., and H.E.B., unpublished data) were derived from a functional HCV H consensus cDNA (38).

overexpression systems [1, 3, 22, 23], indicating that the cellular and viral proteolytic machineries and posttranslational modification pathways were fully functional in these cells (Figure 4). In addition, immunoprecipitation experiments with conformation-sensitive monoclonal antibodies indicated that native envelope glycoprotein complexes were formed in these cells [24].

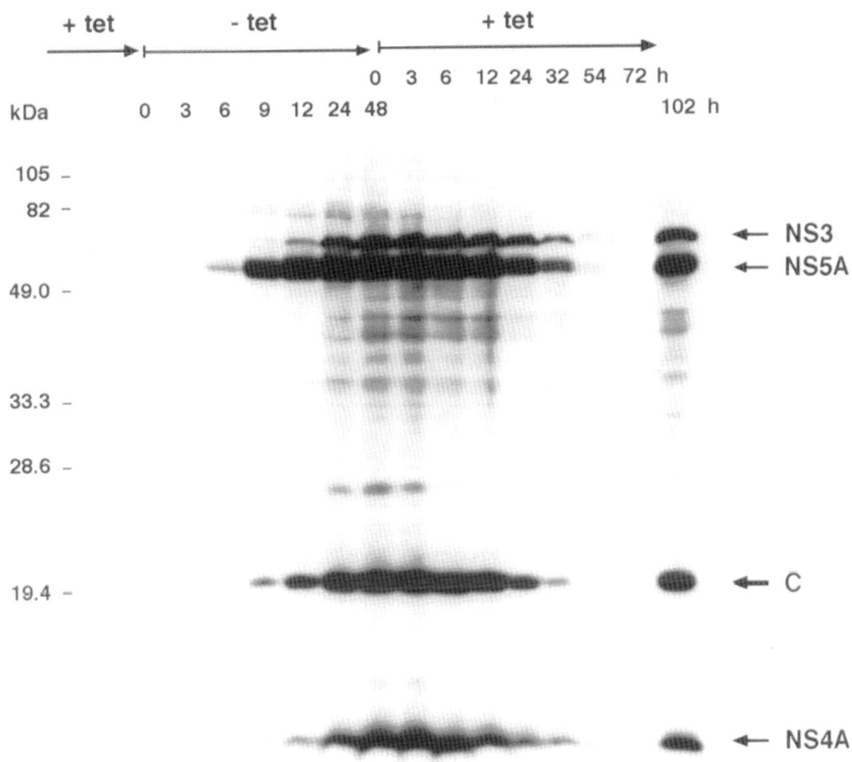

Figure 4. Tightly regulated expression of HCV proteins in UHCV cells [14]. UHCV cells were cultured in the presence of tetracycline until time point 0, when tetracycline was withdrawn from the medium. Subsequently, cells were harvested at the times indicated on top. After 48 h tetracycline was re-added to the medium. In the last lane cells were derepressed for 102 hours. Protein (60 μg per lane) was separated by 12% SDS-PAGE and analyzed by immunoblot with a pool of monoclonal antibodies against core, NS3, NS4A, and NS5A.

Carefully selected clones possessed an induction capacity of more than 1000-fold [12]. More importantly, HCV gene expression could not only be switched on and off, but the steady state expression level could be regulated over a broad range by the concentration of tetracycline in the culture medium [13, 14]. This unique feature may allow for the verification of structural and functional properties of HCV proteins not only at highly overexpressed levels, but also at low levels that may more closely reflect natural HCV infection.

Viral life cycle

Cell lines that allow the regulated expression of HCV proteins may be useful to study selected aspects of the viral life cycle, including polyprotein processing, interactions of viral proteins with each other and with cellular proteins and pathways, and, possibly, the requirements for HCV morphogenesis, in a well-defined and highly reproducible cellular context. In this regard, we found, e.g., that the 54 amino acid polypeptide cofactor NS4A profoundly influenced the subcellular localization, stability, and *trans*-cleavage competence of the HCV NS3-4A complex [15] (Figure 5). These and other recent observations [25, 26] demonstrate the importance of studying HCV proteins in the context of the entire polyprotein. However, the current generation of inducible cell lines, designed to be handled under P1 or P2 (S1 or S2) biosafety conditions, does not allow the study of HCV RNA replication and will not produce infectious virus.

Virus-host interactions

The tetracycline-regulated gene expression system may be particularly suited to study virus-host interactions. In this context, we found that expression of HCV proteins in UHCV cells inhibited IFN-α–induced signal transduction through the Jak-STAT pathway [20] (Figure 6). Inhibition occurred downstream of STAT tyrosine phosphorylation and resulted in an impaired upregulation of IFN target genes. Interference of HCV with IFN signaling could contribute to the resistance to IFN-α therapy observed in the majority of patients and may represent a general escape strategy of HCV contributing to viral persistence and pathogenesis of chronic liver disease.

The HCV nonstructural protein NS5A [27, 28] and the envelope glycoprotein E2 [29] have recently been reported to interfere with the activity of the double-stranded RNA-activated protein kinase (PKR). Interestingly, expression of HCV proteins in UHCV cells in the context of the entire polyprotein interfered with the antiviral action of IFN-α, however, independently from PKR-mediated control of protein synthesis [30].

Humoral and cellular immune response

Interactions of HCV with MHC class I processing and presentation pathways as a potential mechanism of immune evasion have been difficult to investigate due to the lack of a suitable cell culture system [31]. In this context, HLA-A2-positive U-2 OS-derived cell lines expressing HCV proteins in a tetracycline-regulated manner were found to efficiently process and present endogenously synthesized viral proteins *via* MHC class I [21] (Figure 7). The use of tetracycline-regulated cell lines as target cells

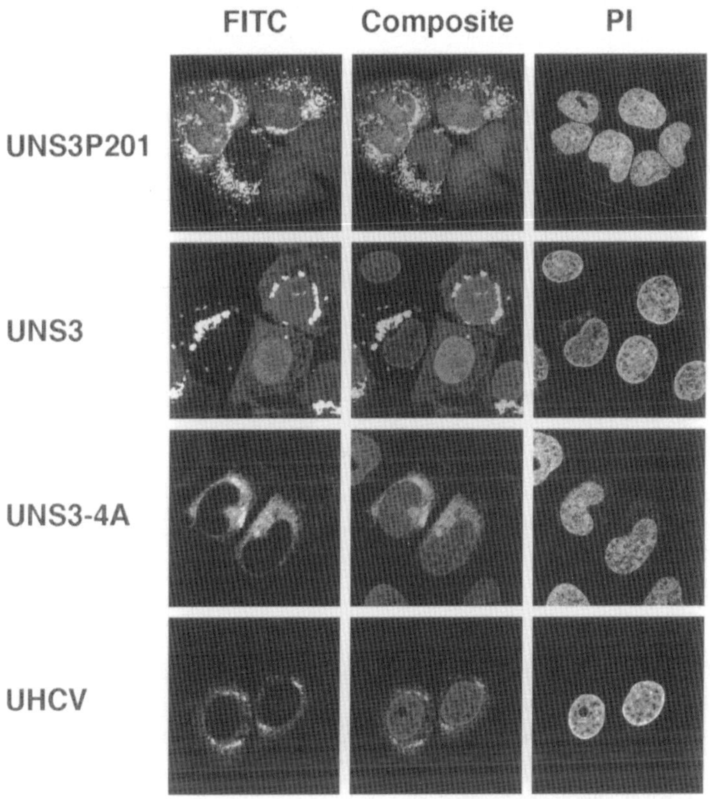

Figure 5. Subcellular localization of the HCV NS3-4A complex. UNS3P201, UNS3, UNS3-4A, and UHCV cells were cultured for 24 h in the absence of tetracycline and subsequently processed for confocal laser scanning microscopy using a monoclonal antibody directed against the NS3 serine protease domain. Cells were counterstained with propidium iodide (PI) to visualize nuclei. Horizontal sections taken through the center of the nuclei are shown. Images recorded in green (FITC) and red (PI) channels are presented separately on the left and on the right, respectively, and composite images are shown in the middle. Adapted from [15] with permission of the American Society for Microbiology.

for HCV-specific human CTL will allow us to analyze potential interactions between viral proteins and the MHC class I processing and presentation pathways, to identify novel and genuinely immunodominant CTL epitopes in an unbiased fashion, and to isolate naturally processed MHC class I ligands. Such studies may ultimately lead to the development of novel immunotherapeutic strategies against HCV infection.

Apart from studies of the cellular immune response, immunofluorescence analyses with sera from HCV-infected patients suggested that cell lines inducibly expressing viral proteins may be used as highly sensitive and specific tools for the immunodiagnosis of

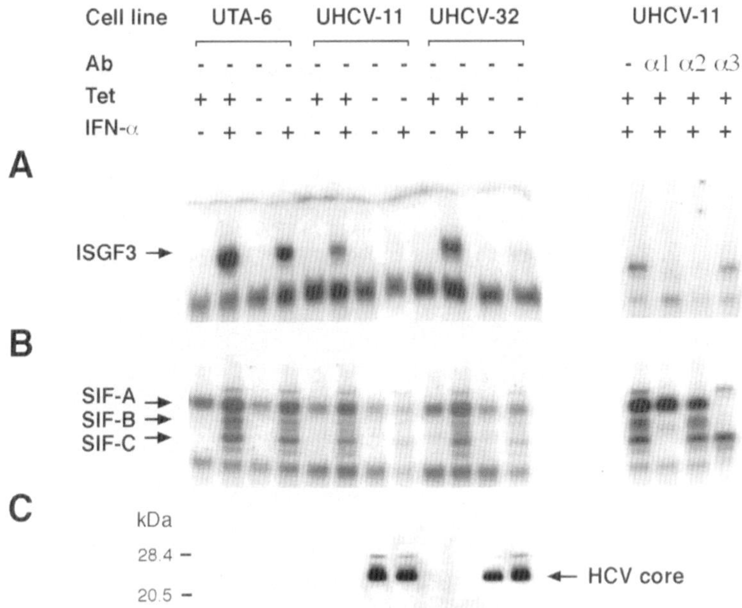

Figure 6. Expression of HCV proteins in UHCV cells inhibits IFN-α-induced signal transduction through the Jak-STAT pathway. UTA-6 founder cells and UHCV-11 and UHCV-32 cells, which inducibly express the entire HCV open reading frame, were cultured in the presence or absence of tetracycline, as indicated. Cells were then either left untreated or stimulated with 500 U/ml IFN-α for 30 min. **(A)** Electrophoretic mobility shift assay with nuclear extracts and the interferon stimulated response element (ISRE) oligonucleotide probe. The position of interferon stimulated gene factor 3 (ISGF3) is indicated by an arrow. In cells expressing HCV proteins, the induction of ISGF3 by IFN-α is inhibited. Antibodies to stat1 (α1) and Stat2 (α2) interfere with ISGF3, resulting in the disappearance of the gel shift signals. Stat3 specific serum (α3) has no effect. **(B)** The same extracts were tested with an m67 oligonucleotide probe. The position of serum inducible factor A (SIF-A), SIF-B and SIF-C are indicated. IFN-α-induced formation of Stat1 and Stat3 complexes is impaired in cells expressing viral proteins. Antiserum to Stat1 supershifts SIF-B and SIF-C. Antiserum to Stat3 supershifts SIF-A and SIF-B. **(C)** Western blot with a monoclonal antibody against the HCV core protein with the corresponding cytoplasmic extracts. Viral proteins are expressed only in UHCV-11 and UHCV-32 cells that were cultured in the absence of tetracycline. Molecular weight markers in kDa are indicated on the left. Adapted from [20] with permission of the American Society for Microbiology.

HCV infection [D.M. and H.E.B., unpublished data].

Novel antiviral strategies

The cell lines described here should allow the evaluation of novel antiviral strategies, particularly those targeting viral gene expression and polyprotein processing. The proteolytic

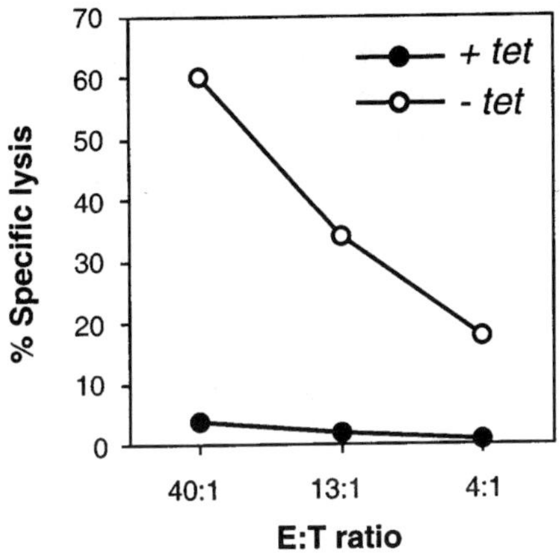

Figure 7. HLA-A2-restricted, HCV-specific human CTL lines recognize HCV proteins endogenously processed in U-2 OS-derived inducible cell lines (21). UNS3-4A cells were cultured in the presence (open circles) or absence (filled circles) of tetracycline and subjected to a ^{51}Cr-release assay with a human CTL line specific for HCV amino acid positions 1073-1081. E:T ratio, effector to target-cell ratio.

events mediated by the NS3 serine protease are essential for viral replication *in vivo* [32]. This biochemically well-characterized viral enzyme, therefore, has become a major target for the development of novel antiviral agents [33, 34]. UHCV cells will be a unique tool to evaluate candidate inhibitor compounds of the NS3 serine protease. Also, nucleic acid-based antiviral strategies such as antisense oligodeoxynucleotides have successfully been evaluated in this system [12].

Conclusions

In conclusion, we have established and characterized a comprehensive panel of continuous human cell lines allowing the tightly regulated expression of HCV structural and nonstructural proteins. The cellular and viral proteolytic machineries and post-translational modification pathways were found to be fully functional in these cell lines. These cell lines represent a unique model system to study structural and functional properties of HCV proteins, their interactions with cellular proteins and pathways, and, possibly, the requirements for viral morphogenesis. In addition, these cell lines should prove useful for the evaluation of novel antiviral strategies against HCV in a well-defined and highly reproducible cellular context.

Acknowledgments

This work was supported by grants Mo 799/1-1 and 799/1-2 from the Deutsche

Forschungsgemeinschaft to D.M. and H.E.B., grant KFS 922-09-1999 from the Swiss Cancer League and grant 32-54973.98 from the Swiss National Science Foundation to M.H.H., and grant 32-59564.99 from the Swiss National Science Foundation to A.C. C.M.R. was supported by National Institutes of Health grants from the U.S. Public Health Service (NCI and NIAID) and the Center for the Study of Hepatitis C.

Note added in proof

UNS4Bcon, and UHCVcon cell lines (Figure 3) are now described in detail in refs. 39 and 40.

References

1. Bartenschlager R and Lohmann V. Replication of hepatitis C virus. *Journal of General Virology* 2000;**81**:1631-1648.
2. Kato N and Shimotohno K. Systems to culture hepatitis C virus. *Current Topics in Microbiology and Immunology* 2000;242:261-278.
3. Reed KE and Rice CM. Overview of hepatitis C virus genome structure, polyprotein processing, and protein properties. *Current Topics in Microbiology and Immunology* 2000;242:55-84.
4. Mizuno M, Yamada G, Tanaka T, Shimotohno K, Takatani M and Tsuji T. Virion-like structures in HeLa cells transfected with the full-length sequence of the hepatitis C virus genome. *Gastroenterology* 1995;109:1933-1940.
5. Yoo BJ, Selby MJ, Choe J, Suh BS, Choi SH, Joh JS, Nuovo GJ, Lee H-S, Houghton M and Han JH. Transfection of a differentiated human hepatoma cell line (Huh7) with *in vitro*-transcribed hepatitis C virus (HCV) RNA and establishment of a long-term culture persistently infected with HCV. *Journal of Virology* 1995;69:32-38.
6. Lohmann V, Körner F, Koch J-O, Herian U, Theilmann L and Bartenschlager R. Replication of subgenomic hepatitis C virus RNAs in a hepatoma cell line. *Science* 1999;285:110-113.
7. Sells M, Chen M-L and Acs G. Production of hepatitis B virus particles in HepG2 cells transfected with cloned hepatitis B virus DNA. *Proceedings of the National Academy of Sciences of the USA* 1987;84:1005-1009.
8. Weiss L, Kekulé A, Jakubowski U, Bürgelt E and Hofschneider PH. The HBV-producing cell line HepG2-4A5: a new *in vitro* system for studying the regulation of HBV replication and for screening anti-hepatitis B virus drugs. *Virology* 1996;216:214-218.
9. Kim DW, Suzuki R, Harada T, Saito I and Miyamura T. *Trans*-suppression of gene expression by hepatitis C viral core protein. *Japanese Journal of Medical Sciences and Biology* 1994;47:211-220.
10. Ray RB, Steele R, Meyer K and Ray R. Transcriptional repression of p53 promoter by hepatitis C virus core protein. *Journal of Biological Chemistry* 1997;272:10983-10986.
11. Kato T, Ahmed M, Yamamoto T, Takahashi H, Oohara M, Ikeda T, Aida Y, Katsuki M, Arakawa Y, Shikata T and Esumi M. Inactivation of hepatitis C virus cDNA transgene by hypermethylation in transgenic mice. *Archives of Virology* 1996;141:951-958.
12. Moradpour D, Englert C, Wakita T and Wands JR. Characterization of cell lines allowing tightly regulated expression of hepatitis C virus core protein. *Virology* 1996;222:51-63.

13. Moradpour D, Wakita T, Wands JR and Blum HE. Tightly regulated expression of the entire hepatitis C virus structural region in continuous human cell lines. *Biochemical and Biophysical Research Communications* 1998;246:920-924.
14. Moradpour D, Kary P, Rice CM and Blum HE. Continuous human cell lines inducibly expressing hepatitis C virus structural and nonstructural proteins. *Hepatology* 1998;28:192-201.
15. Wölk B, Sansonno D, Kräusslich H-G, Dammacco F, Rice CM, Blum HE and Moradpour D. Subcellular localization, stability and *trans*-cleavage competence of the hepatitis C virus NS3-NS4A complex expressed in tetracycline-regulated cell lines. *Journal of Virology* 2000;74:2293-2304.
16. Gossen M and Bujard H. Tight control of gene expression in mammalian cells by tetracycline-responsive promoters. *Proceedings of the National Academy of Sciences of the USA* 1992;89:5547-5551.
17. Shockett PE and Schatz DG. Diverse strategies for tetracycline-regulated inducible gene expression. *Proceedings of the National Academy of Sciences of the USA* 1996;93:5173-5176.
18. Blau HM and Rossi FM. Tet B or not tet B: advances in tetracycline-inducible gene expression. *Proceedings of the National Academy of Sciences of the USA* 1999;96:797-799.
19. Englert C, Hou X, Maheswaran S, Bennett P, Ngwu C, Re GG, Garvin AJ, Rosner MR and Haber DA. WT1 suppresses synthesis of the epidermal growth factor receptor and induces apoptosis. *EMBO Journal* 1995;14:4662-4675.
20. Heim MH, Moradpour D and Blum HE. Expression of hepatitis C virus proteins inhibits signal transduction through the Jak-STAT pathway. *Journal of Virology* 1999;73:8469-8475.
21. Moradpour D, Grabscheid B, Kammer A, Schmidtke G, Groettrup M, Blum HE and Cerny A. Expression of hepatitis C virus proteins does not interfere with major histocompatibility complex class I processing and presentation *in vitro*. Hepatology 2001; 33: 1282-1287.
22. Grakoui A, Wychowski C, Lin C, Feinstone SM and Rice CM. Expression and identification of hepatitis C virus polyprotein cleavage products. *Journal of Virology* 1993;67:1385-1395.
23. Shimotohno K, Tanji Y, Hirowatari Y, Komoda Y, Kato N and Hijikata M. Processing of the hepatitis C virus precursor protein. *Journal of Hepatology* 1995;22 (Suppl 1):87-92.
24. Duvet S, Pillez A, Cocquerel L, Cacan R, Verbert A, Moradpour D, Wychowski C and Dubuisson J. Hepatitis C virus glycoprotein complex localization in the endoplasmic reticulum involves a determinant for retention and not retrieval. *Journal of Biological Chemistry* 1998;273:32088-32095.
25. Koch JO and Bartenschlager R. Modulation of hepatitis C virus NS5A hyperphosphorylation by nonstructural proteins NS3, NS4A, and NS4B. *Journal of Virology* 1999;73:7138-7146.
26. Neddermann P, Clementi A and De Francesco R. Hyperphosphorylation of the hepatitis C virus NS5A protein requires an active NS3 protease, NS4A, NS4B, and NS5A encoded on the same polyprotein. *Journal of Virology* 1999;73:9984-9991.
27. Gale M, Jr, Korth MJ, Tang NM, Tan S-L, Hopkins DA, Dever TE, Polyak SJ, Gretch DR and Katze MG. Evidence that hepatitis C virus resistance to interferon is mediated through repression of the PKR protein kinase by the nonstructural 5A protein. *Virology* 1997;230:217-227.
28. Gale M, Jr., Blakely CM, Kwieciszewski B, Tan SL, Dossett M, Tang NM, Korth MJ, Polyak SJ, Gretch DR and Katze MG. Control of PKR protein kinase by hepatitis C virus nonstructural 5A protein: molecular mechanisms of kinase regulation. *Molecular Cell Biology* 1998;18:5208-18.
29. Taylor DR, Shi ST, Romano PR, Barber GN and Lai MMC. Inhibition of the interferon-inducible protein kinase PKR by HCV E2 protein. *Science* 1999;285:107-110.
30. François C, Duverlie G, Rebouillat D, Khorsi H, Castelain S, Blum HE, Gatignol A, Wychowski C, Moradpour D and Meurs EF. Expression of hepatitis C virus proteins interferes with the antiviral action of interferon independently of the PKR-mediated control of protein synthesis. *Journal of Virology*

2000;74:5587-5596.

31. Cerny A and Chisari FV. Pathogenesis of chronic hepatitis C: immunological features of hepatic injury and viral persistence. *Hepatology* 1999;30:595-601.
32. Kolykhalov AA, Mihalik K, Feinstone SM and Rice CM. Hepatitis C virus-encoded enzymatic activities and conserved RNA elements in the 3' nontranslated region are essential for virus replication *in vivo*. *Journal of Virology* 2000;74:2046-2051.
33. Yao N, Reichert P, Taremi SS, Prosise WW and Weber PC. Molecular views of viral polyprotein processing revealed by the crystal structure of the hepatitis C virus bifunctional protease-helicase. *Structure* 1999;7:1353-1363.
34. Dymock BW, Jones PS and Wilson FX. Novel approaches to the treatment of hepatitis C virus infection. *Antiviral Chemistry and Chemotherapy* 2000;11:79-96.
35. Honda M, Brown EA and Lemon SM. Stability of a stem-loop involving the initiator AUG controls the efficiency of internal initiation of translation on hepatitis C virus RNA. *RNA* 1996;2:955-968.
36. Kolykhalov AA, Feinstone SM and Rice CM. Identification of a highly conserved sequence element at the 3' terminus of hepatitis C virus genome RNA. *Journal of Virology* 1996;70:3363-3371.
37. Blight KJ and Rice CM. Secondary structure determination of the conserved 98-base sequence at the 3' terminus of hepatitis C virus genome RNA. *Journal of Virology* 1997;71:7345-7352.
38. Kolykhalov AA, Agapov EV, Blight KJ, Mihalik K, Feinstone SM and Rice CM. Transmission of hepatitis C by intrahepatic inoculation with transcribed RNA. *Science* 1997;277:570-574.
39. Hügle T, Fehrmann F, Bieck E, Kohara M, Kräusslich H-G, Rice CM, Blum HE, and Moradpour D. The hepatitis C virus nonconstructural protein 4B is an integral endoplasmic reticulum membrane protein. Virology 2001;284:70-81.
40. Schmidt-Mende J, Bieck E, Hügle T, Penin F, Rice CM, Blum HE, and Moradpour D. Determinants for membrane association of the hepatitis C virus RNA-dependent RNA polymerase. J Biol Chem 2001;276:44052-44063.

Novel hepatitis C virus-positive cell line derived from a chimpanzee with chronic HCV infection

BORISLAVA G. PAVLOVA[1,2],
ZSUZSA SCHAFF [3] and GERALD EDER[1]

[1] *Hans Popper Primate Center, Orth/Donau, Austria*
[2] *Ludwig Boltzmann Institute for Leukemia Research and Hematology, Vienna, Austria*
[3] *Semmelweis University, 2nd Institute of Pathology, Budapest, Hungary*

Introduction

The high genetic variability and mutation rate of hepatitis C virus (HCV) and controversies in providing clear evidence of extrahepatic viral reservoirs have hindered the development of therapeutic approaches and vaccine [1-6]. An important issue regarding the pathogenesis of HCV-associated diseases and development of antiviral drugs is to determine the strategy of virus infection, production, sequence mutation and target cell permissiveness. To this end, establishment of *in vitro* cell lines is needed. Culture systems for HCV propagation have been developed from primary hepatocyte cultures, hepatic cell lines and lymphoid cell lines, but the long-term observation of viral growth, persistence and replication remains an unresolved issue [7-11].

Identification of uterine mucosal tissue as a target for HCV

In order to identify new extrahepatic sites capable of supporting HCV replication and permissiveness, we performed an *in situ* RT-PCR analysis for detection of virus presence in uterine mucosal tissue spontaneously excreted during the menstrual cycle of two female chimpanzees (*Pan troglodytes*): E4 with chronic HCV infection after inoculation with a coagulation factor VIII concentrate from an HCV-positive plasma pool including genotypes 1a1b2a2b, and F13 noninfected (negative control) [12-15]. Amplified HCV cDNA was found in the endometrial mucosal cells as well as in the hepatocytes of the liver samples obtained from the E4 chimpanzee. The location of the signals was predominantly in the cell cytoplasm, but some single cells showed whole staining (Figure 1).

Frontiers in Viral Hepatitis Ed. by RF Schinazi, J-P Sommadossi and CM Rice. 187 — 196

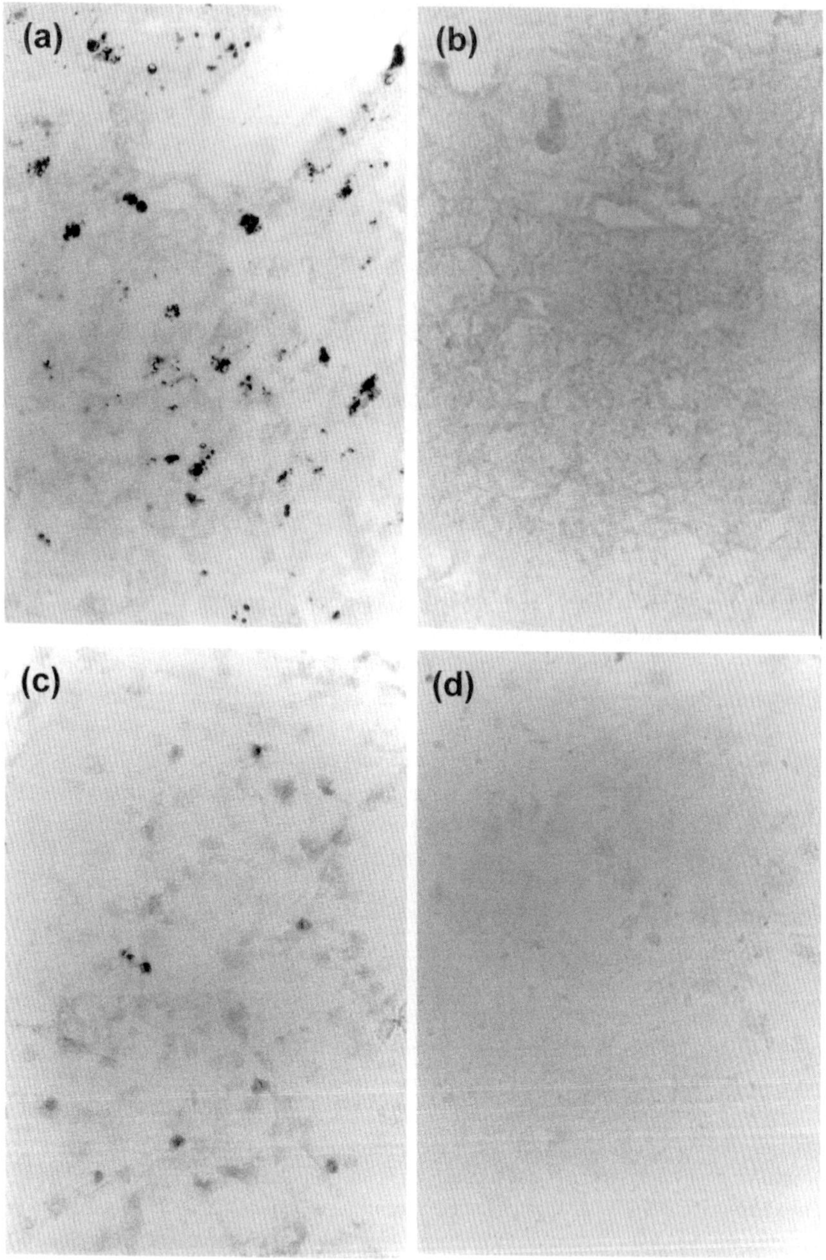

Figure 1. *In situ* HCV RT-PCR with primer for the 5'UTR region of liver and uterine mucosal tissue derived from E4 chronically infected chimpanzee and F13 negative control animal. Amplification of viral cDNA was performed using Dig-labeled nucleotides. Strong positive signals in single cells of both E4 liver (A) and E4 mucosal (C) tissue. No signals were seen in the liver (B) and mucosal (D) samples derived from F13.

Establishment of an endometrial cell line from HCV-positive uterine mucosal tissue

In order to investigate the endometrial cell population as a possible virus reservoir, we set up long-term cultures with mononuclear cells derived from the HCV cDNA-positive uterine mucosal tissue of the E4 chimpanzee and from the HCV negative tissue of the F13 (noninfected) chimpanzee. After one to two months, the fibroblastic cells from the highly confluent areas exhibited a morphology consistent with that of endothelial-like cells (Figure 2). Immunophenotyping of the cultured cells showed a cytokeratin^{neg}/vimentin^{pos} profile, confirming their mesenchymal origin. (Figure 3A, B) [16].

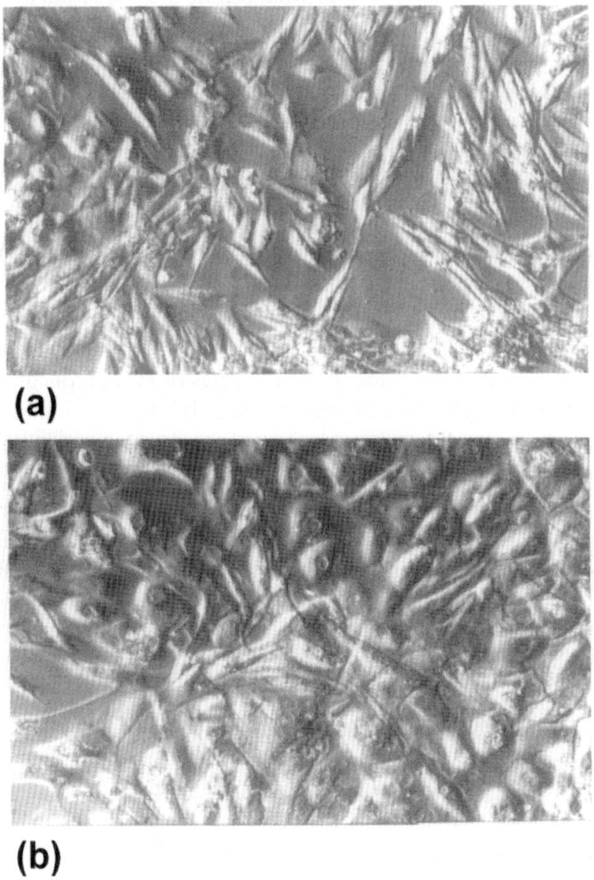

Figure 2. Phase-contrast examination of E4 endometrial cells during *in vitro* cultivation and differentiation. The cultures were initiated with 2x10^7 endometrial cells (separated on a Ficoll-Hypaque gradient) in 10 ml Iscove's modified Dulbecco's medium with 10% horse serum, 10% fetal calf serum, 10-6 mol/L hydrocortisone, 100U/ml penicillin and 100 μg/ml streptomycin, incubated at 37°C (5% CO_2, 100% humidity) and were fed once weekly by replacing 50% of the medium. Switch in cell morphology - from fibroblast-like (A) to endothelial-like (B) phenotype was observed after two months cultivation.

Expression of cell surface CD81 (putative receptor for E2 envelope protein of HCV) was detected in the mucosal tissue and in the cultured cells from both the E4 and F13 chimpanzee (Figure 3C, D) [17, 18].

Cells from the E4 chimpanzee grew in continuous culture without supplementary growth factors for at least 16 months and subsequently became established as a cell line. The F13 cells (from the HCV-negative control animal) started to die after seven months cultivation. Apoptotic cell death was also evaluated on the basis of morphological changes, nuclear DNA fragmentation and high Fas/APO-1 expression.

Detection of HCV-RNA presence and replication in the endometrial cells during cultivation

To analyze the HCV-RNA expression and replication level in the endometrial cells during cultivation, we performed standard nested RT-PCR using primer for the highly conservative 5'UTR region [15]. The level of HCV-RNA in the E4 adherent cells was consistently high and remained constant during cultivation. Amplification of the negative-strand RNA (replication intermediate) was also found to be at a constantly high level in the E4 adherent cell population. In the cell-free supernatant, the level of replicative intermediate appeared to fluctuate, showing transient peaks of detection (Figure 4). Such intermittent detection of HCV genes has been reported both in hepatocyte cultures infected *in vitro* and in chimpanzee and human models, indicating that the E4 cell line closely mimics the intrinsic cycles of HCV replication *in vivo* [7].

The increased viral replication/expression parallel to the inhibited Fas/APO-1 production detected in the E4 culture supernatants could be associated with viral oncogenic activity also responsible for inhibition of the apoptotic mechanism, immortalisation of the E4 cells and establishment of persistent infection. This is consistent with the previously described ability of HCV proteins *in vitro* to transform some cell types to an oncogenic phenotype, to modify the susceptibility of cultured cells to apoptotic signals and to inhibit cisplatin- or c-myc-mediated apoptosis in cell lines [19-23].

Subcellular localization of HCV cDNA

As it was not possible to localize the *in situ* RT-PCR signals — cytoplasmic or nuclear — because of whole staining of some HCV-positive cells, we investigated these reactions by electron microscopy. The amplified Dig-labeled HCV cDNA was identified by binding to anti-Dig Ab and secondary Ab conjugated with gold particles. The intracellular presence of HCV cDNA was visualized by the clustering of gold particles. As with most RNA viruses, cytoplasmic localization along the membrane of the endoplasmic reticulum where virus replication occurred was found in the cultured E4 endometrial cells (Figure 5) as well as in the mucosal tissue [24-26]. No nuclear localization of gold particles was found.

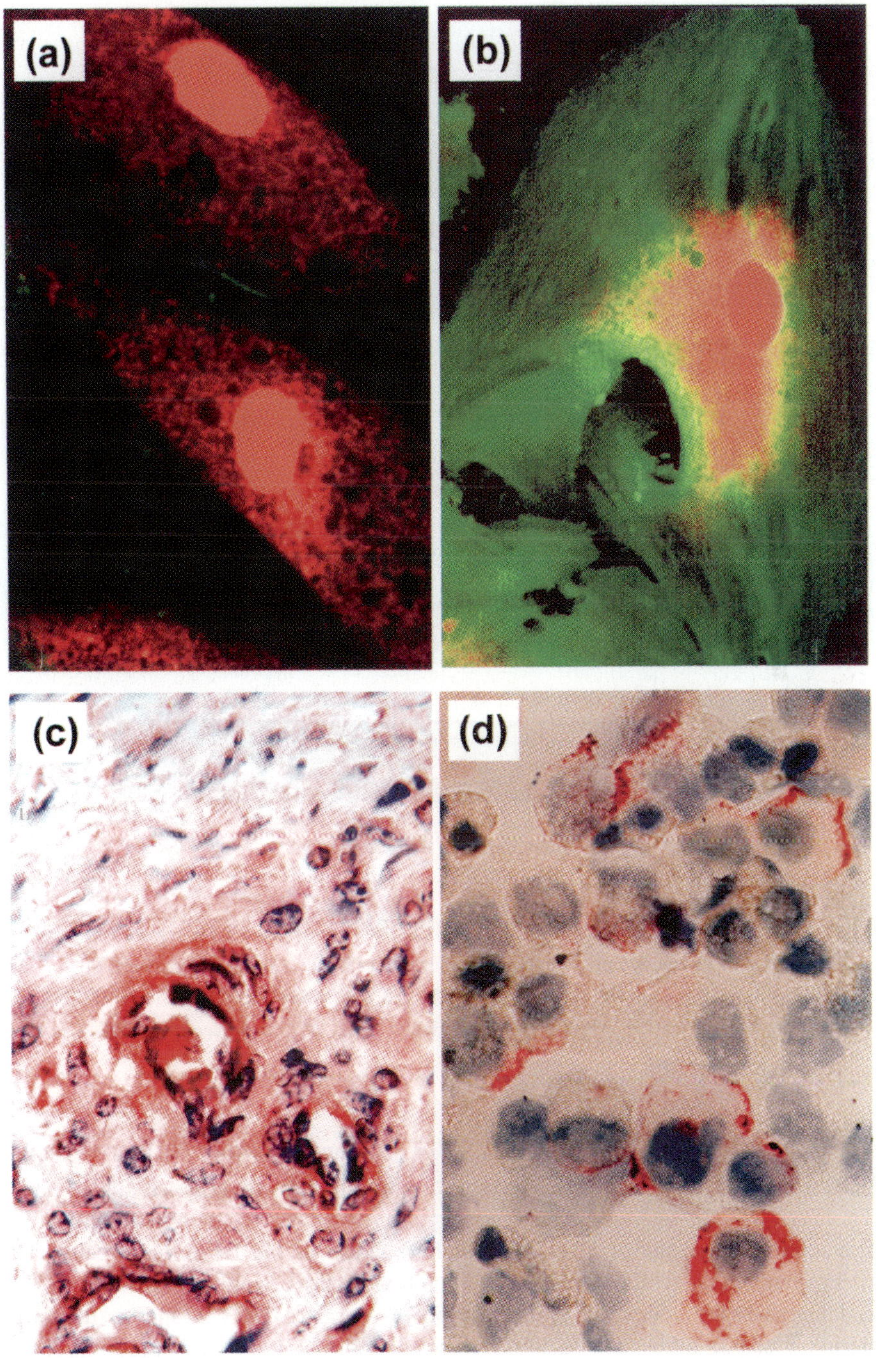

Figure 3. Immunophenotyping of cultured E4 endometrial cells. (A) Staining for cytokeratin-negative reaction, (B) Staining for vimentin-positive reaction - confirmed the mesenchymal origin of the cells, (C) Expression of cell surface CD81 in E4 mucosal tissue, (D) CD81 expression in cultured E4 cells.

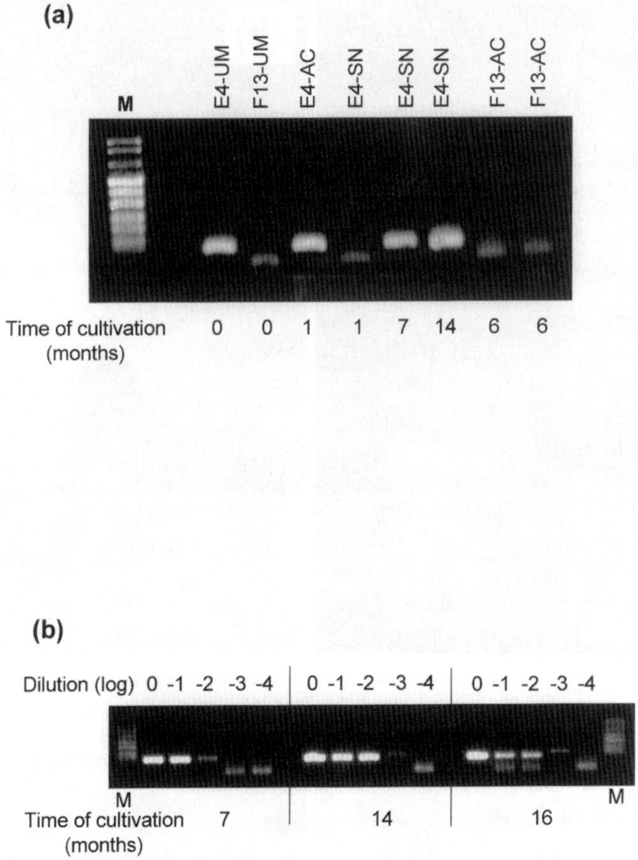

Figure 4. Amplification products of nested RT-PCR with primer for 5'UTR region. (A) Detection of HCV RNA in E4/F13 mucosal tissue, cultured endometrial cells and cell-free supernatants; M, size marker; UM, uterine mucosal tissue; AC, adherent cells; SN, cell free supernatant. (B) Dilution of RNA (log10) isolated from E4 supernatants which showing maximum levels of viral sequences by RT-PCR. Time of cultivation is given in months.

Detection of tissue-specific HCV adaptation and *in vitro* divergence

The sequence analysis of 5'UTR RT-PCR products of the E4 cultured cells showed in the first passages 100% homology, but two to three single nucleotide exchanges in later passages compared to the prototype sequence HCV-1 and to the original uterine mucosal tissue and factor VIII concentrate [27]. The substitutions observed increased to six exchanges in the later passages (14th and 16th months) and remained unchanged in the last passage, which showed that they had not originated from random misincorporation during the PCR.

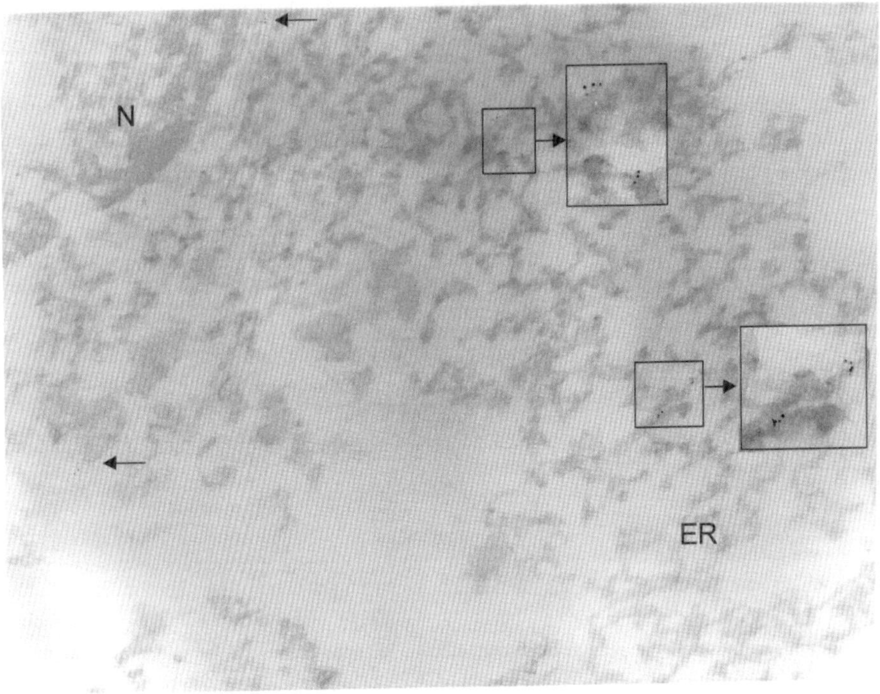

Figure 5. Detection of intracellular presence and localization of HCV cDNA in E4 endometrial cell line using combined *in situ* RT-PCR in suspension and immunogold electron microscopy. Post-*in situ* RT-PCR analysis of intracellular HCV cDNA localization by immunogold electron microscopy showed cytoplasmic accumulation of gold particles (arrows and insets) along the endoplasmic reticulum (not contrasted) (x18000). The insets show higher magnification (x27500) of the regions containing gold particles bound to amplified HCV cDNA. N, nucleus; ER, endoplasmic reticulum.

It was previously observed that in cases of multiple infection, the genotypes identified in the serum of HCV-infected patients may not reflect the genotypes of viral sequences found in the liver or in the peripheral blood cells of the same patients [28, 9]. HCV genotype-specific differences were assessed in different tissues from the E4 chimpanzee, inoculated with two HCV genotypes (1, 2) and four subtypes (1a, b; 2a, b) [30]. The putative HCV-replicative tissue — the liver — expressed the combination of 1b2a2b types, and the mucosal tissue showed a combination of 1b2a types (Figure 6). In both liver and endometrial mucosa, as well as in the cultured E4 endometrial cells, which expressed only the 2a type, the negative replicative HCV strand was found. Serum and mononuclear cells, which were negative for 2a, showed no detectable intermediate replicative strand.

Thus, the presence of type 2a only in tissues and cells containing a replicative virus strand provide evidence for its responsibility for HCV replication. The selection of only one detectable virus type (2a) in the cultured cells, which *in vivo* showed favored tropism to uterine mucosal and liver tissue, might be a result of endometrial cell-specific virus adaptation associated with loss of non-specific types. Similarly, cell tropism differences as an important selection mechanism in the generation of cell- or tissue-specific HCV diversity have been observed [3, 31-33]. Our data support the idea that the host immune pressure is not necessarily involved in genesis of genomic

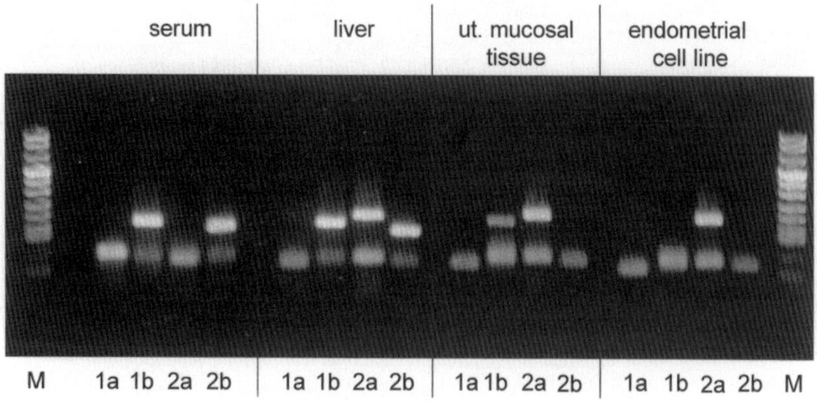

Figure 6. Comparison of the genotype/subtype selection between tissue and serum samples *in vivo* and cultured E4 endometrial cells *in vitro*. Amplification products of nested RT-PCR with primer for core region specific for different virus types (1a1b, 2a2b).

heterogeneity and selection of viral types and subtypes [34].

Concluding remarks

The fact that multipotential cells of mesenchymal origin could be permissive for HCV provides the opportunity to study events associated with viral presence in multiple tissues at various anatomic sites [35]. The capacity of HCV to enter and replicate in immature endometrial cells could also explain the tracking of extrahepatic viral sequences. In conclusion, we believe that this system provides an important tool in understanding the biology of HCV, its life cycle and presence in multiple tissues. This model may be particularly well suited for studying new antiviral agents, because (i) the HCV-positive endometrial cells represent an immortalized, permanent population useful for prolonged drug screens, (ii) the level of viral replication permits easy detection and (iii) the intermittent replication associated with cell-specific virus adaptation mimics the intrinsic replicative cycles and genomic divergence *in vivo*.

References

1. Dusheiko G, Schmilovitz-Weiss H, Brown D, McOmish F, Pong-Lee Y, Sherlock S, McIntire N, Simmons P. Hepatitis C Virus Genotypes. An Investigation of type-specific differences in geographic origin and diseases. *Hepatology* 1994; 19:13-18.
2. Wilson JJ, Polyak SJ, Day TD, Gretch DR. Characterisation of simple and complex hepatitis C virus quasispecies by heteroduplex gel shift analysis: Correlation with nucleotide sequencing. *Journal of General Virology* 1995; 76:1763-1771.
3. Maggi F, Fornai C, Morrica A, Vatteroni ML, Giorgi M, Marchi S, Ciccorossi P. Divergent evolution of hepatitis C virus in liver and peripheral blood mononuclear cells of infected patients. *Journal of Medical Virology* 1999; 57:57-63.
4. Lerat H, Rumin S, Habersetzer F, Berby F, Trabaut MA, Trepo C, Inchauspe G. *In vivo* tropism of hepatitis C virus genomic sequences in hematopoietic cells: Influence of viral load, viral genotype and cell phenotype. *Blood* 1998; 10:3841-3849.
5. Luppi M, Longo G, Ferrari MG, Ferrara L, Marasca R, Barozzi P, Morselli M. Additional neoplasms and HCV infection in low-grade lymphoma of MALT type. *British Journal of Haematology* 1996; 94:373-375.
6. Bukh J, Miller RH, Purcell RH. Genetic heterogeneity of hepatitis C virus: Quasispecies and genotypes. *Seminars in Liver Diseases* 1995; 1:41-63
7. Rumin S, Berthillon P, Tanaka E, Kiyosawa K, Trabaud MA, Bizollon T, Gouillat C. Dynamic analysis of hepatitis C virus replication and quasispecies selection in long-term cultures of adult human hepatocytes infected *in vitro*. *Journal of General Virology* 1999; 80:3007-3018.
8. Iacovacci S, Sarglacomo M, Parolini I, Ponzetto A, Peschle C, Carloni G. Replication and multiplication of hepatitis C virus genome in human foetal liver cells. *Research in Virology* 1993; 144:275-279.
9. Lanford RE, Sureau C, Jacob JR, White R, Fuerst TR. Demonstration of *in vitro* infection of chimpanzee hepatocytes with hepatitis C virus using strand-specific RT/PCR. *Virology* 1994; 202:606-614.
10. Nakajima N, Hijikata M, Yoshikura H, Shimizu YK. Characterisation of long-term cultures of hepatitis C virus. *Journal of Virology* 1996; 70:3325-3329.
11. Shimizu YK, Iwamoto A, Hijikata M, Purcell RH, Yoshiikura H. Evidence for *in vitro* replication of hepatitis C virus genome in a human T cell line. *Proceedings of the National Academy of Sciences, USA* 1992; 89:5477-5481.
12. Nuovo G, Lidonnici K, MacConnell P, Lane B. Intracellular localisation of polymerase chain reaction (PCR)-amplified hepatitis C cDNA. *American Journal of Surgical Pathology* 1993; 17:683-690.
13. Cheng J, Nuovo G. Utility of reverse transcriptase (RT) in situ polymerase chain reaction (PCR) in the diagnosis of viral infections. *Journal of Histotechnology* 1994; 17:247-251.
14. Lau J, Davis G. Detection of hepatitis C virus RNA genome in liver tissue by nonisotopic in situ hybridisation. *Journal of Medical Virology* 1994; 42:268-271.
15. Thaler MM, Park CK, Landers DV, Wara DW, Houghton M, Veereman-Wauters G, Sweet RL, Han JH. Vertical transmission of hepatitis C virus. *Lancet* 1991; 338:17-18.
16. Cordell JL, Falini B, Erber WN, Ghosh AK, Abdulaziz Z, MacDonald S, Pulford KA, Stein H, Mason DY. Immunoenzymatic labeling of monoclonal antibodies using immune complexes of alkaline phosphatase and monoclonal anti-alkaline phosphatase (APAAP complexes). *Journal of Histochemistry and Cytochemistry* 1984; 32:219-229
17. Pileri P, Uematsu Y, Campagnoli S, Galli G, Falugi F, Petracca R, Weiner A, Houghton M, Rosa D, Grandi G, Abrignani S. Binding of hepatitis C virus to CD81. *Science* 1998; 282:938-941.

18. Flint M, Maidens C, Loomis-Price L, Shotton C, Dubuisson J, Monk P, Higinbottom A, Levy S, McKeating JA. Characterisation of hepatitis C virus E2 glycoprotein interaction with a putative cellular receptor, CD81. *Journal of Virology* 1999; 73:6235-6244.
19. Ray RB, Lagging LM, Meyer K, Ray R. Hepatitis C virus core protein cooperates with ras transforms primary rat embryo fibroblasts to tumorigenic phenotype. *Journal of Virology* 1996; 70:4438-4443.
20. Ruggieri A, Harada T, Matsuura Y, Miyamura T. Sensitization to fas-mediated apoptosis by hepatitis C virus core protein. *Virology* 1997; 229:68-76.
21. Ray RB, Meyer K, Ray R. Suppression of apoptotic cell death by hepatitis C virus core protein. *Virology* 1996; 226:176-182.
22. Chang J, Yang SH, Cho YG, Hwang SB, Hahn YS, Sung YC J. Hepatitis C core from two different genotypes has an oncogenic potential but is not sufficient for transforming primary rat embryo fibroblasts in cooperation with the H-ras oncogene. *Journal of Virology* 1998; 72:3060-3065.
23. Ray RB, Lagging LM, Meyer K, Steele R, Ray R. Transcriptional regulation of cellular and viral promoters by the hepatitis C virus core protein. *Virus Research* 1995; 37:209-220.
24. Shimizu YK, Feinstone SM, Kohara M, Purcell RH, Yoshikura H. Hepatitis C virus: detection of intracellular virus particles by electron microscopy. *Hepatology* 1996; 23:205-209.
25. Kim JE, Song WK, Chung KM, Back SH, Jang SK. Subcellular localization of hepatitis C viral proteins in mammalian cells. *Archives of Virology* 1999; 144:329-343.
26. Barba G, Harper F, Harada T, Kohara M, Goulinet S, Matsuura Y, Eder G. *Proceedings of the National Academy of Sciences, USA* 1997; 4:1200-1205.
27. Choo QL, Richman KH, Han JH, Berger K, Lee C, Dong C, Gallegos C. Genetic organisation and diversity of the hepatitis C virus. *Proceedings of the National Academy of Sciences, USA* 1991; 88:2451-2455
28. Shimizu YK, Igarashi H, Kanematu T, Fujiwara K, Wong D, Purcell RH, Yoshikura H. Sequence analysis of the hepatitis C virus genome recovered from serum, liver, and peripheral blood mononuclear cells of infected chimpanzees. *Journal of Virology* 1997; 71:5769-5773.
29. Jarvis JM, Watsoon HJ, McOmish F, Peuthere JF, Ludlam CA, Simmonds P. Frequent reinfection and reactivation of hepatitis C virus genotypes in multitransfused hemophiliacs. *Journal of Infectious Diseases* 1994; 70:1018.
30. Okamoto H, Sugiyama Y, Okada S, Kurai K, Akahane Y, Sugai Y, Tanaka T. Typing hepatitis C virus by polymerase chain reaction with type specific primers: Application to clinical surveys and tracing infectious sources. *Journal of General Virology* 1992; 73:673.
31. Navas S, Martin J, Quiroga JA, Castillo I, Carreno V. Genetic diversity and tissue compartmentalisation of the hepatitis C virus genome in blood mononuclear cells, liver, and serum from chronic hepatitis C patients. *Journal of Virology* 1997; 72:1640-1646.
32. Maggi F, Fornai C, Vatteroni ML, Giorgi M, Morrica A, Pistello M, Cammarota G et al. Differences in hepatitis C virus quasispecies composition between liver, peripheral blood mononuclear cells and plasma. *Journal of General Virology* 1997; 78:1521-1525.
33. Kurosaki M, Enomoto N, Marumo F, Sato C. Evolution and selection of hepatitis C virus variants in patients with chronic hepatitis C. *Virology* 1994; 205:161-169.
34. Weiner AJ, Geysen M, Christopherson C, Hall JE, Mason TJ, Saracco G, Bonino F et al. Evidence for immune selection of hepatitis C virus (HCV) putative envelope glycoprotein variants: potential role in chronic HCV infections. *Proceedings of the National Academy of Sciences, USA* 1992; 89:3468-3472.
35. Pittenger M, Mackay A, Beck S, Jaiswal R, Douglas R, Mosca J, Moorman M et al. Multilineage potential of adult human mesenchymal stem cells. *Science* 1999; 284:143-147.

A transgenic mouse lineage useful for testing antivirals targeting hepatitis B virus

P.L. MARION[1, 2], F.H. SALAZAR[2], K. LIITTSCHWAGER[1], B.B. BORDIER[1], C. SEEGER[3], M.A. WINTERS[2], A.D. COOPER[4] and J.M. CULLEN[5]

[1] *Stanford University, Stanford, CA*
[2] *Hepadnavirus Testing, Inc., Mountain View, CA*
[3] *Fox Chase Cancer Center, Philadelphia, PA*
[4] *Palo Alto Medical Foundation, Palo Alto, CA*
[5] *North Carolina State University, Raleigh, NC*

Abstract

To test novel therapeutics for efficacy against hepatitis B virus (HBV), we have made a lineage of transgenic mice which has serum HBV DNA levels of 10^6 to 10^8 viral genome equivalents/ml. Of 135 offspring derived from FVB mouse embryos injected with HBV DNA constructs similar to those used by Guidotti et al. [1], two produced readily detected viral DNA and HBsAg in their sera. Mice from the lineage producing the highest levels of HBV markers were further developed. Endogenous DNA polymerase activity was present in particles pelleted from serum, and the product of this reaction migrated in agarose gelss like HBV DNA from human serum, indicating that whole virus is present in the mouse serum. HBV replicative intermediates were observed in the liver by Southern blotting. HBV core antigen was detected by immunohistochemistry in the nuclei and the cytoplasm of hepatocytes and the renal tubular epithelial cells of all mice. The antigen was also found in the nuclei of the exocrine pancreatic cells of most mice, and pancreatic islet cells were stained less frequently. HBV surface antigen was detected in the cytoplasm of a minority of hepatocytes only. There was no evidence of inflammation in the liver, kidney, or pancreas in mice less than four months of age. The only lesions seen in mice up to 20 months of age occurred in the liver, but the lesions were similar to those seen in age-matched non-transgenic control mice. In the majority of mice, viral DNA and HBsAg titers of these mice decline slowly (approximately two- to threefold) after one month of age, then appear to stabilize. The effects of two nucleoside analogues, lamivudine and entecavir, provided by R. J. Colonno of Bristol-Myers Squibb, were evaluated. Treatment with 200 mg/kg/day lamivudine or with 2 mg/kg/day entecavir resulted in similar 2.0 $\log_{10}$ drops in serum HBV DNA levels after three weeks of treatment, while treatment with vehicle alone resulted in a 0.7 $\log_{10}$ drop. After a two-week follow-up, viral DNA levels of vehicle- and lamivudine-treated mice increased to 27 and 17% of pretreatment levels, respectively,

Frontiers in Viral Hepatitis Ed. by RF Schinazi, J-P Sommadossi and CM Rice. 197 — 210

while those of the entecavir-treated mice remained at 1% of pretreatment levels. These results indicate that this model system can be used to evaluate the efficacy of inhibitors of viral DNA replication.

Introduction

More than 300 million people worldwide are at high risk of developing chronic liver disease and liver cancer as a result of chronic infection with HBV. There is presently no adequate antiviral treatment for chronic HBV infection. Because of the limited host range of HBV, it has been difficult to find suitable *in vivo* models of infection with which to study the potential of antivirals targeting HBV-specific nucleic acid sequences or amino acid residues, or to study the effect of combining reverse transcriptase (RT) inhibition and specific stimulation of an adequate immune response. While the HBV-related woodchuck, squirrel, and duck viruses exhibit sensitivities to RT inhibitors similar to those of HBV, the components and characteristics of their host immune systems are less characterized than those of more established laboratory animals. Chisari, Guidotti and colleagues [1] have made mouse lineages which express HBV at levels approaching those found in many human carriers. Serum virus is reduced in the 1.3.32 lineage mice treated with lamivudine, a pyrimidine dideoxynucleoside analogue that has been shown to reduce HBV replication in controlled clinical trials, indicating that RT inhibitors are effective in these mice [2].

The development of transgenic mice that express the entire HBV genome also creates an opportunity to study the effects of viral protein expression on hepatocyte health and hepatic carcinogenesis. These lineages can be manipulated to study the immunopathogenesis of hepatic inflammation and hepatocellular carcinoma, including studies using chemical carcinogens, genetically altered mice with increased susceptibility to cancer (i.e., p53 hemizygous knockout mice), or adoptive transfer of immune cells.

We have made an additional transgenic lineage which secretes high and relatively stable levels of HBV viral DNA. The efficacy of lamivudine in reducing levels of viremia was evaluated and compared to that of entecavir, one of a number of compounds currently under investigation for therapeutic use against HBV. Entecavir (BMS-200475) is a cyclopentyl 2'-deoxy-guanosine nucleoside which is in clinical development for treatment of chronic HBV infections. It inhibits HBV replication in 2.2.15 cells [3] and is active against woodchuck hepatitis virus in woodchucks [4] and duck hepatitis B virus (DHBV) in ducks [4a].

Methods

Construction of transgenic mice

A plasmid construct, pTHBV2, was made which included 4.1 kb of HBV DNA, containing the entire ayw genome [5] plus a redundancy for the sequences between 1067 and 1996 (see Figure 1). Embryos of FVB-strain mice were injected with the HBV

DNA excised from pTHBV2 using digestion with HindIII and KpnI, and implanted into pseudopregnant mice of the same strain. Offspring were screened for the presence of HBsAg, then for HBV DNA as described below. Two of 135 offspring, both males, were positive by both criteria and served as founders of two lineages, STC and PAMF. Animal use was in compliance with the Stanford University Institutional Animal Care and Use Committee.

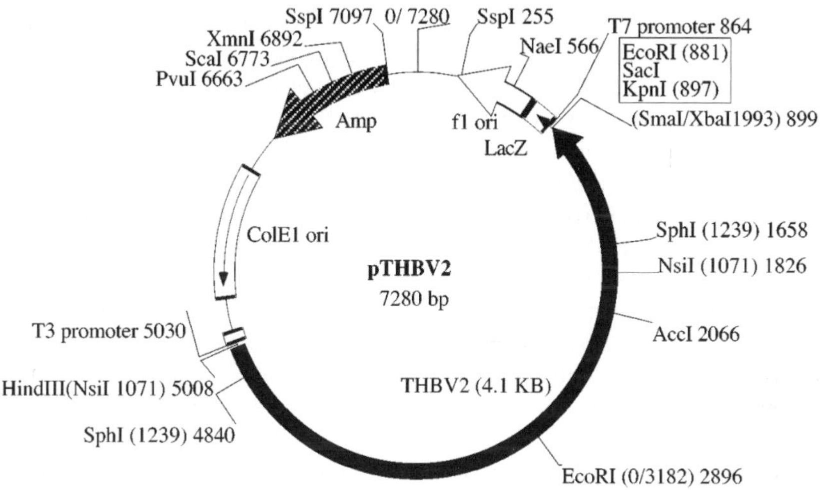

Plasmid name: pTHBV2
Plasmid size: 7280 bp
Constructed by: Kurt Liittschwager
Construction date: June 1996
Comments/References: HBV ayw construct for producing HBV-secreting transgenic mice. 5' HindIII-SphI (5008-4840) is PCR sequence, remaining sequence from pFC80 [genome length SphI fragment (4840-1658) and SphI - XbaI(fill) (1658-899)]. Removed as H indIII-KpnI frag.

Figure 1. pTHBV2 plasmid construct for producing HBV-secreting transgenic mice. HBV DNA sequences are shown as the thick arrow arc and labeled as THBV2 (4.1 KB).

Assays for viral antigens

HBsAg and HBeAg levels in sera were measured using commercial assays (Auszyme Monoclonal and HBe (rDNA) EIA, Abbott Laboratories) after diluting individual sera 20-100 fold in phosphate-buffered saline with 10% fetal calf serum.

HBV DNA quantification and analysis

HBV DNAs were quantified initially by PCR assay using the Roche Amplicor HBV Monitor system generously provided by Roche Diagnostics. Later measurement of HBV DNA levels was by an in-house, semi-quantitative HBV DNA PCR ELISA. In this assay, mouse serum samples were diluted in PBS containing 10% fetal bovine serum and denatured with an equal volume of 0.2 N sodium hydroxide. After incubation at 60°C for 30-60 minutes, the mixture was neutralized with 0.2M Tris-HCl (pH 8.0) and added to a PCR master mix containing buffer, 2.5 mM magnesium chloride, 200 μM dNTP, 2.5 units Taq DNA polymerase (Life Technologies, Gaithersburg, MD), and 30 pmol each of primers HBV-1 (GGA GTG TGG ATT CGC ACT) and biotinylated HBV-2 (TGA GAT CTT CTG CGA CGC) [ref. 6]. Serial 0.5 log dilutions of hepatitis B genome-containing plasmid were amplified in parallel, along with in-house prepared mouse serum standards. The PCR product was then quantified by capturing the product onto avidin-coated 96-well plates, probing with a digoxigenin-labeled HBV oligonucleotide (HBV-3: 5'-TAG AAG AAG AAC TCC CTC GCC TCG CAG ACG-3') followed by a peroxidase-labeled anti-digoxigenin antibody (Boehringer-Mannheim). After reaction with substrate, the optical density (OD) of each well was read. HBV DNA levels were calculated from a standard curve generated using known amounts of HBV DNA determined by methods previously described [7].

Forty-three serum samples were tested in two to four different assays to assess the reproducibility of the in-house HBV DNA assay. Results showed a median 0.17 log difference (mean = 0.23 ± 0.207 log DNA copies/ml, n = 115 comparisons) between replicate evaluations of serum samples. Comparison of the results of the in-house HBV DNA assay with the Roche Amplicor assay is shown in Figure 2. There was a highly significant correlation between the two assays ($r = 0.851$, $p < 0.0001$, $n = 71$).

HBV particles were pelleted from 1 ml of pooled sera from one- to two-month-old STC mice, and the viral DNA radiolabeled using the endogenous DNA polymerase [8], and analyzed by agarose gel electrophoresis. HBV particles pelleted from a pool of human and chimpanzee sera [9] were treated in the same fashion to serve as a control. For Southern blot analysis of replicative DNA forms of HBV, DNA was extracted from viral cores purified from liver homogenates as previously described [10].

Histopathology and Immunohistochemistry

A variety of tissues including liver, kidney, pancreas, spleen, lung, and salivary glands from the mice were fixed in either buffered formalin or zinc formalin overnight at room temperature and were processed routinely into paraffin for histologic review or immunohistochemistry. Sections for histology were stained with hematoxylin and eosin. Immunohistochemical staining for hepatitis B viral antigens was performed on fixed, paraffin-embedded sections of liver and other tissues. A polyclonal rabbit anti-HBcAg antibody (Cortex Biochem, San Leandro, CA) was used as a primary antibody at a 1:200 dilution. Primary antibody binding was detected using a BioGenex Supersensitive Streptavidin peroxidase kit (San Ramon, CA) with goat anti-rabbit antibody following manufacturer's directions with AEC as the chromagen. For detection of HBsAg a

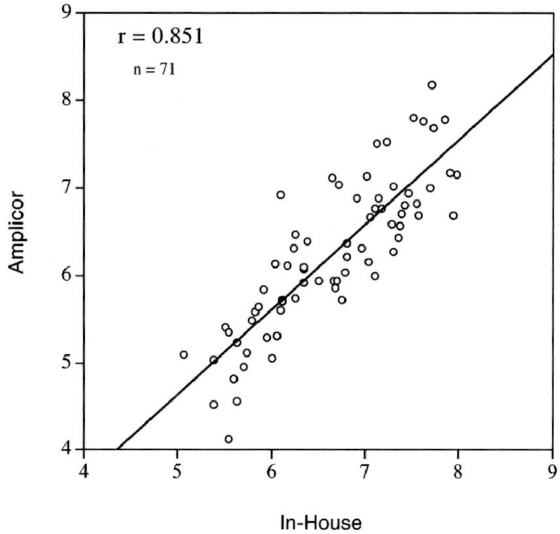

Figure 2. Correlation between Roche Amplicor and an in-house HBV DNA assay of mouse serum samples. Results are expressed as log HBV DNA copies per ml of serum.

polyclonal rabbit antibody conjugated to biotin (Cortex Biochem, San Leandro, CA) was used at a 1:200 dilution. Streptavidin peroxidase (BioGenex, San Ramon, CA) was applied to detect bound primary antibody. HBV-infected human liver was used as positive control tissue. Replacement of primary antibody with non-immune sera served as the negative control.

Treatment of HBV-producing mice with drugs

To evaluate the effect of RT inhibitors against HBV produced in STC lineage mice, 200 mg/kg (600 mg/m^2/day) lamivudine were administered once daily by intraperitoneal injection (IP) to eight STC mice for 31 days. Two additional groups of mice were given 2 mg/kg/day entecavir either orally by gavage or IP, and another eight received vehicle (0.1% carboxymethyl cellulose) alone IP. Serum samples were taken at -two, six, 13, 20, and 31 days of treatment and at 38 and 46 days during a two-week follow-up period. HBV DNA levels were quantified by in-house HBV DNA PCR assay.

Results

Replication of HBV in STC and PAMF lineages of transgenic mice

Two lineages, STC and PAMF, were derived from two HBV-positive founder males. Progeny have been healthy and fertile. Serum levels of HBsAg and HBeAg in the

F1 generation of the STC mice reflected the viral DNA levels (Figure 3A and data not shown). Unlike the 1.3.32 lineage, there did appear to be a difference in HBeAg levels between male and female mice (data not shown). After four generations of interbreeding, the STC lineage, like the founder, had serum HBV DNA levels of 10^6 to 10^8 viral genome equivalents (vge)/ml in 70% of offspring tested at 30 days of age, with the remainder producing virus at lower levels (Figure 3B). Levels of HBV DNA in the urine ranged up to 10^6 vge/ml (data not shown). After eight generations, all offspring have levels of viral DNA in the serum which appear to be higher by tenfold or greater

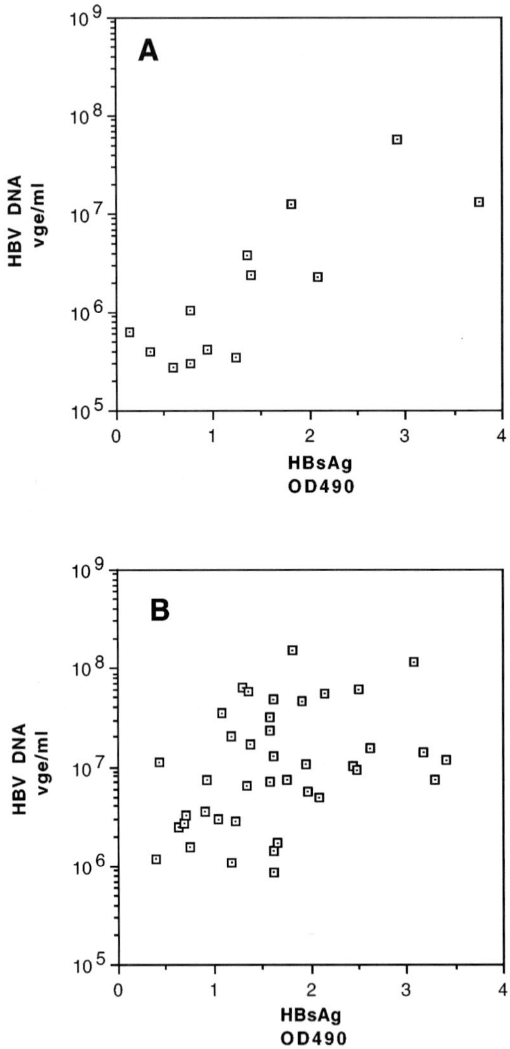

Figure 3. Scatter plots of levels of HBV DNA in viral genome equivalents per ml (vge/ml) vs levels of HBsAg in sera of individual mice of the F1 generation (A) and the F5 generation (B). Dilutions of sera for HBsAg analysis were 20-fold for the F1 generation and 100-fold for the F5 generation.

than those of the 1.3.32 lineage [2]. An endogenous DNA polymerase activity is present in particles pelleted from serum, and the product of this reaction migrates on agarose gels like HBV DNA from human serum, indicating that whole virus is present in the mouse serum (Figure 4). Replicative forms of HBV DNA can be observed in DNA extracted from the liver and analyzed by Southern blotting (Figure 5). The HBV DNA titers of untreated or vehicle-treated STC mice drop about 0.5-0.7 logs from day 30 to ~day 55 after birth (Figure 6), but titers generally remain constant at least to five months of age (data not shown).

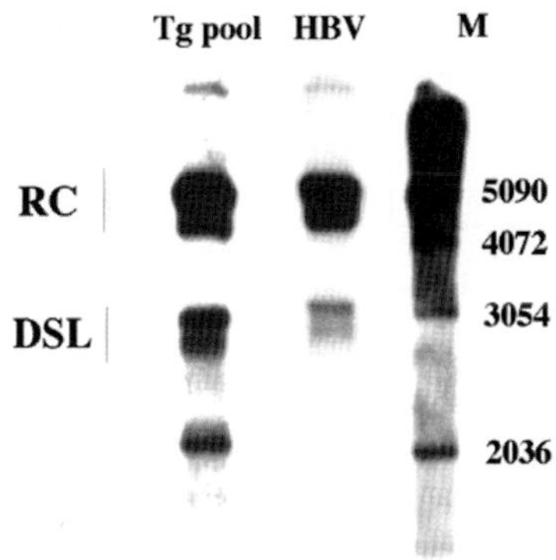

Figure 4. Gel electrophoretic analysis of ^{32}P-radiolabeled products of DNA polymerase reactions from particles pelleted from a pool of serum from the STC lineage (Tg pool) or a pool of human and chimpanzee sera from HBV chronic carriers (HBV). M = DNA size markers, RC = migration location of relaxed circular DNA, DSL = migration location of double stranded linear DNA.

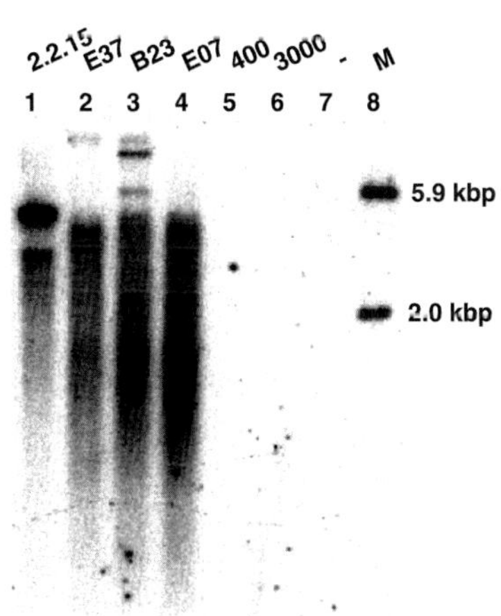

Figure 5. Southern blot analysis of HBV DNA replicative forms extracted from the livers of three mice of the STC lineage (E37, B23, and E07) and two mice of the PAMF lineage (400 and 3000) and compared to those extracted from the HBV-producing 2.2.15 cells (2.2.15). M = DNA size markers. The amount of DNA in each lane was that extracted from nucleocapsids prepared from 25 mg of liver.

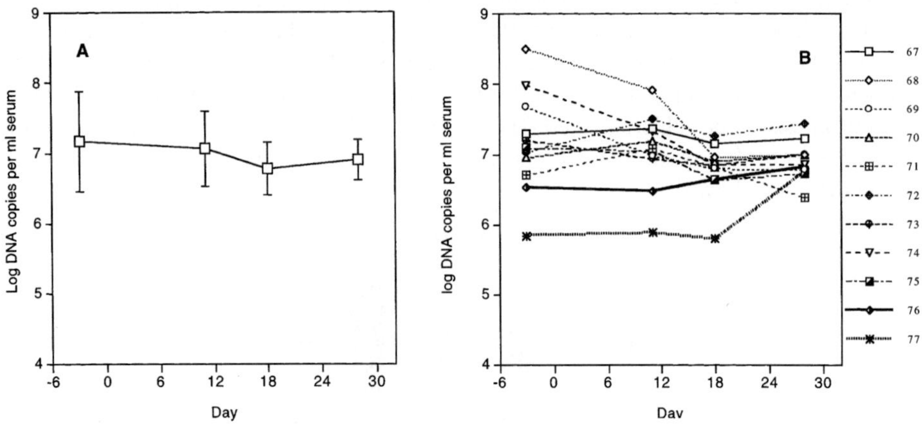

Figure 6. Serum HBV DNA levels during daily oral dosing of STC mice with 0.1% carboxymethylcellulose as vehicle. A. Mean levels of 11 mice, with standard deviation, B. Individual mice, indicated by numbers 67-77.

Less viral DNA is detected in the serum of the PAMF lineage (average ~10^5 to 10^6 vge/ml) than the STC lineage, but higher levels of HBsAg are observed in some of the mice (data not shown).

Immunohistochemistry of the STC lineage

HBcAg was detected in the nuclei of approximately 50% of hepatocytes, but was evident in the cytoplasm of hepatocytes significantly less often (Figure 7). Hepatocytic cytoplasmic staining was most frequent in the region surrounding the central vein, as was previously noted in the 1.3.32 lineage [1]. HBcAg was also detected in the nuclei of proximal renal tubular epithelial cells in a lower proportion of cells than in the liver (Figure 8). Cytoplasmic staining was infrequent, but when present affected the inner portions of the renal cortex. Staining was also evident in low numbers of nuclei from cells of the exocrine pancreas and islets of Langerhans (Figure 9). Staining intensity was increased in the Zn formalin-fixed tissues. HBsAg was detected in a small proportion of centrilobular hepatocytes only.

Histology

No histologic lesions have been identified in liver, kidney, or other tissues in either lineage of mice up to four months of age. Inflammation was found in older mice. Ten (5M/5F) STC lineage mice aged 13-17 months and nine PAMF lineage mice (4M/5F) aged 11-20 months had evidence of scattered foci of lymphocytes and occasional macrophages in the hepatic parenchyma, often associated with individual

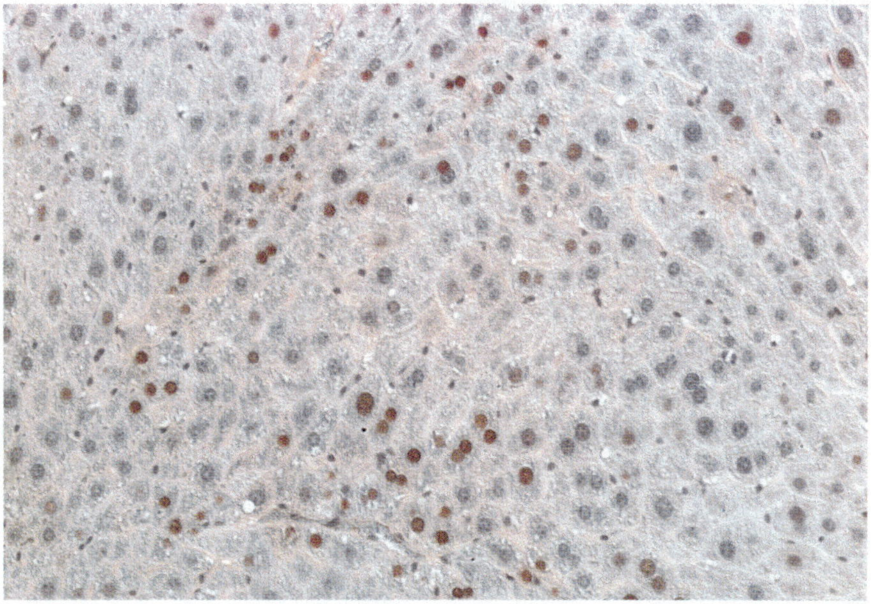

Figure 7. Anti-HBcAg immunohistochemical stain of an STC lineage mouse. Stained hepatocellular nuclei are scattered throughout the parenchyma.

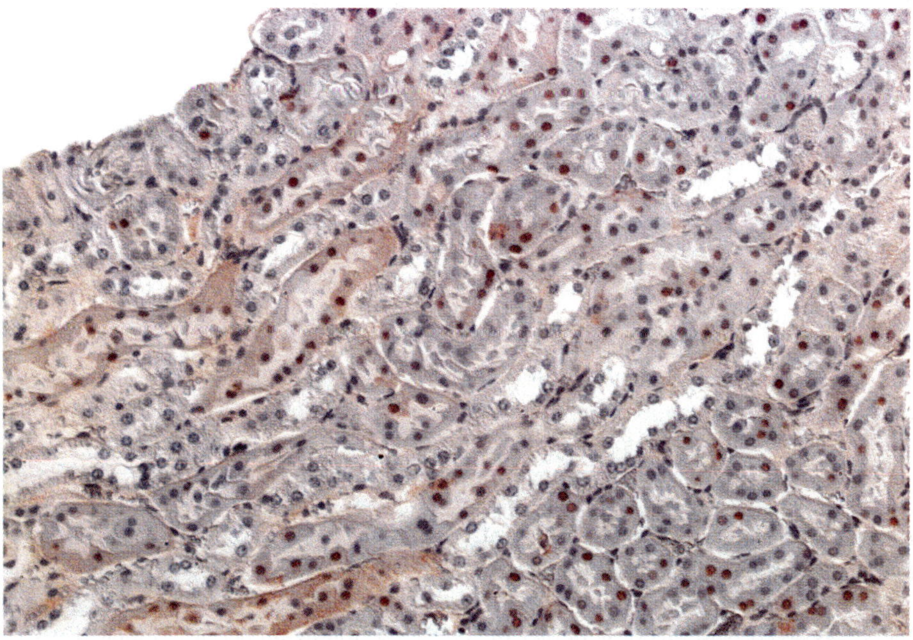

Figure 8. Anti-HBcAg immunohistochemical stain of STC lineage mouse kidney. Numerous stained nuclei are evident in the renal tubular epithelium.

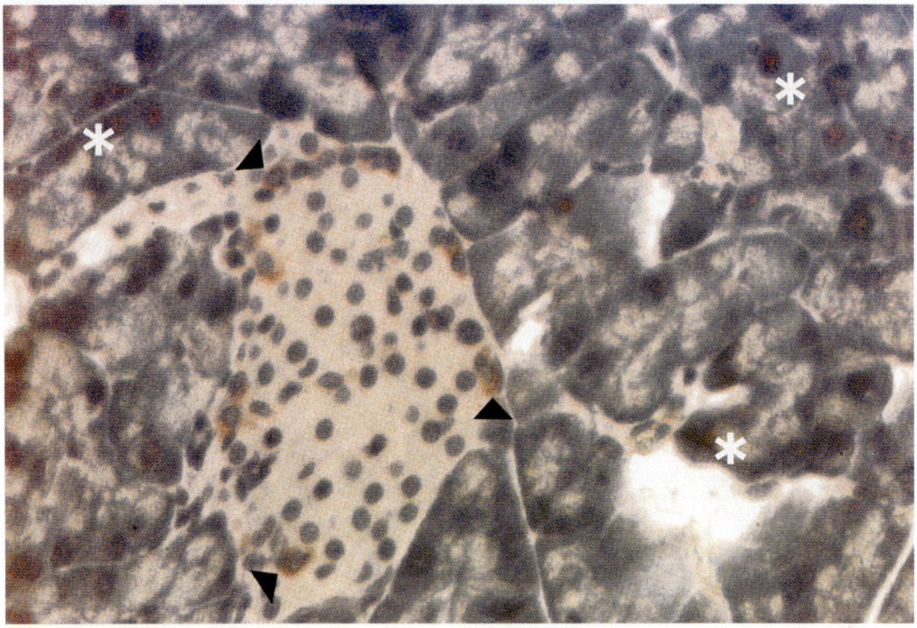

Figure 9. Anti-HBcAg immunohistochemical stain of STC lineage mouse pancreas. Stained nuclei in the exocrine pancreas (∗) and stained nuclei and cytoplasm of Sislet cells (▲) are evident.

necrotic hepatocytes (Figure 10). However, age-matched non-transgenic FVB/N mice had similar lesions with the same frequency, and the lesions could not be attributed to the presence of HBV.

Treatment of HBV-producing mice with entecavir, lamivudine or vehicle

Mice of the STC lineage were treated with antiviral compounds known to be active against HBV in culture. As seen in Figure 11, treatment with lamivudine resulted in a mean drop in HBV DNA per ml of 2.0 logs at three weeks and 1.7 logs at the end of treatment, with a mean rebound of 1 log. No toxicity was observed in that the weights of the mice were similar to those of the controls at the end of treatment, and no morbidity was noted. The serum HBV DNA titers of mice treated with vehicle also dropped, but by an average 1.0 log at the end of treatment, with a slight rebound (0.3 logs) after the follow-up period.

Treatment of mice in the same experiment with 2 mg/kg/day entecavir resulted in a mean reduction of viral titers similar to those seen with the lamivudine treatment (Figure 11), again with no apparent toxicity. Similar results were obtained with oral (shown in Figure 11) and IP delivery (not shown), though less variability during the course of treatment was seen with oral delivery. Interestingly, no rebound of virus titers was noted with this drug during the two-week follow-up period. Similar patterns of reductions of virus titers and absence of rebound were seen in two additional experiments with 1 and 2 mg/kg/day entecavir.

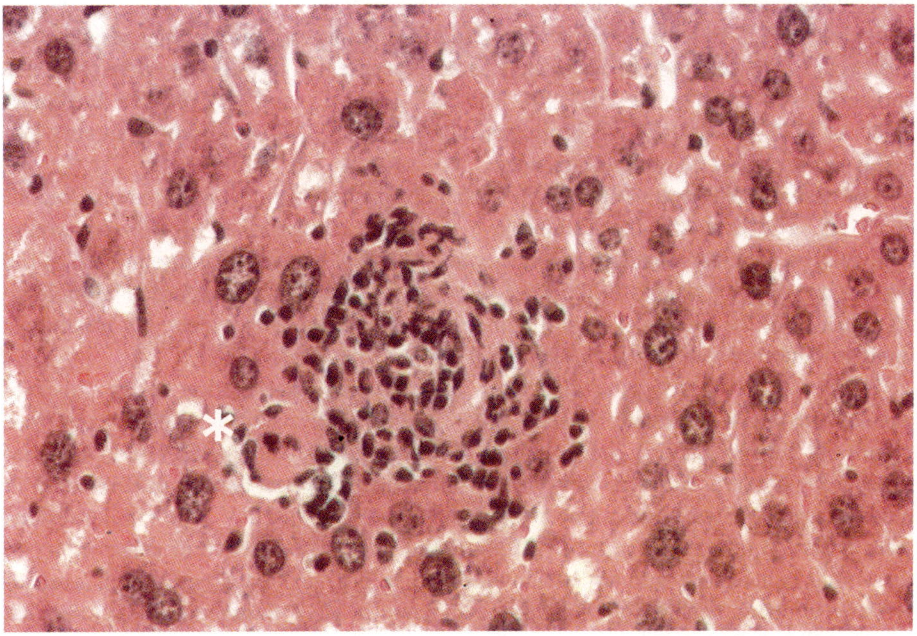

Figure 10. Focal lymphocytic hepatic parenchymal aggregates in a 14-month-old STC mouse. Apoptotic hepatocytes (*). These lesions were found in STC mice and in non-transgenic FVB/N controls.

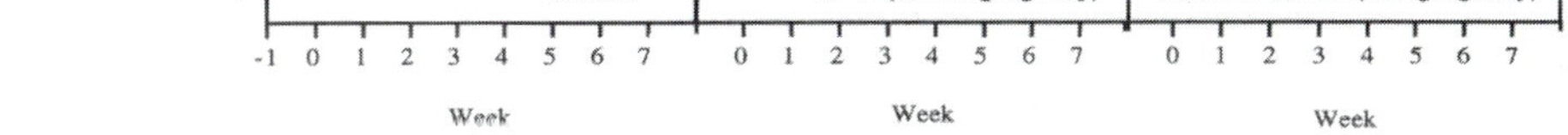

Figure 11. Mean serum levels of HBV DNA in STC mice treated with vehicle, lamivudine (3TC), or entecavir (BMS 200, 475). Bars indicate the standard deviation.

Discussion

We have made a lineage of transgenic mice that produces levels of hepatitis B virus in sera that equal or exceed those of existing lineages [2, 11]. The STC mouse lineage is immunocompetent, like the 1.3.32 lineage [1, 2] and in contrast to that developed in

SCID mice [11]. As with the other HBV-producing transgenic mouse lineages, the viral life cycle is not complete because there is no evidence for the susceptibility of mouse hepatocytes to infection by HBV [9]. The STC lineage is unlikely to have detectable levels of CCC DNA, since this replicative form of HBV DNA is absent or in very low levels in previously constructed lineages.

The tissue distribution of HBcAg in these mice is similar to that reported by Guidotti et al. [1]. The liver and the kidney have the greatest proportion of cells containing core antigen. Nuclear staining is more frequent than cytoplasmic staining in both of the organs, and may be related to the level of virus production in the organs. The biologic significance of the presence of viral antigen in the pancreas is not clear, but it parallels the distribution of viral antigens seen in DHBV-infected ducks [12].

There was no histologic evidence of inflammation, degeneration or apoptosis in any of the HBV-expressing tissues (liver, kidney and pancreas) taken from four month old transgenic mice, indicating the non-cytopathic nature of HBV (and apparent immunologic tolerance of the host to the viral antigens). Focal hepatic inflammation in older transgenic mice could not be attributed to expression of HBV since similar lesions were observed in non-transgenic FVB/N control mice. The absence of tissue injury in these mice is in accord with findings in other transgenic mice that produce high levels of HBV. In contrast, hepatic inflammation is apparent in HBV transgenic SCID mice that have been engrafted with lymphocytes from non-transgenic syngeneic mice [11].

Treatment of the STC lineage with 2 mg/kg/day entecavir caused a reduction in viremia similar to that resulting from treatment with 200 mg/kg/day lamividine. This observation is in concordance with previous studies comparing the two drugs in other experimental systems. Entecavir has been shown to have a 50% effective concentration (EC_{50}) over 30-fold lower than that of lamivudine in HBV-producing tissue culture cells [3]. In WHV-infected woodchucks 20 μg/kg/day entecavir was more effective in reducing viremia than 5 mg/kg/day lamivudine [4]. The delay in rebound after the end of treatment seen in entecavir-treated STC mice is similar to that seen in WHV-infected woodchucks treated with the same drug. This delayed or absent rapid recovery in virus levels contrasts sharply with the rapid rebound that is seen with lamivudine treatment of hepadnavirus infection in both transgenic mice and woodchucks. While the exact mechanism for the delay in rebound is not known, the delay is more likely to be due to the longer intracellular half-life of entecavir rather than a curing of individual cells. The latter is unlikely to occur in such a brief treatment period and in the transgenic model where virus is copied from integrated rather than episomal DNA.

Recently several mouse models have been devised that permit infection of grafted human hepatocytes with HBV [9, 13]. These models should be very useful in studies in which the complete viral life cycle is required, or for infection by viruses like HCV for which *in vivo* models are limited. However, they are less suited to most studies of inhibition of HBV replication than transgenic mice in that levels of viremia are relatively low (~10^5 HBV genome equivalents/ml) and of limited duration, and the mice are more difficult to produce, requiring surgical intervention on each mouse as well as the availability of suitable human liver for implantation. The STC lineage of transgenic mice, with mean serum HBV titers of 10^7 HBV genome equivalents/ml, provides a small animal model in which reductions of HBV viremia of 3-4 logs can be readily observed if therapeutic treatment is successful.

Acknowledgments

This work was supported in part by Public Health grant AI-20551. Funding by Digestive Diseases core grant DK38707 provided part of the resources for creating the transgenic mice.

References

1. Guidotti L, Matzke B, Schaller H and Chisari FV. High-level hepatitis B virus replication in transgenic mice. *Journal of Virology*, 1995, 69:6158-6169.
2. Morrey JD, Korba BE and Sidwell RW. Transgenic mice as a chemotherapeutic model for hepatitis B virus infection. *Antiviral Therapy*, 1998; 3:59-68.
3. Innaimo SF, Seifer M, Bisacchi GS, Standring DN, Zahler R and Colonno RJ. Identification of BMS-200475 as a potent and selective inhibitor of hepatitis B virus. *Antimicrobial Agents and Chemotherapy*, 1997, 41:1444-1448.
4. Genovesi EV, Lamb L, Medina I, Taylor D, Seifer M, Innaimo S, Colonno RJ, Standring DN and Clark JM. Efficacy of the carbocyclic 2'-deoxyguanosine nucleoside BMS-200475 in the woodchuck model of hepatitis B virus infection. *Antimicrobial Agents and Chemotherapy*, 1998, 42:3209-3217.

4a. Marion PL, Salazar FH, Winters MA and Colonno RJ. Potent efficacy of entecavir in a duck model of hepatitis B virus replication. *Antimicrobial Agents and Chemotherapy*, 2002, 46:82-88.

5. Galibert F, Mandart E, Fitoussi F, Tiollais P and Charnay P. Nucleotide sequence of the hepatitis B viral genome (subtype ayw) cloned in *E. coli*. *Nature*, 1979; 281:646.
6. Erhardt A, Schaefer S, Athanassiou N, Kann M and Gerlich WH. Quantitative assay of PCR-amplified hepatitis B virus DNA using a peroxidase-labelled DNA probe and enhanced chemiluminescence. *Journal of Clinical Microbiology*, 1996; 34:1885-1891.
7. Winters MA, Tan LB, Katzenstein DA and Merigan TC. Biological variation and quality control of plasma human immunodeficiency type 1 RNA quantitation by reverse transcriptase polymerase chain reaction. *Journal of Clinical Microbiology*, 1993, 31(11):2960-2966.
8. Radziwill G, Tucker W and Schaller H. Mutational analysis of the hepatitis B virus P gene product: domain structure and RNase H activity. *Journal of Virology*, 1990; 64:613-620.
9. Ohashi K, Marion PL, Nakai H, Meuse L, Cullen JM, Bordier BB, Schwall R, Greenberg HB, Glenn JS and Kay MA. Sustained survival of human hepatocytes in mice: A model for *in vivo* infection with human hepatitis B and hepatitis delta viruses. *Nature Medicine*, 2000, 6:327-331.
10. Condreay LD, Wu TT, Aldrich CE, Delaney MA, Summers J, Seeger C and Mason WS. Replication of DHBV genomes with mutations at the sites of initiation of minus- and plus-strand DNA synthesis. *Virology*, 1992, 188:208-216.
11. Larkin J, Clayton M, Sun B, Perchonock CE, Morgan JL, Siracusa LD, Michaels FH and Feitelson MA. Hepatitis B virus transgenic mouse model of chronic liver disease. *Nature Medicine*, 1999, 5:907-912.
12. Cullen JM, Marion PL andNewbold JM. A sequential histologic and immunohistochemical study of duck hepatitis B virus infection in Pekin ducks. *Veterinary Pathology*, 1989, 26:164-172.

13. Ilan H, Burakova T, Dagan S, Nussbaum O, Lubin I, Eren R, Ben-Moshe O, et al. The hepatitis B virus-Trimera Mouse: A model for human HBV infection and evaluation of anti-HBV therapeutic agents. *Hepatology*, 1999, 29:553-562.

Evaluation of therapies for hepatitis B virus in the HBV transgenic SCID mouse model

MILIND KAMKOLKAR[1], MARCIA M. CLAYTON[1],
SHU MIN ZHANG[1], PAUL BLACK[2],
RAYMOND F. SCHINAZI[3] and MARK A. FEITELSON[1,4]

[1] *Department of Pathology, Anatomy and Cell Biology, Thomas Jefferson University, Philadelphia, PA 19107*
[2] *QuadPharma, Inc., 1860 Montreal Road, Suite 217, Tucker, GA 30084*
[3] *Department of Pediatrics, VA Medical Center, Emory University, Medical Research Service #151H, 1670 Clairmont Road, Decatur, GA 30033*
[4] *Department of Microbiology and Immunology, Kimmel Cancer Center, Thomas Jefferson University, Philadelphia, PA*

Abstract

Hepatitis B virus (HBV) transgenic SCID mice support virus gene expression and replication. Following adoptive transfer, these mice develop acute and chronic hepatitis. In order to exploit this system for screening the next generation of antiviral compounds, these mice were treated with nucleoside analogs having known antiviral activities against HBV. When groups of mice were treated for six days with lamivudine (3TC), [-]-FTC, [+/-]-FTC, L-FMAU, or D-D4FC, which were active against HBV, HBsAg and/or HBV DNA were partially or completely cleared from blood. Virus markers reappeared in some mice within a week after the end of therapy. In contrast, AZT and D4T, which lack antiviral activity against HBV, were largely inactive in these mice. The results are an important step in validating the HBV transgenic mouse model for screening compounds for activity against HBV *in vivo*.

Introduction

Chronic carriers of hepatitis B are at high risk for the development of hepatitis, cirrhosis and hepatocellular carcinoma (HCC) [1, 2]. These diseases carry with them considerable morbidity and mortality, especially in light of the more than 300 million carriers worldwide [2]. Chronic hepatitis, for example, often recurs over the course of many years or decades, resulting in repeated hospitalizations. Cirrhosis may be fatal, especially when accompanied by decompensation. HCC is one of the most frequent cancers worldwide, with up to a million new cases annually [3]. The survival rate

Frontiers in Viral Hepatitis Ed. by RF Schinazi, J-P Sommadossi and CM Rice. 211 — 222

for HCC is less than 3% over five years. Interferon-α, the first drug approved for the treatment of hepatitis B, is expensive and only benefits 20-25% of treated carriers; and it has serious side effects at the high doses needed for clinical efficacy [4, 5]. More recently, lamivudine (3TC) has been approved for use. Although lamivudine treatment results in the partial or total clearance of virus from blood and in the improvement of liver histology in most patients [6, 7], prolonged treatment is associated with the appearance of drug-resistant mutants in up to 20% of patients per year [8-10]. Other drugs, such as adefovir dipivoxil [11], are effective against lamivudine-resistant mutants [12, 13], and may play a role in future combination therapies.

A number of new nucleoside analogs have been shown to be effective against HBV in cell lines that support viral replication. In addition to lamivudine [(-)-β-L-2', 3'-dideoxy-3'-thiacytidine or 3TC] [14-16], these include *cis*-5-fluoro-1-(2-(hydroxymethyl)-1, 3-oxathiolan-5-yl)-cytosine (emtricitabine or [-]-FTC), the 5-fluorinated derivative of lamivudine [17-19], 2'-fluoro-5-methyl-β-L-arabinofuranosyluracil (L-FMAU) [20-22], and β-D-2', 3'-didehydro-2', 3'-dideoxy-5-fluorocytidine (D-D4FC) [23-26], among others [27]. Lamivudine [28], [-]-FTC [29], and L-FMAU [30] also have antiviral activities against HBV-related viruses in ducks and woodchucks. On the other hand, 3'-azido-3'-deoxythmidine (zidovudine or AZT) and 2', 3'-didehydro-2', 3'-dideoxythymidine (stavudine or D4T) are active against human immunodeficiency virus type 1 (HIV-1) but not against HBV [31, 32]. The antiviral characteristics of these compounds are important in the development and validation of new models of HBV infection and disease, since their application in new biological models will determine the utility of such models for screening new drug candidates.

Part of the problem in developing new drugs against HBV is the lack of suitable *in vivo* models in which both the virus and associated liver disease can be targeted. Given the very narrow host range of HBV, it is impractical to test antivirals in HBV infected chimpanzees, due to cost and limited availability. HBV-like viruses exist in ground squirrels, woodchucks and ducks [33-35], and these systems have been successfully used to screen for new drugs with activity against hepadnaviruses [36-38]. HBV transgenic mice that support virus replication have also been used for testing putative antiviral compounds *in vivo* [39], although these mice are tolerant to the virus and do not develop chronic liver disease. The recent development of chronic liver disease in HBV transgenic SCID mice following adoptive transfer of syngeneic, unprimed splenocytes [40] represents a unique model for antiviral drug evaluation against both HBV and liver disease. In this report, several nucleoside analogs with known activities against HBV have been evaluated in the HBV transgenic SCID mouse model. The results show that compounds with activity against HBV (3TC, FTC, L-FMAU, and D-D4FC) in tissue culture, in other animal models (e.g., ducks and woodchucks), and in human clinical trials are also active against HBV in the HBV transgenic SCID mice. In addition, nucleoside analogs with little activity against HBV (D4T and AZT) also have little activity against the virus in the HBV transgenic mouse model.

Materials and methods

HBV transgenic SCID mice were bred and tested for the levels of HBV DNA in blood by semiquantitative PCR, exactly as described [40]. Transgenic mice approximately three months of age with virus levels in blood ranging from 4-20 x 10^5 virus genome equivalents/ml were used. For drug evaluation, groups containing five mice each were injected intraperitoneally (i.p.) once a day with 100 mg/kg for each of six days. The drugs used were lamivudine (3TC), [-]-FTC, [±]-FTC, L-FMAU, D-D4FC, D4T and AZT. An additional group of five mice were injected with an equivalent volume of phosphate-buffered saline (PBS) containing no drug. In addition to the prebleed (day 0), mice were bled on days 3, 5, and 8, and then exsanguinated on day 12. All injections and analyses of sera were conducted blindly by animal number. Serum samples from each time point were tested for alanine aminotransferase (ALT) using a commercially-available kit (ALT/AST 50, Sigma Chemical Co., St. Louis, MO). HBV DNA was semiquantitated in each serum sample exactly as described [40]. Serum samples were then tested for the presence of hepatitis B surface antigen (HBsAg) in a commercially-available EIA (Auszyme kit, Abbott Labs., North Chicago, Il) with modifications [40]. All mice were housed in a BL-3 facility and treated by trained personnel in accordance with university policy and approved animal protocols.

Results

Prior to treatment, HBV transgenic SCID mice were verified to have circulating HBV DNA in the range of 4-20 x 10^5 virus genome equivalents/ml in prebleed samples. These mice were also verified to have detectable HBsAg in blood by specific EIA. Prebleeds were also tested for ALT to exclude nonspecific causes of liver injury. Only animals with ALT values < 20 units/liter (U/L) were entered into the treatment protocol. These mice were then injected i.p. with drugs at a dose of 100 mg/kg/day for each of six days, and then allowed to recover for an additional seven days prior to sacrifice. The compounds used were 3TC, [-]-FTC, [±]-FTC, L-FMAU, D-D4FC, D4T and AZT. An additional group of five mice was injected with an equivalent volume of PBS.

Freshly acquired blood samples collected on days 0, 3, 5, 8 and 12 (bleedout sample) were tested for ALT. All animals had ALT levels in the normal range (< 20 U/L) at all time points, indicating that the drugs were not directly toxic to the liver of the mice at the doses used (data not shown). These findings suggested that decreased virus titers were due to the antiviral activity of each drug and not due to nonspecific hepatotoxicity caused by these drugs.

Overall, there were three types of outcomes to drug treatment. A complete response was characterized by the clearance of HBsAg and HBV DNA in the serum of animals within three to five days of treatment. Given that all mice started with an initial virus concentration of 4-20 x 10^5 virus genome equivalents/ml, failure to detect HBV DNA during or after treatment corresponded to a 4-5 log drop. In a partial response, HBsAg became undetectable, but the viral DNA either remained positive throughout the period of observation or became undetectable and then reappeared. In mice that were nonresponders, or that were injected with PBS, HBsAg persisted throughout the period of observation, while differences in the levels of HBV DNA reflected variation within the PCR assay used.

Among animals treated with lamivudine (3TC), one animal (no. 5) became HBsAg negative by day 3, while another three animals became negative by day 8 (Table 1). PCR analysis showed a similar trend, where one animal (no. 5) had undetectable HBV DNA by day 3. This animal remained PCR-negative for the remainder of the experiment, indicating that viral clearance was sustained for a week after the end of treatment (Table 1). Two other animals in this group (nos. 1 and 2) cleared virus from blood by day 8, and this clearance was apparently sustained through day 12. In the remaining two mice, HBV DNA was found to persist in one animal (no. 3) for the entire observation period, while in the other (no. 4), it became undetectable by day 12. Hence, by the end of the experiment, four out of five treated mice (80%) were negative for both HBsAg and HBV DNA. These trends were confirmed by semiquantitative PCR, where titers dropped by up to 3 logs in two mice (nos. 1 and 5) by day 3, and in another mouse (no. 2) by day 5 (Figure 1A). A partial rebound in virus was observed in the remaining two mice (nos. 3 and 4) by day 5. Together, these results suggest that lamivudine is effective against HBV in these mice.

When another group of mice was treated with emtricitabine ([-]-FTC), two mice (nos. 9 and 10) had undetectable HBsAg by day 3, while an additional two mice (nos. 6 and 7) cleared HBsAg by day 5, and the remaining mouse (no. 8) cleared HBsAg by day 8 (Table 1). The PCR signals dropped tenfold in all [-]-FTC-treated mice by day 3 of treatment (Figure 1B). By day 8, none of the mice had detectable HBV DNA by PCR, but by day 12, a single mouse (no. 8) had detectable PCR to about one tenth the pretreatment levels. Similar results were obtained when a third group of mice were treated with a racemic mixture of emtricitabine ([±]-FTC). In two mice (nos. 14 and 15; Table 1) HBsAg became undetectable by day 3, and by day 8, HBsAg was undetectable in all animals. Although virus DNA was undetectable in the same two

Table 1. HBsAg EIA and Semiquantitative PCR of HBV DNA in the Sera of HBV Transgenic SCID Mice Treated with Selected Drugs

Drug	Mouse	HBV PCR / HBsAg EIA				
		prebleed	day 3	day 5	day 8	day 12
3TC	1	+/+	+/+	+/+	-/-	-/-
	2	+/+	+/-	+/+	-/-	-/-
	3	+/+	-/+	+/+	+/+	+/+
	4	+/+	+/+	+/+	+/-	-/-
	5	+/+	-/-	-/-	-/-	-/-
[-]-FTC	6	+/+	+/+	+/-	-/-	-/-
	7	+/+	+/+	+/-	-/-	-/-

Table 1. Continued

		HBV PCR / HBsAg EIA				
Drug	Mouse	prebleed	day 3	day 5	day 8	day 12
[-]-FTC	8	+/+	+/+	+/+	-/-	+/-
	9	+/+	+/-	+/-	-/-	-/-
	10	+/+	+/-	+/-	-/-	-/-
[+/-]-FTC	11	+/+	+/+	+/+	-/-	-/-
	12	+/+	+/+	+/+	-/-	+/+
	13	+/+	+/+	+/+	-/-	-/-
	14	+/+	-/-	+/-	-/-	-/-
	15	+/+	-/-	-/-	-/-	-/-
L-FMAU	16	+/+	+/+	+/+	+/+	-/-
	17	+/+	+/+	-/-	-/-	-/-
	18	+/+	+/+	+/+	+/+	-/-
	19	+/+	+/+	-/-	-/-	-/-
	20	+/+	+/+	+/+	-/-	-/-
D-D4FC	21	+/+	+/+	+/+	-/-	-/-
	22	+/+	+/+	+/+	+/-	+/+
	23	+/+	+/+	+/+	-/-	-/-
	24	+/+	+/+	-/-	-/-	-/-
	25	+/+	+/+	+/+	+/+	-/-
AZT	26	+/+	+/+	+/+	+/+	+/-
	27	+/+	+/+	+/+	+/+	+/+
	28	+/+	+/+	+/+	+/-	+/-
	29	+/+	+/+	+/+	+/+	+/+
	30	+/+	+/+	+/+	+/+	+/+
D4T	31	+/+	+/+	+/+	+/+	+/+
	32	+/+	+/+	+/+	+/+	+/+
	33	+/+	+/+	+/+	+/+	+/+
	34	+/+	+/+	+/+	+/+	+/+
	35	+/+	+/+	+/+	+/+	+/+
PBS	36	+/+	+/+	+/+	+/+	+/+
	37	+/+	+/+	+/+	+/+	+/+
	38	+/+	+/+	+/+	+/+	+/+
	39	+/+	+/+	+/+	+/+	+/+
	40	+/+	+/+	+/+	+/+	+/+

mice that cleared HBsAg by day 3, virus DNA was detectable again by day 5, and then became undetectable again for the remainder of the observation period (Table 1). Interestingly, when the levels of HBV DNA were quantitated in these animals, four of the five mice had evidence of a transient rebound on day 5 (Figure 1C), and in one of these (no. 12), both HBsAg and HBV DNA reappeared on day 12. Although the results of [-]-FTC and [±]-FTC are distinct (compare Figure 1B to 1C), it is clear that both of these treatment protocols demonstrate strong antiviral effects upon HBV in this model system.

When a fourth group of mice was treated with L-FMAU, both HBsAg and HBV DNA became undetectable in three of the five mice by day 8, although both markers were cleared in all mice by day 12 (Table 1). At the level of semiquantitative PCR, decreases in the levels of viral DNA of at least tenfold were observed in two mice (nos. 19 and 20) by day 3, and in another two mice (nos. 16 and 18) by day 5 (Figure 1D). The remaining mouse (no. 17) cleared approximately 3 logs of virus by day 5, and then cleared virus DNA from serum for the remainder of the experiment. These results suggest that L-FMAU is also active against HBV in this animal model, although clearance appears to be delayed in some animals in comparison to FTC.

Delayed virus clearance was also characteristic of another group of animals that were treated with D-D4FC. One mouse (no. 24) demonstrated clearance of HBsAg and viral DNA by day 5 of treatment. An additional two mice (nos. 21 and 23) had undetectable HBsAg and HBV DNA by day 8 (Table 1). Another mouse (no. 25) cleared virus only by day 12, while the last mouse in this group (no. 22) did not clear virus at all. When these mice were analyzed for HBV DNA by semiquantitative PCR, levels dropped 1-2 logs by day 5 of treatment (nos. 21 and 24), while another mouse showed a twofold decrease on the same day (no. 23) (Figure 1E). The remaining two mice (nos. 22 and 25) showed detectable decreases in virus DNA by day 8. One of these mice (no. 22) relapsed by day 12, since HBsAg again became positive (Table 1) and HBV DNA titer increased (Figure 1E).

A separate group of mice was treated with zidovudine (AZT). The results show that one mouse (no. 28) lost HBsAg by day 8 while another (no. 26) lost HBsAg by day 12 (Table 1). None of the animals lost HBV DNA by PCR (Table 1), although two animals experienced a marginal, twofold decrease in HBV DNA during the course of treatment (Figure 1F). Likewise, treatment of an independent group of mice with stavudine (D4T) resulted in no loss of HBsAg or HBV DNA in any of the mice (Table 1, Figure 1G). Exactly the same results were obtained in mice injected with PBS (Table 1, Figure 1H). The fluctuations in the PCR signals reported in Figures 1G and 1H are within the limits of the PCR assay, suggesting that they do not represent changes in virus titer. These results indicate that AZT and D4T are ineffective as antiviral agents in HBV transgenic SCID mice.

Discussion

Part of the difficulty in developing and evaluating new antiviral drugs against hepatitis B is the lack of a suitable animal model replicating this human pathogen. Chimpanzees

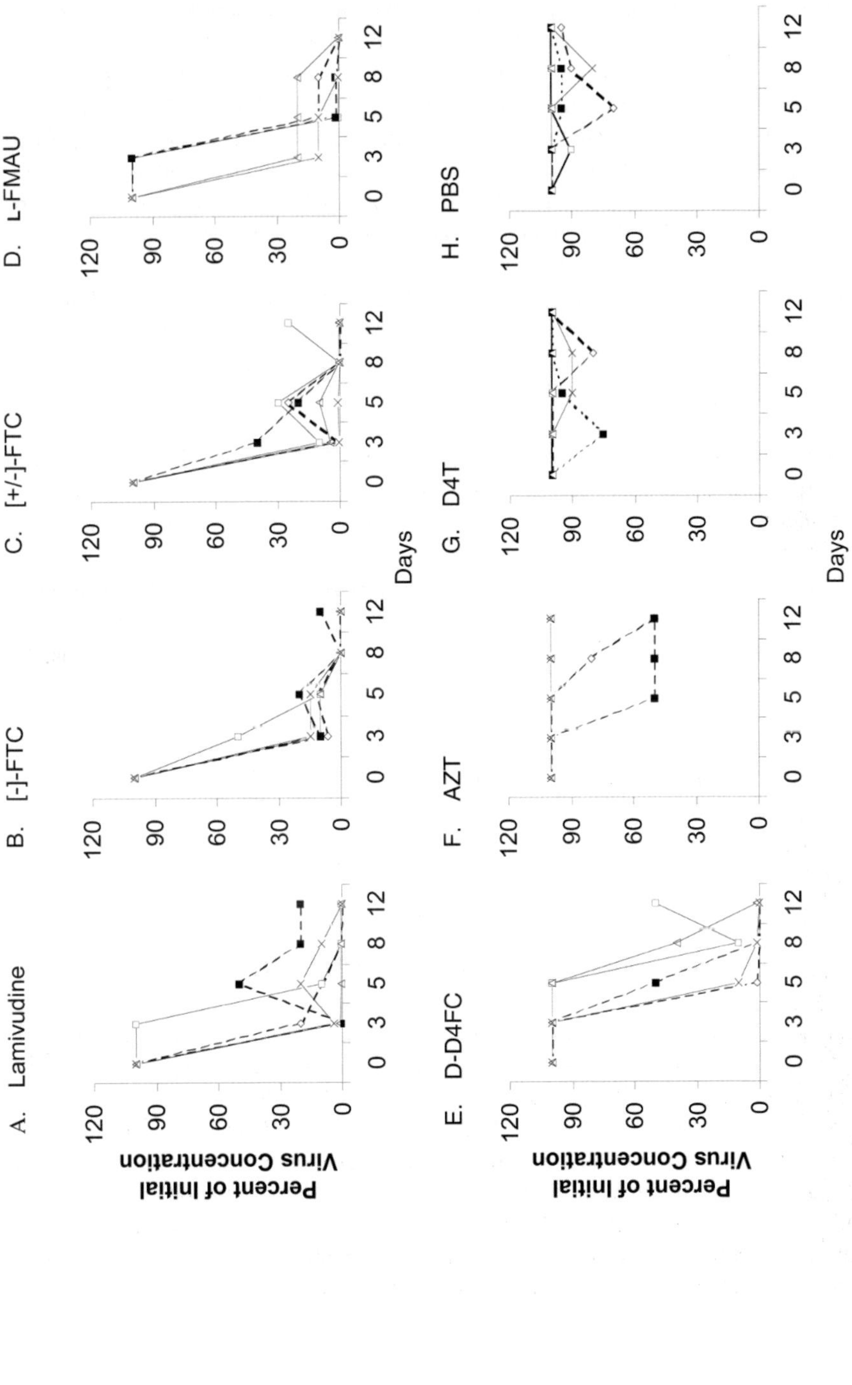
A. Lamivudine
B. [-]-FTC
C. [+/-]-FTC
D. L-FMAU
E. D-D4FC
F. AZT
G. D4T
H. PBS
Percent of initial Virus Concentration
Days
0
3
5
8
12
120
90
60
30
0

Figure 1.

are one of the very few hosts susceptible to HBV infection, although expense and endangered status have precluded their widespread use in the evaluation of HBV therapeutics. Transgenic mice expressing some of the HBV gene products [41-43] or supporting virus replication [44, 45] have been reported, but these have not been used extensively for antiviral drug testing [39]. Alternatively, natural or experimental infections of woodchucks or Pekin ducks with woodchuck hepatitis virus (WHV) or duck hepatitis B virus (DHBV), respectively, have been very useful as preclinical models for the development of HBV therapeutics [20, 28-30, 36, 37]. However, WHV and DHBV are not human pathogens, nor are the animal models easily manipulated to evaluate combination therapies. In addition, antiviral and immunomodulatory activities of compounds, important in the design of combination therapies, cannot be independently evaluated in these models of natural infection. The HBV transgenic SCID mouse model represents the first time a transgenic mouse system supporting HBV replication also develops chronic liver disease following the adoptive transfer of normal, syngeneic splenocytes [40]. The system is easy to manipulate, cost-effective, and can be used to evaluate single or combination therapies against the virus or disease. To achieve this goal, nucleoside analogs with known activities against HBV were tested in these mice, to validate the system for the evaluation of less characterized compounds.

Lamivudine was highly effective against HBV in tissue-culture cells [14, 5] and in clinical trials, where it reduced serum HBV DNA by 4-6 logs, normalized transminases, and improved histopathology in 60-70% of treated patients [6, 7, 8, 46]. However, the relapse rate was high after the end of therapy. In HBV transgenic mice, four out of five animals had a reduction in HBV DNA levels of approximately 3 logs during treatment. Two of the four animals in this group that responded to lamivudine within the first three days of treatment (nos. 3 and 4) partially relapsed by day 5 and still had detectable HBV DNA on day 8 (Figure 1A). One or these mice (no. 4) cleared HBV DNA from serum by day 12, suggesting a sustained response in three of the five mice (60%) during the week after the end of treatment. Hence, the outcome for the clearance of HBV DNA from blood is similar in mice and patients, although the clearance of HBsAg from serum in all of the lamivudine-treated mice (Table 1) is quite distinct from that observed among patients, where HBsAg clearance is rare.

Emtricitabine, or [-]-FTC, is a nucleoside analog with a very high selectivity index for HBV that is currently in clinical trials [17-19]. These trials have demonstrated a greater than 3-log reduction in viral DNA and normalization of transaminases among responders. Both [-]-FTC and [+]-FTC enantiomers have been shown to be active against HBV in tissue-culture cells supporting virus replication, although the former is the much more potent enantiomer, while the latter is more toxic [17, 18]. Among HBV transgenic mice, treatment with [-]-FTC resulted in clearance of HBsAg in two mice by day 3 of treatment, and in four out of five by day 5. HBV DNA levels were depressed by 1-2 logs during treatment. By day 8, both HBsAg and HBV were undetectable in all mice. The latter corresponded to a 5-6 log drop in virus titer. These results suggest that [-]-FTC was highly effective in clearance of virus from the circulation. In contrast to lamivudine, there was no sign of rebound in the levels of HBV DNA during the course of treatment (Figure 1B). However, when mice were treated with a racemic mixture of FTC, the partial rebound phenomenon at day 5 was observed in four out of the five mice.

However, [+/-]-FTC treatment cleared HBsAg and viral DNA from serum in all treated animals by day 8 (Figure 1C), which was observed with [-]-FTC, but with no other drug tested. Hence, FTC is active against HBV replicating in tissue-culture cells, in chronically infected patients, and in HBV transgenic SCID mice.

L-FMAU has been shown to be an inhibitor of HBV replication in tissue-culture cells [20-22], of WHV replication in woodchucks [20], and of DHBV replication in ducklings [30]. In HBV transgenic mice, only three of the five mice in this group cleared HBsAg and HBV DNA from serum by day 8, unlike the lamivudine- and FTC-treated animals. By day 12, however, both HBsAg and HBV DNA were undetectable in all mice, demonstrating that L-FMAU is effective in HBV transgenic SCID mice, as in other models, although complete clearance is somewhat delayed in L-FMAU treated animals compared to those treated with lamivudine and FTC.

D-D4FC has demonstrated activity against both HIV and HBV [23-26]. Among HBV transgenic mice, all mice were responsive to this drug, although clearance of virus markers began on day 5, which was later than in animals treated with lamivudine, FTC or L-FMAU (Figure 1). In addition, only three of the five animals in the D-D4FC-treated group had a sustained response for up to one week after the end of treatment. Therefore, viral replication in HBV transgenic mice was also sensitive to this antiviral compound, although clearance was delayed and incomplete relative to the other compounds tested above.

The results of this study show that all of the nucleoside analogs (3TC, FTC, L-FMAU, and D-D4FC) that are known to be active against HBV were also active in HBV transgenic mice to differing extents. When additional animals were treated with either AZT or D4T, which are known to be inactive against HBV, none showed even a single log decrease in virus DNA, nor a sustained clearance of HBsAg (Figure 1). The combined results demonstrate that active nucleoside analogs have direct antiviral activities *in vivo*, since they were evaluated in animals that were not adoptively transferred and that had not developed antiviral immunity. In addition, these results validate the HBV transgenic SCID mice as a preclinical model for the testing of promising compounds directed against the polymerase as well as other targets in the virus. Additional work is now underway to ask whether the antiviral activities shown above also translate into activity against chronic liver disease in transgenic mice treated after adoptive transfer.

Acknowledgments

These studies were supported from NIH grant CA79512 and through a grant from QuadPharma, Inc. to MAF.

References

1. Szmuness W. Hepatocellular carcinoma and hepatitis B virus: Evidence for a causal association. *Progress in Medical Virology* 1978; 24:40-69.

2. Tiollais P, Pourcel C, and Dejean A. The hepatitis B virus. *Nature* 1985; 317:489-495.
3. Feitelson MA. Hepatitis B virus in Hepatocarcinogenesis. *Journal of Cellular Physiology* 1999; 181:188-202.
4. Perrillo RP. Antiviral therapy of chronic hepatitis B: past, present, and future. *Journal of Hepatology* 1993; 17(Suppl 3):S56-S63.
5. Lok ASF. Treatment of chronic viral hepatitis. *Journal of Viral Hepatitis* 1994; 1:105-124.
6. Hunt CM, Brown NA, and Rubin M. Lamivudine therapy of chronic hepatitis B. *Advances in Experimental Medicine and Biology* 1999; 458:11-21.
7. Suzuki Y, Kumada H, Ikeda K, Chayama K, Arase Y, Saitoh S, Tsubota A, Kobayashi M, Koike M, Ogawa N, and Tanikawa K. Histological changes in liver biopsies after one year of lamivudine treatment in patients with chronic hepatitis B infection. *Journal of Hepatology* 1999; 30:743-748.
8. Dienstag JL, Schiff ER, Mitchell M, Casey DE, Jr., Gitlin N, Lissoos T, Gelb LD, Condreay L, Crowther L, Rubin M, and Brown N. Extended lamivudine retreatment for chronic hepatitis B: maintenance of viral suppression after discontinuation of therapy. *Hepatology* 1999; 30:1082-1087.
9. Tipples GA, Ma MM, Fischer KP, Bain VG, Kneteman NM, and Tyrell DLJ. Mutation in the HBV RNA-dependent DNA polymerase confers resistance to lamivudine *in vivo*. *Hepatology* 1996; 24:714-717.
10. Bartholomew MM, Jansen RW, Jeffers LJ, Reddy KR, Johnson LC, Bunzendahl H, Condrey LD, Tzakis AG, Schiff ER, and Brown NA. Hepatitis B virus resistance to lamivudine given for recurrent infection after orthotopic liver transplantation. *Lancet* 1997; 349:20-22.
11. Gilson RJC, Chopra KB, Newell AM, Murray-Lyon IM, Nelson MR, Rice SJ, Tedder RS, Toole J, Jaffe HS, and Weller IVD. A placebo-controlled phase I/II study of adefovir dipivoxil in patients with chronic hepatitis B virus infection. *Journal of Viral Hepatitis* 1999; 6:387-395.
12. Xiong X, Flores C, Yang H, Tooke JJ, and Gibbs, CS. Mutations in hepatitis B DNA polymerase associated with resistance to lamivudine do not confer resistance to adefovir *in vitro*. *Hepatology* 1999; 28:1669-1673.
13. Perillo R, Schiff E, Magil A, and Murry A. *In vivo* demonstration of sensitivity of YMDD variants to adefovir (abstr.) *Hepatology* 1999; 30(Suppl. 1):122.
14. Doong S, Tsai C, Schinazi R, Liotta D, and Cheng Y. Inhibition of the replication of hepatitis B virus *in vitro* by 2', 3'-dideoxy-3'thiacytidine and related analogues. *Proceedings of the National Academy of Sciences of the United States of America* 1991; 88:8495-8499.
15. Chang CN, Doong S, Zhou J, Beach J, Jeong L, Chu C, Tsai C, Cheng Y, Liotta D, and Schinazi R. Deoxycytidine deaminase-resistant stereoisomer is the active form of (+/-)2', 3'-dideoxy 3'-thiacytidine in the inhibition of hepatitis B virus replication. *Journal of Biological Chemistry* 1992; 267:13938-13942.
16. Delaney WE, Miller TG, and Isom HC. Use of the hepatitis B virus recombinant baculovirus-HepG2 system to study the effects of (-) 2', 3'-dideoxy-3'-thiacytidine on replication of hepatitis B virus and accumulation of covalently closed circular DNA. *Antimicrobial Agents and Chemotherapy* 1999; 36:1688-1694.
17. Furman PA, Davis M, Liotta DC, Paff M, Frick LW, Nelson DJ, Dornsife RE, Wurster JA, Wilson LJ, and Fyfe JA. The anti-hepatitis B virus activities, cytotoxicities, and anabolic profiles of the (-) and (+) enantiomers of cis-5-fluoro-1-(2-[hydroxymethyl]-1, 3-oxythiolan-5-yl)-cytosine (FTC). *Antimicro-bial Agents and Chemotherapy* 1992; 36:2686-2692.
18. Cui L, Schinazi RF, Gosselin G, Imbach JL, Chu CK, Rando RF, Revankar GR, and Sommadossi JP. Effect of beta-enantiomeric and racemic nucleoside analogues on mitochrondrial functions in HepG2 cells. Implications for predicting drug hepatotoxicity. *Biochemical Pharmacology* 1996; 52:1577-1584.

19. Paff MT, Averett DR, Prus KL, Miller WH, and Nelson DJ. Intracellular metabolism of (-) and (+)-cis-5-fluoro-1-[2-(hydroxymethyl)-1, 3-oxathiolan-5-yl]cytosine in HepG2 derivative 2.2.15 (subclone P5A) cells. *Antimicrobial Agents and Chemotherapy* 1994; 38:1230-1238.
20. Chu CK, Boudinot FD, Peek SF, Hong JH, Choi Y, Korba BE, Gerin JL, Cote PJ, Tennant BC, and Cheng YC. Preclinical investigation of L-FMAU as an anti-hepatitis B virus agent. *Antiviral Therapy* 1998; 3(Suppl 3):113-121.
21. Pai SB, Liu SH, Zhu YL, Chu CK, and Cheng YC. Inhibition of hepatitis B virus by a novel L-nucleoside, 2'-fluoro-5-methyl-β-L-arabinofuranosyl uracil. *Antimicrobial Agents and Chemotherapy* 1996; 40:380-386.
22. Chu CK, Ma T, Shanmuganathan K, Wang C, Xiang Y, Pai SB, Yao GQ, Sommadossi JP, and Cheng YC. Use of 2'fluoro-5-methyl-β-L-arabinofuranosyluracil as a novel antiviral agent for hepatitis B virus and Epstein-Barr virus. *Antimicrobial Agents and Chemotherapy* 1995; 39:979-981.
23. Schinazi RF, Ma L, Shi J, Horwitz SJ, Schlueter Wirtz S, Kupfer S, Juodawalkis A, McAtee J, Liotta DC, McClure HM, Faraj A, and Sommadossi JP. Nucleosides with dual anti-HIV and HBV activity. 1998; abst. 629, p 198. *In* Fifth Conference on Retrovirus and Opportunistic Infections.
24. Ussery MA, Wood OL, Kunder SC, Bacho MA, Broud DD, Papermaster SF, Hall BE, Ciaverella A, Nielsen CJ, and Schinazi RF. Anti-HIV activity in the HuPBMC SCID mouse model of six novel nucleoside analogs: (-)-FTC, (±)-FTC, D-DAPD, D-D4FC, CS-92 and CS-87. *Antiviral Research* 1998; 37:A49 (abst. 33).
25. Ma L, Hurwitz SJ, Shi J, Mcatee JJ, Liotta DC, McClure HM, and Schinazi RF. Pharmacokinetics of the antiviral agent D-D4FC I rhesus monkeys. *Antimicrobial Agents and Chemotherapy* 1999; 43:381-384.
26. Shi J. McAtee JJ. Schlueter Wirtz S. Tharnish P. Juodawlkis A. Liotta DC. and Schinazi RF. Synthesis and biological evaluation of 2', 3'-didehydro-2', 3'-deoxy-5-fluorocytidine (D4FC) analogues: discovery of carbocyclic nucleoside triphosphates with potent inhbibitory activity against HIV-1 reverse transcripase. *Journal of Medicinal Chemistry* 1999; 42:859-867.
27. De Clercq, E. Perspectives for the treatment of hepatitis B virus infections. *International Journal of Antimicrobial Agents* 1999; 12:81-95.
28. Mason WS, Cullen J, Moraleda G, Saputelli J, Aldrich CE, Miller DS, Tennant B, Frick L, Averett D, Condreay LD, and Jilbert AR. Lamivudine therapy of WHV-infected woodchucks. *Virology* 1998; 245:18-32.
29. Cullen JM, Smith SL, Davis MG, Dunn SE, Botteron C, Cecchi A, Linsey D, Linzey D, Frick L, Paff MT, Goulding A, and Biron K. *In vivo* antiviral activity and pharmacokinetics of (-)-*cis*-5-fluoro-1-[2-(hydroxymethyl)-1, 3-oxathiolan-5-yl]cytosine in woodchuck hepatitis virus infected woodchucks. *Antimicrobial Agents and Chemotherapy* 1997; 41:2076-82.
30. Aguesse-Germon S, Liu SH, Chevallier M, Pichoud C, Jamard C, Borel C, Chu CK, Trepo C, Cheng YC, and Zoulim F. Inhibitory effect of 2'-fluoro-5-methyl-β-L-arabinofuranosyluracil on duck hepatitis B virus replication. *Antimicrobial Agents and Chemotherapy* 1998; 42:369-76.
31. Hurst M, and Noble S. Stavudine: an update of its use in the treatment of HIV infection. *Drugs* 1999; 58:919-949.
32. Crouch RA, and Arras JD. AZT trials and tribulations. *Hastings Center Report* 1998; 28:26-34.
33. Marion PL, Oshiro LS, Regnery DC, Scullard GH, and Robinson WS. A virus in Beechey ground squirrels that is related to hepatitis B virus of humans. *Proceedings of the National Academy of Sciences of the United States of America* 1980; 77:2941-2945.
34. Summers J, Smolec JM, and Snyder R. A virus similar to human hepatitis B virus associated with

hepatitis and hepatoma in woodchucks. *Proceedings of the National Academy of Sciences of the United States of America* 1978; 75:4533-4537.

35. Mason WS, Seal G, and Summers J. Virus of Pekin ducks with structural and biological relatedness to human hepatitis B virus. *Journal of Virology* 1980; 36:829-836.
36. Tsiquaye KN, Sutton D, Maung M, and Boyd MR. Antiviral activities and pharmacokinetics of penciclovir and famciclovir in Pekin ducks chroncally infected with duck hepatitis B virus. *Antiviral Chemistry and Chemotherapy* 1996; 7:153-159.
37. Korba BE, Xie H, Wright KN, Hornbuckle WE, Gerin JL, Tennant BC, and Hostetler KY. Liver targeted antiviral nucleosides: enhanced antiviral activity of phosphatidyl-dedeoxyguanosine *versus* dideoxyguanosine in woodchuck hepatitis *in vivo. Hepatology* 1996; 23:958-963.
38. Nicoll A, Colledge D, Toole J, Angus P, Smallwood R, and Locarnini S. Inhibition of duck hepatitis B virus replication by 9[2-phosphonylmethoxyethyl]adenine, an acyclic phosphonate nucleoside analogue. *Antimicrobial Agents and Chemotherapy* 1998; 42:3130-1335.
39. Nagahata T, Araki K, Yamamura KI, and Matsubara K. Inhibition of intrahepatic hepatitis B virus replication by antiviral drugs in a novel transgenic mouse model. *Antimicrobial Agents and Chemotherapy* 1992; 36:2042-2045.
40. Larkin J, Clayton MM, Sun B, Perchonock CE, Morgan JL, Siracusa LD, Michaels F, and Feitelson MA. Hepatitis B virus transgenic SCID mouse model of chronic liver disease. *Nature Medicine* 1999; 5:907-912.
41. Babinet C, Farza H, Morello D, Hadchouel M, and Pourcel C. Specific expression of hepatitis B surface antigen (HBsAg) in transgenic mice. *Science* 1985; 230:1160-1163.
42. Burk RD, DeLoia JA, ElAwady MK, and Gearhart JD. Tissue preferential expression of the hepatitis B virus (HBV) surface antigen gene in two lines of HBV transgenic mice. *Journal of Virology* 1988; 62:649-654.
43. Chisari FV, Klopchin K, Moriyama T, Pasquinelli C, Dunsford HA, Sell S, Pinkert CA, Brinster RL, and Palmiter RD. Molecular pathogenesis of hepatocellular carcinoma in hepatitis B virus transgenic mice. *Cell* 1989; 59:1145-1156.
44. Araki K, Miyazaki JL, Hino O, Tomita N, Chisaka O, Matsubara K, and Yamamura KI. Expression and replication of hepatitis B virus genome in transgenic mice. *Proceedings of the National Academy of Sciences of the United States of America.* 1989; 86:207-211.
45. Farza H, Hadchouel M, Scotto J, Tiollais P, Babinet C, and Pourcel C. Replication and gene expression of hepatitis B virus in a transgenic mouse that contains the complete viral genome. *Journal of Virology* 1988; 62:4144-4152.
46. Lai C, Chien R, Leung N, Chang T, Guan R, Tai D, Ng K, Wu P, Dent J, Barber J, Stephenson S, and Gray D. A one-year trial of lamivudine for chronic hepatitis B. Asia Hepatitis Lamivudine Study Group. *New England Journal of Medicine* 1998; 339:61-68.

DRUG DISCOVERY AND DEVELOPMENT: NOVEL THERAPEUTICS FOR HEPATITIS B AND C

Novel approaches in the management of chronic HBV infection

ANGELINE BARTHOLOMEUSZ[1], PHILLIP FURMAN[2] and STEPHEN LOCARNINI[1]

[1] *Victorian Infectious Diseases Reference Laboratory, 10 Wreckyn Street, North Melbourne, Victoria, 3051, Australia*
[2] *Triangle Pharmaceuticals, 4611 University Drive, 4 University Place, Durham, NC, 27717-0530, USA*

Abstract

The two main goals in the treatment of chronic hepatitis B are:
1. Prevention of liver fibrosis, which requires long-term suppression of HBV replication, and
2. Prevention of hepatocellular carcinoma, where treatment needs to be initiated before HBV DNA integration into host cell DNA has occurred.

The management of chronic hepatitis B should be based on an understanding of the pathogenesis of the disease. There are three key elements here: the virus, the hepatocyte and the immune response. Thus, the best therapeutic approach would be based on at least one or all of the following: (a) immune modulation with cytokines and therapeutic vaccines; (b) blocking viral replication using antiviral agents and cytokines; (c) preventing re-infection by neutralising antibodies.

Current antiviral therapy includes agents such as interferon alpha, lamivudine (LMV), famciclovir (FCV), adefovir dipivoxil (ADV), entecavir, emtricitabine (FTC), clevudine (L-FMAU) and DAPD/DXG. Similarly, immunomodulatory therapy can consist of either the use of nonspecific immunotherapy with interferon alpha, HBIg and cytokines such as IL-2, IL-12 and thymosin-α1, or active immuno-therapy comprising peptides, viral envelope proteins and adjuvants in the form of therapeutic vaccines, HBsAg-Ab complexes, DNA vaccines and particular viral vectors. Current approved therapy consists of interferon alpha and/or lamivudine. Adefovir dipivoxil, emtricitabine, clevudine and entecavir are in various stages of clinical development.

Overall, the three major aims of a successful therapeutic strategy in hepatitis B should be:
1. To decrease viral load to undetectable levels
2. To decrease rate of disease progression, and
3. To decrease rate of emergence of drug-resistant HBV.

These aims can be readily achieved using combination chemotherapy.

Frontiers in Viral Hepatitis Ed. by RF Schinazi, J-P Sommadossi and CM Rice. 225 — 243

Introduction

Almost 400 million people will be infected with hepatitis B virus (HBV) by the end of the year 2000 [40, 64, 66]. This is equivalent to about 5% of the world's population and more than ten times the number infected with the human immunodeficiency virus (HIV). Up to half of these hepatitis B surface antigen (HBsAg)-positive individuals will succumb due to the development of liver failure and/or hepatocellular carcinoma, clinical sequelae developed as a consequence of persistent HBV carriage [58].

Hepatitis B virus can cause both acute and chronic liver disease. The outcome depends on the interplay between the virus, the hepatocyte, and the host's immune response [18]. Under most circumstances, HBV is not cytopathic and it is the infected host's immune response that is responsible for the liver damage during infection [33]. In specialized circumstances, such as after orthotopic liver transplantation, viral infection may cause unique histopathological damage resulting in fibrosing cholestatic hepatitis (FCH) [57]. Before the advent of specific antiviral therapy [3], FCH was invariably fatal.

Thus, antiviral chemotherapy remains the major treatment option for controlling chronic HBV infection, with the immune modulating agent interferon alpha and the antiviral compound lamivudine (LMV) being the only two FDA-approved treatments. The registration of LMV was only a recent event, and a number of new deoxynucleoside analogues and derivatives are in various stages of clinical development. These include entecavir, famciclovir, clevudine, emtricitabine and adefovir dipivoxil. These new anti-HBV drugs are capable of reducing viral loads very rapidly, but the initial response is invariably followed by a very much slower elimination of residual virus [92]. The long-term treatment which is required to eliminate residual virus may carry with it increased risks for cumulative toxicity and drug resistance. Fortunately, experience to date indicates that toxicity is not a major problem with these newer nucleoside analogues, so emergence of drug resistance during the slower phase of HBV elimination appears most likely to become the single significant obstacle in the eventual control of chronic infection [85].

Molecular virology of HBV

HBV is a small DNA-containing virus with four overlapping open-reading frames. The four genes encoded are core (pre-core and core proteins), surface (pre-S1, pre-S2 and S proteins), X and polymerase. The core gene encodes the core nucleocapsid protein and the secreted, soluble hepatitis Be antigen (HBeAg) protein. The surface gene encodes pre-S1, pre-S2 and S protein, yielding the large-, middle- and small-surface proteins, respectively. The X gene encodes the X protein, which has transactivating properties and may be important in hepatic carcinogenesis. The polymerase gene encodes a large protein with functions critical for DNA replication and packaging (Figure 1) [10, 34].

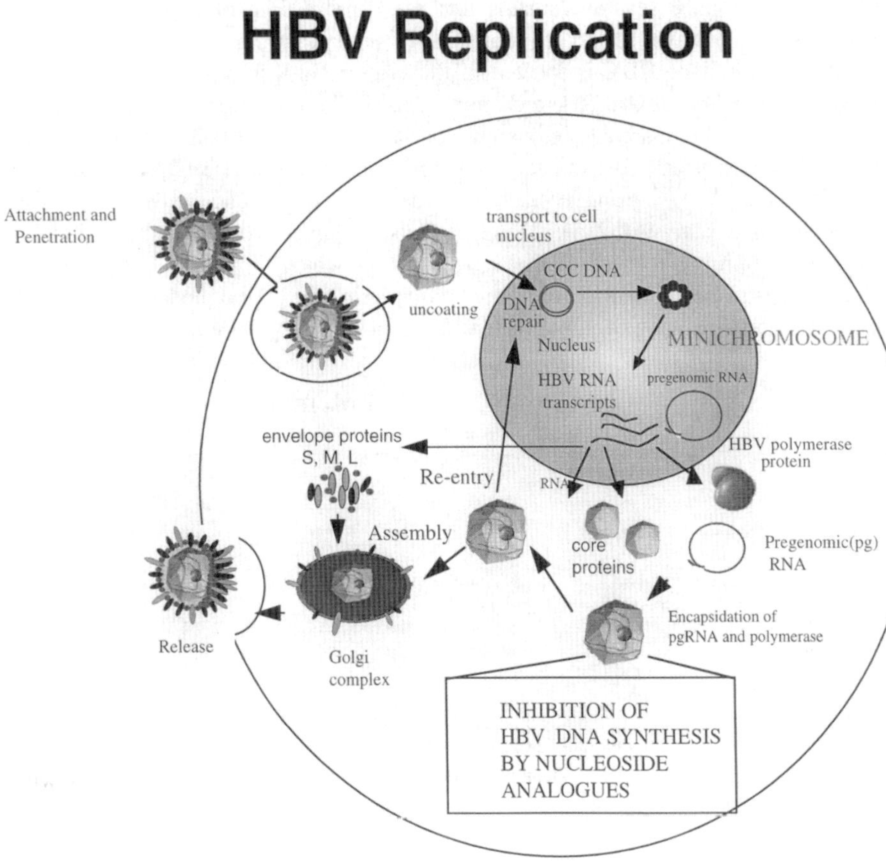

Figure 1. Hepatitis B virus replication cycle. The virus in the serum adheres to the surface of the hepatocytes through a receptor. Through the process of endocytosis the virus enters the cell and is uncoated to remove the envelope proteins. The viral core particles bind to the nuclear pore and the HBV genome enters the nucleus. In the nucleus the HBV DNA is repaired and chromatinized to form a minichromosome. The minichromosome is used as the transcriptional template for RNA synthesis by RNA Polymerase II. The HBV RNA is transported into the cytoplasm where the viral proteins are made. The pre-genomic RNA is encapsidated. In the viral RNA cores DNA synthesis occurs through a process of reverse transcription and also DNA synthesis. The viral cores can be either transported back into the nucleus for further genomic amplification, or are enveloped and secreted into the blood.

HBV polymerase

The HBV polymerase gene encodes for a protein which has four functional regions: The terminal protein (TP), Spacer region, Reverse Transcriptase (RT) and RNAse H.

The HBV RT contains several domains that are conserved in other RNA-dependent polymerases which have designated domains F, and A to E (Figure 2), [83, 59]. The "YMDD" motif of HBV is located in the C domain. The polymerase protein of HBV has not been crystallized. There is amino acid similarity with HIV in the conserved domains, and these comparable regions may be involved in NTP binding and substrate recognition. It was proposed from the analysis of the X-ray crystal structure of HIV that the domains A, C, D and F may participate directly in nucleotide triphosphate (NTP) binding and catalysis [52, 51]. Domains B and E may be involved in the positioning of the template-primer relative to the active site, in which domain B forms part of the "template grip" and domain E forms the "primer grip" [68]. Two models for the HBV RT catalytic domains have been published [2, 8] based on the HIV structure.

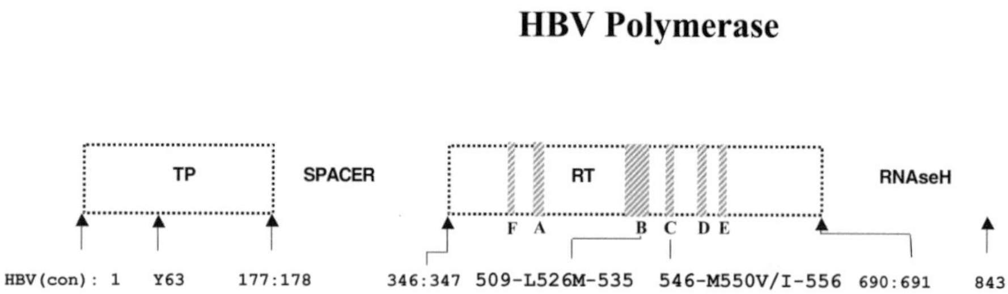

Figure 2. Organisation of the HBV polymerase. The different domains of the terminal protein (TP), Spacer region, Reverse Transcriptase (RT) and RNAse H domain of the HBV polymerase are indicated with a dotted line. The conserved domains within the Reverse Transcriptase are indicated by shaded boxes. The numbering for HBV consensus sequence in which the methionine in the "YMDD" motif is designated 550 is shown, and this corresponds to the numbering for genotypes B, C and F. This figure was modified from Stuyver et al. 2000.

HBV antiviral resistance

In HBV, LMV resistance is usually associated with a change of the methionine in the "YMDD" motif in the C domain to either valine (at M550V) or isoleucine (at M550I). The numbering for HBV polymerase varies with the different genotypes. In this study the methionine in the "YMDD" motif is designated 550, and this corresponds to the numbering for genotypes B, C and F (Table 1) [9, 2, 72]. M550I usually occurs as a single codon change, whereas the M550V is detected with a second codon change at L526M in the B domain [2, 72]. These mutations have been confirmed to be associated with LMV resistance using *in vitro* cell culture assays and also polymerase enzyme assays [2, 30, 54, 97, 98]. The M550I and the M550V + L526M dual mutant both result in

Table 1. Mutations in HBV polymerase protein associated with drug resistance to LMV and FCV with the corresponding change in HBsAg

LMV Mutations		HBsAg Mutations
I399S		not published
F512L	B Domain	A157D
V519L	B Domain	E164D
L526M/V	B Domain	no change
T530S		not published
A546V		not published
M550I	C Domain	W196S, W196L
M550V	C Domain	I195M
V553I	C Domain	M198I/W199S
S559T		not published
S565P		S210R
L575V		not published
FCV Mutations		HBsAg Mutations
H436N/Y	A Domain	no change
V519L	B Domain	E164D
P523L	B Domain	no change
L526M/V	B Domain	no change
T530S		not published
V553I	C Domain	W199 Stop/no change
N/S/H584K	D Domain	After end HBsAg
R588K	D Domain	After end HBsAg
ADV Mutations	None to date	

a greater than 10,000-fold increase in the IC_{50} levels of the antiviral effect of LMV against HBV. In enzyme assays with LMV-triphosphate (TP), the HBV polymerase containing these mutations (M550I, or M550V + L526M) were associated with an 8.0- or 25.2-fold increase in the K_i, respectively (Xiong et al. 2000) (Table 2). The other mutations which are associated with LMV resistance are discussed below (Section 6 compensatory mutations).

Resistance to famciclovir (FCV) is associated with two mutations at L526M and V519L [6]. The HBV isolated from the serum of a patient with HBV encoding these mutations had a reduced sensitivity to penciclovir (PCV)-TP in the endogenous

Table 2. Inhibition of HBV DNA polymerases expressing LMV- or FCV-associated mutations (from Xiong et al. Hepatology 1998;28:1669, Xiong et al., Hepatology 2000;31:219)

Enzyme	Lamivudine (3TCTP)		Famciclovir (PCVTP)		Adefovir (ADVDP)	
	K_i (μM)[a]	Fold increase[b]	K_i (μM)[a]	Fold increase[b]	K_i (μM)[a]	Fold increase[b]
Wild type	0.25±0.03	1.0	4.8±0.1	1	0.10±0.01	1.0
F512L	1.5±0.03	6.0	ND*	-	0.19±0.03	1.9
M550I	2.0±0.1	8.0	5.9±1.1	1.2	0.13±0.03	1.3
M550V	4.9±0.4	19.6	11.3±2.2	2.4	0.22±0.02	2.2
L526M	0.64±0.04	2.6	18.7±2.8	3.9	0.23±0.04	2.3
L526M/M550V	6.3±2.4	25.2	11.9±1.7	2.5	0.079±0.018	0.79
L526M/M550I	3.8±1.0	15.2	ND*	-	0.18±0.03	1.8
F512L/526M	2.6±0.5	10.4	ND*	-	0.11±0.04	1.1
V519L	0.31±0.06	1.2	15.1±5.1	3.1	0.15±0.04	1.5
P523L	0.89±0.06	3.6	11.0±2.5	2.3	0.23±0.06	2.3
T530S	0.60±0.05	2.4	7.7±2.0	1.6	0.18±0.03	1.8
V553I	0.87±0.13	3.6	29.7±5.8	6.2	0.19±0.01	1.9

a. All inhibition constants (K_i) are the average of three separate experiments K_i values are means ± S.D.

b. Fold increase = (mutant K_i)/(wild-type K_i)

* ND = Not done

HBV DNA polymerase assay [6]. This patient subsequently responded clinically and virologically to LMV, but LMV resistance emerged within six months [63]. A mutation at V553I has been reported to occur transiently in chronically infected patients treated with FCV [82]. Virus containing this mutation was resistant to PCV in *in vitro* assays, but remained sensitive to LMV. This change in the HBV polymerase gene did result in a stop codon in the overlapping HBsAg reading frame, which may alter the replication competence of this virus and account for it being detected only transiently.

The inhibition constants of PCV-TP were measured for the wild-type HBV polymerase and the HBV polymerase containing either V519L, P523L, L526M, T530S or V553I. In these enzyme assays there was only a modest increase in the K_i with the polymerase containing the mutation at V553I (approximately sixfold) and only a threefold increase in the K_i with HBV polymerase encoding the mutation at either codon V519L or codon L526M (Table 2). These mutations were tested individually in these assays and multiple mutations such as V519L + L526M may need to be examined to determine if there is a greater increase in the resistance profile [6, 82].

Compensatory mutations

Other mutations within the catalytic domain have been detected in association with the LMV resistance mutations M550I/V, which may function as compensatory mutations. HBV containing the L526M mutation alone confers a fivefold increase in the IC_{50} for LMV compared to the wild-type [17]. The L526M mutation is also associated with resistance to FCV [6]. The HBV polymerase containing the L526M mutation showed a 2.6-fold increase in the K_i value for LMV-5'triphosphate (TP) (0.64 ± 2.4) compared to wildtype polymerase (0.25 ± 0.03) [97, 98]. The M550V/L526M double mutant showed a 25.2-fold increase in the K_i value for LMVTP compared to a 19.6-fold increase in the K_i obtained for LMVTP with the M550V mutant polymerase. A mutation adjacent to the L526M at A527T was also reported recently [99]. HBV encoding this mutation emerged as the major population during LMV treatment in three patients and replaced HBV encoding M550V/L526M as the major population.

The M550I mutation has been detected in conjunction with the L526M mutation in HBV from HBV/HIV co-infected patients receiving "highly active anti-retroviral therapy" (HAART). The appearance of these mutations in this patient population may be due to antiviral selection pressure from the antiviral agents including LMV with which the patients are being treated [88]. This mutation was also detected in HBV isolated from patients on long-term LMV therapy and replaced HBV encoding M550V/L526M as the major population [99].

[89] reported that a patient on HBIg and LMV therapy had high HBV DNA levels while on LMV therapy. This was confirmed using transient transfection studies of HBV DNA encoding HBIg selected mutations at codons P120T or G145R, in addition to the LMV resistant mutations [11]. In cells transfected with HBV DNA encoding the HBIg and LMV mutations, greater amounts of replicative intermediates were detected in the presence of LMV compared to HBV encoding the mutations at M550I/V alone. These HBIg mutations at codons P120T and G145R occur with the concomitant mutations in the overlapping polymerase gene at codons P474N and R/W449Q, respectively. Both polymerase mutations are located in the region between domains A and B.

Patients infected with HBV encoding a mutation at codons L426V/I or L428V in addition to the mutation at M550I, had higher DNA levels than pre-LMV therapy [74]. These mutations are located in the A domain of the polymerase and are likely located near the mutation at YMDD on the proposed models of the HBV polymerase.

Cross-resistance/sensitivity

The LMV-resistant virus with mutations at M550I and M550V + L526M are sensitive to adefovir, lobucavir and ganciclovir, as demonstrated in cell culture experiments using a transient transfection assay [97, 76, 77, 98]. The antiviral activity of the M550V HBV mutant (without the corresponding mutation at L526M) and wild-type virus was determined for a number of new antiviral compounds which are in various stages of development. This assay employed cells stably transfected with a 1.5 genome length of either wild-type HBV (AD38 cells) or HBV containing the M550V mutation (AD79 cells). Virus replication was under the control of the tetracycline-responsive promoter. In this assay system the M550V virus was resistant to LMV, and was sensitive to penciclovir, lobucavir, dioxalane guanine [DXG], 1-β-2,6-diaminopurine dioxalane [DAPD], L-FMAU, adefovir and tenofovir [100]. The FCV associated mutations at V519L, L526M, V553I are sensitive to LMV and ADV [97, 98].

Principals of antiviral resistance

To reduce the rate of emergence of drug-resistant virus, viral and host cellular factors, as well as the treatment regimen, all need to be considered. In particular:

(a) The emergence of mutations and viral quasi-species within a host is a dynamic process which likely results from lack of proofreading ability of the HBV polymerase. Thus, naturally occurring variants resistant to nucleoside analogues may preexist and are selected for during antiviral therapy.

(b) The dynamics of viral clearance during antiviral treatment may influence the overall treatment protocol. Partial suppression of the virus will promote antiviral resistance and thus decrease the time to the detection of resistant virus. Antiviral strategies that significantly reduce the viral load and inhibit viral replication may prolong the time before antiviral resistant virus is detected.

(c) Host cellular factors may also be involved in the development of antiviral resistance.

(a) Generation of resistance mutations

As outlined earlier, the error rate, or the rate for nucleotide substitutions that occur during HBV replication, is approximately 1.4 to 3.2 x 10^{-5} substitutions/site/year [75, 78]. In the liver transplant setting, it is almost 100-fold higher, in the range of 1.1 x 10^{-2} to 5.9 x 10^{-3} substitutions/site/year (Sterneck et al. 1997). In comparison, the HIV retroviral RT error rate is 3 x 10^{-3} substitutions/site/year. The lower error rate in HBV in comparison to HIV may be due to the constraints in the overlapping reading frames [75, 86]. The much higher substitution rate in the liver transplant setting may be due to a number of factors, including possible infection of the liver after the graft by a different subpopulation of the virus that may have been present in extra hepatic sites. Infection of the new liver also occurs at a very rapid rate, which may result in an increased mutation rate for the virus. The high substitution rate may also be influenced by the immunosuppression regime associated with the transplant, or by the treatment with HBIg.

HBV LMV resistance requires either a single nucleotide change to alter the codon at M550I, or two nucleotide changes to alter the codon at M550V + L526M. The probability of a single or a double spontaneous mutation occurring in a single HBV genome chronic infection is 2.6 x 10^{-4}/day or 6.76 x 10^{-16}, respectively. The total daily production of HBV has been estimated to be approximately 10^{11} particles in a viral dynamic study [73]. Thus, the chance of the generation of HBV mutants encoding a single error in chronically infected patients is approximately 10^{7} per day, whereas the chance of two spontaneous mutations arising is approximately 10^{-5} to 10^{-6} per day. These values do not take into consideration that certain regions of the genome may contain "hot spots" or "hyper-variable regions" which have a higher mutation rate (such as in HCV), and they do not take into account the viability or the replication fitness of the virus generated. In addition, these calculations estimate the chance of spontaneous mutations occurring in a virus in a single day. It does not take into account that viable virus with a selective advantage may re-infect the host and serve as the template for the generation of virus with multiple mutations on sequential days. In other viruses, silent mutations which alter the third nucleotide position of the codon would have a limited effect on viability. However, in HBV the genome encodes for four overlapping reading frames, and silent mutations which do not affect one or more of the overlapping reading frames are likely to be rare. Thus, the number of HBV particles encoding a single mutation, which are able to infect new cells and replicate, would be considerably lower than the estimated figure of 10^7 HBV mutants generated per day. The estimation of the probability of a pre-existing variant which is resistant to a single antiviral agent depends not only on the mutation rate per virion and the total rate of production of virus within the host, but also on the number of mutations required to convey high-level antiviral resistance. [21] have predicted that it is highly likely for a pre-existing resistant variant to emerge as the major viral species when a single antiviral is used in HIV treatment. It is unlikely that pre-existing resistance occurs with three or more antivirals in the case of HAART.

In antiviral naïve patients with HIV, naturally occurring HIV variants which contain mutations associated with resistance have been reported [67, 24]. HIV encoding resistance to LMV has a higher fidelity than wild-type virus [50]. In HBV isolated from patients treated with antiviral agents, the HBV error rate may be affected by the antiviral treatment. In both HIV and HBV *in vitro* studies, the fidelity of replication by viral polymerase may be affected by the concentration of the intracellular deoxynucleotide triphosphate pools [35]. There are no published studies of HBV LMV resistant mutants detected in antiviral naïve patients. The lack of detection of pre-existing resistant HBV variants may be due to the poor sensitivity in the detection methods. Direct sequencing of HBV isolated from patients can only ascertain the sequence of the predominate quasi-species. Antiviral resistant variants or other mutations can only be detected by direct sequencing when they comprise greater than 20% of the total HBV quasi-species in the serum. In studies which have cloned and sequenced PCR-amplified HBV DNA, only a limited number of clones have been analyzed. HBV variants that represent less than 1% of the total population may not have been detected. New methods for the detection of resistance mutations have been published. These include LiPA [87], real-time PCR with molecular probes [14] and molecular beacons [81]. The molecular beacon technology has a sensitivity of 0.01% [93]. The rate of change in the proportion of LMV-resistant virus to wild-type during antiviral selection pressure has not been determined for HBV. The fidelity of the HBV polymerase encoding the LMV-resistant mutations has not been determined.

(b) Management of HBV resistance and viral clearance dynamics

In longitudinal studies of patients with HBV encoding the LMV-resistant mutation, following the cessation of antiviral treatment, the wild-type emerged as the predominant quasi-species [16]. On re-treatment, the LMV-resistant virus once again becomes the predominant species. In studies with HIV, partial suppression of the virus by inadequate antiviral treatment promotes resistance. Sanctuary sites such as the brain also need to be considered [39]. Inhibiting virus replication and reducing the total viral load can increase the time to detection of resistant variants. In HIV-infected patients, suppression of viral load to <20 copies/ml provided maximal antiviral response [62].

The rate of HBV viral clearance in antiviral treated patients has been examined, and mathematical models of viral dynamics have been developed. These models may be useful to monitor the progression of HBV and to predict the duration of treatment required to decrease viral loads to a level which may be sufficient to induce seroconversion [73, 92, 53]. Three main parameters are included in the models; (a) the population of susceptible uninfected cells, (b) the population of cells which are infected and are capable of producing virus, and (c) the level of circulating virus in the serum. The clearance of HBV is proposed to be biphasic [92, 53]. There is a large initial reduction of virus produced prior to the inhibition of viral replication. The second, slower reduction may reflect the replication of virus from the covalently closed circular (CCC) DNA template, or death of infected cells [85]. During LMV treatment in patients with chronic HBV, there was a 10^3-fold decrease in viral load in the serum [12]. However, in the same patients the intrahepatic viral load did not alter dramatically and was only reduced approximately two- to threefold [12]. Colledge, *et al.* examined CCC DNA in DHBV-infected cells treated with LMV and PCV. LMV did not affect the stability of CCC DNA, whereas there was a decrease in CCC DNA in infected cells treated with PCV+LMV. The turnover of hepatocytes and the number of hepatocytes which can be infected with LMV-resistant virus may affect the rate of emergence of resistant virus as the predominant species in the serum.

The total reduction in viral load after 12 weeks of ADV 30-mg treatment in humans was 4.1 $\log_{10}$ [92]. The half-life of the virus in infected cells was calculated to be 11-30 days and 10-100 days by [92, 73], respectively. In comparison, the viral half-life in cells infected with HIV was estimated to be 1.6 days [80]. [92] have estimated that with the biphasic pattern of viral clearance and the reduction in viral load during ADV treatment, it would take 517 days to get the total plasma viral load from 1 x 10^8 copies/ml to 1 copy/ml. However, it should be noted that the extreme variability in viral loads will affect these calculations. Furthermore, detection limits of the current assays for HBV DNA may affect the calculations [103]. The type of test and the lower limit of detection of HBV DNA used to measure viral loads should be considered. The Amplicor HBV DNA Monitor test with COBAS modification has a lower detection limit of 200 genomes/ml [103].

(c) Host mechanisms involved in antiviral resistance

In clinical trials with the nucleoside analogue FCV, partial response and non-response to the antiviral drug were noted [26, 82]. This may be due to patients not metabolising FCV or the presence of a naturally FCV-resistant HBV variant. In cell culture, it has been established that a number of antiviral compounds are not efficiently metabolised [4]. Recently, [84], have shown an increase in the transcription of the MRP4 gene in cells in viral cultures resistant to adefovir. The MRP4 protein and MRP5 protein may be involved in the transport or efflux of the antiviral nucleoside out of the cell [84, 94]. Increased transcription of this gene in HIV patients on adefovir treatment was also noted.

New antivirals and combination testing

A number of new antiviral nucleoside analogues have been identified and are undergoing late pre-clinical or phase I-II clinical trial evaluation. Amongst these compounds are found: adefovir dipivoxil, Emtricitabine (FTC), Clevudine (L-FMAU) and Entecavir.

a) Adefovir dipivoxil (bis-POM PMEA or 9-[2-bis(pivaloyloxymethyl) phosphonyl methoxyethyl]adenine)

Adefovir dipivoxil is a phosphonated acyclic purine nucleoside with broad spectrum antiviral activity and is a potent inhibitor of HBV replication [26]. PMEA, the active component, is poorly absorbed and the addition of the bis(pivaloyloxymethyl) group produces the prodrug adefovir dipivoxil (bis-POM PMEA), which greatly increases oral bioavailability [26]. PMEA is monophosphorylated. After cellular uptake, it is then converted to the triphosphate form by mitochondrial adenylate kinase [26]. Adefovir dipivoxil has greater inhibitory effects on viral polymerases than on host cell DNA polymerases α, β and γ [4, 26] and acts by competitive inhibition of the viral polymerase with dATP and viral DNA chain termination [4, 7, 26]. Adefovir dipivoxil may also stimulate natural killer cells and endogenous α-interferon production [4, 13, 26].

Adefovir dipivoxil inhibits replication of hepadnaviruses both *in vitro* and *in vivo* [102, 37, 38, 101, 32, 71]. The IC_{50} of PMEA-DP for HBV in stably transfected human hepatoma cell lines is 0.05 μg/ml, while the cytotoxic IC_{50} is approximately 15 μg/ml, giving a selectivity index of 300 [101]. Treatment of ducks congenitally infected with DHBV with adefovir dipivoxil produces marked reductions in all viral markers of replication, including pregenomic RNA, pre-S and core proteins and CCC DNA, but only whilst on treatment [37, 71]. In a phase I/II study in humans chronically infected with HBV, adefovir dipivoxil treatment resulted in a rapid and marked reduction in serum HBV DNA, with minimal toxicity [96, 36]. Serum HBV DNA fell by 99.99%, or 4 $\log_{10}$ from baseline, and up to 27% lost HBeAg [36]. PMEA also retains its antihepadnaviral activity *in vitro* against HBV variants that have become resistant to lamivudine and famciclovir [96]. Adefovir dipivoxil may therefore be an effective nucleoside analogue for the treatment of HBV.

b) FTC (5-fluoro-thiacytidine)

Fluorcytidine (FTC) is a pyrimidine analogue with activity against HBV and HIV [15, 29]. FTC is similar to lamivudine in that it also exists as two enantiomers, both forms having activity against HBV. Phosphorylation of (-)-FTC (emtricitabine) to the triphosphate ((-)-FTC-TP) is performed by cytoplasmic cytidine kinase, and the mode of action of (-)-FTC-TP is as a competitive inhibitor for dCTP [15, 60, 31]. FTC has excellent oral bioavailability of 60-90% and is excreted unchanged in urine [15]. In contrast to (-)-FTC, which does not affect mitochondrial DNA synthesis, (+)-FTC is 20 times more toxic on cell growth and 12 times more potent at inhibiting mitochondrial DNA polymerase γ [15, 60]. The (-)-FTC is a more potent inhibitor of HBV with an IC_{50} of 0.03 μM, while that of (+)-FTC is 0.72 μM [15, 31, 55]. Cross-resistance between lamivudine and FTC in DHBV has been reported [29] and may limit the usefulness of FTC in patients who have prior treatment failure with lamivudine. Phase I clinical studies of FTC are currently in progress.

c) L-FMAU (2'-fluoro-5-methyl-β-L-arabinofuranosyluracil)

L-FMAU is a pyrimidine analogue with antiviral activity against HBV and EBV, but not HSV 1 or 2, nor HIV [19, 79, 95]. L-FMAU is phosphorylated to the triphosphate form intracellularly, and L-FMAU-TP is removed slowly from cells, thus exerting a sustained inhibitory antiviral activity [95]. L-FMAU-TP is not incorporated into host cell DNA and is not a substrate for DNA polymerase α, β, γ, and ε [1]. In contrast to D-FMAU, FIAU and ddC, L-FMAU does not increase lactate production [19, 1, 95]. The drug is relatively well absorbed with an oral bioavailability of 20-60% [95]. The IC_{50} of L-FMAU for HBV *in vitro* is 0.1μM, while the cytotoxic IC_{50} is greater than 100-200 μM [19]. In HBV transfected cell culture, L-FMAU produces a dose-dependent inhibition of HBV DNA, but not of HBV RNA [19, 79, 95], and a similar reduction in serum DHBV DNA is also observed in ducks, although CCC DNA is not affected [1]. Treatment of ducks for eight days with 40 mg/kg resulted in a 72% inhibition of DHBV and no rebound of viremia was detected in a two-week follow-up period [1]. In pre-clinical studies L-FMAU (10 mg/kg daily) was given to four woodchucks chronically infected with WHV for 50 weeks. There was a greater than 1000-fold decrease in viraemia within two weeks [19]. At the end of the treatment period there was a further decrease in WHV replicative intermediates. Toxicity studies in both ducks and woodchucks treated with L-FMAU showed no change in body weight. These results suggest that L-FMAU may be a promising antiviral agent for the treatment of HBV.

Combination antiviral therapy

The use of single agent nucleoside analogues in the treatment of chronic hepatitis B, although welltolerated, has not resulted in clearance of infection [27, 28, 65, 91, 70, 55]. In addition, long-term treatment has resulted in the emergence of resistance to famciclovir and lamivudine [5, 61, 69, 90, 9]. The use of lamivudine and penciclovir in combination has been evaluated *in vitro* [22]. These authors investigated the antiviral efficacy of lamivudine and penciclovir alone and in combination, in primary duck hepatocytes from DHBV congenitally-infected ducks [22]. Penciclovir was found to be slightly more potent than lamivudine in inhibiting DHBV. In addition, penciclovir inhibited CCC DNA and pre-S antigen production, while lamivudine had no effect [22]. The combination of these two nucleoside analogues resulted in additive and synergistic inhibition of DHBV [22]. The results of this study suggest that the use of combination antiviral nucleoside analogues may be more effective than single agent therapy. The use of combinations of nucleoside analogues may delay, or possibly even prevent, the development of resistance to single agents. The use of combination therapy has revolutionized the management of HIV [25, 23, 56], and with evidence now emerging demonstrating synergistic activity of famciclovir and lamivudine HBV [22], the use of combination antiviral nucleoside analogues for the treatment of chronic hepatitis B infection warrants further investigation.

Conclusion

The treatment of chronic hepatitis B infection is currently restricted to α-interferon and a small number of nucleoside analogues, with infrequent clearance of infection. The failure to eradicate chronic infection and the development of resistance may limit their usefulness in the long-term.

Antiviral nucleoside analogues are effective and convenient therapeutic agents, but do not eradicate chronic infection. The use of extended treatment courses with single agents has seen the emergence of antiviral resistant-variants of HBV over relatively short periods of time. The widespread use of these agents, with the emergence of drug-resistant variants, may substantially reduce the long-term efficacy of nucleoside analogues. It is highly unlikely that the use of single agent chemotherapy will result in the clearance, or even the long-term suppression, of chronic hepatitis B infection. Given this limitation of nucleoside analogues, the study of these antiviral drugs in combination should now be considered. The efficacy of combinations of nucleoside analogues and cross-resistance patterns can be studied using *in vitro* techniques, such as transient transfections of infectious HBV clones into HepG2 cells, stably transfected HBV producing HepG 2.2.15 cells and polymerase assay using recombinant baculovirus-expressed HBV polymerase. Animal models, in particular DHBV, will be useful in determining whether combinations of antiviral agents have additive or synergistic effects, and whether long-term therapy results in increased toxicity. These *in vitro* and *in vivo* models will provide invaluable information on combination nucleoside analogue therapy for chronic hepatitis B infection and help guide future clinical trials of combinations of antiviral, antisense and immune modulating therapeutics.

References

1. Aguesse S, Borel C, Chevalier M, Liu S, Chu C, Cheng Y, Trepo C, Zoulim F. Inhibitory effect of 2'-fluoro-5-methyl-″-L-arabinosyluracil (L-FMAU), a novel L-nucleoside analog, on duck hepatitis B virus replication. *Hepatology* 1996;24: A372.
2. Allen MI, Deslauriers M, Andrews CW, Tipples GA, Walters KA, Tyrrell DL, Brown N, Condreay LD. Identification and characterisation of mutations in hepatitis B virus resistant to lamivudine. Lamivudine Clinical Investigation Group. *Hepatology* 1998;27: 1670-7.
3. Angus P, Richards M, Bowden S, Ireton J, Sinclair R, Jones B, Locarnini S. Combination chemotherapy controls severe post-liver transplant recurrence of hepatitis B virus infection. *J. Gastroenterology and Hepatology* 1993;8: 353-7.
4. Aoki-Sei S, O'Brien MC, Ford H, Fujii H, Gilbert DA, Cooney DA, Johns DG, Broder S, Mitsuya H (). *In vitro* inhibition of hepatitis B virus replication by 2', 3'- dideoxyguanosine, 2', 3'-dideoxy-inosine, and 3'-azido-2', 3'- dideoxythymidine in 2.2.15 (PR) cells. *J Infect Dis* 1991;164: 843-51.
5. Aye T, Bartholomeusz A, Shaw T, Breschkin A, Gronen L, Bowden D, McMillan Jea (1996). Hepatitis B virus polymerase mutations during famciclovir therapy in patients following liver transplantation. *Hepatology* 24 285A.
6. Aye TT, Bartholomeusz A, Shaw T, Bowden S, Breschkin A, McMillan J, Angus P, Locarnini S. Hepatitis B virus polymerase mutations during antiviral therapy in a patient following liver transplantation. *J Hepatol* 1997;26: 1148-53.
7. Balzarini J, Hao Z, Herdewijn P, Johns D, De Clercq E. Intracellular metabolism and mechanism of anti-retrovirus action of 9-(2-phosphonylmethoxyethyl)adenine, a potent anti-human immunodeficiency virus compound. *Proc Natl Acad Sci USA* 1991;88: 1499-503.
8. Bartholomeusz A, Groenen L, Locarnini SA. Clinical experience with famciclovir against Hepatitis B virus and development of resistance. *Intervirology* 1998;40: 337-42.
9. Bartholomew M, Jansen R, Jeffers L, Reddy K, Johnson L, Bunzendhl H, Condreay L, Tzakis A, Schiff E, Brown N. Hepatitis B virus resistance to lamivudine given for recurrent infection after orthotopic liver transplantation. *Lancet* 1997;349: 20-2.
10. Blum HE. Variants of hepatitis B, C and D viruses: molecular biology and clinical significance. *Digestion* 1995;56: 85-95.
11. Bock T, Torresi J, Tillmann H, Locarnini S, Manns M, Trautwein C. Replication and fitness of hepatitis B virus polymerase mutants after antiviral treatment following liver transplantation. *Hepatology* 1999;30: 79A.
12. Cacciola I, Pollicino T, Squadrito G, Cerenzia G, Villari D, de Franchis R, Santantonio T, Brancatelli S, Colucci G, Raimondo G. Quantification of intrahepatic hepatitis B virus (HBV) DNA in patients with chronic HBV infection. *Hepatology* 2000;31: 507-12.
13. Calio R, Villani N, Balestra E, Sesa F, Holy A, Balzarini J, De Clercq E, Perno CF, Del Gobbo V. Enhancement of natural killer activity and interferon induction by different acyclic nucleoside phosphonates. *Antiviral Research* 1994;23: 77-89.
14. Cane PA, Mutimer D, Ratcliffe D, Cook P, Beards G, Elias E, Pillay D. Analysis of hepatitis B virus quasispecies changes during emergence and reversion of lamivudine resistance in liver transplantation. *ntivir Ther* 1999;4: 7-14.
15. Chang C, Doong S, Zhou J, Beach J, Jeong L, Chu C, Tsai C, Cheng Y, Liotta D, Schinazi R. Deoxycytidine deaminase-resistant stereoisomer is the active form of (+/-)-2', 3'-dideoxy-3'-thiacytidine in the inhibition of hepatitis B virus replication. *Biol Chem* 1992;267: 13938-42.

16. Chayama K, Suzuki Y, Kobayashi M, Kobayashi M, Tsubota A, Hashimoto M, Miyano Y, Koike H, Kobayashi M, Koida I. Emergence and takeover of YMDD motif mutant hepatitis B virus during long-term lamivudine therapy and re-takeover by wild-type after cessation of therapy. *Hepatology* 1998;27: 1711-6.
17. Chin R, Torresi J, Earnest-Silveira L, Bock T, Manns M, Trautwein C, Furman P, Cleary D, Locarnini S. Two novel antiviral agents, DAPD and L-FMAU, which are active against wild-type and lamivudine-resistant HBV. *Hepatology* 1999;30: 421A.
18. Chisari F, Ferrari C. Hepatitis B virus immunopathogenesis. *Ann Rev Immunol* 1995, 13: 29-60.
19. Chu CK, Boudinot FD, Peek SF, Hong JH, Choi Y, Korba BE, Gerin JL, Cote PJ, Tennant BC, Cheng Y-C. Preclinical investigation of L-FMAU as an anti-hepatitis B virus agent. 1998 In: Schinazi RF, Sommadossi J-P, Thomas HC eds. *Therapies for Viral Hepatitis.* London: International Medical Press; p 303-12.
20. Chu CK, Ma T, Shanmuganathan K, Wang C, Xiang Y, Pai SB, Yao GQ, Sommadossi JP, Cheng YC (1995). Use of 2'-Fluoro-5-Methyl-b-L-Arabinofuranosyluracil as a Novel Antiviral Agent for Hepatitis B Virus and Epstein-Barr Virus. *Antimicrobial Agents and Chemotherapy* 39: 979-81.
21. Colgrove R, Japour A. A combinatorial ledge: reverse transcriptase fidelity, total body viral burden, and the implications of multiple-drug HIV therapy for the evolution of antiviral resistance. *Antiviral Res* 1999;41: 45-56.
22. Colledge D, Locarnini S, Shaw T. Synergistic Inhibition of Hepadanaviral Replication by Lamivudine in Combination With Penciclovir *In Vitro*. *Hepatology* 1997;26: 216-25.
23. Corey L, Holmes KK. Therapy for human immunodeficiency virus infection - what have we learned? *N Engl J Med* 1996;335: 1142-4.
24. Cornelissen M, van den Burg R, Zorgdrager F, Lukashov V, Goudsmit J. Pol gene diversity of five human immunodeficiency virus type 1 subtypes: evidence for naturally occurring mutations that contribute to drug resistance, limited recombination patterns, and common ancestry for subtypes B and D. *J Virol* 1997;71: 6348-58.
25. De Jong MD, Boucher CAB, Galasso GJ, Hirsch MS, Kern ER, Lange JMA, Richman DD. Consensus symposium on combination therapy. *Antiviral Research* 1995;29: 5-29.
26. De Man RA, Bartholomeusz A, Niesters HGM, Zondervan PE, Locarnini S. The sequential occurrence of viral mutations in a liver transplant recipient re-infected with hepatitis B virus: Hepatitis B Immune Globulin Escape, Famciclovir Non-Response, followed by lamivudine resistance resulting in graft loss. *Journal of Hepatology* 1998;29: 669-75.
27. Dienstag J, Perrillo R, Schiff E, Bartholomew M, Vicary C, Rubin M. A preliminary trial of lamivudine for chronic hepatitis B infection. *N Engl J Med* 1995;333: 1657-61.
28. Dienstag J, Schiff E, Mitchell M, Gitlin N, Lissoos T, Condreay L, Garrett L, Rubin M, Brown N. Extended lamivudine retreatment for chronic hepatitis B. *Hepatology* 1996;26: A245.
29. Fischer K, Cheng Y-C, Tyrrell D. The mutation in duck hepatitis B polymerase which confers resistance to lamivudine (″-L-(-)-thiacytidine, 3TC) also confers cross-resistance to ″-L-dideoxy-5-fluorocytidine. *Hepatology* 1996;24: A246.
30. Fu L, Cheng YC. Role of additional mutations outside the YMDD motif of hepatitis B virus polymerase in L(-)SddC (3TC) resistance. *Biochem Pharmacol* 1998;55: 1567-72.
31. Furman P, Painter G. The role of absolute configuration in the anti-HIV and anti-HBV activity of nucleoside analogues. *International Antiviral News* 1995;3: 74-7.
32. Gilson R, Chopra K, Murray-Lyon I, Newell A, Nelson M, Tedder R, Toole J, Jaffe H, Hellmann N, Weller I. A placebo-controlled phase I/II study of Adefovir Dipivoxil (bis-POM PMEA) in patients with

chronic hepatitis B infection. *Hepatology* 1996;24: 281A.

33. Guidotti LG, Rochford R, Chung J, Shapiro M, Purcell R, Chisari FV. Viral clearance without destruction of infected cells during acute HBV infection. *Science* 1999;284: 825-9.
34. Gunther S, Fischer L, Pult I, Sterneck M, Will H. Naturally occurring variants of hepatitis B virus. *Adv Virus Res* 1999;52: 25-137.
35. Gunther S, Sommer G, Pilkat U, Iwanska A, Wain--Hobson S, Will H, Meyerhans A. Naturally occurring hepatitis B virus genomes bearing the hallmarks of retroviral G to A hypermutation. *Virology* 1997;235: 104-8.
36. Heathcote EJ, Jeffers L, Wright T, Sherman M, Perrillo R, Sacks S, Carithers R, Rustgi V, Di Bisceglie A, Balan V. Loss of serum HBV DNA and HBeAg seroconversion following short-term (12 weeks) adefovir dipivoxil therapy in chronic hepatitis B: two placebo-controlled Phase II studies. *Hepatology* 1998;28: A620.
37. Heijtink R, De Wilde G, Kruining J, Berk L, Balzarini J, De Clercq E, Holy A, Schalm S. Inhibitory effect of 9-(2-phosphonoyl-methoxyethyl)-adenine (PMEA) on human and duck hepatitis B virus infection. *Antiviral Res* 1993;21: 141-53.
38. Heijtink R, Kruining J, de Wilde G, Balzarini J, de Clercq E, Schalm S. Inhibitory effects of acyclic nucleoside phosphonates on human hepatitis B virus and duck hepatitis B virus infections in tissue culture. *Antimicrob Agents Chemother* 1994;38: 2180-2.
39. Hoetelmans RM. Sanctuary sites in HIV-1 infection. *Antivir Ther* 1998;3: 13-7.
40. Hollinger F, Ed. Hepatitis B Virus. In: Fields Virology, 3rd Edition. 1996 Philadelphia, Lippincott-Raven Publishers.
50. Hsu M, Inouye P, Rezende L, Richard N, Li Z, Prasad VR, Wainberg MA. Higher fidelity of RNA-dependent DNA mispair extension by M184V drug-resistant than wild-type reverse transcriptase of human immunodeficiency virus type 1. *Nucleic Acids Res* 1997;25: 4532-6.
51. Huang H, Chopra R, Verdine GL, Harrison SC. Structure of a covalently trapped catalytic complex of HIV-1 reverse transcriptase: implications for drug resistance. *Science* 1998;282: 1669-75.
52. Jacobo-Molina A, Ding J, Clark AD, Lu X, Tantillo C, Williams RL, Kamer G, Ferria AL, Clark P. Crystal structure of human immunodeficiency virus type 1 reverse transcriptase complexed with double-stranded DNA at 3.0 A resolution shows bent DNA. *Proc National Acad of Sci, USA* 1993;90: 6320-4.
53. Ka-Kit G, Lau K, Tsiang M, Hou J, Yuen S, Carman WF, Zhang L, Gibbs CS, Lam S. Combination therapy with lamivudine and famciclovir for chronic hepatitis B-infected chinese patients: A viral dynamics study. *Hepatology* 2000;32: 394-9.
54. Ladner SK, Miller TJ, King RW. The M539V polymerase variant of human hepatitis B virus demonstrates resistance to 2'-deoxy-3'-thiacytidine and a reduced ability to synthesize viral DNA. *Antimicrob Agents Chemother* 1998;42: 2128-31.
55. Lai C, Chien R, Leung N, Chang T, Guan R, Tai D, Ng K, Wu P, Dent J, Barber J. A one-year trial of lamivudine for chronic hepatitis B. Asia Hepatitis Lamivudine Study Group. *N Engl J Med* 1998;339: 61-8.
56. Larder BA, Kemp SD, Harrigan PR. Potential mechanism for sustained antiviral efficacy of AZT-3TC combination therapy. *Science* 1995;269: 696-9.
57. Lau JY, Bain VG, Davies SE, O'Grady JG, Alberti A, Alexander GJ, Williams R. High-level expression of hepatitis B viral antigens in fibrosing cholestatic hepatitis. *Gastroenterology* 1992;102: 956-62.
58. Lee W (1997). Hepatitis B virus infection. *N Engl J Med* 337: 1733-45.
59. Lesburg CA, Cable MB, Ferrari E, Hong Z, Mannzino F, Weber C. Crystal structure of the RNA-

dependent RNA polymerase from hepatitis C virus reveals a fully encircled active site. *Nature America* 1999;6: 937-43.

60. Lin TS, Luo MZ, Liu MC, Pai SB, Dutschman GE, Cheng YC. Antiviral activity of 2', 3'-dideoxy-beta-L-5-fluorocytidine (beta-L-FddC) and 2', 3'-dideoxy-beta-L-cytidine (beta-L-ddC) against hepatitis B virus and human immunodeficiency virus type 1 *in vitro*. *Biochem Pharmacol* 1994;47: 171-4.
61. Ling R, Mutimer D, Ahmed M, Boxall EH, Elias E, Dusheiko GM, Harrison TJ. Selection of mutations in the hepatitis B virus polymerase during therapy of transplant recipients with lamivudine. *Hepatology* 1996;24: 711-3.
62. Locarnini S, Birch C. Antiviral chemotherapy for chronic hepatitis B infection: Lessons learned from treating HIV infected patients. *Journal of Hepatology* 1999;30: 536-50.
63. Locarnini SA, Aye TT, De Man R, Angus PW, McCaughan GW, Bartholomeusz AI. The emergence of famciclovir resistant mutants in the hepatitis B virus polymerase during therapy in patients following liver transplantation. *Hepatology* 1997;26: 368A.
64. Mahoney FJ. Update on diagnosis, management, and prevention of hepatitis B virus infection. *Clin Microbiol Rev* 1999;12: 351-66.
65. Main J, Brown J, Howells C, Galassini R, Crossey M, Karayiannis P, Georgiou P, Atkinson G, Thomas H. A double blind, placebo-controlled study to assess the effect of famciclovir on virus replication in patients with chronic hepatitis B virus infection. *J Viral Hep* 1996;3: 211-5.
66. Mast EE, Alter MJ, Margolis HS. Strategies to prevent and control hepatitis B and C virus infections: a global perspective. *Vaccine* 1999;17: 1730-3.
67. Najera I, Holguin A, Quinones-Mateu ME, Munoz-Fernandez MA, Najera R, Lopez-Galindez C, Domingo E. Pol gene quasispecies of human immunodeficiency virus: mutations associated with drug resistance in virus from patients undergoing no drug therapy. *J Virol* 1995;69: 23-31.
68. Nanni R, Ding J, Jocobo-Molina A, Hughes S, Arnold E. Review of HIV-1 reverse transcriptase three dimensional structure: Implications for drug design. *Perspectives Drug Discovery Design* 1993;1: 129-50.
69. Naoumov NV, Chokshi S, Smith H, Williams R. Emergence and characterisation of lamivudine resistant hepatitis B virus variant. *Hepatology* 1996;24: 282A.
70. Neuhaus P, Mannus M, Atkinson G. Safety and efficacy of famciclovir for the treatment of recurrent hepatitis B infection in liver transplant recipients. *Hepatology* 1997;26: A528.
71. Nicoll A, Colledge D, Wang Y, Toole J, Dean J, Angus P, Smallwood R, Locarnini S. PMEA, an acyclic phosphonate nucleoside analogue with activity against duck hepatitis B virus *in vitro*. *Hepatology* 1996;24: A375.
72. Niesters HG, Honkoop P, Haagsma EB, de Man RA, Schalm SW, Osterhaus AD. Identification of more than one mutation in the hepatitis B virus polymerase gene arising during prolonged lamivudine treatment. *J Infect Dis* 1998;177: 1382-5.
73. Nowak MA, Bonhoeffer S, Hill AM, Boehme R, Thomas HC, McDade H. Viral dynamics in hepatitis B virus infection. *Proc Natl Acad Sci USA* 1996;93: 4398-402.
74. Ogata N, Fujii K, Takigawa S, Nomoto M, Ichida T, Asakura H. Novel patterns of amino acid mutations in the hepatitis B virus polymerase in association with resistance to lamivudine therapy in japanese patients with chronic hepatitis B. *J Med Virol* 1999;59: 270-6.
75. Okamoto H, Imai M, Kametani M, Nakamura T, Mayumi M. Genomic heterogeneity of hepatitis B virus in a 54-year-old woman who contracted the infection through materno-fetal transmission. *Jpn J Exp Med* 1987;57: 231-6.
76. Ono-Nita SK, Kato N, Shiratori Y, Lan K-H, Yohida H, Carrilho FJ, Omata M. Susceptibility of lamivudine-

resistant hepatitis B virus to other reverse transcriptase inhibitors. *J Clin Invest* 1999;103: 1635-40.

77. Oon CJ, Chen WN, Lim N, Koh S, Lim GK, Leong AL, Tan GS. Hepatitis B virus variants with lamivudine-related mutations in the DNA polymerase and the 'a' epitope of the surface antigen are sensitive to ganciclovir. *Antiviral Res* 1999;41: 113-8.
78. Orito E, Mizokami M, Ina Y, Moriyama EN, Kameshima N, Yamamoto M, Gojobori T. Host-independent evolution and a genetic classification of the hepadnavirus family based on nucleotide sequences. *Proc Natl Acad Sci USA* 1989;86: 7059-62.
79. Pai S, Liu S-H, Zhu Y-L, Chieng C. Inhibition of hepatitis B virus by a novel L-nucleoside 2'-fluoro-5-methyl-″-L-arabinofuranosyl uracil. *Antimicrob Agents Chemotherap* 1996;40: 380-6.
80. Perelson AS, Neumann AU, Markowitz M, Leonard JM, Ho DD. HIV-1 dynamics *in vivo*: virion clearance rate, infected cell life-span, and viral generation time. *Science* 1996;271: 1582-6.
81. Piatek AS, Telenti A, Murray MR, El-Hajj H, Jacobs WR Jr., Kramer FR, Alland D. Genotypic analysis of Mycobacterium tuberculosis in two distinct populations using molecular beacons: implications for rapid susceptibility testing. *Antimicrob Agents Chemother* 2000;44: 103-10.
82. Pichoud C, Seigneres B, Wang Z, Trepo C, Zoulim F. Transient selection of a hepatitis B virus polymerase gene mutant associated with a decreased replication capacity and famciclovir resistance. *Hepatology* 1999;29: 230-7.
83. Poch O, Sauvaget I, Delarue M, Tordo N. Identification of four conserved motifs among the RNA-dependent polymerase encoding elements. *European Molecular Biology Organisation* 1989;8: 3867-74.
84. Schuetz JD, Connelly MC, Sun D, Paibir SG, Flynn PM, Srinivas RV, Kumar A, Fridland A. MRP4: A previously unidentified factor in resistance to nucleoside-based antiviral drugs. *Nat Med* 1999;9: 1048-51.
85. Shaw T, Locarnini S. Combination Chemotherapy for Hepatitis B Virus: The Final Solution? *Hepatology* 2000;32: 430-2.
86. Sterneck M, Gunther S, Gerlach J, Naoumov NV, Santantonio T, Fischer L, Rogiers X, Greten H, Williams R, Will H. Hepatitis B virus sequence changes evolving in liver transplant recipients with fulminant hepatitis. *J Hepatol* 1997;26: 754-64.
87. Stuyver L, Van Geyt C, De Gendt S, Van Reybroeck G, Zoulim F, Leroux-Roels G, Rossau R. Line probe assay for monitoring drug resistance in hepatitis B virus-infected patients during antiviral therapy. *J Clin Microbiol* 2000;38: 702-7.
88. Thibault V, Benhamou Y, Seguret C, Bochet M, Katlama C, Bricaire F, Opolon P, Poynard T, Agut H. Hepatitis B virus (HBV) mutations associated with resistance to lamivudine in patients coinfected with HBV and human immunodeficiency virus. *J Clin Microbiol* 1999;37: 3013-6.
89. Tillmann HL, Trautwein C, Bock T, Boker KWH, Jackel E, Glowienka M, Oldhafer K, Bruns J, Condreay LD, Raab HR. Mutational analysis of hepatitis B virus on sequential therapy with famciclovir and lamivudine in patients with hepatitis B virus reinfection occuring under HBIg immunoglobulin after liver transplantation. *epatology* 199930: 244-56.
90. Tipples A, Ma MM, Fischer KP, Bain VG, Kneteman NM, Tyrrell DL. Mutation in HBV RNA-dependent DNA polymerase confers resistance to lamivudine *in vivo*. *Hepatology* 1996;24: 714-7.
91. Trepo C, Jezek P, Atkinson G, Boon R. Efficacy of famciclovir in chronic hepatitis B: Results of a dose finding study. *Hepatology* 1996;24: A188.
92. Tsiang M, Rooney JF, Toole JJ, Gibbs CS. Biphasic clearance kinetics of hepatitis B virus from patients during adefovir dipivoxil therapy. *Hepatology* 1999;29: 1863-9.
93. Vet JA, Majithia AR, Marras SA, Tyagi S, Dube S, Poiesz BJ, Kramer FR. Multiplex detection of four pathogenic retroviruses using molecular beacons. *Proc Natl Acad Sci USA* 1999;96: 6394-9.

94. Wijnholds J, Mol CAAM, van Deemter L, de Haas M, Scheffer GL, Baas F, Beijnen JH, Scheper RJ, Hatse S, De Clercq E. Multidrug-resistance protein 5 is a multispecific organic anion transporter able to transport nucleotide analogs. *Proc NY Acad Sci* 2000;97: 7476-81.
95. Witcher J, Boudinot F, Baldwin B, Ascenzi M, Tennant B, Du J, Chu C. Pharmacokinetics of1-(2-fluoro-5-methyl-beta-L-arabinofuranosyl) uracil in woodchucks. *Antimicrob Agents Chemother* 1997;41: 2184-7.
96. Xiong X, Flores C, Gibbs C, Toole I. Lack of cross resistance to PMEA for human hepatitis B DNA polymerase which expresses lamivudine resistance codons. *Hepatology* 1997;26: A1211.
97. Xiong X, Flores C, Yang H, Toole JJ, Gibbs CS. Mutations in hepatitis B DNA polymerase associated with resistance to lamivudine do not confer resistance to adefovir *in vitro*. *Hepatology* 1998;28: 1669-73.
98. Xiong X, Yang H, Westland C, Zou R, Gibbs C. *In vitro* evaluation of hepatitis B virus polymerase mutations associated with famciclovir resistance. *Hepatology* 2000;31: 219-24.
99. Yeh CT, Chien RN, Chu CM, Liaw YF. Clearance of the original hepatitis B virus YMDD-motif mutants with emergence of distinct lamivudine-resistant mutants during prolonged lamivudine therapy. *Hepatology* 2000;31: 1318-26.
100. Ying C, De Clercq E, Nicholson W, Furman P, Neyts J. Inhibition of the replication of the DNA polymerase M550V mutation variant of human hepatitis B virus by adefovir, tenofovir, L-FMAU, DAPD, penciclovir and lobucavir. *J Viral Hepat* 2000;7: 161-5.
101. Yokota T, Konno K, Shigeta S, Holy A, Balzarini J, De Clerq E. Inhibitory effects of acyclic nucleoside phosphonate analogues on hepatitis B virus DNA synthesis in HB G11 cells. *Antiviral Chem Chemother* 1994;5: 57-63.
102. Yokota T, Mochizuki S, Konno K, Mori S, Shigeta S, De Clercq E. Inhibitory effects of selected antiviral compounds on human hepatitis B virus DNA synthesis. *Antimicrob Agents Chemother* 1991;35: 394-7.
103. Yuen M-F, Lai C-L. Debates in Hepatitis: How to assess HBV DNA reductions in association with therapy. *Viral Hepatitis Reviews* 1999;5: 159-75.

Antiviral β-L-nucleosides specific for hepatitis B virus infection

MARTIN L. BRYANT[1], EDWARD G. BRIDGES[1], LAURENT PLACIDI[2], ABDESSLEM FARAJ[3], ANNA-GIULIA LOI[3], CLAIRE PIERRA[3], SAMIRA BENZARIA[3], DAVID DUKHAN[3], GILLES GOSSELIN[4], JEAN-LOUIS IMBACH[4], BRENDA HERNANDEZ[2], AMY JUODAWLKIS[1], BUD TENNANT[5], BRENT KORBA[6], PAUL COTE[6], ERIKA CRETTON-SCOTT[1], RAYMOND F. SCHINAZI[7], MAUREEN MYERS[1] and JEAN-PIERRE SOMMADOSSI[1]

[1] *Idenix, Inc., 125 CambridgePark Dr., Cambridge, MA 02140, USA*
[2] *Department of Pharmacology and Toxicology, Division of Clinical Pharmacology, The Liver Center, University of Alabama at Birmingham, Birmingham, AL 35294, USA*
[3] *Idenix, SARL, Immeuble "La Vigie", 170 Rue Leon Blum, 34000, Montpellier, France*
[4] *Laboratoire de Chimie Bioorganique, CNRS UMR 5625, Universite de Montpellier II, Place Eugene Bataillon, 34095 Cedex 5 Montpellier, France*
[5] *Department of Clinical Sciences, College of Veterinary Medicine, Cornell University, Ithaca, NY 14853, USA*
[6] *Division of Molecular Virology and Immunology, Georgetown University College of Medicine, Rockville, MD 20852, USA*
[7] *Laboratory of Biochemical Pharmacology, Department of Pediatrics, Emory University School of Medicine and Veterans Affairs Medical Center, Decatur, GA 30033, USA*

Introduction

Several therapeutic strategies have been evaluated for the treatment of chronic HBV infection with the goal of eliminating persistent viral replication and preventing progression to chronic active hepatitis, cirrhosis and hepatocellular carcinoma (HCC). Currently, the only approved treatment options are interferon-α (IFN) and lamivudine (3TC, β-L-2', 3'-dideoxy-3'-thiacytidine). The response rate to IFN is low and drug-associated side effects are significant. Individuals who are immunosuppressed [e.g., transplant recipients or those co-infected with the human immunodeficiency virus (HIV)] rarely respond to IFN therapy. Lamivudine is an example of the class of "unnatural" β-L-nucleoside analogs that have recently drawn considerable attention as antiviral and anticancer agents. Similar to IFN, however, a complete antiviral response, as assessed by HBe seroconversion, is seen in only a minority of patients after one year

Frontiers in Viral Hepatitis Ed. by RF Schinazi, J-P Sommadossi and CM Rice. 245 — 261

of treatment. In addition, cessation of lamivudine therapy frequently leads to a marked rebound in viral replication (hepatitis flare), which can be life threatening in HIV-HBV co-infected patients. With long-term survival increasing for HIV-infected patients, chronic HBV infection is becoming an important determinant of disease outcome in the co-infected patient population. Also, lamivudine resistance is now recognized in 16-32% of HBV-infected patients after one year of treatment, and in as much as 58% after two to three years [1, 2].

Other nucleoside analogs currently under evaluation for the treatment of HBV infection are listed in Table 1. These include adefovir dipivoxil (an oral prodrug of PMEA), which may be beneficial against lamivudine-resistant mutants, and emtricitabine [(-)-FTC], which is similar to lamivudine. Development of famciclovir (an oral prodrug of penciclovir) and lobucavir have been discontinued due to limited antiviral activity and adverse side effects, respectively. Two other potent nucleoside analogs, L-FMAU and BMS200-458, are currently in human trials, although clinical data have not yet been reported.

Table 1. Nucleosides approved or in development for HBV therapy

Compound	Company	Originally Developed for	HBV Development Status
lamivudine	GlaxoSmithKline	HIV	Approved
adefovir dipivoxil	Gilead	HIV	Phase IIb/IIIa
emtricitabine	Triangle	HIV	Phase I/II
lobucavir	Bristol-Myers Squibb	CMV, HSV	Discontinued (adverse side effects)
famciclovir	GlaxoSmithKline	HSV-1, HSV-2, VZV	Discontinued (limited activity)
DAPD	Triangle	HIV	preclinical
L-FMAU	Triangle	HBV	(clinical ex-US)
L-dA (NV-02A)	Idenix	HBV	preclinical
L-dT (NV-02B)	Idenix	HBV	Phase I/II
L-dC (NV-02C)	Idenix	HBV	Phase I/II
L-D4FC	Achillion	HIV	preclinical
D-D4FC	Pharmasset	HIV	preclinical
BMS200-475	Bristol-Myers Squibb	HSV	Phase I/II

Structure-activity relationships identify new class of β-L-nucleosides specific for hepadnaviruses

Now, through an extensive structure-activity analysis, a unique series of simple, β-L-nucleosides that specifically inhibit hepatitis B virus (HBV) replication has been discovered. The most potent, selective and specific members of the class are L-dA, L-dC, and L-dT (Figure 1).

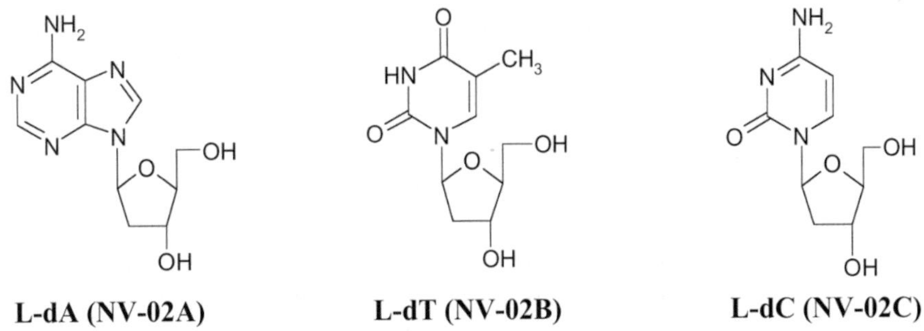

Figure 1. Structures of β-L-nucleoside compounds

The structure–activity relationship (SAR) established among the β-L-2'-deoxycytidine, -thymidine and –deoxyadenosine series are presented in Table 2. These molecules have in common a hydroxyl group (-OH) in the 3'-position of the β-L-2'-deoxyribose sugar that confers antiviral activity specifically against hepadnaviruses. Replacement of the 3'-OH broadens activity to other viruses. Substitution in the base decreases antiviral potency and selectivity.

Substitution of a halogen atom at the 5-position (R1) in the pyrimidine ring of L-dC, without modification of the deoxyribose sugar (e.g., β-L-2'-deoxy-5-fluorocytidine, L-5-FdC; β-L-2'-deoxy-5-chlorocytidine, L-5-CldC), decreased the potency against HBV but did not affect the antiviral specificity for HBV. In contrast, analogs of L-dC which lacked the 3'-OH group (R3) on the deoxyribose sugar (e.g., β-L-2', 3'-dideoxycytidine, L-ddC; β-L-2', 3'-dideoxy-3'-thiacytidine, 3TC; β-L-2', 3'-didehydro-2', 3'-dideoxycytidine, L-d4C) lost antiviral specificity for HBV and showed activity against HIV. Similarly, replacement of the 3'-OH group with a 3'-fluoro moiety (e.g., β-L-2', 3'-dideoxy-3'-fluorocytidine, L-3'-FddC) eliminated the antiviral specificity, although antiviral potency against HBV and HIV was retained.

In addition, substitutions at the 5-position (R1) of the pyrimidine base of β-L-2', 3'-dideoxycytidine lacking the 3'-OH group (e.g., β-L-2', 3'-dideoxy-5-fluorocytidine, L-5-FddC; β-L-2', 3'-dideoxy-5-chlorocytidine, L-5-ClddC; β-L-2', 3'-dideoxy-3'-thia-5-fluorocytidine, FTC; β-L-2', 3'-didehydro-2', 3'-dideoxy-5-fluorocytidine, L-d4FC; β-L-2', 3'-dideoxy-3'-fluoro-5-fluorocytidine, L-3'-F-5-FddC; β-L-2', 3'-dideoxy-3'-azido-5-fluorocytidine, L-3'-azido-5-FddC) further affected the antiviral potency of these analogs against HBV, as well as HIV. These studies suggest that the 3'-OH of the β-L-2'-deoxyribose of L-dC plays a crucial role in inhibiting virus replication, possibly by specific interruption of the DNA dependant DNA polymerase step.

The structure-activity relationships for the L-dT and L-dA series (Table 2) were similar to that observed for the L-dC series. The specific anti-HBV activity of L-dT and L-dA was lost upon removal or substitution of the 3'-OH group (R3). β-L-2'-deoxy-xylo-thymidine (L-xylo-dT), which is identical to L-dT except for the 3'-OH group in the opposite orientation (R2), also lost anti-HBV activity, further emphasizing the importance of the 3'-OH group in the inhibition of HBV replication. An L-dT analog with a fluorine

Table 2. Structure-activity relationship of β-L-2'-deoxynucleosides

	R1	R2	R3	X	EC_{50} (μM)[a] anti-HBV 2.2.15 cells	anti-HIV PBM cells
L-dC	H	H	OH	CH	0.24±0.08	>200
L-5-FdC	F	H	OH	CH	5	>100
L-5-CldC	Cl	H	OH	CH	10	>100
L-ddC	H	H	H	CH	0.1	0.26
3TC	H	H	–	S	0.05±0.01	0.002
L-3'-azido-5-FddC	F	H	N_3	CH	0.11±0.09	0.05
L-3'-FddC	H	H	F	CH	0.5	82
FTC	F	H	–	S	0.04	0.008
L-5-ClddC	Cl	H	H	CH	10	>100
L-d4C	H	–	–	CH	<0.1	1.0
L-d4FC	F	–	–	CH	<0.1	0.034
L-3'-F-5-FddC	F	–	F	CH	4	>100
L-5-FddC	F	–	–	CH	0.10±0.05	0.021
L-dT		H	OH		0.19±0.09	>200
L-ddT		H	H		>10	>100
L-3'-FddT		H	F		>10	>100
L-3'-azido-ddT		H	N_3		>10	>100
L-3'-amino-ddT		H	NH_2		>10	>10
L-d4T		–	–		>10	>100
L-xylo-dT		OH	H		>10	>10
L-dA	H	H	OH		0.10-1.9	>10
L-2-CldA	Cl	H	OH		>10	>10
L-ddA	H	H	H	5	>10	
L-d4A	H	–	–		0.80±0.10	0.38
L-3'-azido-ddA	H	H	N_3	5	>10	
L-3'-amino-ddA	H	H	NH_2		>10	>10
L-3'-fluoro-ddA	H	H	F		>10	>100
L-ddAMP-bis(tbutylSATE)	H	H	H		0.08±0.03	0.002
L-3'-azido-d4A	H	–	N_3		>10	>100

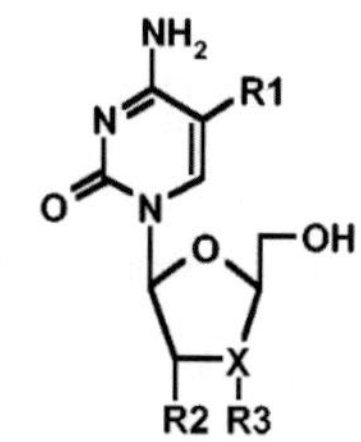

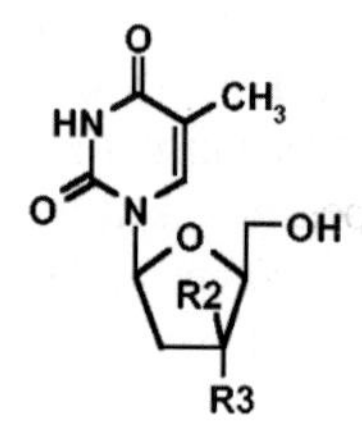

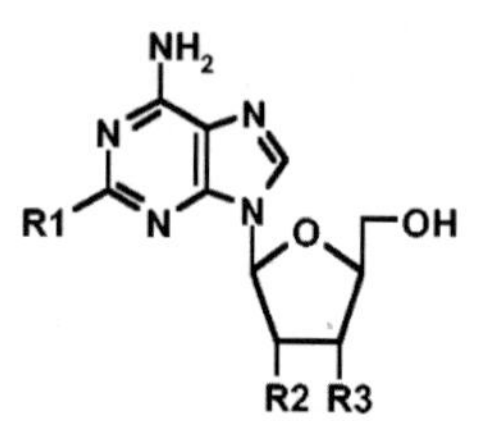

[a] Antiviral 50% effective concentration (EC_{50}). The *greater than* symbol (>) is used to indicate the highest concentration at which the compounds were tested. Values are presented as means of at least three independent experiments. Anti-HIV data for L-ddC, 3TC, FTC, L-5-FddC, L-d4FC from references [3-5]. L-d4T, L-ddA and L-d4A data from references [6, 7].

substitution at the 2' up-position (L-FMAU, β-L-2'-deoxy-2'-fluoro-5-methyl-arabinofuranosyl uracil) has been reported to have activity against both HBV and EBV [8]. Thus, it is possible that modification of the 2'-position in addition to the 3'-position of L-dT may also change antiviral specificity for HBV.

Substitution at the 2-position (R1) on the purine base of L-dA (e.g., β-L-2'-deoxy-2-chloroadenosine, L-2-CldA) had a negative effect on anti-HBV activity. The analogs of L-dA lacking the 3'-OH group with or without further modification of the deoxyribose sugar lost specificity and were not as potent against HBV. The marginal antiviral activity of β-L-2', 3'-dideoxyadenosine (L-ddA), despite its potent inhibitory activity against both HIV reverse transcriptase (HIV-RT) and woodchuck hepatitis (WHV) DNA polymerase [9], can be explained by the low intracellular concentrations of the phosphorylated form due to rapid and extensive catabolism [10]. This conclusion is also supported by recent studies that demonstrated potent antiviral activity of an L-ddA 5'-monophosphate prodrug (β-L-2',3'-dideoxy-adenosine-5'-monophosphate-t-butyl-S-acyl-2-thioethyl; L-ddAMP-bis-(tbutyl-SATE)). The prodrug form decreases the intracellular catabolism of the parent molecule [11] and releases the 5'-monophosphate derivative inside the cell. When used in this pronucleotide form, L-ddA was active against both HIV and HBV, further supporting the importance of the 3'-OH group for antiviral specificity. As in the L-dC and L-dT series, unmodified β-L-2'-deoxyadenosine most potently and specifically inhibited HBV replication.

Demonstration that L-dNTP analogs can inhibit HBV reverse transcriptase/DNA polymerase activity does not preclude other mechanisms of action. Inhibition of other important activities of the polymerase (which include RNaseH activity, priming of reverse transcription and co-ordination of intracellular virion assembly), or the possibility of internal incorporation of L-dNMP into viral DNA as a mechanism of inhibition are currently under investigation.

The β-L-deoxynucleoside series is specific for hepatitis B virus

To further assess their antiviral specificity, L-dC, L-dT and L-dA were screened against 15 different RNA and DNA viruses (Table 3).

The antiviral potencies of L-dA, L-dT and L-dC were measured by the magnitude of the reduction of extracellular HBV DNA and intracellular replicative intermediates compared to untreated HBV-expressing hepatoma 2.2.15 cells. The β-L-2'-deoxynucleosides inhibited hepadnavirus replication as previously defined by the SAR, but had no activity against HIV-1, HSV-1, HSV-2, VZV, EBV, HCMV, adenovirus type-1, influenza A and B, measles virus, parainfluenza type-3, rhinovirus type-5 and RSV type-A at concentrations as high as 100 μM. Potent antiviral activity against the woodchuck hepatitis B virus (WHV) is described later using an *in vivo* model of chronic hepatitis B virus infection. Thus, the unmodified β-L-2'-deoxynucleosides, L-dC, L-dT and L-dA, are uniquely specific for the hepadnaviruses HBV, DHBV, and WHV.

Table 3. Antiviral activity and cytotoxicity levels of L-dC, L-dT and L-dA

		EC_{50} (μM)[b]			CC_{50} (μM)[b]		
Virus[a]	Cell line	L-dC	L-dT	L-dA	L-dC	L-dT	L-dA
HBV	2.2.15	0.24	0.19	0.10	>2000	>2000	>1000
DHBV	PDH	0.87	0.18	0.15	nd[c]	nd	nd
HIV-1	PBMC	>100	>100	>100	>100	>100	>100
HSV-1	HFF	>20	>200	>100	>60	>200	>100
HSV-2	HFF	>100	>100	>100	>100	>100	>100
VZV	HFF	>100	45.2	>100	>100	18.6	>100
EBV	Daudi	>50	>50	5.7	>50	>50	23.1
HCMV	HFF	>100	>100	>100	>100	>100	>100
adenovirus type-1	A549	>100	nd	>100	>100	nd	>100
influenza A	MDCK	>100	>100	>100	>100	>100	>100
influenza B	MDCK	>100	>100	>100	>100	>100	>100
measles	CV-1	>100	>100	>100	>100	>100	>100
parainfluenza type-3	MA-104	>100	>100	>100	>100	>100	>100
rhinovirus type-5	KB	>100	nd	>100	>100	nd	>100
RSV type-A	MA-104	>100	>100	>100	>100	>100	>100

a The specific antiviral activity of L-dC, L-dT and L-dA was confirmed using a panel of viruses tested by the NIH NIAID Antiviral Research and Antimicrobial Chemistry Program.

b Antiviral 50% effective concentration (EC_{50}) and 50% cytotoxic concentration (CC_{50}). PDH, primary duck hepatocytes; PBMC, peripheral blood mononuclear cells; HFF, human foreskin fibroblast; Daudi, Burkitt's B-cell lymphoma; A549, human lung carcinoma; MDCK, canine kidney epithelial cells; CV-1, African green monkey kidney fibroblast cells; MA-104, Rhesus monkey kidney epithelial cells; KB, human nasopharyngeal carcinoma.

c nd, not determined.

Intracellular activation, metabolism, and pharmacology

The metabolic pathways shown in Figure 2 for L-dT and Figure 3 for L-dC are based on intracellular accumulation and decay data, and on competition experiments using the corresponding endogenous D-nucleosides.

L-dC, L-dT and L-dA were efficiently metabolized (activated) to their respective 5'-triphosphate derivatives in HepG2 cells and human hepatocytes in primary culture [12]. The intracellular triphosphate concentrations should well exceed the antiviral EC_{90} for most wild-type and mutant HBV. The metabolic profiles obtained after a 24-hour exposure of HepG2 cells to 10 μM [^{3}H]-L-dT and [^{3}H]-L-dC are shown in Figure 4 (Accumulation and Decay). The phosphorylation pattern in primary hepatocytes of

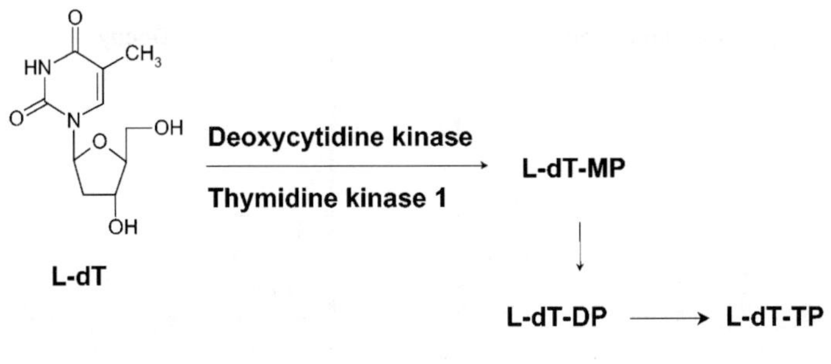

Figure 2. Proposed metabolic pathway for L-dT.

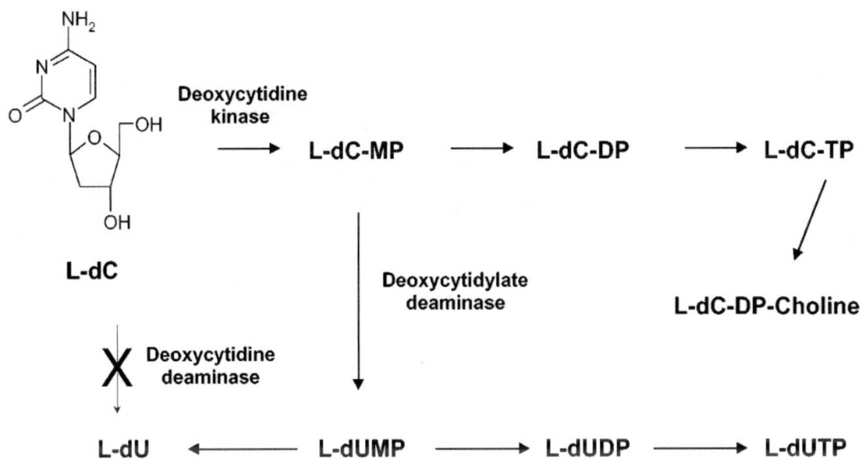

Figure 3. Proposed metabolic pathway for L-dC.

human and animal origin is qualitatively and quantitatively similar for the activated 5'-TP form of each compound. This is in contrast to earlier studies reporting limited intracellular activation of L-dT [13, 14]. The 5'-triphosphates of L-dC, L-dT and L-dA inhibited WHV DNA polymerase with a 50% inhibitory concentration (IC_{50}) of 0.24–1.82 μM. In addition, exposure of HepG2 cells to L-dC led to a second 5'-triphosphate derivative, i.e., β-L-2'-deoxyuridine 5'-triphosphate (L-dUTP), which also inhibited WHV DNA polymerase with an IC_{50} of 5.26 μM [12, 15]. Similar to β-L-cytidine analogs [16-19], L-dC was not a substrate for cytosolic cytidine deaminase, suggesting that the 5'-monophosphate metabolite of L-dC is probably susceptible to deamination through deoxycytidylate deaminase. The apparent intracellular half-lives of the L-dT-5'-TP and L-dC-5'-TP were ≥14 hours, which correlated with the prolonged antiviral activity following drug withdrawal in virus rebound experiments (data not shown).

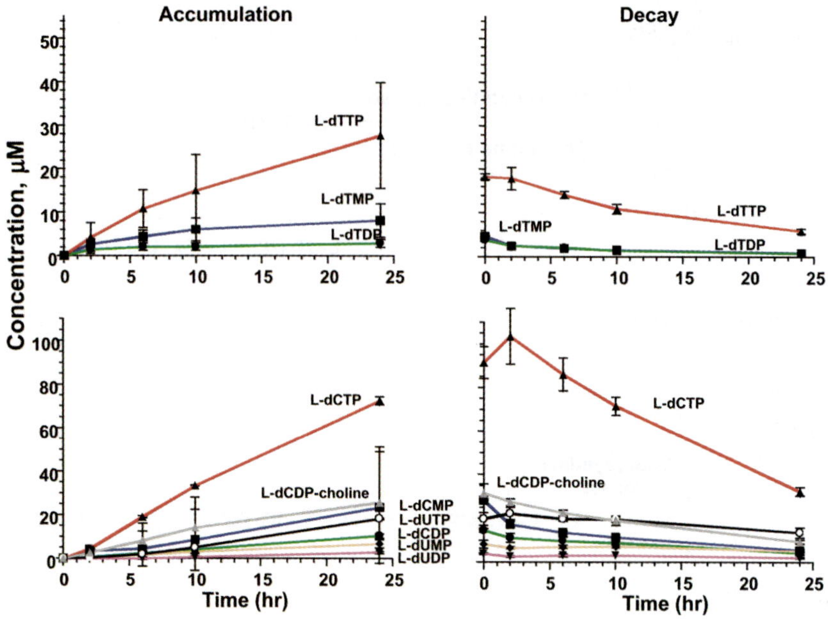

Figure 4. Intracellular accumulation and decay of metabolites after exposure of HepG2 cells to 10 µM L-dT or L-dC (24 hr).

Pharmacokinetic profiles

The pharmacokinetic profile of L-dT in the monkey is presented in Figure 5.

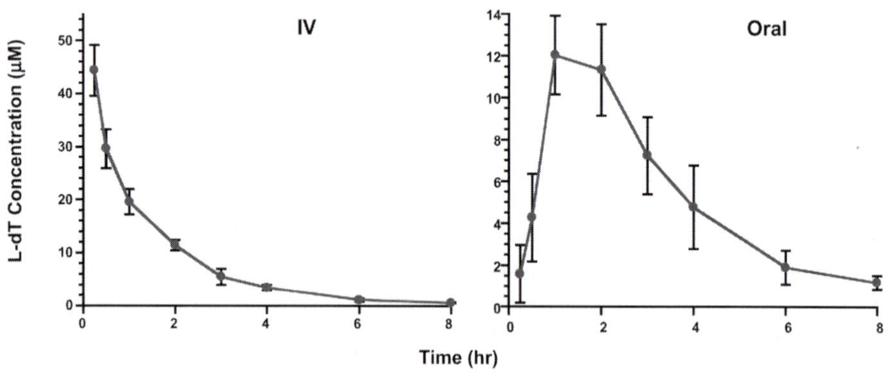

Figure 5. Plasma concentration in monkeys after administration of 10 mg/kg L-dT.

The data are the mean (± SD) from three animals per group. Following i.v. administration, plasma concentrations of L-dT in monkeys declined in a bi-exponential manner, and it was not detectable after eight hours. The estimated terminal phase half-life was shorter in monkeys (1.33 hr) than in woodchucks (3.99 hr). The total clearance was higher in monkeys (0.74 l/hr/kg) than in woodchucks (0.20 l/hr/kg). The apparent volume of distribution (V_d) indicated good intracellular distribution in both species. Oral absorption of L-dT in monkeys, and in woodchucks, was slow, with peak concentrations occurring one to four hours after dosing. The F for L-dT was high in monkeys (68.6%) and in woodchucks (38.3%).

The oral bioavailability (F) of L-dC was lower and more variable than L-dT in woodchucks (9.6%) and monkeys (16.4%). The elimination of L-dC was approximately fourfold faster in rats than woodchucks. Absorption of L-dC in rats after oral administration was also slow, with peak plasma concentrations occurring one hour post dosing. The elimination half-life of L-dC was shorter in rats, and the V_d was similar to that observed in woodchucks and monkeys. The oral bioavailability of L-dC was higher in rats (15.4%) than in woodchucks. Low plasma levels of L-dU were detected in woodchucks: 0.75 μM and 0.19 μM after intravenous and oral administration, respectively. L-dU was detected in plasma after L-dC administration to monkeys and rats at detectable but not quantifiable levels (<0.1 μM). L-dU was detected in urine in all three species. The pharmacokinetic parameters for L-dT and L-dC were consistent among the three species, with the exception of a slower elimination rate for both compounds in woodchucks.

Because the oral bioavailability of L-dC was low (F in monkeys 16%), a series of ester prodrugs was synthesized. The oral bioavailability of the 3', 5' ester prodrug of L-dC in cynomologus monkeys increased at least threefold in monkeys compared to L-dC.

Antiviral activity and safety in the woodchuck chronic hepatitis model

Woodchucks chronically infected with WHV are widely accepted as a model of HBV infection and have proven useful in the evaluation of anti-HBV agents. Antiviral activity in this model has been a positive predictor of antiviral activity in human chronic HBV infection [20-22]. The serum levels of WHV DNA during four weeks of daily treatment with L-dT or L-dC and eight weeks of follow-up were determined. The dosing of L-dT, L-dC and L-dA (0.01-10 mg/kg orally, three animals per compound-treatment group, four animals in placebo group) for 28 days in chronically infected woodchucks showed a dose-related, potent inhibition of viral replication in each case (data for L-dT shown in Figure 6).

The serum levels of WHV DNA during four weeks of drug treatment and eight weeks of post-treatment follow-up were determined by DNA dot-blot hybridization (detection limit approximately 10^7 genome equivalents/ml serum) and by quantitative PCR (detection limit approximately 300 genome equivalents/ml serum). The WHV DNA replication was significantly inhibited within the first few days of treatment and was maintained throughout the treatment period. Notably, serum WHV DNA levels (HBV viremia)

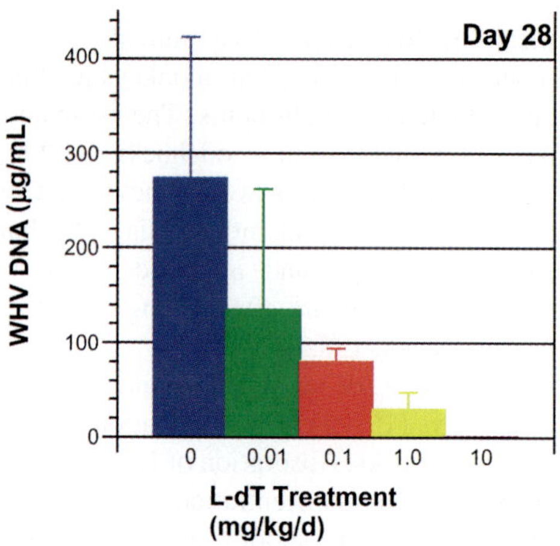

Figure 6. Reduction of serum virus load in the woodchuck chronic-HBV model (dose response).

decreased up to 8 logs, to below the limit of detection by PCR in the L-dT treated animals (Figure 7), and decreased by up to 6 logs in the majority of L-dC treated animals (not shown). The ester prodrug of L-dC, which had an oral bioavailability of three times that of L-dC, has not yet been tested in the woodchuck model, but would be expected to show antiviral activity similar to that of L-dT.

WHV DNA levels rebounded to near pre-treatment levels by eight weeks following drug withdrawal. Viral rebound was detected within the first week post-treatment. In addition a decline in WHV surface antigen, as measured using the method of Cote, et al. [23], paralleled the marked reduction in viral load. The onset of the response was delayed by at least one week but continued to fall for several weeks after drug removal.

The cytidine analog lamivudine (10 mg/kg/d), used for comparison to the L-dC treatment group, reduced the HBV genome equivalents/ml in serum by 0.5 to 1.0 log. This reduced effect is consistent with previous studies using similar doses of lamivudine [24]. Higher doses (40–200 mg/kg) are required to produce significant antiviral activity in this model [25]. The low activity of lamivudine in the woodchuck model has been explained in part by the low conversion of lamivudine and other cytidine analogs to their active 5'-triphosphate forms in woodchuck liver compared to that in human liver. In addition, the oral bioavailability of lamivudine in woodchucks was reported to be 18%-54%, whereas the oral bioavailability observed in humans was 82% [26, 27]

The woodchuck model was also valuable for the preclinical toxicological evaluation of nucleoside analogs. This model identified the delayed, severe hepatocellular toxicity induced by FIAU (fialuridine, 1, 2'-deoxy-2'-fluoro-1-β-D-arabinofuranosly-5-iodo-uracil) in humans, which was not seen in preclinical evaluation in rats, dogs or monkeys [28, 29]. The FIAU-induced toxicity observed in woodchucks, including significant weight loss, wasting and hepatocellular damage seen on liver biopsy, was identified beginning six to eight weeks from onset of treatment and was similar to that observed in the treated HBV-infected patients [30].

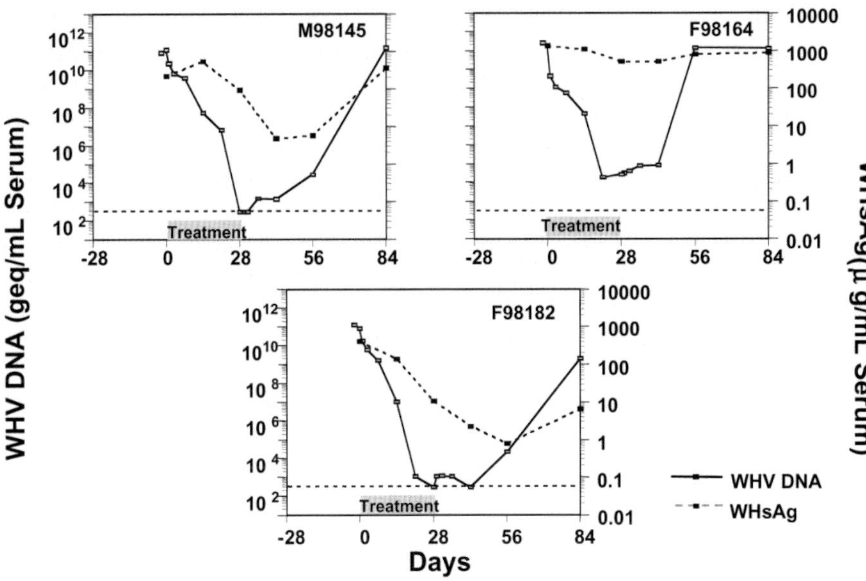

Figure 7. Reduction of serum virus load and WHsAg by L-dT (10 mg/kg) in the woodchuck chronic-HBV model.

In a separate 12-week study in the woodchuck model, the combination of 1 mg/kg/day L-dT and 1 mg/kg/day L-dC reduced viral load to levels significantly lower than either agent alone. This combination of L-dT and L-dC (each at one-tenth the concentration of monotherapy) reduced viral load to the limit of detection (10^3 genome equivalents per ml serum). Following drug removal, the time to viral rebound was markedly prolonged when L-dT and L-dC were administered in combination. A dramatic decrease in hepatitis B surface antigen, as a marker of viral replication, was also seen. In both the 28-day study and the 12-week study, no toxicity was seen at the highest dose tested. All animals gained weight compared to placebo treated control animals, and end-of-treatment liver biopsies from the animals in the 12 week study were normal, without evidence of microvesicular steatosis.

Selectivity and lack of cellular toxicity

Since long-term treatment is expected for chronic HBV infection, drug selectivity and lack of cytotoxicity is a critical issue. Toxic side effects have also been a major limitation for the clinical use of some nucleoside analogs [31-34].

The 5'-triphosphates of L-dC, L-dT and L-dA do not inhibit human DNA polymerases α, β and γ at concentrations up to 100 μM. Krayevsky and coworkers also reported that the 5'-triphosphates of L-dC and L-dT were not substrates for human DNA polymerases [35].

L-dC, L-dT and L-dA had no cytotoxic effect on the human hepatoma cell line 2.2.15 (CC_{50} values > 2,000 μM), in primary human peripheral blood mononuclear cells (PBMC), human foreskin fibroblasts (HFF), or other cell types of mammalian origin (Table 2). In addition, studies by Verri, et al. [19], demonstrated that L-dC was not cytotoxic toward lymphoblastoid T cells.

Human bone marrow stem cells in primary culture have been shown to be a good predictor of potential nucleoside analog-induced hematotoxicity in patients [36, 37]. Granulocyte-macrophage (CFU-GM) and erythroid (BFU-E) precursors exposed to L-dC, L-dT and L-dA in clonogenic assays, which routinely detect the cellular toxicity of ZDV, were not affected [Table 4]. These results suggest that L-dC, L-dT and L-dA are highly selective, and their phosphorylated forms will be non-toxic *in vivo*.

Table 4. Human bone marrow toxicity of L-dA, L-dT and L-dC in granulocyte macrophage progenitor and erythrocyte precursor cells

Compound	CFU-GM[a] IC_{50} (μM)	BFU-E[b] IC_{50} (μM)
L-dA	> 40	> 10
L-dT	> 40	> 10
L-dC	> 40	> 10
ZDV	1.9±1.2	0.6±0.5

[a] CFU-GM: Granulocyte macrophage progenitor cells, colony forming units.

[b] BFU-E: Erythrocyte precursor cells, burst forming units.

Nucleoside analogs used in AIDS therapy, such as zidovudine (AZT, β-D-3'-azido-3'-deoxythymidine), stavudine (d4T, β-L-2', 3'-didehydro-2', 3'-dideoxythymidine), didanosine (ddI, β-D-2', 3'-dideoxyinosine) and zalcitabine (ddC, β-D-2', 3'-dideoxycytidine), have shown clinically limiting delayed toxicities, such as peripheral neuropathy, myopathy, and pancreatitis [31-34]. These adverse effects are attributable to decreased mitochondrial DNA (mtDNA) content and altered mitochondrial function leading to increased lactic acid production and hepatic steatosis [38-44]. Concomitant morphological changes in mitochondria (e.g., loss of cristae, matrix dissolution and swelling, and lipid droplet formation) can be observed with ultrastructrual analysis using transmission electron microscopy [40, 45, 46]. For example, fialuridine (FIAU) toxicity was shown to be associated with an irreversible intracellular event which decreased mitochondrial respiratory function, resulting in decreased mitochondrial ATP production and fatty acid metabolism. This form of mitochondrial toxicity can be initially identified in cell culture by increased lactic acid production and intracellular lipid droplet formation. In HepG2 cells incubated with 10 μM FIAU, a substantial increase in lactic acid production was observed (Table 3). Electron micrographs of these cells showed the presence of enlarged mitochondria with morphological changes consistent with mitochondrial dysfunction. Lamivudine (10 μM) did not effect mitochondrial structure or function. Using similar conditions, exposure of HepG2 cells to 10 μM L-dC, L-dT or L-dA for 14 days had no effect on lactic acid production, mitochondrial DNA content or morphology (Table 5).

Table 5. Effect of L-dC, L-dT and L-dA on mitochondria in HepG2 cells

Compound	Conc. (μM)	Cell Density	L-Lactate	mtDNA	Lipid Droplet Formation	Mitochondrial Morphology
			% of control			
Control		100	100	100	neg[a]	normal
L-dC	0.1	102 12	100 4	105 11	nd[b]	nd
	1.0	100 6	101 ± 6	99 ± 10	nd	nd
	10	101 ± 10	101 ± 2	107 ± 8	neg	normal
L-dT	0.1	103 ± 7	102 ± 2	103 ± 4	nd	nd
	1.0	106 ± 8	99 ± 2	101 ± 7	nd	nd
	10	97 ± 7	105 ± 2	97 ± 4	neg	normal
L-dA	0.1	103 ± 14	99 ± 3	97 ± 14	nd	nd
	1.0	102 ± 14	102 ± 3	92 ± 8	nd	nd
	10	100 ± 14	103 ± 5	88 ± 18	neg	normal
Lamivudine[c]	0.1	101 ± 2	99 ± 5	107 ± 8	nd	nd
	1.0	99 ± 1	101 ± 3	96 ± 9	nd	nd
	10	99 ± 1	98 ± 3	98 ± 10	neg	normal
FIAU[c]	0.1	83 ± 6	119 ± 5	101 ± 2	nd	nd
	1.0	73 ± 9	134 ± 9	118 ± 5	nd	nd
	10	37 ± 10	203 ± 13	86 ± 4	positive	abnormal

HepG2 cells were treated with the indicated concentrations of L-dT, L-dC or L-dA for 14 days. Values are presented as means and standard deviations of three independent experiments.

[a] neg, negative.

[b] nd, not determined.

[c] Data from reference [34, 43].

In acute (50-2000 mg/kg single oral dose) and subchronic (500-2000 mg/kg/day orally for 28 days) toxicology studies in rats and monkeys, there were no overt signs of toxicity, nor were there any L-dT related effects on body weight, food consumption, or clinical pathology parameters (hematology and serum chemistry). In addition, there were no macroscopic lesions observed at necropsy, nor were there any microscopic findings on histomorphological analysis attributable to L-dT. Based on the results of these studies, the no observed adverse effect level (NOAEL) for L-dT following a single oral dose, or repeated dosing for 28 days by oral gavage in the Sprague-Dawley rat and cynomologus monkey, was 2000 mg/kg.

In normal, healthy woodchucks or woodchucks chronically infected with hepatitis B virus, no toxicity was observed during acute (10 mg/kg single dose IV and PO) and subchronic (28 days at 10 mg/kg/day orally and 12 weeks at 1 mg/kg/day orally) studies. There was no weight loss in the L-dT treatment groups compared to control animals, clinical pathology parameters (hematology and serum chemistry) were in the normal range, and end- of- treatment liver biopsies in the 12-week study showed no evidence of fatty change (microvesicular steatosis).

L-dT and L-dC were not mutagenic in the *S. typhimurium* or *E. coli* plate incorporation mutagenicity assay, at concentrations up to a maximum of 5000 μg/plate tested. There was no evidence of chromosomal aberrations in the Chinese hamster ovary (CHO) assay after exposure to L-dT or L-dC at concentrations up to a maximum of 5000 μg/mL (20.6 mM). In the mouse micronucleus assay, L-dT and L-dC were not clastogenic to male or female animals (maximum dose tested 2000 mg/kg).

These investigational agents, used alone or in combination, are expected to offer new therapeutic options for patients with chronic hepatitis B virus infection.

(Since presentation at the International Conference on Therapies for Viral Hepatitis, Maui, 1999, much of this work has been published in *Antimicrobial Agents and Chemotherapy* 45: 229-235, 2001.)

References

1. Lai, C.L., Chien, R.N., Leung, N.W., Chang, T.T., Guan, R., Tai, D.I., Ng, K.Y., Wu, P.C., Dent, J.C., Barber, J., Stephenson, S.L., and Gray, D.F. 1998. A one-year trial of lamivudine for chronic hepatitis B. Asia Hepatitis Lamivudine Study Group. New England Journal of Medicine 339(2):61-8.
2. Dienstag, J.L., Schiff, E.R., Mitchell, M., Casey, D.E., Gitlin, N., Lissoos, T., Gelb, L.D., Condreay, L., Crowther, L., Rubin, M., and Brown, N. 1999. Extended lamivudine retreatment for chronic hepatitis B: maintenance of viral suppression after discontinuation of therapy. Hepatology 30(4):1082-7.
3. Gosselin, G., Mathe, C., Bergogne, M.C., Aubertin, A.M., Kirn, A., Schinazi, R.F., Sommadossi, J.P., and Imbach, J.L. 1994. Enantiomeric 2', 3'-dideoxycytidine derivatives are potent human immunodeficiency virus inhibitors in cell culture. C R Acad Sci III 317:85-9.
4. Schinazi, R.F., McMillan, A., Cannon, D., Mathis, R., Lloyd, R.M., Peck, A., Sommadossi, J.-P., St. Clair, M., Wilson, J., Furman, P.A., Painter, G., Choi, W.-B., and Liotta, D.C. 1992. Selective inhibition of human immunodeficiency viruses by racemates and enantiomers of *cis*-5-fluoro-1-[2-hydroxymethyl)-1, 3-oxatiolan-5-yl]cytosine. Antimicrobial Agents and Chemotherapy 36(11):2423-31.
5. Shi, J., McAtee, J.J., Schlueter Wirtz, S., Tharnish, P., Juodawlkis, A., Liotta, D.C., and Schinazi, R.F. 1999. Synthesis and biological evaluation of 2', '-didehydro-2', 3'- dideoxy-5- fluorocytidine (D4FC) analogues: discovery of carbocyclic nucleoside triphosphates with potent inhibitory activity against HIV-1 reverse transcriptase. Journal of Medicinal Chemistry 42(5):859-67.
6. Bolon, P.J., Wang, P., Chu, C., Gosselin, G., Boudou, V., Pierra, C., Mathe, C., Imbach, J.L., Faraj, A., Alaoui, A., Sommadossi, J.-P., Pai, S.B., Zhu, Y.L., Lin, J.S., Cheng, Y.C., and Schinazi, R.F. 1996. Anti-human immunodeficiency and anti-hepatitis B virus activities of beta-L-2', 3'-dideoxy purine nucleosides. Bioorg Med Chem Lett 6(14):1657-1662.
7. Gosselin, G., Boudou, V., Griffon, J.F., Pavia, G., Pierra, C., Imbach, J.L., Aubertin, A.M., Schinazi, R.F., Faraj, A., and Sommadossi, J.P. 1997. New unnatural L-nucleoside enantiomers: From their stereoselective synthesis to their biological activities. Nucleosides and Nucleotides 16(7-9):1389-98.
8. Chu, C.K., Boudinot, F.D., Peek, S.F., Hong, J.H., Choi, Y., Korba, B.E., Gerin, J.L., Cote, P.J., Tennant, B.C., and Cheng, Y.C. 1998. Preclinical investigation of L-FMAU as an anti-hepatitis B virus agent,

p. 303-312. *In* R. F. Schinazi, J.-P. Sommadossi, and H. C. Thomas (ed.), Therapies for Viral Hepatitis. International Medical Press, London.

9. Placidi, L., Faraj, A., Loi, A.G., Pierra, C., Egron, D., Cretton-Scott, E., Gosselin, G., Perigaud, C., Martin, L.T., Schinazi, R.F., Imbach, J.L., El Kouni, M.H., Bryant, M.L., and Sommadossi, J.-P. 2000. Antiviral activity and intracellular metabolism of bis(tbutylSATE) phosphotriester of β-L-2', 3'-dideoxyadenosine, a potent inhibitor of HIV and HBV replication. Antivir Chem Chemother submitted.
10. Placidi, L., Cretton-Scott, E., Gosselin, G., Pierra, C., Schinazi, R.F., Imbach, J.L., el Kouni, M.H., and Sommadossi, J.P. 2000. Intracellular metabolism of ≤-L-2', 3'-dideoxyadenosine: relavance to its limited antiviral activity. Antimicrobial Agents and Chemotherapy 44(4):853-8.
11. Faraj, A., Placidi, L., Perigaud, C., Cretton-Scott, E., Gosselin, G., Martin, L.T., Pierra, C., Schinazi, R.F., Imbach, J.L., and Sommadossi, J.-P. 1999. Intracellular metabolism of b-L-ddAMP-bis(tbutylSATE), a potent inhibitor of hepatitis B virus replication. Nucleosides and Nucleotides 18(4&5):987-8.
12. Placidi, L., Hernández, B., Cretton-Scott, E., Faraj, A., Bryant, M., Imbach, J.-L., Gosselin, G., Pierra, C., Dukhan, D., and Sommadossi, J.-P. 1999. Cellular pharmacology of ≤-L-thymidine (L-dT, NV-02B) and ≤-L-2'-deoxycytidine (L-dC, NV-02C) in HepG2 cells and primary rat, monkey and human hepatocytes. Antiviral Therapy 4(Supplement 4):A122.
13. Focher, F., Maga, G., Bendiscioli, A., Capobianco, M., Colonna, F., Garbesi, A., and Spadari, S. 1995. Stereospecificity of human DNA polymerases alpha, beta, gamma, delta and epsilon, HIV-reverse transcriptase, HSV-1 DNA polymerase, calf thymus terminal transferase and Escherichia coli DNA polymerase I in recognizing D- and L-thymidine 5'-triphosphate as substrate. Nucleic Acids Res 23(15):2840-7.
14. Spadari, S., Maga, G., Focher, F., Ciarrocchi, G., Manservigi, R., Arcamone, F., Capobianco, M., Carcuro, A., Colonna, F., Iotti, S., and et al. 1992. L-thymidine is phosphorylated by herpes simplex virus type 1 thymidine kinase and inhibits viral growth. J Med Chem 35(22):4214-20.
15. Faraj, A., Loi, A.G., Cui, L., Xie, M.-Y., Bryant, M., Bridges, E.G., Juodawlkis, A., Pierra, C., Dukhan, D., Gosselin, G., Imbach, J.L., Schinazi, R.F., Pai, B., Korba, B., Marion, P.L., and Sommadossi, J.-P. 1999. β-L-Thymidine and β-L-2'-deoxycytidine are potent, selective and specific anti-hepatitis B virus agents. Antiviral Therapy 4(Supplement 4):A119.
16. Chang, C.N., Doong, S.L., Zhou, J.H., Beach, J.W., Jeong, L.S., Chu, C.K., Tsai, C.H., Cheng, Y.C., Liotta, D., and Schinazi, R. 1992. Deoxycytidine deaminase-resistant stereoisomer is the active form of (+/-)-2', 3'-dideoxy-3'-thiacytidine in the inhibition of hepatitis B virus replication. Journal of Biological Chemistry 267(20):13938-42.
17. Furman, P.A., Davis, M., Liotta, D.C., Paff, M., Frick, L.W., Nelson, D.J., Dornsife, R.E., Wurster, J.A., Wilson, L.J., Fyfe, J.A., Tuttle, J.V., Miller, W.H., Condreay, L., Averett, D.R., Schinazi, R.F., and Painter, G.R. 1992. The anti-hepatitis B virus activities, cytotoxicities, and anabolic profiles of the (-) and (+) enantiomers of *cis*-5-fluoro-1-[2-(hydroxymethyl)-1, 3-oxathiolan-5-yl]cytosine. Antimicrobial Agents and Chemotherapy 36(12):2686-92.
18. Martin, L.T., Faraj, A., Schinazi, R.F., Gosselin, G., Mathe, C., Imbach, J.-L., and Sommadossi, J.-P. 1997. Effect of stereoisomerism on the cellular pharmacology of beta- enantiomers of cytidine analogs in Hep-G2 cells. Biochem Pharmacol 53(1):75-87.
19. Verri, A., Focher, F., Priori, G., Gosselin, G., Imbach, J.L., Capobianco, M., Garbesi, A., and Spadari, S. 1997. Lack of enantiospecificity of human 2'-deoxycytidine kinase: relevance for the activation of beta-L-deoxycytidine analogs as antineoplastic and antiviral agents. Molecular Pharmacology 51(1):132-8.
20. Tennant, B.C., Peek, S.F., Tochkov, I.A., Baldwin, B.H., Hornbuckle, W.E., Korba, B.E., Cote, P.J., and

Gerin, J.L. 1998. The woodchuck in preclinical assessment of therapy for hepatitis B virus infection, p. 171-176. *In* R. F. Schinazi, J.-P. Sommadossi, and H. C. Thomas (ed.), Therapies for Viral Hepatitis, First ed. International Medical Press, London.

21. Korba, B.E., Cote, P.J., Tennant, B.C., and Gerin, J.L. 1990. Woodchuck hepatitis virus infection as a model for the development of antiviral therapies against HBV, p. 663-5. *In* F. B. Hollinger, Lemon, S.M., Margolis, H. (ed.), Viral hepatitis and liver disease. Williams and Wilkins, Baltimore.
22. Korba, B.E., Cote, P., Hornbuckle, W., Tennant, B.C., and Gerin, J.L. 2000. Treatment of chronic woodchuck hepatitis virus infection in the eastern woodchuck (Marmota monax) with nucleoside analogues is predictive of therapy for chronic hepatitis B virus infection in humans. Hepatology 31(5):1165-75.
23. Cote, R.J., Roneker, C., Cass, K., Schodel, F., Peterson, D., Tennant, B., De Noronha, F., and Gerin, J. 1993. New enzyme immunoassays for the serologic detection of woodchuck hepatitis virus infection. Viral Immunology 6(2):161-9.
24. Genovesi, E.V., Lamb, L., Medina, I., Taylor, D., Seifer, M., Innaimo, S., Colonno, R.J., Standring, D.N., and Clark, J.M. 1998. Efficacy of the carbocyclic 2'-deoxyguanosine nucleoside BMS-200475 in the woodchuck model of hepatitis B virus infection. Antimicrobial Agents and Chemotherapy 42(12):3209-17.
25. Mason, W.S., Cullen, J., Moraleda, G., Saputelli, J., Aldrich, C.E., Miller, D.S., Tennant, B., Frick, L., Averett, D., Condreay, L.D., and Jilbert, A.R. 1998. Lamivudine therapy of WHV-infected woodchucks. Virology 245:18-32.
26. Rajagopalan, P., Boudinot, F.D., Chu, C.K., Tennant, B.C., Baldwin, B.H., and Schinazi, R.F. 1996. Pharmacokinetics of (-)-2'-3'-dideoxy-3'-thiacytidine in woodchucks. Antimicrobial Agents and Chemotherapy 40(3):642-5.
27. van Leeuwen, R., Lange, J.M., Hussey, E.K., Donn, K.H., Hall, S.T., Harker, A.J., Jonker, P., and Danner, S.A. 1992. The safety and pharmacokinetics of a reverse transcriptase inhibitor, 3TC, in patients with HIV infection: a phase I study. AIDS 6(12):1471-5.
28. Richardson, F.C., Engelhardt, J.A., and Bowsher, R.R. 1994. Fialuridine accumulates in DNA of dogs, monkeys, and rats following long-term oral administration. Proc Natl Acad Sci USA 91(25):12003-7.
29. Tennant, B.C., Baldwin, B.H., Graham, L.A., Ascenzi, M.A., Hornbuckle, W.E., Rowland, P.H., Tochkov, I.A., Yeager, A.E., Erb, H.N., Colacino, J.M., Lopez, C., Engelhardt, J.A., Bowsher, R.R., Richarson, F.C., Lewis, W., Cote, P.J., Korba, B.E., and Gerin, J.L. 1998. Antiviral activity and toxicity of fialuridine in the woodchuck model of hepatitis B virus infection. Hepatology 128(1):179-91.
30. McKenzie, R., Fried, M.W., Sallie, R., Conjeevaram, H., Di Bisceglie, A.M., Park, Y., Savarese, B., Kleiner, D., Tsokos, M., Luciano, C., Pruett, T., Stotka, J.L., Straus, S.E., and Hoofnagle, J.H. 1995. Hepatic failure and lactic acidosis due to fialuridine (FIAU), an investigational nucleoside analogue for chronic hepatitis B. New England Journal of Medicine 333(17):1099-1105.
31. Faulds, D., and Brogden, R.N. 1992. Didanosine. A review of its antiviral activity, pharmacokinetic properties and therapeutic potential in human immunodeficiency virus infection. Drugs 44(1):94-116.
32. Hurst, M., and Noble, S. 1999. Stavudine: an update of its use in the treatment of HIV infection. Drugs 58(5):919-49.
33. Whittington, R., and Brogden, R.N. 1992. Zalcitabine. A review of its pharmacology and clinical potential in acquired immunodeficiency syndrome (AIDS). Drugs 44(4):656-83.
34. Wilde, M.I., and Langtry, H.D. 1993. Zidovudine. An update of its pharmacodynamic and pharmacokinetic properties, and therapeutic efficacy. Drugs 46(3):515-78.
35. Semizarov, D.G., Arzumanov, A.A., Dyatkina, N.B., Meyer, A., Vichier-Guerre, S., Gosselin, G.,

Rayner, B., Imbach, J.-L., and Krayevsky, A.A. 1997. Stereoisomers of deoxynucleoside 5'-triphosphates as substrates for template-dependent and -independent DNA polymerases. Journal of Biological Chemistry 272(14):9556-60.

36. Faraj, A., Fowler, D.A., Bridges, E.G., and Sommadossi, J.-P. 1994. Effects of 2',3'-dideoxynucleosides on proliferation and differentiation of human pluripotent progenitors in liquid culture and their effects on mitochondrial DNA synthesis. Antimicrobial Agents and Chemotherapy 38(5):924-930.
37. Sommadossi, J.-P., Carlisle, R., and Zhou, Z. 1989. Cellular pharmacology of 3'-azido-3'-deoxythymidine with evidence of incorporation into DNA of human bone marrow cells. Molecular Pharmacology 36(1):9-14.
38. Chen, C.H., and Cheng, Y.C. 1989. Delayed cytotoxicity and selective loss of mitochondrial DNA in cells treated with the anti-human immunodeficiency virus compound 2',3'- dideoxycytidine. Journal of Biological Chemistry 264(20):11934-7.
39. Cui, L., Locatelli, L., Xie, M.Y., and Sommadossi, J.-P. 1997. Mitochondrial DNA effect of nucleoside analogs on neurite regeneration and mitochondrial DNA synthesis in PC-12 cells. Journal of Pharmacology and Experimental Therapeutics 280:1228-1234.
40. Cui, L., Schinazi, R.F., Gosselin, G., Imbach, J.-L., Chu, C.K., Rando, R.F., Revankar, G.R., and Sommadossi, J.-P. 1996. Effect of β-enantiomeric and racemic nucleoside analogues on mitochondrial funtions in HepG2 cells. Biochemical Pharmacology 52:1577-1584.
41. Cui, L., Yoon, S., Schinazi, R.F., and Sommadossi, J.-P. 1995. Cellular and molecular events leading to mitochondrial toxicity of 1-(2-deoxy-2-fluoro-1-β-D-arabinofuranoxyl)-5-iodouracil in human liver cells. Journal of Clinical Investigation 95:555-563.
42. Dalakas, M.C., Illa, I., Pezeshkpour, G.H., and al., e. 1990. Mitochondrial myopathy caused by long-term zidovudine therapy. New England Journal of Medicine 322(16):1098-1105.
43. Lewis, W., Gonzalez, B., Chomyn, A., and Papoian, T. 1992. Zidovudine induces molecular, biochemical, and ultrastructural changes in rat skeletal muscle mitochondria. J Clin Invest 89(4):1354-60.
44. Pan-Zhou, X.R., Cui, L., Zhou, X.J., Sommadossi, J.-P., and Darley-Usmar, V.M. 1999. Differential effects of antiretroviral nucleoside analogs on mitochondrial function; dual inhibition of citrate synthase and cytochrome c oxidase by AZT. Antimicrobial Agents and Chemotherapy In press.
45. Lewis, W., Levine, E.S., Griniuviene, B., Tankersly, K.O., Colacino, J.M., Sommadossi, J.P., Watanabe, K.A., and Perrino, F.W. 1996. Fialuridine and its metabolites inhibit DNA polymerase gamma at sites of multiple adjacent analog incorporation, decrease mtDNA abundance, and cause mitchondrial structural defects in cultured hepatoblasts. Proceedings of the National Academy of Sciences, USA 93(8):3592-7.
46. Pan-Zhou, X.-R., Cretton-Scott, E., Zhou, X.-J., Yang, M.-X., Lasker, J.M., and Sommadossi, J.-P. 1998. Role of human liver P450s and cytochrome *b5* in the reductive metabolism of 3'-azido-3'-deoxythymidine (AZT) to 3'-amino-3'-deoxythymidine. Biochemical Pharmacology 55:757-766.

Toxicological study of the anti-HBV agent β-L-thymidine

EDWARD G. BRIDGES[1], MARTIN L. BRYANT[1],
LAURENT PLACIDI[2], ABDESSLEM FARAJ[3], ANNA-GIULIA LOI[3],
CLAIRE PIERRA[3], DAVID DUKHAN[3], GILLES GOSSELIN[4],
JEAN-LOUIS IMBACH[4], BRENDA HERNANDEZ[2],
AMY JUODAWLKIS[1], BUD TENNANT[5],
ERIKA CRETTON-SCOTT[1] and JEAN-PIERRE SOMMADOSSI[1]

[1] *Idenix, Inc., 125 CambridgePark Dr., Cambridge, MA 02140, USA*
[2] *Department of Pharmacology and Toxicology, Division of Clinical Pharmacology, The Liver Center, University of Alabama at Birmingham, Birmingham, AL 35294, USA*
[3] *Idenix Pharmaceuticals, SARL*
[4] *Laboratoire de Chimie Bioorganique, CNRS UMR 5625, Universite de Montpellier II, Place Eugene Bataillon, 34095 Cedex 5 Montpellier, FRANCE*
[5] *Department of Clinical Sciences, College of Veterinary Medicine, Cornell University, Ithaca, NY 14853, USA*

Introduction

β-L-Thymidine (L-dT) is an unsubstituted, unmodified β-L-deoxynucleoside with potent antiviral activity against hepadnaviruses *in vitro* and *in vivo*, and a favorable pharmacological profile. As part of its development as a potential oral anti-HBV agent, a series of pre-clinical studies *in vitro* and in laboratory animals were conducted to delineate the cytotoxic, genotoxic, toxicologic and toxicokinetic profile of L-dT.

In vitro cytotoxicity

Effect on various cell types

A major issue limiting the use of some antiviral nucleoside analogs in patients has been drug-associated toxic side effects [1-3]. Drug selectivity is a critical issue in the treatment of patients chronically infected with HBV, since long-term therapy is needed. In cell culture, L-dT was non-cytotoxic (50% cytotoxic concentration, CC_{50} > 2000 μM) to the human hepatoma cell line 2.2.15, routinely used to determine the anti-HBV activity of potential antiviral agents, and was not cytotoxic to human peripheral blood mononuclear cells (CC_{50} >100 μM). In addition, L-dT was non-cytotoxic to numerous

Frontiers in Viral Hepatitis Ed. by RF Schinazi, J-P Sommadossi and CM Rice. 263 — 270

other cell lines of human and mammalian origin, including HFF, Daudi, A549, MDCK, CV-1, MA-104, and KB.

Effect on human bone marrow progenitor cells

The myelosuppressive effects of certain antiviral nucleoside analogs have highlighted the need to test for potential adverse effects on the growth of human bone marrow progenitor cells in clonogenic assays [4]. In particular, anemia and neutropenia are the most common drug-related clinical toxicities associated with the anti-human immunodeficiency virus (HIV) drug zidovudine (ZDV). This toxicity can be modeled in an *in vitro* assay that employs bone marrow cells obtained from healthy volunteers [5]. ZDV has been shown to directly inhibit human granulocyte-macrophage (CFU-GM) and erythroid (BFU-E) lineage colony proliferation at clinically relevant concentrations of 1-2 μM [5-11]. Using human bone marrow clonogenic assays, L-dT had a 50% inhibitory concentration (IC_{50}) in CFU-GM and BFU-E of greater than 10 μM.

Effect on mitochondrial function

Clinically limiting toxicities including peripheral neuropathy, myopathy, and pancreatitis are associated with the anti-HIV drugs ZDV, stavudine (d4T), didanosine (ddI), and zalcitabine (ddC) [4, 12-14]. These clinically adverse events have been attributed to inhibition of mitochondrial function due to reduction in mitochondrial DNA (mtDNA) content and nucleoside analog incorporation into mtDNA. In addition, a particular nucleoside analog, fialuridine (FIAU), caused hepatic failure, pancreatitis, neuropathy, myopathy, and lactic acidosis due to direct mitochondrial toxicity [15].

To assess the potential of L-dT to produce mitochondrial toxicity, several *in vitro* studies were conducted using the human hepatoma cell line HepG2 and normal human hepatocytes. These studies included analysis of lactic acid production, mtDNA content, and determination of changes in morphology (e.g., loss of cristae, matrix dissolution and swelling, and lipid droplet formation) of mitochondrial ultrastructure. In HepG2 cells chronically treated with L-dT for 14 and 28 days, there was no change in mtDNA content and no difference in cellular lactic acid production compared to untreated control cells (Faraj et al., *Antiviral Therapy*, 1999, 4 (suppl 4) A119). Furthermore, the ultrastructure of HepG2 cells, and in particular mitochondria, were examined by transmission electron microscopy. No discernible changes in cell architecture or mitochondrial morphology were detected. The size and organization of mitochondrial cristae were normal. Thus, L-dT had no apparent effect on mitochondrial morphology or function.

Mutagenicity and genotoxicity

Three studies were undertaken to determine the mutagenetic potential of L-dT: *S. typhimurium* and *E. coli* plate incorporation mutation assay and chromosomal aberration assay, and the mouse micronucleus assay.

L-dT was tested for its potential to cause mutations at the histidine operon of four strains of *Salmonella typhimurium* and at the tryptophan operon of *Escherichia coli*. In the bacterial reverse mutation assay, L-dT was tested up to a concentration of 5000 μg/plate. Test strains were exposed to L-dT or control in the absence of exogenous activation and in the presence of induced rat liver S-9 plus cofactors. No substantial increases in the number of revertant colonies were observed for any of the test strains in the presence or absence of induced rat liver S-9. There was no evidence of mutagenicity in the *S. typhimurium* or *E. coli* plate incorporation mutation assay with L-dT concentrations up to 5000 μg/plate.

In the cytogenetic study *in vitro*, there was no indication that L-dT was clastogenic, as evidenced by a lack of chromosomal aberrations in the Chinese hamster ovary (CHO) assay after exposure to L-dT at concentrations up to 5000 μg/mL, either with or without metabolic activation.

L-dT was tested for its potential to induce micronucleated polychromatic erythrocytes (MPCE) in the bone marrow cells of male and female mice. The results of the study indicate that there was no statistically significant increase (defined as a p-value ≤ 0.025, determined by a one-tailed Student's t-test) in the number of MPCE at any timepoint at concentrations up to 2000 mg/kg following a single oral dose. Furthermore, no reduction of more than 20% compared to negative control in the percentage of polychromatic erythrocytes (PCE), as an indication of toxicity, was observed at any timepoint in any L-dT dose group. Thus, L-dT was not clastogenic to male or female animals at doses up to 2000 mg/kg.

Acute toxicity

A protocol was designed to evaluate the potential acute toxicity of L-dT in a rodent and non-human primate species. Rats (Sprague-Dawley) were administered a single oral dose of L-dT at 0, 500, 1000 or 2000 mg/kg of body weight, followed by 15 days of observation and a comprehensive gross necropsy. Cynomologus monkeys (*Macaca fascicularis*) were used to further evaluate the toxicity of L-dT in an oral-dose escalation study at levels of 20, 100, 500, 1000 and 2000 mg/kg body weight over 14 days, followed by a comprehensive gross necropsy on Day 17. Toxicity was assessed by clinical observations, body weights, clinical pathology, organ weights, and macroscopic pathological evaluation.

No overt signs of toxicity were observed in either rats or monkeys during these studies at dosages up to 2000 mg/kg. All animals maintained body weight during the course of the studies, and there were no significant differences between the mean body weights of the L-dT treated animals and control groups. In addition, there were no significant differences in organ weights, both absolute and relative (organ-to-body weight and organ-to-brain weight). No treatment-related effects attributable to L-dT were observed in the clinical pathology parameters (hematology and serum chemistry). Furthermore, macroscopic examination for gross lesions in the organs at necropsy did not reveal any change due to L-dT administration. Based on the results of these acute toxicity studies, there was no demonstrable toxicity attributable to L-dT exposure, and the no observed adverse event level (NOAEL) for L-dT following oral administration in the rat and monkey was 2000 mg/kg.

Subchronic toxicity

The potential for toxicity during 28-day repeated dosing with L-dT was evaluated in rats (Sprague-Dawley) and cynomologus monkeys by oral administration of 0, 500, 1000, or 2000 mg/kg-body-weight/day. Throughout the whole treatment period there were no overt signs of toxicity, nor were there any L-dT-related effects in either rats or monkeys on body weight, food consumption, clinical pathology parameters (hematology and serum chemistry), histopathology, or organ weight (absolute and relative). No macroscopic lesions attributable to L-dT were observed at necropsy, nor were there any microscopic findings considered to be related to L-dT administration in rats or monkeys. It was observed that female rats in the 500 mg/kg and 2000 mg/kg group exhibited greater adrenal gland weights compared to the vehicle control females. There were no histomorphologic correlates to the increased adrenal weights. Based on the results of this study, the no observed adverse event level (NOAEL) for L-dT following repeated dosing for 28 days by oral gavage in rats and monkeys was 2000 mg/kg.

Oral pharmacokinetics

Blood samples were collected on Day 1 and Day 28 from rats and monkeys during the subchronic study for toxicokinetic analysis of drug exposure. The plasma concentration-time data were subjected to non-compartmental analysis using WinNonlin 1.5 (Model 200). The exposure to L-dT appeared to be comparable for male and female rats and monkeys within each dose group on Day 1 and Day 28. The mean C_{max} and AUC increased generally in an apparent dose-proportional manner in both species on each sampling day in males and females. The median T_{max} was determined to be one to two hours for both sexes at all three dose levels on Days 1 and 28 in both rats and monkeys and is indicative of moderately rapid absorption from the gastrointestinal tract.

L-dT was eliminated in an apparent mono-exponential manner in rats and in an apparent bi-exponential manner in monkeys. The estimated terminal-phase mean half-lives ranged from 3.1 to 6.0 hours in rats, irrespective of dose and gender. Similarly, there were no dose or gender differences in the estimated terminal-phase mean half-lives of L-dT in monkeys, but the $t_{1/2}$ ranged from 7.2 to 12.1 hours on Day 1, and from 13.4 to 22.6 hours on Day 28.

Mean plasma concentration-time curves of L-dT for male and female rats (2000 mg/kg dose groups) on Day 1 and Day 28 are illustrated in Figure 1. The mean C_{max} values for male and female rats were similar within each sampling day and dose group. However, there was a tendency toward slightly higher values for female rats on Day 1 for the 2000 mg/kg group and on Day 28 for the 500 mg/kg and 1000 mg/kg groups. C_{max} values for males in each dose group and for females (2000 mg/kg group) were lower on Day 28 compared to Day 1. The C_{max} for females in the 500 mg/kg and 1000 mg/kg

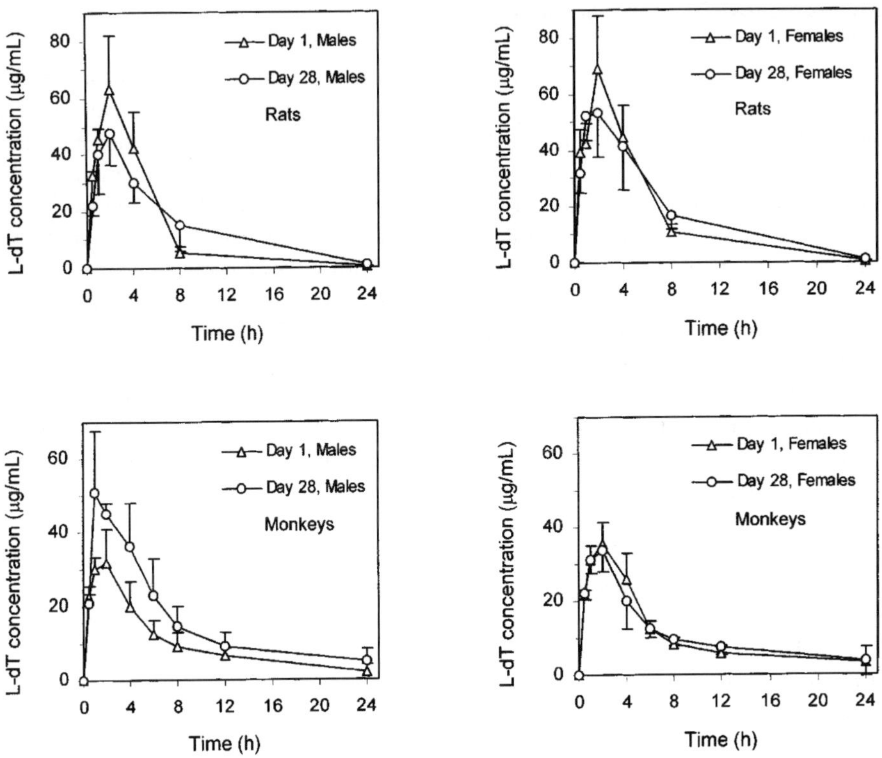

Figure 1. Plasma profiles of L-dT following 1-day and 28-day repeated oral dosing at 2000 mg/kg/day in male and female rats and monkeys (n = 4/sex).

groups were comparable on Day 1 and Day 28. Overall, exposure to L-dT appeared to be comparable for male and female rats within each dose group on Day 1 and Day 28, following 28-day, repeated oral dosing. In addition, exposure appeared to increase in a linear, dose-proportional relationship across the dosage range of 500 to 2000 mg/kg/day.

In monkeys, the C_{max} for the 2000 mg/kg treatment group on Day 28 was greater in males than females (Figure 1). For both male and female monkeys in the 500 mg/kg and 1000 mg/kg groups and the 2000 mg/kg group males, the C_{max} was higher on Day 28 compared to Day 1. The C_{max} values on both sampling days were similar for the 2000 mg/kg group females. In monkeys, the AUC showed trends similar to those noted for C_{max}. Overall, exposure to L-dT appeared to be comparable for male and female monkeys within each dose group on Day 1 and Day 28. In addition, exposure on Day 28 appeared to be greater by 20% to 60% and generally increased in a dose-proportional manner on both Day 1 and Day 28.

Subchronic toxicity in woodchucks

This study in a second rodent species supports the toxicology studies in the rat. The woodchuck model has been valuable for the preclinical toxicological evaluation of nucleoside analogs. This animal model identified the delayed severe hepatocellular toxicity induced by FIAU in humans that is not seen in preclinical evaluation in other rodents or primates [16, 17]. The FIAU-induced toxicity observed in woodchucks was similar to that observed in drug-treated, HBV-infected patients [15, 16]. Toxicity was identified after six to eight weeks of drug exposure for woodchucks and was manifested as significant weight loss, wasting and hepatocellular damage seen on liver biopsy.

Woodchucks received L-dT at doses of 0.01, 0.1, 1.0, or 10.0 mg/kg/day orally for 28 days. No toxicity was observed during the four-week treatment period or eight-week post-treatment follow-up period. Furthermore, all animals gained weight in a fashion similar to control animals during the 84-day protocol. One animal in the 0.1 mg/kg/day group lost weight during the treatment phase of the study but gained weight post-treatment.

L-dT was also tested through 12 weeks of treatment (1 mg/kg/day via the oral route) and 12 weeks of follow-up. L-dT was well tolerated and showed no drug-related toxicity. Animals in the treated groups did not show any weight loss attributable to drug exposure when compared to the control group. Serum chemistries and hematology from all animals were in the normal range before and after 12 weeks of treatment. Liver tissue histomorphology as evaluated by routine light microscopy was normal for all groups. There was no evidence of fatty change (microvesicular steatosis).

Chronic toxicity

Studies are in progress to evaluate the chronic exposure of L-dT in rats (Sprague-Dawley) and cynomologus monkeys. In rats, L-dT dosing occurs over a six-month period by oral drug administration of 0, 100, 500, or 1000 mg/kg-body-weight/day. A subset of animals will be evaluated after 3 months of dosing. Chronic exposure of cynomologus monkeys to L-dT at the same dose levels will be conducted for nine months, with a subset evaluated at three months.

Summary

L-dT is a potent antiviral nucleoside against HBV replication in cell culture and has a favorable *in vitro* toxicity profile. *In vivo* efficacy studies conducted in chronically infected woodchucks indicated that L-dT has potent antihepadnaviral activity, decreasing plasma viral DNA loads by up to 8 logs. L-dT is non-toxic and non-clastogenic at doses much greater than those most likely to be used clinically. No adverse events were observed in acute toxicity studies in rats and monkeys after oral administration of L-dT at concentrations up to 2000 mg/kg of body weight. In subchronic toxicity studies, L-dT showed no toxic effect at doses up to 2000 mg/kg of body weight after

28 days repeated oral administration to rats and monkeys. The potent antiviral efficacy and low toxicity *in vitro* and *in vivo* makes L-dT an attractive candidate for further development as an anti-HBV agent.

References

1. Faulds D and Brogden RN, Didanosine. A review of its antiviral activity, pharmacokinetic properties and therapeutic potential in human immunodeficiency virus infection. *Drugs* 44(1): 94-116, 1992.
2. Whittington R and Brogden RN, Zalcitabine. A review of its pharmacology and clinical potential in acquired immunodeficiency syndrome (AIDS). *Drugs* 44(4): 656-83, 1992.
3. Wilde MI and Langtry HD, Zidovudine. An update of its pharmacodynamic and pharmacokinetic properties, and therapeutic efficacy. *Drugs* 46(3): 515-78, 1993.
4. Richman DD, Fischl MA, Grieco MH, Gottlieb MS, Volberding PA, Laskin OL, Leedom JM, Groopman JE, Mildvan D, Hirsch MS, Jackson GG, Durack DT, Nusinoff-Lehrman S and and the AZT Collaborative Working Group, The toxicity of azidothymidine (AZT) in the treatment of patients with AIDS and AIDS-related complex. A double-blind, placebo-controlled trial. *N Engl J Med* 317(4): 192-7, 1987.
5. Sommadossi J-P and Carlisle R, Toxicity of 3'-azido-3'-deoxythymidine and 9-(1, 3-dihydroxy-2-propoxymethyl)guanine for normal human hematopoietic progenitor cells *in vitro*. *Antimicrobial Agents and Chemotherapy* 31(3): 452-454, 1987.
6. Berman E, Duigou-Osterndorf R, Krown SE, Fanucchi MP, Chou J, Hirsch MS, Clarkson BD and Chou TC, Synergistic cytotoxic effect of azidothymidine and recombinant interferon alpha on normal human bone marrow progenitor cells. *Blood* 74(4): 1281-6, 1989.
7. Yoshida Y and Yoshida C, Reversal of azidothymidine-induced bone marrow suppression by 2', 3'- dideoxythymidine as studied by hemopoietic clonal culture. *AIDS Res Hum Retroviruses* 6(7): 929-32, 1990.
8. Lerza R, Castello G, Mela GS, Arboscello E, Cerruti A, Bogliolo G, Mencoboni M, Ballarino P and Pannacciulli I, *In vitro* synergistic inhibition of human bone marrow hemopoietic progenitor growth by a 3'-azido-3'-deoxy-thymidine, 2', 3'- dideoxycytidine combination. *Exp Hematol* 25(3): 252-5, 1997.
9. Dornsife RE and Averett DR, *In vitro* potency of inhibition by antiviral drugs of hematopoietic progenitor colony formation correlates with exposure at hemotoxic levels in human immunodeficiency virus-positive humans. *Antimicrob Agents Chemother* 40(2): 514-9, 1996.
10. Kurtzberg J and Carter SG, Differential toxicity of carbovir and AZT to human bone marrow hematopoietic progenitor cells *in vitro*. *Exp Hematol* 18(10): 1094-6, 1990.
11. Weinberg RS, Chusid ED, Galperin Y, Thomson JC, Cheung T and Sacks HS, Effect of antiviral drugs and hematopoietic growth factors on *in vitro* erythropoiesis. *Mt Sinai J Med* 65(1): 5-13, 1998.
12. Browne MJ, Mayer KH, Chafee SB, Dudley MN, Posner MR, Steinberg SM, Graham KK, Geletko SM, Zinner SH, Denman SL, Dunkle LM, Kaul S, McLaren C, Skowron G, Kouttab NM, Kennedy T, Weitberg AB and Curt GA, 2', 3'-didehydro-3'-deoxythymidine (d4T) in patients with AIDS or AIDS-related complex: a phase I trial. *J Infect Dis* 167(1): 21-9, 1993.
13. Fischl MA, Olson RM, Follansbee SE, Lalezari JP, Henry DH, Frame PT, Remick SC, Salgo MP, Lin AH, Nauss-Karol C, Lieberman J and Soo W, Zalcitabine compared with zidovudine in patients with advanced HIV-1 infection who received previous zidovudine therapy. *Ann Intern Med* 118(10): 762-9, 1993.

14. Yarchoan R, Pluda JM, Thomas RV, Mitsuya H, Brouwers P, Wyvill KM, Hartman N, Johns DG and Broder S, Long-term toxicity/activity profile of 2', 3'-dideoxyinosine in AIDS or AIDS-related complex. *Lancet* 336(8714): 526-9, 1990.
15. McKenzie R, Fried MW, Sallie R, Conjeevaram H, Di Bisceglie AM, Park Y, Savarese B, Kleiner D, Tsokos M, Luciano C, Pruett T, Stotka JL, Straus SE and Hoofnagle JH, Hepatic failure and lactic acidosis due to fialuridine (FIAU), an investigational nucleoside analogue for chronic hepatitis B. *New England Journal of Medicine* 333(17): 1099-1105, 1995.
16. Tennant BC, Baldwin BH, Graham LA, Ascenzi MA, Hornbuckle WE, Rowland PH, Tochkov IA, Yeager AE, Erb HN, Colacino JM, Lopez C, Engelhardt JA, Bowsher RR, Richarson FC, Lewis W, Cote PJ, Korba BE and Gerin JL, Antiviral activity and toxicity of fialuridine in the woodchuck model of hepatitis B virus infection. *Hepatology* 128(1): 179-91, 1998.
17. Richardson FC, Engelhardt JA and Bowsher RR, Fialuridine accumulates in DNA of dogs, monkeys, and rats following long-term oral administration. *Proc Natl Acad Sci USA* 91(25): 12003-7, 1994.

Pharmacokinetics of β-L-thymidine and β-L-2'-deoxycytidine in woodchucks and monkeys

ERIKA CRETTON-SCOTT[1], EDWARD G. BRIDGES[1],
BUD C. TENNANT[2], AMY JUODAWLKIS[1], GILLES GOSSELIN[3],
JEAN-LOUIS IMBACH[3], CLAIRE PIERRA[4], DAVID DUKHAN[4],
MARTIN L. BRYANT[1] and JEAN-PIERRE SOMMADOSSI[1]

[1] *Idenix Pharmaceuticals, Inc., 125 CambridgePark Dr., Cambridge, MA 02140, USA*
[2] *Department of Clinical Sciences, College of Veterinary Medicine, Cornell University, Ithaca, NY 14853, USA*
[3] *Laboratoire de Chimie Bioorganique CNRS UMR 5625, Universite de Montpellier II, Place Eugene Bataillon, 34095 Cedex 5 Montpellier, France*
[4] *Idenix Pharmaceuticals, SARL, Immeuble "La Vigie", 170 Rue Leon Blum, 34000, Montpellier, France*

Introduction

Chronic hepatitis B virus (HBV) infection is a major global health problem, affecting approximately 5% of the world's population and up to one million people in the United States. It is estimated that more than 2 billion people worldwide have been infected with HBV and that 350 million are chronically infected and at risk of death from cirrhosis and liver cancer. The development of an effective vaccine to prevent HBV infection should lead to the eventual eradication of the virus, however, antiviral therapy still remains the only therapeutic approach to delay or prevent the progression of this disease in chronically infected individuals.

Currently, the only approved treatment options include α-interferon (INF) and lamivudine (3TC, β-L-2', 3'-dideoxy-3'-thiacytidine). Response rates with INF are low, and use of the drug is associated with side effects that can lead to discontinuation of therapy [1, 2]. In addition, response to INF therapy in immunosuppressed patients such as transplant recipients or those co-infected with the human immunodeficiency virus (HIV) is rare [3]. Lamivudine is a nucleoside analog with the unnatural β-L sugar configuration, which has been in use for the treatment of HIV since its approval for this disease in 1995. However, similar to INF therapy, complete antiviral response to lamivudine is seen only in a small fraction of HBV patients after one year of therapy [4]. Further limitations of lamivudine therapy include a rapid rebound in viral replication upon cessation of therapy that can be life threatening in HIV-HBV co-infected individuals [5] and the rapid emergence of lamivudine resistance [4, 6].

Frontiers in Viral Hepatitis Ed. by RF Schinazi, J-P Sommadossi and CM Rice. 271 — 279

Since the approval of lamivudine for the treatment of HIV in 1995 and HBV in 1998, the search for other unnatural L-nucleosides with antiviral activity has been intense. Several such nucleosides are in various stages of development as potential antiviral agents, including the 5-fluoro congener of lamivudine, (-)-2'-deoxy-5-fluoro-3'-thiacytidine (FTC) [7] and 2'-fluoro-5-methyl-β-L-arabinofuranosyl-uracil (L-FMAU) [8]. Recently, β-L-thymidine (L-dT) and β-L-2'-deoxycytidine (L-dC), two representatives of β-L-2'-deoxynucleosides, were shown to be potent, selective and specific inhibitors of HBV replication both *in vivo* and *in vitro* (EC_{50} = 0.19-0.24 μM in 2.2.15) [9]. Neither compound exhibits cellular or mitochondrial toxicity, and neither inhibits human cellular DNA polymerase α, β, or γ at concentrations as high as 100 μM [10]. Thus, both nucleosides appear to have promise as anti-HBV agents.

To assess the preclinical pharmacokinetics of L-dT and L-dC, intravenous and oral cross-over studies were conducted in woodchucks (*Marmota monax*) and monkeys (*Macaca fascicularis*). The woodchuck is a useful animal model for studying anti-HBV agents due to the many similarities between woodchuck hepatitis virus (WHV) and HBV, hence providing important information on the *in vivo* efficacy of anti-HBV candidates [11, 12]. Likewise, monkeys have been well-established as an animal model that is predictive of the metabolic disposition of a number of antiviral agents in humans [13-15].

Pharmacokinetics

Woodchuck

Healthy woodchucks, negative for WHV infection, received 10 mg/kg of L-dT or L-dC with a radiolabeled tracer as a single intravenous dose. Following a four-week washout period, the same animals received an identical oral dose of L-dT or L-dC. Plasma and urine samples were collected and analyzed by HPLC.

Plasma concentration-versus-time curves following intravenous and oral administration of L-dT and L-dC are illustrated in Figures 1 and 2. Plasma levels declined in a biexponential manner for both compounds following intravenous administration, with mean apparent terminal half-life ($t_{1/2}$) values of 3.99 ± 0.69 h for L-dT and 2.85 ± 1.30 h for L-dC. The pharmacokinetic parameters of L-dT and L-dC generated by model-independent methods are summarized in Tables 1 and 2. The area under the plasma concentration-time curve (AUC) values for both compounds were similar, averaging 216 ± 46.2 μM*h for L-dT and 174 ± 117 μM*h for L-dC. Peak plasma concentrations of L-dT averaged 162 ± 8.75 μM and 112 ± 32.7 μM for L-dC. Both compounds were detectable 24 hours after drug administration. The apparent total clearance (CL) was moderate, with mean values of 0.20 ± 0.47 and 0.39 ± 0.34 L/h/kg for L-dT and L-dC, respectively. The apparent volume of distribution (V_d) for L-dT averaged 1.13 ± 0.23 L/kg, which is greater than the total volume of water in woodchucks, indicating intracellular distribution. Similarly, L-dC demonstrated intracellular distribution with a mean V_d of 1.17 ± 0.36 L/kg.

Plasma L-dT and L-dC concentrations following oral administration were lower than those after intravenous administration. Absorption was slow with peak plasma

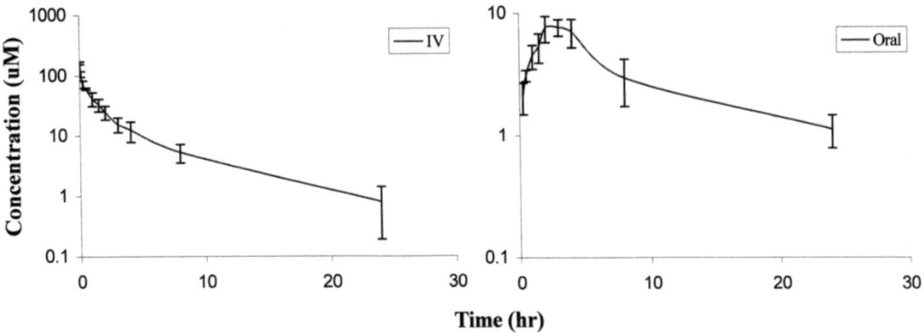

Figure 1. Plasma profile of L-dT (10 mg/kg) in woodchucks; mean (±SD) n=3.

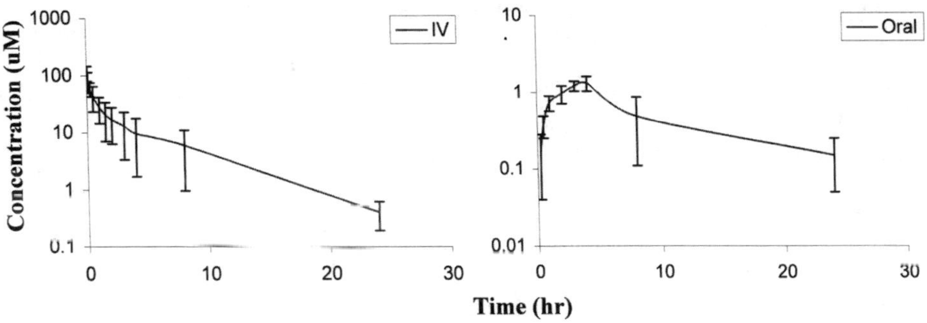

Figure 2. Plasma profile of L-dC (10 mg/kg) in Woodchcucks; mean (±SD) n=3.

concentrations (C_{max}) of 8.58 ± 1.02 μM and 1.37 ± 0.22 μM for L-dT and L-dC, respectively, occurring three to four hours following dose administration. Both L-dT and L-dC were still detectable after 24 hours following drug administration. The elimination $t_{1/2}$ values for both compounds were substantially higher than values observed after intravenous administration (Tables 1 and 2) due to prolonged oral absorption. L-dT exhibited good oral bioavailability (F), ranging from 34.9 to 43.4%. No metabolites of L-dT were detected in plasma. In contrast, absorption of L-dC was limited, with an average F of 9.57 ± 6.36%.

The metabolic fate of L-dT and L-dC was examined after both intravenous and oral administration. Low levels (at the limit of detection of 0.1 μM) of the deaminated derivative of L-dC, -L-2'-deoxyuridine (L-dU), were detected in plasma

Table 1. Pharmacokinetics of L-dT (10 mg/kg) in woodchucks

Woodchuck	Sex	AUC (μM*h)	$t_{1/2}$ (h)	C_{max} (μM)	T_{max} (h)	CL (L/h/Kg)	Vd (L/Kg)	MRT (h)	F (%)
IV									
98255	M	246	3.57	158	0	0.17	0.88	3.97	
98262	M	163	3.61	172	0	0.25	1.32	3.47	
98331	F	239	4.78	157	0	0.17	1.20	5.48	
Mean		216	3.99	162	0	0.20	1.13	4.31	
(± SD)		(46.2)	(0.69)	(8.75)		(.47)	(0.23)	(1.05)	
Oral									
98255	M	76.9	7.29	7.35	4.0			10.5	34.9
98262	M	57.7	6.95	9.50	2.0			10.4	36.6
98331	F	92.4	8.38	8.90	3.0			12.5	43.4
Mean		75.7	7.54	8.58	3.0			11.2	38.3
(± SD)		(14.4)	(0.75)	(1.02)	(1.0)			(1.18)	(4.5)

Table 2. Pharmacokinetics of L-dC (10 mg/kg) in woodchucks

Woodchuck	Sex	AUC (μM*h)	$t_{1/2}$ (h)	C_{max} (μM)	T_{max} (h)	CL (L/h/Kg)	Vd (L/Kg)	MRT (h)	F (%)
IV									
98254	M	181	3.55	108	0	1.23	1.11	4.64	
98272	M	288	3.66	147	0	0.79	0.68	4.52	
98333	F	54	1.35	82	0	1.50	1.02	1.32	
Mean		174	2.85	112	0	1.17	0.94	3.49	
(± SD)		(117)	(1.30)	(32.7)	0	(0.36)	(0.23)	(1.88)	
Oral									
98254	M	9.61	5.55	1.19	2.0			7.61	5.60
98272	M	16.6	7.72	1.32	4.0			11.59	6.20
98333	F	7.76	2.38	1.61	3.0			4.19	16.90
Mean		11.32	5.22	1.37	3.0			7.80	9.57
(± SD)		(4.66)	(2.69)	(022)	(1.0)			(3.70)	(6.36)

after intravenous and oral administration of L-dC. To determine the metabolic pathway involved in the formation of L-dU, human liver cytosolic and plasma (sources of cytidine deaminase) were exposed to L-dC. Deamination of L-dC to L-dU did not occur at any time point examined (data not shown). Interestingly, when intact human liver cells were exposed to L-dC, deamination of its 5'-monophosphate derivative (L-dCMP) to the 5'-monophosphate derivative of L-dU (L-dUMP) with subsequent degradation to L-dU was demonstrated [16], suggesting that the low levels of L-dU detected in plasma may be derived from the intracellular deamination of L-dCMP.

Formal urinary excretion was not determined in this study, however L-dT and L-dC were detected unchanged, and minor amounts of L-dU were also identified in the L-dC treatment group.

Monkey

Healthy non-naïve cynomologus monkeys received 10 mg/kg of L-dT or L-dC with a radiolabeled tracer as a single intravenous dose. Following a six-week washout period, the same animals received an identical oral dose of L-dT or L-dC. Plasma and urine samples were collected and analyzed by HPLC.

The mean plasma profiles of L-dT and L-dC in cynomologus monkeys after intravenous and oral administrations are illustrated in Figures 3 and 4. Both L-dT and L-dC concentrations in plasma declined rapidly following intravenous administration, with mean $t_{1/2}$ values of 1.33 ± 0.04 h and 1.59 ± 0.09 h, respectively. In contrast to the woodchuck, both L-dT and L-dC were below the lower limit of quantitation after eight hours post-dose. Further studies will evaluate the terminal half-life in humans. The pharmacokinetic parameters of L-dT and L-dC after intravenous and oral administrations are presented in Tables 3 and 4. AUC and C_{max} values for L-dC were slightly higher than those observed for L-dT following intravenous drug administration. Total CL was moderate, averaging 0.74 ± 0.10 L/h/kg for L-dT and 0.53 ± 0.04 L/h/kg for L-dC. Mean V_d values (Tables 3 and 4) indicate intracellular distribution for both compounds. Following oral administration, peak plasma concentrations of L-dT and L-dC were observed within two hours after administration. Apparent terminal $t_{1/2}$ values observed for Ld-T and L-dC following oral administration were not significantly

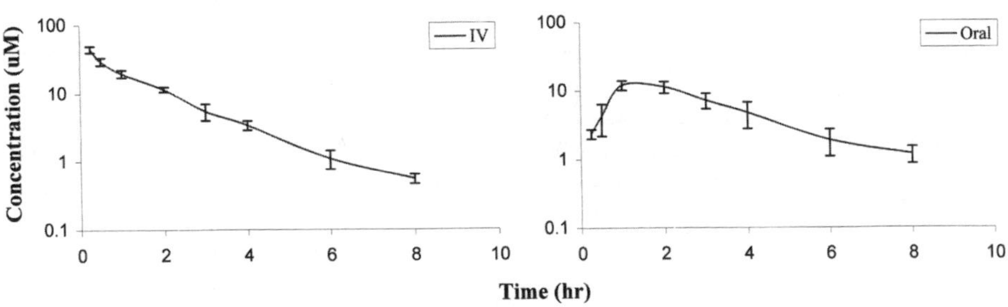

Figure 3. Plasma profile of L-dT (10 mg/kg) in Monkeys mean (±SD) n=3.

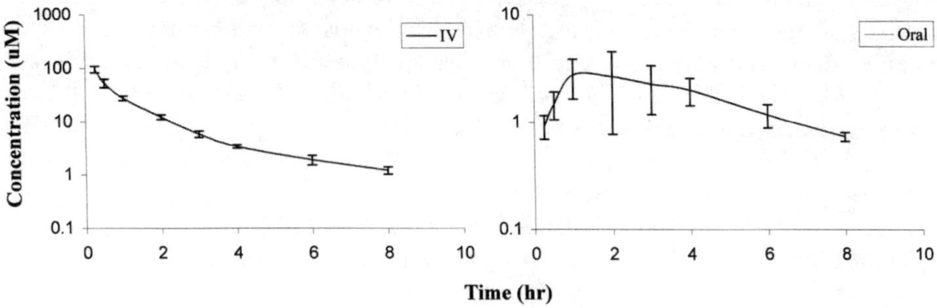

Figure 4. Plasma profile of L-dC (10 mg/kg) in Monkeys mean (±SD) n=3.

Table 3. Pharmacokinetics of L-dT (10 mg/kg) in cynomologus monkeys

Monkey	Sex	AUC (μM*h)	$t_{1/2}$ (h)	C_{max} (μM)	T_{max} (h)	CL (L/h/Kg)	Vd (L/Kg)	MRT (h)	CL_R (L/h/kg)	f_e	F (%)
IV											
1001	M	63.04	1.37	49.78	0	0.64	1.27	1.56	0.42	0.65	
1002	M	55.83	1.32	40.67	0	0.75	1.43	1.59	0.53	0.70	
1003	M	49.23	1.30	42.06	0	0.84	1.58	1.39	0.75	0.89	
Mean		56.03	1.33	44.35	0	0.74	1.43	1.51	0.57	0.75	
(± SD)		(6.91)	(0.04)	(4.80)	0	(0.10)	(0.16)	(0.11)	(0.17)	(0.13)	
Oral											
1001	M	48.77	1.87	12.35	2.0			3.60		0.55	69.38
1002	M	39.02	1.78	12.83	2.0			3.29		0.29	67.34
1003	M	36.46	1.67	13.71	1.0			2.87		0.26	69.05
Mean		41.40	1.77	12.97	1.67			3.25		0.37	68.59
(± SD)		(6.50)	(0.10)	(0.69)	(0.58)			(0.37)		(0.16)	(1.09)

different from those observed after intravenous administration. L-dT was readily absorbed, exhibiting a mean F of 68.59 ± 1.09%. No metabolites of L-dT were detected in plasma after either intravenous or oral administration. As observed in the woodchuck, the oral absorption of L-dC was significantly lower than L-dT, with F averaging 16.38 ± 5.00%. As reported in the woodchuck studies, low levels (below quantitation) of L-dU were detectable in monkey plasma following both intravenous and oral administrations of L-dC.

Table 4. Pharmacokinetics of L-dC (10 mg/kg) in cynomologus monkeys

Monkey	Sex	AUC (μM*h)	$t_{1/2}$ (h)	C_{max} (μM)	T_{max} (h)	CL (L/h/Kg)	Vd (L/Kg)	MRT (h)	CL_R (L/h/kg)	f_e	F (%)
IV											
2001	M	80.84	1.48	85.37	0	0.53	1.13	1.34	0.31	0.83	
2002	M	75.55	1.64	91.55	0	0.57	1.35	1.32	0.33	0.89	
2003	M	86.96	1.65	110.05	0	0.50	1.19	1.29	NA*	NA	
Mean		81.12	1.59	95.66	0	0.53	1.22	1.32	0.32	0.86	
(± SD)		(5.71)	(0.09)	(12.84)	0	(0.04)	(0.11)	(0.03)	(0.01)[2]	(0.04)[2]	
Oral											
2001	M	18.31	2.34	4.82	2.0			4.15		0.08	21.40
2002	M	13.09	2.04	2.54	4.0			4.63		0.11	16.33
2003	M	9.72	4.47	2.79	1.0			7.00		0.08	11.40
Mean		13.71	2.95	3.38	2.33			5.26		0.09	16.38
(± SD)		(4.33)	(1.32)	(1.25)	(1.53)			(1.53)		(0.02)	(5.00)

* NA Not Available.

[2] Mean of two animals.

Urinary excretion of L-dT was rapid, with the majority of the recovered dose being excreted within 24 hours following intravenous administration. The mean fraction of L-dT excreted in urine within 24 h was 0.75 ± 0.13 and 0.37 ± 0.16 after intravenous and oral administration, respectively. L-dT was detected unchanged in the urine, and no metabolites were detected. Apparent renal CL (CL_R) averaged 0.57 ± 0.17 L/h/kg after intravenous administration. CL_R accounted for 77% of total CL of L-dT, suggesting that renal excretion is the major route of elimination for this L-nucleoside. Urinary excretion of L-dC was also rapid, with the majority of the recovered dose being excreted in urine within 24 hours following intravenous administration. Due to incomplete urine sampling, the fraction excreted unchanged in urine (f_e) and CL_R after intravenous administration for animal #2003 could not be determined. The mean fraction of L-dC excreted within 24 hours was 0.86 ± 0.04 (n = 2) and 0.09 ± 0.02 (n = 3) after intravenous and oral administration, respectively. Mean CL_R was 0.32 ± 0.01 L/h/kg following intravenous which accounts for 60% of total L-dC CL, suggesting that renal excretion is the major route of elimination.

Deamination to L-dU was detected in urine after both oral and intravenous administration of L-dC. However, over the entire two-week urine collection period, L-dU accounted for only 2.87 ± 0.56% of the total recovered dose after intravenous administration and 2.76 ± 0.64% of the total recovered dose after oral administration. These observations further suggest that L-dU is generated from the deamination of L-dCMP with subsequent breakdown to L-dU, accounting for such low levels of the latter in both plasma and urine.

Summary

Pharmacokinetic studies in woodchucks and monkeys indicated that the disposition of L-dT is comparable to the pharmacokinetic characteristics of other nucleoside analogs after administration to these animals. The compound has good oral bioavailability and is eliminated, unchanged, in urine. In contrast, L-dC exhibited lower oral bioavailability in both species. Several pro-drugs, which improve the oral bioavailability of L-dC, are currently under evaluation. It should be noted, however, that despite an oral bioavailability of approximately 10% in woodchucks, efficacy studies conducted in woodchucks chronically infected with WHV indicated that L-dC (10 mg/day/kg for four weeks) reduced viral load 4-6 logs and was considered a potent antiviral agent [9]. In this same study, L-dT reduced viral load up to 8 logs. In conclusion, potent *in vitro* and *in vivo* efficacy coupled with favorable pharmacokinetic disposition make both L-dT and L-dC promising antiviral candidates for the treatment of chronic HBV infection, warranting their further development.

References

1. Wong DK, Cheung AM, O'Rourke K, Naylor CD, Detsky AS and Heathcote J, Effect of alpha-interferon treatment in patients with hepatitis B e antigen-positive chronic hepatitis B. A meta-analysis. *Annals of Internal Medicine* 119(4): 312-23, 1993.
2. Hoofnagle JH and di Bisceglie AM, The treatment of chronic viral hepatitis. *New England Journal of Medicine* 336(5): 347-56, 1997.
3. Davis GL, Interferon treatment of viral hepatitis in immunocompromised patients. *Seminars in Liver Disease* 9(4): 267-72, 1989.
4. Lai CL, Chien RN, Leung NW, Chang TT, Guan R, Tai DI, Ng KY, Wu PC, Dent JC, Barber J, Stephenson SL and Gray DF, A one-year trial of lamivudine for chronic hepatitis B. Asia Hepatitis Lamivudine Study Group. *New England Journal of Medicine* 339(2): 61-8, 1998.
5. Liaw YF, Chien RN, Yeh CT, Tsai SL and Chu CM, Acute exacerbation and hepatitis B virus clearance after emergence of YMDD motif mutation during lamivudine therapy. *Hepatology* 30(2): 567-72, 1999.
6. Dienstag JL, Schiff ER, Wright TL, Perrillo RP, Hann HL, Goodman Z, Crowther L, Condreay LD, Woessner M, Rubin M, Brown NA and for the US Lamivudine Investigator Group, Lamivudine as initial treatment for chronic hepatitis B in the United States. *New England Journal of Medicine* 341(17): 1256-1263, 1999.
7. Cullen JM, Smith SL, Davis MG, Dunn SE, Botteron C, Cecchi A, Linsey D, Linzey D, Frick L, Paff MT, Goulding A and Biron K, *In vivo* antiviral activity and pharmacokinetics of (-)-*cis*-5-fluoro-1-[2-(hydroxymethyl)-1, 3-oxathiolan-5-yl]cytosine in woodchuck hepatitis virus infected woodchucks. *Antimicrobial Agents and Chemotherapy* 41(10): 2076-82, 1997.
8. Chu CK, Boudinot FD, Peek SF, Hong JH, Choi Y, Korba BE, Gerin JL, Cote PJ, Tennant BC and Cheng YC, Preclinical investigation of L-FMAU as an anti-hepatitis B virus agent. *Antiviral Therapy* 3: 113-21, 1998.
9. Bryant ML, Bridges EG, Placidi L, Faraj A, Loi AG, Pierra C, Dukhan D, Gosselin G, Imbach JL, Hernandez B, Juodawlkis A, Tennant B, Korba B, Cote P, Marion P, Cretton-Scott E, Schinazi RF, and

Sommadossi JP, Antiviral L-nucleosides specific for Hepatitis B virus infection. *Antimicrobial Agents and Chemotherapy* 45: 229-235, 2001.

10. Sommadossi JP, Bryant ML, Gosselin G, Schinazi RF and Imbach J-L, Anti-hepatitis B virus specific L-nucleosides. *Antiviral Therapy* 4: A19, 1999.
11. Fourel I, Hantz O, Watanabe KA, Jacquet C, Chomel B, Fox JJ and Trepo C, Inhibitory effects of 2'-fluorinated arabinosyl-pyrimidine nucleosides on woodchuck hepatitis virus replication in chronically infected woodchucks. *Antimicrobial Agents and Chemotherapy* 34(3): 473-5, 1990.
12. Korba BE, Cote P, Hornbuckle W, Tennant BC and Gerin JL, Treatment of chronic woodchuck hepatitis virus infection in the eastern woodchuck (Marmota monax) with nucleoside analogues is predictive of therapy for chronic hepatitis B virus infection in humans. *Hepatology* 31(5): 1165-75, 2000.
13. Boudinot FD, Schinazi RF, Gallo JM, McClure HM, Anderson DC, Doshi KJ, Kambhampathi PC and Chu CK, 3'-Azido-2', 3'-dideoxyuridine (AzddU): comparative pharmacokinetics with 3'-azido-3'-deoxythymidine (AZT) in monkeys. *AIDS Research and Human Retroviruses* 6(2): 219-28, 1990.
14. Schinazi RF, Boudinot FD, Doshi KJ and McClure HM, Pharmacokinetics of 3'-fluoro-3'-deoxythymidine and 3'-deoxy-2', 3'-didehydrothymidine in rhesus monkeys. *Antimicrobial Agents and Chemotherapy* 34(6): 1214-9, 1990.
15. Cretton EM, Zhou Z, Kidd LB, McClure HM, Kaul S, Hitchcock MJ and Sommadossi JP, *In vitro* and *in vivo* disposition and metabolism of 3'-deoxy-2',3'- didehydrothymidine. *Antimicrob Agents Chemother* 37(9): 1816-25, 1993.
16. Placidi L, Hernandez B, Cretton-Scott E, Faraj A, Bryant ML, Imbach J-L, Gosselin G, Pierra C, Dukhan D and Sommadossi JP, Cellular pharmacology of β-L-thymidine and β-L-2'-deoxycytidine in HepG2 cells and primary rat, monkey and human hepatocytes. *Antiviral Therapy* 4: A122, 1999.

Clevudine: A novel 1-β-L nucleoside analogue in clinical development for the treatment of HBV infection

GEORGE R. PAINTER, LAWRENCE C. TROST,
M. ROBERT BLUM, GEORGE M. SZCZECH and
PHILLIP A. FURMAN

Triangle Pharmaceuticals, 4611 University Dr.,
Durham, NC 27717, USA

Introduction

Dose-limiting toxicities and viral resistance have fueled the search for novel, structurally diverse nucleoside analogues for the treatment of HBV. Advances in synthetic methodology and the application of modern separation technologies have made it possible to study chirality and its influence on the pharmacology of antiviral drugs. As a result, a number of nucleosides possessing the unnatural 1-β-L stereochemistry have been synthesized and reported to have anti-HBV activity [1-10]. Some of these L nucleosides are more potent and less toxic than their enantiomers that possess the natural 1-β-D stereochemistry [1-3, 7, 8].

Ma et al. [11] reported the synthesis of a series of 2'-fluoro-substituted 1-β-L 2'-deoxyarabino pyrimidines including 1-(2-deoxy-2-fluoro-β L-arabinofuranosyl)-5-methyluracil (L-FMAU, clevudine, Figure 1). Clevudine possesses potent activity against HBV and EBV *in vitro* [8, 11-14] and against hepatitis virus *in vivo* [15-19].

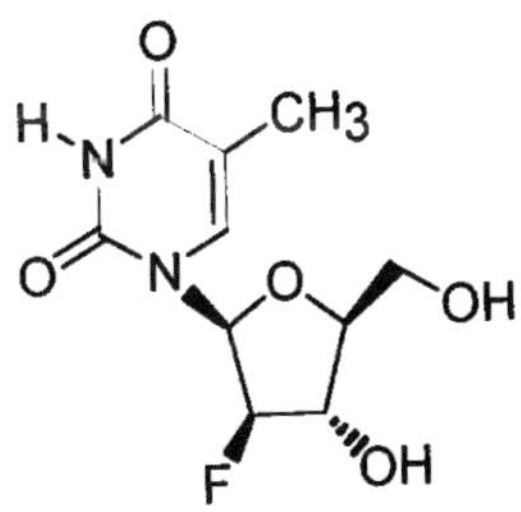

Figure 1. Clevudine, 1-(2-deoxy-2-fluoro-β-L-arabinofuranosyl)-5-methyluracil [7].

Prior to the synthesis of clevudine a series of 1-β-D-2'-deoxy-2'-fluro-arabino pyrimidines, including D-FMAU (1-(2-deoxy-2-fluoro-5-methyl-β-D-arabinofuranosyl)uracil, D-FEAU (1-(2-deoxy-2-fluoro-5-ethyl-β-D-arabinofuranosyl)uracil) and D-FIAU (1-(2-

Frontiers in Viral Hepatitis Ed. by RF Schinazi, J-P Sommadossi and CM Rice. 281 — 300

deoxy-2-fluoro-5-iodo-β-D-arabinofuranosyl)uracil), had been shown to possess potent activity against herpesvirus (D-FMAU) and HBV (D-FEAU and D-FIAU) [7, 8, 12]. D-FMAU and D-FIAU entered clinical trials, D-FMAU for the treatment of cancer [20] and FIAU for treatment of HBV infection [21]. Both caused significant morbidity and mortality. Because of this experience there has been concern regarding the safety of 2'-deoxy-2'-fluoro arabinofuranosyl nucleoside analogues in general. However, all of the available preclinical antiviral and toxicological data suggest that, because of the change in chirality, clevudine is readily distinguishable from its enantiomer D-FMAU. The profound impact absolute stereochemistry can have on biological activity and toxicology has been observed in other classes of drugs [22]. In this report we present an extensive review of the antiviral data that has motivated the further development of clevudine and the toxicological data that has supported the introduction of the compound into the clinic. Clevudine is in Phase I clinical trials and will soon enter a Phase I/II multiple dose trial.

In vitro anti-HBV activity

Clevudine produces a dose-dependent inhibition of HBV replication in the 2.2.15, subclone P5A cell line, a HepG2 derivative. Results of *in vitro* testing by several groups are compiled in Table 1.

Table 1. Comparison of the anti-HBV activity of clevudine with other nucleoside analogues.

Compound	*Anti-HBV Activity in 2.2.15 Cells* [a]	
	EC_{50}, μM	EC_{90}, μM
Clevudine	0.1, 0.49	1.55
D-FMAU	2.0	ND
(-)-FTC	0.05	0.15
DAPD	0.06	0.23
DXG	0.25	1.1
Penciclovir	1.04	3.5
3TC	0.08	0.19

[a] Data taken from reference 7, 8, 11, 12

The EC_{50} value of 0.1 μM determined for clevudine against HBV is 20-fold lower than the EC_{50} value determined for D-FMAU [7, 8, 11, 12]. Using the method of Korba and Gerin [23], the anti-HBV activity of clevudine was compared directly with that of 3TC, penciclovir, FTC, DAPD and DXG. A somewhat higher median EC_{50} of 0.49 μM was determined using this method, and the EC_{90} value was found to be 1.55 μM (Table 1). These values are approximately tenfold higher than the corresponding values obtained for 3TC, FTC, and DAPD, and three- to fourfold lower than the EC_{50} and EC_{90} values obtained for penciclovir. The EC_{50} and EC_{90} values of clevudine are comparable to those obtained for DXG.

The effects of clevudine in combination with other anti-HBV compounds were investigated in the 2.2.15 assay. Analysis of synergism, additivity, or antagonism was performed using the CalcuSyn™ program (Biosoft, Inc.) and isobologram analysis. Results showed clevudine to be synergistic with FTC, DAPD, penciclovir, adefovir and lamivudine [24].

The inhibitory effect of clevudine on viral replication has also been investigated using cultures of primary hepatocytes from chronically DHBV-infected ducklings [15]. Quantitation of virion DNA released into the culture supernatant by dot blot hybridization showed a concentration dependent inhibitory effect of clevudine with an EC_{50} of 0.1 μM. At concentrations above 1 μM, the effect reached a plateau of 80-90% inhibition. Southern blot analysis of intracellular duck hepatitis B virus DNA using a ^{32}P-labeled DNA probe for the complete viral genome showed a dramatic decrease in the amount of replicative intermediates at the end of treatment. However, DHBV cccDNA was still detectable, which suggests that clevudine did not directly affect cccDNA in the primary culture. Removal of clevudine from the medium resulted in a rebound in the level of replicative intermediates; however, the level did not return to that seen in the control cultures. This pattern was most apparent in cells treated with the highest dose used in the study, 10 μM.

Inhibition of HBV resistant to lamivudine

Treatment of HBV-infected patients with lamivudine for greater than 12 months has been associated with the development of resistance [25]. In a recent study, Chin et al. [26] compared the activity of clevudine against wild-type HBV and the lamivudine-resistant mutants, L526M, M550I and L526M/M550V. The EC_{50} value for both clevudine and lamivudine against wild-type HBV, determined by measuring the dose-response of drugs on viral replicative intermediates and extracellular virus, was calculated to be 0.1 μM. Against the L526M variant the EC_{50} for clevudine, determined by the reduction in extracellular virus, was similar to that of wild-type virus (0.5 μM). However, the EC_{50} value for the same mutant, based on quantification of replicative intermediates, increased to greater than 100 μM, indicating strong resistance. EC_{50} values for the M550I mutant, determined using extracellular virus and replicative intermediates increased to 57 μM and greater than 100 μM, respectively. In the stably transformed AD79 cells, which express HBV containing only the M550V mutation, no resistance was seen to clevudine compared to wild type. Fu et al. [27] found in a transient transfection assay that HBV containing lamivudine-resistant mutations in the polymerase gene (L526M, V553I, and A546V alone or in combination with M550V/I) was also resistant to clevudine. These results, based on quantification of replicative intermediates, are in agreement with the results of Chin et al. [26]. Thus, there is the possibility of partial cross-resistance of clevudine to certain lamivudine-resistant viruses. Additional studies need to be done to clarify this issue.

In vivo activity

The anti-hepatitis virus activity of clevudine *in vivo* has been extensively examined in the woodchuck [7, 8, 16, 17]. In a dose-escalation study [7, 8, 16, 17], 28 adult woodchucks chronically infected with WHV were randomly assigned to groups of four animals. Six of the seven groups were treated orally with clevudine at doses ranging from 0.03 to 10.0 mg/kg/day for four weeks. The seventh group received sterile water as placebo. Serum WHV DNA was quantitated by slot blot hybridization and PCR analysis on samples taken on days 0, 1, 2, 3, 5, 7; weekly for the remainder of the treatment periods and at 1, 2, 4, 6, 8, 10, and 12 weeks posttreatment. During treatment, there was a marked, prompt and dose-dependent reduction in serum WHV DNA. At the 10 mg/kg dose, viremia was depressed 10- to 200-fold from baseline levels in 24 hours, and 5 x 10^6 to 10^9-fold by the end of treatment. At low doses, following drug withdrawal, a dose-dependent return in viremia was observed. However, at the two highest doses, WHV DNA in some animals remained significantly below pretreatment levels for the duration of the post-dose follow up period. Viremia in two of the four animals receiving 10 mg/kg remained 1000- to one millionfold below pretreatment levels for as long as 25 weeks posttreatment. This observation, along with the rapid rate of decline in viremia, is one of the most compelling virologic reasons for the clinical development of clevudine.

In a subsequent study [7, 8, 16, 17], four chronic WHV carrier adult woodchucks were dosed orally for 12 weeks with clevudine at 10 mg/kg/day. Serum WHV DNA was measured by slot blot hybridization weekly for the first month of therapy and biweekly thereafter until the end of treatment. Biweekly WHV DNA quantification was continued for a total of 56 weeks following drug withdrawal, after which the animals died due to hepatocellular carcinoma. Within seven days of initiating treatment, a greater than 1000-fold reduction in serum WHV DNA was observed. Viremia in three of the four animals remained at levels that were greater than 100,000-fold below pretreatment levels throughout the post-dose period. Viremia in the fourth animal remained suppressed for approximately 20 weeks posttreatment. By the end of treatment, WHV replicative intermediates were reduced more than 10,000-fold and WHV RNA was reduced more than 100-fold. Serum WhsAg began to decline after four to six weeks of treatment in all four animals and remained suppressed during the posttreatment period at levels that were 100- to 1000-fold below pretreatment values. Whc and Whs antigens in liver biopsy specimens also declined to levels that were essentially undetectable by immunohistochemical staining by 12 weeks posttreatment. By the end of the 12-week treatment period, serum ALT and GGT had dropped to normal levels in all four animals, and marked histologic improvement in the degree of hepatitis was observed. An analysis of WHV cccDNA in the terminal liver samples showed a marked reduction when compared to pretreatment levels in the three animals with sustained low levels of viral replication.

Zhu et al. [18] also examined the impact of clevudine on cccDNA *in vivo*. In their study, chronically infected woodchucks were dosed orally with 10 mg/kg/day of clevudine for 12 weeks. The effect on replicative DNA levels, cccDNA, and the percent of infected hepatocytes were evaluated. DNA replication intermediates were virtually undetectable after the first six weeks of therapy. In contrast, cccDNA levels declined more slowly with a half-life of approximately 33 to 50 days. PCNA staining indicated a correlation between the decline in cccDNA levels and hepatocyte turnover. The loss of cccDNA occurred at a rate comparable to that expected from the estimated half-life of hepatocytes in woodchucks, suggesting that death of infected hepatocytes was one of the major routes for clearance of cccDNA.

Jacob et al. [19] showed in a similar study that clevudine (10 mg/kg/day) caused a rapid decrease in WHV replicative intermediates, from an average of 2800 copies/cell to essentially undetectable after 12 weeks of treatment. However, compared to the results of Zhu et al. [18], the impact of drug treatment on cccDNA levels appears somewhat more rapid. The hepatic WHV cccDNA in the clevudine-treated animals decreased from an average of 30 copies/cell to 4 copies/cell after 4 weeks of treatment and to approximately one copy/cell after eight weeks of treatment. The $t_{1/2}$ for hepatic cccDNA was about 11 days during the 12 weeks of treatment. In the absence of hepatic cccDNA, WHV RNA was not detected. It was concluded that the sustained antiviral effect of clevudine after drug withdrawal in chronic WHV carriers was the result of the significant reduction in cccDNA.

The *in vivo* efficacy of orally administered clevudine has also been studied in experimentally DHBV-infected ducklings [15]. Five-day old Pekin ducklings were inoculated intravenously with infectious DHBV-containing serum. Each duckling received 1.5 x 10^7 viral genome equivalents. Clevudine was administered starting at three days post-infection. Animal weight and lactic acid levels were monitored daily during the study period. In an experiment designed to determine the appropriate dosing frequency, clevudine was administered orally for four days at 20 mg/kg b.i.d. and 40 mg/kg-qd [15]. Both doses gave a similar antiviral effect, as evidenced by decreases in extracellular DHBV DNA. A rebound of viremia after cessation of treatment occurred in both treatment groups. Whether the rate and extent of rebound was dependent on dosing regimen was not discussed.

In the second phase of the study, antiviral efficacy of a more prolonged administration of clevudine was examined [15]. Four ducklings received a 40 mg/kg qd oral dose for five days; four received the same dose for eight days, and four served as untreated controls. Administration of clevudine for five days resulted in a 55% inhibition of DHBV viremia, followed by a weak, transient rebound of viremia five days after cessation of treatment. Eight days of treatment resulted in a 72% inhibition of DHBV viremia, with no rebound of viremia during the two-week posttreatment follow-up. The mean area under the curve for viremia in the eight-day treatment group was significantly reduced for the clevudine treated animals compared to the control animals ($P = 0.0482$; Wilcox-Mann Whitney test, Monte Carlo modification for small numbers). DNA sequence analysis of the DHBV polymerase gene showed no amino acid sequence variation in the viral polymerase isolated by PCR from virus at the end of the eight days of clevudine treatment. Analysis for viral replicative intermediates 16 days after cessation of treatment showed the persistence of DHBV single-stranded and relaxed circular DNAs, as well as viral cccDNA. These results indicate that short-term treatment with clevudine does not clear DHBV infection from the liver of ducklings, but does produce a substantial drop in the level of viremia. Western blot analysis performed on liver samples showed a similar reduction in the expression of DHBV core proteins in clevudine-treated and control ducklings. An ELISA assay for anti-pre-S antibody did not show the appearance of antibody, indicating that an immune response was not responsible for clearance of circulating virus. Determination of lactic acid levels in the plasma of animals clevudine for eight days showed no significant increase compared with the levels in the control animals, indicating a lack of effect on mitochondria.

Mechanism of action

Using HBV particles isolated from the medium of 2.2.15 cell cultures, Pai et al. [14] demonstrated that the 5'-triphosphate of clevudine inhibits the activity of the endogenous HBV polymerase in a concentration-dependent manner. Liu et al. [28] reported that clevudine 5'-triphosphate acts as a potent inhibitor of HBV DNA polymerase with a K_i of 0.12 μM.

Taken as a whole, the available data indicate that clevudine is a specific inhibitor of viral DNA synthesis. Studies with DHBV polymerase expressed in a reticulocyte lysate system showed an inhibitory effect of clevudine 5'-triphosphate on the incorporation of radiolabeled thymidine 5'-monophosphate during viral minus-strand DNA synthesis [15]. Inhibition of thymidine 5'-monophosphate incorporation suggests that clevudine 5'-triphosphate is an inhibitor of reverse transcription [15]. Clevudine 5'-triphosphate was also shown to cause a time-dependent inhibition of the synthesis of the short DNA primer required for DHBV replication. In a transient transfection assay in which DNA replicative intermediates were isolated from HBV-infected HuH7 cells and separated using gel electrophoresis, clevudine proved to be a weak inhibitor of single-strand DNA synthesis, and a strong inhibitor of double-strand DNA synthesis [29]. Thus the 5'-triphosphate of clevudine may act as an inhibitor of viral replication by specifically inhibiting the DNA-dependent DNA polymerase activity of HBV polymerase.

Although clevudine is a potent inhibitor of HBV DNA replication, it does not inhibit the generation of the various species of HBV RNA [14]. A six-day treatment of 2.2.15 cells with either 0.5 or 1.0 μM clevudine had no significant effect on the transcription of HBV or host cell genetic information, as judged by comparison with the level of transcription of a cellular housekeeping enzyme, glyceraldehyde-3-phosphate dehydrogenase [14]. Measurement of HBV surface antigen in the medium of treated cells showed that clevudine had no significant dose-dependent inhibitory effect on HBsAg or HBcAg in the treated cultures, as determined by Western blot analysis [14]. These results support the conclusion that the effect of clevudine is specific for the DNA synthetic component of HBV replication.

In vitro metabolism

Clevudine, which is phosphorylated to its 5'-triphosphate by host cell kinases [14, 28], acts (*vide supra*) as a competitive inhibitor of HBV polymerase. The enzymes responsible for the first step in the phosphorylation of clevudine have been identified [28]. Unlike other thymidine or deoxycytidine analogues, clevudine is phosphorylated by cytosolic thymidine kinase, cytosolic deoxycytidine kinase, and mitochondrial deoxypyrimidine kinase. When the efficiency (V_{max}/K_m) of clevudine as a substrate for all three enzymes was examined, it was found to be within the same order of magnitude as those of natural substrates.

Pai et al. [14] examined the metabolism of clevudine in hepatoma cells. HepG2 2.2.15 cells were treated with tritium-labeled clevudine, lysed with perchloric acid and the acid soluble sample fractionated by high performance liquid chromatography for identification of metabolites. Treating the cells for 24 hours with 5 μM [^{3}H]-clevudine resulted in the rapid intracellular formation of the 5'-mono-, 5'-di-, and 5'-triphosphates. Formation of phosphorylated clevudine species occurred as early as two hours after treatment, with maximal metabolite levels being reached at eight hours after treatment. The major metabolite was the 5'-triphosphate. In washout experiments to determine the half-life of the 5'-triphosphate, cells were treated with clevudine for 24 hours. Following removal of compound, the decline in the levels of 5'-mono-, 5'-di-, and 5'-triphosphate did not appear to follow first-order kinetics. In the initial phase, the levels of the metabolites dropped rapidly, with about 50% of the 5'-triphosphate disappearing in four to five hours, and 90% of the 5'-triphosphate disappearing in the first eight hours. In the subsequent 16 hours, the 5'-triphosphate levels declined at a slower rate, with a small amount still present at 24 hours.

Cytotoxicity

The cytotoxicity of clevudine has been evaluated in several *in vitro* growth inhibition assays [7, 8, 11-14]. In each of the cell lines tested, clevudine has shown no cytoxicity (Table 2). However, the 1-β-D enantiomer D-FMAU is cytotoxic as indicated by the substantially lower CC_{50} values. The CC_{50} values of FTC and 3TC are included in Table 2 for comparison.

Table 2. Comparison of the cytotoxicity of clevudine with other nucleoside analogues.

Compound	*Cell Line (CC_{50}, μM)*[a]			
	2.2.15	*MT2*	*CEM*	*Hl*
Clevudine	>200, 984	100	>100, >200	913 ± 70, 1000 ± 80
D-FMAU	50	8-9	–	<10
3TC	2007	ND	>100	ND
FTC	2137	>100	>1000	ND

a. Data taken from references 7, 8, 11, 12

Because of the apparent correlation between toxicity to bone marrow progenitor cells *in vitro* and bone marrow suppression *in vivo* seen for other nucleosidde analogues clevudine was assayed for bone marrow toxicity using a colony formation assay. Cells were exposed to compound (0.1-100 μM) for 14 to 18 days. The CC_{50} values for clevudine were greater than the highest concentration tested for both progenitor cell types (Table 3), indicating clevudine was not toxic to bone marrow progenitor cells. CC_{50} values for AZT, 2'-CDG, FTC and 3TC are included in Table 3 for comparison.

Table 3. Effect of clevudine on human bone marrow progenitor cells.

Compound	BFU-ECC_{50}(μM)	CFU-GMCC_{50}(μM)
Clevudine	>100	>100
AZT[a]	0.3 ± 0.06	10 ± 0.3
2'-CDG[a]	4 ± 2	0.4 ± 0.3
FTC	220 ± 8	300 ± 40
3TC[a]	180 ± 2	250 ± 8

a. Data taken from reference 4

Several of the toxicities associated with nucleoside analogs can be attributed to their incorporation into nuclear DNA [30, 31, 32]. In addition, long-term treatment with these drugs can interfere with mitochondrial DNA synthesis, resulting in delayed toxicity [32, 33]. The liver toxicity of D-FIAU, for example, has been attributed to mitochondrial toxicity [32, 33]. The incorporation of clevudine and D-FMAU into cellular DNA was studied by Yao et al. [13]. H1 cells were exposed to [^{3}H]-clevudine (10 μM) or [^{14}C]-D-FMAU (0.2 μM), and the nucleic acid was isolated and analyzed for incorporation of either compound using cesium sulfate isopycnic ultracentrifugation. A substantial amount of D-FMAU (greater than 10 pmol/10^6 cells) was incorporated into DNA, while little or no clevudine (less than 0.1 pmol/10^6 cells) was incorporated into DNA. In addition, treating H1 cells with 1 mM clevudine for six days resulted in no decrease in mitochondrial DNA content.

In a study performed by Pai et al. [14], 2.2.15 cells were treated with 1 μM clevudine or with 1 μM 2', 3'-dideoxycytidine (ddC) as a positive control for mitochondrial DNA damage. Clevudine had no effect on the mitochondrial DNA content. In a separate study, the effect of clevudine on mitochondrial function in 2.2.15 cells was examined by measuring the concentrations of lactic acid in extracellular medium, measuring mitochondrial DNA content, and by examining the cells using electron microscopy to detect structural abnormalities. The results of this study showed that clevudine had no effect on cell growth or lactic acid production up to the highest concentration tested, 10 μM (Table 4). Mitochondrial DNA content was not affected by clevudine at concentrations up to and including 10 μM (Table 4). Finally, electron microscopic evaluation indicated that no morphological changes in mitochondria occurred following exposure of cells to clevudine.

Table 4. Effect of clevudine on cell proliferation, and mitochondrial function and morphology in HepG2 cells.

Clevudine (μM)	Cell Density ($\times 10^4$/ml)	L-Lactate (mg/10^6 Cells)	% of mtDNA Content to Control	Lipid Droplet Formation	Mitochondrial Morphology
0	17.9 ± 0.6	2.47 ± 0.11	100	æ	normal
0.1	18.3 ± 1.2	2.39 ± 0.14	106 ± 11	ND	ND
1	17.7 ± 0.6	2.46 ± 0.04	96 ± 10	ND	ND
10	17.8 ± 0.5	2.45 ± 0.05	101 ± 14	æ	normal

One of the principal mechanisms by which nucleoside analogues interfere with cellular and/or mitochondrial DNA synthesis is their 5'-triphosphate acting as an alternative substrate inhibitor for endogenous polymerases. Yao et al. [13] and Kukhanova et al. [34] examined the ability of human DNA polymerase α, β, γ and δ to utilize the 5'-triphosphates of clevudine and D-FMAU as substrates for DNA replication. Both clevudine 5'-triphosphate (1-100 μM) and D-FMAU 5'-triphosphate (0.5-10 μM) were analyzed for their incorporation into the 3'-terminus of a phage DNA primer-template complex. The 5'-triphosphate of clevudine was not incorporated into the template primer by any of the four human DNA polymerases. In contrast, D-FMAU 5'-triphosphate was utilized efficiently as a substrate by the four human DNA polymerases. The results are consistent with the lack of impact on cellular and mitochondrial DNA levels, and the lack of cellular and mitochondrial toxicity for clevudine as shown by the data in Tables 2, 3 and 4.

Toxicology

Severe preclinical [21, 35, 37, 40] and fatal clinical toxicities [36] were encountered in the development of the nucleoside analogue D-FIAU for the treatment of HBV infection. Multiorgan toxicity was observed in subchronic toxicology studies in woodchucks [37], dogs and rodents [21]. The toxicity, manifested as microvesicular hepatic steatosis, was attributed to apparently irreversible effects on mitochondria [33, 38, 39]. Two comprehensive reports produced by an FDA-appointed panel [40] and the Institute of Medicine [21] provide a thorough review of D-FIAU development.

Because of this experience, clevudine was tested extensively in preclinical safety studies prior to the first clinical trial. Numerous additions to standard toxicology protocols were made to detect potential adverse effects on mitochondria. Results of chronic treatment with clevudine, six months in both rats and monkeys, supported the administration of single escalating doses in the first Phase I trial [43]. Nevertheless, the chronic toxicology studies were continued, so that dosing of rats for nine months and of monkeys for 12 months was completed before the trial was initiated. Finally, the results of pharmacokinetic, safety pharmacology, mutagenicity, and single-dose toxicology studies were also available in advance of the first human exposure and were uniformly negative.

Pharmacokinetic studies

Pharmacokinetic parameters were carefully examined in the rodent and non-rodent species employed in the toxicology studies to insure that exposure levels would be adequate to achieve appropriate multiples of the proposed human dose. Extensive pharmacokinetic work had previously been reported [43, 44, 45].

Two groups of male CD rats (24 per group) were given an oral or intravenous dose of 50 mg/kg clevudine. Cynomolgus monkeys (four males) also received 50 mg/kg clevudine by the oral route and by the intravenous route after a two-week washout. Timed blood samples were collected for determination of plasma clevudine levels. Calculated pharmacokinetic parameters are presented in Table 5.

Table 5. Summary of pharmacokinetic parameters in rats and cynomolgus monkeys after administration of 50 mg/kg clevudine.

Route	C_{max} (µg/mL)	T_{max} (h)	$AUC_{0-\infty}$ (h•µg/mL)	$t_{1/2}$ (h)	Cl (L/h/kg)	F (%)
Rats						
i.v.	76.4	0.08	64.7	6.8	0.77	-
p.o.	11.8	2.0	43.8	5.9	-	67.7
Cynomolgus Monkeys						
i.v.	58.4	0.08	60.1	4.1	0.85	-
p.o.	6.8	1.6	26.5	9.7	-	43.7

Abbreviations: $AUC_{0-\infty}$, area under the concentration vs time curve; Cl, clearance; C_{max}, maximum plasma concentration; F, bioavailability; i.v., intravenous; p.o., oral; $t_{1/2}$, half-life of elimination; T_{max}, time of maximum plasma concentration

The results show that adequate plasma levels of clevudine can be achieved in rats and monkeys by the oral route.

Safety pharmacology and receptor binding studies

In vivo (single dose administration) and *in vitro* studies were performed with clevudine to test for undesirable pharmacological effects on general behavior, and on neurologic, autonomic, central nervous system, pulmonary, cardiovascular, renal, gastrointestinal, and smooth muscle function. Clevudine caused no significant secondary pharmacologic effects. Clevudine was also tested in a panel of *in vitro* receptor binding assays, the Spectrum Screen from PanLabs, and found to have no affinity for any of the receptors tested.

Genetic toxicology studies

Clevudine was tested in three standard assays for mutagenicity: the bacterial reverse mutation (Ames) assay, the chromosomal aberrations assay in Chinese hamster ovary cells, and the micronucleus assay in rats. Clevudine was not mutagenic in these experiments.

Acute toxicity

The approximate oral LD_{50} was greater than 5000 mg/kg in mice and greater than 3000 mg/kg in rats. These were the highest doses tested.

Dose-range-finding toxicology studies

Four groups of five male and five female CD-1 rats were given oral doses of clevudine of 0, 100, 300 and 900 mg/kg/day for nine days. Due to lack of toxicity, the rats dosed at 300 mg/kg/day were necropsied on day 10, and the 100 and 900 mg/kg/day doses were increased to 1500 and 3000 mg/kg/day, respectively, from day 10 to study completion on day 21. Clinical chemistry and hematology were evaluated on day 10 and prior to necropsy on day 21. Histopathology was performed on all rats. Toxicokinetics sampling demonstrated linear and dose-proportional increases in exposure to clevudine, with no significant differences between female and male rats, or between the first and last dose day at a given dose. The $AUC_{0\text{-}24}$ at the 3000 mg/kg/day dose averaged 1344 μg•hr/mL, and the C_{max} averaged 104.3 μg/mL. No toxicity was observed.

In the non-rodent species, four groups of two cynomolgus monkeys, each group consisting of one female and one male, were given oral doses of clevudine of 0, 100, 300 or 900 mg/kg/day for 14 days. Again, due to lack of toxicity, monkeys given 300 mg/kg/day were necropsied on day 14, and the 100 and 900 mg/kg/day doses were increased to 1500 and 3000 mg/kg/day, respectively. This dosing regimen was continued from day 14 to completion of the study on day 25. Serum biochemical and hematological tests were performed on day 14 and prior to necropsy on day 25. Timed plasma samples for toxicokinetics were collected on days 1, 14, and 24. Systemic exposure was dose-dependent, with no significant differences between sexes, or between the first and last dose day at a given dose. At 3000 mg/kg/day the $AUC_{0\text{-}24}$ averaged 505 μg•hr/mL and the C_{max} averaged 57.5 μg/mL. Signs of toxicity were limited to the two monkeys given 3000 mg/kg/day from day 14 to day 25 and included loose white stools (presumed to contain unabsorbed clevudine), anemia, increased values for serum enzymes (male only), and extramedullary hematopoiesis in liver. The male monkey also had an enlarged spleen and splenic extramedullary hematopoiesis.

Chronic toxicology studies

Chronic toxicology studies conducted for 39 weeks in rats and 52 weeks in monkeys were designed to detect effects of clevudine on mitochondria in addition to monitoring conventional endpoints for toxicity. Determination of lactic acid was included in the biochemistry screens. Electron microscopy was performed on sections of heart, skeletal muscle, liver and kidney to look for changes in mitochondrial morphology. Electrophysiology assessments were conducted to detect peripheral nervous system toxicity. There was no toxicity seen in rats given clevudine at daily oral doses of 0, 25, 100 and 400 mg/kg for nine months. Toxicokinetics sampling at regular intervals indicated systemic exposures that were dose-dependent and similar between male and females.

Clevudine was well tolerated when given for six months to cynomolgus monkeys at daily oral doses of 0, 25, 100 and 400 mg/kg. However, one high-dose (400 mg/kg/day) female exhibited persistent anorexia and related body weight loss that was first noted at dose week 17. This monkey was sacrificed in poor physical condition during week 26; histopathology revealed moderate bilateral nephrosis of uncertain relationship to treatment with clevudine. In the remaining high-dose monkeys, there was no evidence of treatment-related effects on physical condition, electrocardiograms, ophthalmologic examinations, clinical pathology values, organ weights, the incidence of gross or histopathologic lesions, or the morphology of mitochondria in heart, liver and skeletal muscle. Although the difference, as compared to control values, was not significant, body weight gains were slightly retarded in high dose males after 26 weeks of dosing. The only other observation after six months of dosing was a slight decrease in the amplitude of the peroneal nerve response in high-dose monkeys. Amplitudes were normal in the median motor and sural nerves, and nerve conduction velocities were normal.

Electrophysiology measurements were repeated during week 39 and revealed decreased amplitude for the peroneal nerve response in monkeys at the mid-dose (100 mg/kg/day), and a further decrease from week-26 values for the high-dose group (400 mg/kg/day). Nerve conduction velocities remained normal. The continued decrease in peroneal amplitude prompted a neuropathology study in one high-dose male. Due to signs of overt toxicity, this particular monkey was selected for perfusion fixation and subsequent neuropathological evaluation. Representative histologic sections of 44 sites in the peripheral and central nervous systems were examined by light microscopy. No treatment-related neuropathologic lesions were observed.

Anorexia, lethargy, a decline in body weight, altered clinical pathology values and poor physical condition necessitated a dose reduction in the high-dose (400 mg/kg/day) monkeys during week 39. In four monkeys (two male, two female) dosing was suspended, and in the remaining four monkeys (two male and two female) the dose was reduced to 200 mg/kg/day for the remainder of the 52-week study. The 25 and 100 mg/kg/day doses were not changed. The four monkeys judged to be in the poorest physical condition at week 39 were the ones for which dosing was suspended. These monkeys were selected to study the reversibility of the toxicity and were subsequently re-dosed. The re-dose phase was essentially a second chronic toxicology study at 200 mg/kg/day clevudine as described below. A third high dose monkey (female) was sacrificed because of deteriorating physical condition during week 39.

This monkey had multiple internal abscesses in liver, spleen and other sites. The poor physical condition was attributed to septicemia, confirmed by light microscopy, and was considered unrelated to treatment with clevudine.

After the change in the dosing regimen at week 39 in the high-dose group, feed consumption resumed within days, both in the monkeys being administered the reduced dose of 200 mg/kg/day and in those for which dosing was suspended. Body weight gains and a prompt return to normal physical activity were observed in both groups. Clinical pathology values also returned to normal by 7 weeks after the dose modification.

All monkeys were sacrificed during week 52, with the exception of the control animals and the high-dose monkeys for which dosing was suspended at week 39. There were no consistent treatment-related findings in laboratory values, electrocardiograms, organ weights, or morphology of mitochondria in heart, liver, kidney, and skeletal muscle examined by electron microscopy. Concentrations of myelin basic protein in cerebrospinal fluid collected from control and high-dose (400/200 mg/kg/day) monkeys were comparable. The only treatment-related histopathologic alteration in tissues was minimal skeletal muscle myopathy. The incidence appeared to be dose-related and was observed in skeletal muscle from three of six low-dose monkeys, and in six of six monkeys in the mid- and high-dose groups. A small increase in AST was observed in high-dose monkeys. Widely scattered necrosis of individual myofibers, lack of inflammatory response and the presence of occasional myocytes with multiple nuclei clustered at the sarcolemma characterized this subtle myopathy. The latter were interpreted as regenerating myocytes.

To investigate the potential mechanism for the skeletal muscle myopathy observed at one year in the chronic monkey study, *in vitro* experiments were performed in rat smooth and skeletal muscle cell cultures to study the potential for direct effects of clevudine on muscle. Rat cardiac and striated muscle cells were incubated in the presence of 100 μM clevudine for four weeks (seven passages), followed by 200 μM for one week (one passage). Clevudine had no effect on cell growth or viability, mitochondrial DNA synthesis, or total nucleic acid content.

The control and high-dose monkeys not sacrificed at week 52 are being treated as follows. After a 30 week post-dose observation period, dosing was reinitiated at 200 mg/kg/day. Laboratory values were normal and comparable to control values at weeks four and 26 and 32 of the new dosing period. In addition, the activity, body weights and physical condition of the re-dose monkeys has been normal for 34 weeks. This re-dosing phase will be extended to nine months of dosing at 200 mg/kg/day.

Importantly, as was true for woodchucks dosed with clevudine for 12 weeks [16], there was no sign of microvesicular hepatic steatosis in any monkeys at any observation period in the chronic toxicology study. Values for ALT and serum lactate were marginally increased for high-dose monkeys, but only associated with inappetence and overt toxicity observed during week 39. Values for bilirubin, lipase and amylase were normal at all sampling intervals, regardless of the dose of clevudine administered or the duration for which it was given. There were no treatment-related liver lesions (histopathology and electron microscopy) at either six months or one year.

To conclude, doses of 25 and 100 mg/kg/day were essentially no-effect doses when given to monkeys for 12 months. The 400 mg/kg/day dose produced overt toxicity at week 39, but there was prompt recovery on dose reduction to 200 mg/kg/day for the balance of a one year exposure. The exposures produced by these doses of clevudine were dose-proportional in female and male monkeys and comparable at weeks 13, 26, 39 and 52. At week 26 the average AUC_{0-24} at the 400 mg/kg/day dose was 176.9 μg•hr/mL, and the average C_{max} was 24.3 μg/mL.

Phase I clinical trial

The objectives of the phase I trial were to establish the safety and tolerability of a single escalating dose of clevudine, and to determine the single-dose pharmacokinetics [46]. In addition, a preliminary evaluation of the effect of food on the bioavailability of clevudine was made.

Twelve healthy male subjects received single, escalating oral doses of 10, 300, 600, 900 and 1200 mg of clevudine, with a minimum one-week washout interval between doses. At all dosing levels except 600 mg, nine subjects were randomized to receive active drug and three subjects to receive placebo in a double-blind fashion under fasting conditions. At the 600 mg dose, subjects were randomized to take the 600 mg dose following an overnight fast or a high-fat breakfast. For each dose, clevudine pharmacokinetics were evaluated for 24 hours post-dose, with collections of blood samples pre-dose and 0.25, 0.50, 0.75, 1, 1.5, 2, 3, 4, 6, 8, 12, 16 and 24 hours post-dose. Urine was collected over the intervals of 0-6, 6-12 hours and 12-24 hours post-dose. Standard clinical assessments, including vital signs and ECG, were made pre-dose and at approximately 1, 2, 4, 8, 12 and 24 hours post-dose. Standard laboratory assessments (hematology, clinical chemistry and urinalysis) were made pre-dose and 24-hours post-dose.

The pharmacokinetic parameters from the study are shown in Table 6.

Table 6. Clevudine pharmacokinetic parameters by dose[a].

Dose (mg)	Subjects	C_{max} (μg/mL)	t_{max} (hr)	$AUC_{0\text{-}inf}$ (hr*μg/mL)	$t_{1/2}$ (hr)	CL/F (mL/min)	Urinary Recovery[b]
150	9	0.62 (34)	1.4 (53)	2.3 (21)	12.4 (43)	1137 (23)	20.8 (33)
300	9	1.11 (47)	1.9 (56)	5.3 (35)	10.3 (26)	1052 (34)	21.7 (32)
600	12	2.60 (32)	2.1 (37)	17.4 (30)	8.4 (14)	636 (38)	29.9 (24)
600 fed	12	1.93 (16)	2.9 (36)	16.8 (18)	8.1 (24)	614 (17)	29.0 (17)
900	9	3.10 (36)	1.6 (57)	23.6 (30)	10.6 (19)	688 (30)	31.1 (28)
1200	9	4.66 (18)	1.9 (55)	34.3 (14)	9.9 (14)	594 (15)	31.0 (7)

[a] mean (%CV)

[b] % dose excreted as unchanged clevudine

Strict dose proportionality is observed between 600 and 1200 mg. Reasonable linearity in $AUC_{o\text{-}inf}$ and C_{max} is observed over the entire dose range. As demonstrated by the 600 mg dose, a high-fat meal did not affect the extent of absorption. Even though $t_{1/2}$ may be underestimated due to the short evaluation period (24 hours), the reported values are sufficiently long to support a once-daily dosing schedule.

Clinical and laboratory evaluation indicated that clevudine was well tolerated. Adverse events and laboratory toxicities (grade 2 and above) are shown in Table 7. Four subjects reported a total of five adverse events. All were mild and resolved spontaneously. Four grade 2 laboratory toxicities were reported. A grade 3-lipase elevation was reported in one subject following the 150 mg dose. No other abnormalities were observed for this patient at the higher doses.

Table 7. Safety results.

Adverse Events

Subject	Adverse Event	Onset Day Relative to Dose
1	Blood spot in stool	5 days after 150 mg
1	Swollen lymph node	3 days after 1250 mg
7	Headache	On day of placebo dose
9	Run of 3 ventricular beats	On day of placebo dose
10	Loose stool	On day of placebo dose

Laboratory Toxicities.

Laboratory Test	Grade 2	Grade 3	Grade 4
Creatine Kinase[a]	3	0	0
Triglycerides	1	0	0
Lipase	0	1[b]	0

[a] Elevated in 1 subject after the 150-mg dose, and in 2 subjects after the 300 mg dose.

[b] Grade 3-lipase elevation following 150 mg dose; normal values after all other doses.

In summary, clinical and laboratory evaluations indicate that clevudine was well tolerated following single-dose administration at doses up to and including 1200 mg.

Discussion

The overall activity and chronic toxicological profile of clevudine supports the rapid development of this compound. The ability of the drug to arrest HBV replication, most probably by inhibition of the DNA-dependent DNA polymerase activity, and produce a significant drop in viral load has been clearly demonstrated [15, 16, 17, 29]. Two of the most intriguing properties of clevudine are the rate at which viral load is reduced and the low level at which circulating WHV DNA can be maintained over extended dosing periods in the woodchuck model. It has become very clear from the clinical experience with HIV that to control disease progression and the emergence of resistant virus, viral replication must be held in check at extremely low levels. The ability to maintain suppression results is related to the durability of response. Clearly clevudine holds the promise of fitting this criterion.

Another significant result of treatment with clevudine in animal-model studies has been the lack of recrudescence [16, 17]. In some woodchuck studies, serum WHV DNA levels have been observed to remain as much as 1000- to one millionfold below pretreatment levels for as long as 25 weeks after drug treatment was stopped. This effect may be another manifestation of the powerful antiviral activity of clevudine. The work of Zhu et al. [18] and Jacobs et al. [19] suggests that when the rate of viral replication is lower than the rate of hepatocyte turnover, then there is an apparent reduction in cccDNA due to dilution. This loss of cccDNA could account for the sustained antiviral effect. The hope is that this type and level of activity will also be observed in humans, and will translate into a longer interval of suppression before the emergence of resistant virus.

Before introducing clevudine into clinical trials it was imperative to clearly and definitively differentiate the toxicological profile from that of D-FMAU and D-FIAU. The results of comprehensive preclinical *in vivo* testing have provided a large body of data that confirms clevudine to be different. In chronic toxicology studies there was no toxicity in rats dosed for nine months. Monkeys also tolerated a high dose for six months. When toxicity appeared in chronic studies at week 39, it was unlike the toxicity encountered with substantially lower doses of D-FIAU or D-FMAU. It reversed very rapidly with dose reduction or cessation. All of these features clearly separate clevudine from both D-FIAU and D-FMAU, where irreversible multiorgan toxicity appeared with very low doses in multiple species well before 12 weeks. Thus the data give reasonably strong assurance about the safety of clevudine and support the idea that the L enantiomer represents a distinct class of nucleoside analogue.

Although it is very early in the development program, the initial clinical experience with clevudine is very promising. The pharmacokinetic profile is dose proportional, and the exposure levels are more than adequate to anticipate good antiviral activity based on preclinical *in vitro* and *in vivo* data. In addition, the drug is thus far well tolerated. These results are extremely compelling when one considers that the minimum cumulative dose that each subject received was 2500 mg, more than twice the average cumulative dose of FIAU that led to morbidity. The outcome of the Phase I trial and the extensive preclinical toxicology program support the initiation of the Phase I/II program. If the level of suppression and durability of response seen in the woodchuck model is observed in the human trials, clevudine could become an important new drug for the treatment of HBV infection.

References

1. Furman PA, Wilson JE, Reardon JE, & Painter GR. The effect of absolute configuration on the anti-HIV and anti-HBV activity of nucleoside analogues. Antiviral Chemistry and Chemotherapy 1995; 6:345-355.
2. Coats JAV, Inggall HG, Pearson BA, Penn CR, Storer R, Williamson C, & Cameron JM. Carbovir: The (-) enantiomer is a potent and selective antiviral agent against human immunodeficiency virus replication *in vitro*. Antiviral Research 1991; 15:161-168.
3. Coats JAV, Cammack N, Jenkinson HJ, Jowett AJ, Jowett MI, Pearson BA, Penn CR, Rouse PL, Viner KC, & Cameron JM. (-) 2'-Deoxy-3'-thiacytidine is a potent, highly selective inhibitor of human immunodeficiency type 1 and type 2 replication *in vitro*. Antimicrobial Agents and Chemotherapy 1992; 36:733-739.
4. Furman PA, Davis M, Liotta DC, Paff M, Frick LW, Nelson DJ, Dornsife RE, Wurster JA, Wilson LJ, Fyfe JA, Tuttle JV, Miller WH, Condreay L, Averett DR, Schinazi RF, & Painter GR. The anti-hepatitis B virus activity, cytotoxicity and anabolic profile of the (-) and (+) enantiomers of cis-5-fluoro-1-[2-(hydroxymethyl)-1, 3-oxathiorlan-5-yl] cytosine. Antimicrobial Agents and Chemotherapy 1992; 36:2686-2692.
5. Lin T-S, Luo M-Z, Lui M-C, Pai SB, Dutschman GE, & Cheng Y-C. Synthesis and biological evaluation of 2'3'-dideoxy-L-pyrimidine nucleosides as potential antiviral agents against human immunodeficiency virus (HIV) and hepatitis B virus (HBV). Journal of Medicinal Chemistry 1994; 37:798-803.
6. Graciet J-CG & Schinazi RF. From D-to L-nucleoside analogs as antiviral agents. In Advances in Drug Design, 1999; vol 3, pp1-68. JAI Press Inc.
7. Chu CK, Hong JH, Cho Y, Du J, Lee K, Chen BK, Boudinot DF, Peek SF, Korba BE, Tennant BC & Cheng YC. L-FMAU. Drugs of the Future 1998; 23:821-826.
8. Chu CK, Boudinot DF, Peek SF, Hong JH, Choi Y, Korba BE, Cote PJ, Tennant BC, & Cheng Y-C. Preclinical investigation of L-FMAU as an anti-hepatitis B virus agent. In Therapies for Viral Hepatitis, 1998;pp 303-312. Edited by RF Schinazi, J-P Sommadossi and HC Thomas. Atlanta: International Medical Press.
9. Dukhan D, Pierra C, Bryant M, Sommadossi J-P, Imbach JL & Gosselin G. β-L-2'-deoxynucleosides as potent anti-HBV agents (Part 1): Large-scale stereospecific synthesis of β-L-2'-deoxyadenosine. 13th International Conference on Antiviral Research, Baltimore Maryland, 16-21 April 2000; Abstract 89.
10. Pierra C, Bryant M, Sommadossi J-P, Inbach J-L & Gosselin G. β-L-2'-Deoxynucleosides as potent Anti-HBV agents (Part II): Large-scale stereospecific synthesis of β-L-thymidine. 13th International Conference on Antiviral Research, Baltimore, Maryland, 16-21 April 2000; Abstract 90.
11. Ma T, Lin JS, Gary Newton M, Cheng Y-C & Chu CK. Synthesis and anti-hepatitis B virus activity of 9-(2-deoxy-2-fluoro-β-L-arabinofuranosyl)-purine nucleosides. Journal of Medicinal Chemistry 1997; 40:2750-2754.
12. Chu CK, Ma TW, Shanmuganathan K, Wang CG, Xiang YJ, Pai SB, Yao GQ, Sommadossi J-P & Cheng Y-C. Use of 2'-fluoro-5-methyl-β-D arabinofuranosyl-uracil as a novel antiviral agent for hepatitis B virus and Epstein-Barr virus. Antimicrobial Agents and Chemotherapy 1995; 39:979-981.
13. Yao G-Q, Lin SH, Chou E, Kukhanova M, Chu CK & Cheng Y-C. Inhibition of Epstein-Barr virus replication by a novel L-nucleoside, 2'-fluoro-5-methyl-β-L arabinofuranosyl uracil. Biochemical Pharmacology 1996; 51:941-947.
14. Pai SB, Lui SH, Zhu YL, Chu CK & Cheng Y-C. Inhibition of hepatitis B virus: A novel L-nucleoside, 2'-fluoro-5-methyl-β-L-arabinofuranosyl uracil. Antimicrobial Agents and Chemotherapy

1996; 40:380-386.

15. Aguesse-Germon S, Lui SH, Chevallier M, Pichoud C, Jamard C, Borel C, Chu CK, Trepo C, Cheng Y-C & Zoulim F. Inhibition effect of 2'-fluoro-5-methyl-β-L-arabinofuranosyl uracil on duck hepatitis B virus replication. Antimicrobial Agents and Chemotherapy 1998; 42:369-376.
16. Peek SF, Jacob JR, Tochkov IA, Korba BE, Gerin JL, Chu CK & Tennant BC. Sustained antiviral activity of 1-(2-fluoro-methyl-β-L arabinofuranosyl) uracil (L-FMAU) in the woodchuck model of hepatitis B virus (HBV) infection. Hepatology 1997; 26:1187.
17. Korba BE, Peek SF, Baldwin B, Cote PJ, Tochkov IA, Jacob JR, Chu CK, Gerin JL & Tennant BC. Antiviral activity of 1-(2-fluoro-5-methyl-β-L-arabinofuranosyl) uracil (L-FMAU) against WHV replication and gene expression in chronically infected woodchucks. The Molecular Biology of Hepatitis B Viruses, San Diego, California, 30 August - 3 September 1998, Abstract 151.
18. Zhu Y, Cullen J, Saputelli J, Aldrich C, Schinazi R, Furman P & Mason W. L-FMAU treatment of woodchucks chronically infected with WHV. 50th American Association for the Study of Liver Diseases, Dallas, Texas, 5-9 November 1999, Abstract 738.
19. Jacob JR, Korba BE, Peek SF, Fullmer CS, Tochkov I, Chu CK, Cote PJ, Gerin JL & Tennant BC. Pharmacodynamics of 1-(2-fluoro-5-methyl-β-L arabinofuranosyl) uracil (L-FMAU) in the woodchuck model of hepatitis B virus (HBV) infection. The Molecular Biology of Hepatitis Viruses, Santa Cruz, California, 18-22 July 1999, Abstract 149.
20. Abbruzzese JL, Schmidt S, Raber MN, Levy JK, Castellanos AM, Legha SS & Krakoff IH. Phase I trial of 1-(2'-deoxy-2'-fluoro-1-beta-D-arabinofuranosyl)-5-methyl uracil (FMAU) terminated by severe neurologic toxicity. Investigational New Drugs 1989; 7:195-201.
21. Manning FJ, Swartz M & *Editors.* Review of the Fialuridine (FIAU) Clinical Trials. Committee to Review the Fialuridine (FIAU/FIAC) Clinical Trials Division of Health Sciences Policy. Institute of Medicine. 1995 National Academy Press, Washington DC.
22. Beckett AH. Chirality and its importance in drug development. Biochemistry Society Transactions 1991; 19:443-446.
23. Korba BE & Gerin JL. Use of standardized cell culture assay to assess activities of nucleoside analogs against hepatitis B virus replication. Antiviral Research 1992; 19:55-70.
24. Korba BE, Chu CK, Hill E & Furman PA. Effectiveness of combination therapies against hepatitis B Virus (HBV) replication *in vitro.* The Molecular Biology of Hepatitis Viruses, Santa Cruz, California, 18-22 July 1999, Abstract 152.
25. Allen MI, Deslauriers M, Andrews CW, Tipples GA, Walters KA, Tyrrell D L-J & Brown N. For The Lamivudine Clinical Investigation Group, and Condreay LD. Identification and Characterization of Mutations in Hepatitis B Virus Resistant to Lamivudine. Hepatology 1998; 27:1670-1677.
26. Chin R, Torresi J, Earnest-Silveira L, Trautwein C, Bock T, Manns MP, Furman PA, Cleary D & Locarnini SA. Two novel antiviral agents, DAPD and L-FMAU, which are active against wild type and lamivudine-resistant HBV. 50th American Association for the Study of Liver Diseases, Dallas, Texas, 5-9 November 1999, Abstract 1041.
27. Fu L, Lin SH & Cheng Y-C. Sensitivity of L- (-) 2, 3-deoxythiacytidine resistant hepatitis B virus to other antiviral nucleoside analogues. Biochemical Pharmacology 1999; 57:1351-1359.
28. Lui SH, Grove KL & Cheng Y-C. Unique metabolism of a novel antiviral L-nucleoside analogue, L-FMAU: A substrate for both thymidine kinase and deoxycytidine kinase. Antimicrobial Agents and Chemotherapy 1998; 42:833-839.
29. Seigneres B, Pichoud C, Germon S, Furman P, Trepo C & Zoulim F. Inhibitory activity of new nucleoside analogs on wild type and YMDD mutants of the Hepadnavirus reverses transcriptase. 13th International

Conference on Antiviral Research, Baltimore, Maryland, 16-21 April 2000; Abstract 68.

30. Dayan AD & Anderson D. Toxicity of Antiviral Compounds. In Antiviral Agents: The Development and Assessment of Antiviral Chemotherapy Volume I, 1998; pp 111-125. Edited by HJ Field. Boca Raton, Florida: CRC Press.
31. Wagar MA, Evans MJ, Manly KF, Hughes RG & Huberman JA. Effects of 2'-2'-dideoxynucleosides on mammalian cells and viruses. Journal of Cellular Physiology 1984; 121:402-408.
32. Chen C-H, Vazquez-Padua M & Cheng Y-C. Effect of anti-human immunodeficiency virus nucleoside analogs on mitochondrial DNA and its implication for delayed toxicity. Molecular Pharmacology 1991; 39:345-355.
33. Parker WB & Cheng Y-C. Mitochondrial toxicity of antiviral nucleoside analogs. The Journal of NIH Research 1994; 6:57-61.
34. Kukhanova M, Lin ZY, Yas'co M & Cheng Y-C. Unique inhibitory effect of 1-(2'deoxy-2'-fluoro-β-L-arabinofuranosyl)-5-methyluracil 5'-triphosphate on Epstein-Barr virus and human DNA polymerases. Biochemical Pharmacology 1998; 55:1181-1187.
35. Fourel I, Hantz O, Watanabe KA, Jacquet C, Chomel B, Fox JJ & Trepo C. Inhibitory effects of 2'-fluorinated arabinosyl-pyrimidine nucleosides on woodchuck hepatitis virus replication in chronically infected woodchucks. Antimicrobial Agents and Chemotherapy 1990; 34:473-475.
36. McKenzie RC, Fried MW, Sallie R, Conjeevaram H, Bisceglie AM, Park Y, Savarese B, Kleiner D, Tsokos M, Luciano C, Pruett T, Stotka JL, Straus SE & Hoofnagle JH. Hepatic failure and lactic acidosis due to filauridine (FIAU), an investigational nucleoside analog for chronic HBV. NEJM. 1995; 333:1099-1105.
37. Tennant BC, Baldwin BH, Graham LA, Ascenzi MA, Hornbuckle WE, Rowland PH, Tochkov IA, Yeager AE, Erb HN, Colacino JM, Lopez C, Englehardt JA, Bowsher RR, Richardson FC, Lewis W, Cote PJ, Korba BE & Gerin JL. Antiviral activity and toxicity of fialuridine in the woodchuck model of hepatitis B virus. Hepatology 1998; 28:179-191
38. Lewis W, Griniuviene B, Tankersley KO, Levine ES, Montione R, Engelman L, de Courten-Meyers G, Ascenzi MA, Hornbuckle WE, Gerin JL & Tennant B. Depletion of mitochondrial DNA, destruction of mitochondria, and accumulation of lipid droplets result from filauridine treatment in woodchucks (Marmota monax). Laboratory Investigation 1997; 76:77-87.
39. Halvering LM, Richardson KA, Englehardt JA & Richardson FC. Fialuridine (FIAU) depletes mitochondrial DNA in the liver and heart of rat, dog, and monkey during long-term oral administration. American Association of Cancer Research 1995; 36:358.
40. Report of a FDA Task Force. Fialuridine: Hepatic and Pancreatic Toxicity. Food and Drug Administration, November 1993.
41. Cui L, Schinazi RF, Gosselin G, Imbach JL, Chu CK, Rando RF, Revankar GR & Sommadossi J-P. Effect of β-enantiomeric and racemic nucleoside analogues on mitochondrial functions in HepG2 cells. Biochemical Pharmacology 1996; 52:1577-1584.
42. Zhou XRP, Cui L, Zhou XJ, Sommadossi J-P & Darley-Urmar VM. Differential Effects of antiretroviral nucleoside analogs on mitochondrial function in HepG2 cells. Antimicrobial Agents and Chemotherapy 2000; 44:496-503.
43. Wright JD, Ma T, Chu CK & Boudinot FD. Pharmacokinetics of 1-(2-deoxy-2-fluoro-β-L-arabinofuranosyl)-5-methyl uracil (L-FMAU) in rats. Pharmaceutical Research 1998; 12:1350-1353.
44. Wright JD, Ma T, Chu CK & Boudinot FD. Discontinuous oral absorption pharmacokinetic model and bioavailability of 1-(2-fluoro-5-methyl-β-L-arabinofuranosyl)-uracil (L-FMAU) in rats. Biopharmaceutics and Drug Disposition 1996; 17:197-207.

45. Witcher JW, Boudinot FD, Baldwin BH, Ascenzi MA, Tennant BC, Du JF & Chu CK. Pharmacokinetics of 1-(2-fluoro-5-methyl-β-L-arabinofuranosyl)-uracil (L-FMAU) in woodchucks. Antimicrobial Agents and Chemotherapy 1997; 41:2184-2187.
46. Blum R, Chittick G, Wang L, Fang L, Szczech G & Rousseau F. Phase I Pharmacokinetic and Safety Evaluation of Clevudine (L-FMAU), a new agent under development for the treatment of hepatitis B virus (HBV) infection. 2000, L-FMAU 101 Abstract ICCAC.

Glucosidase/protein folding inhibitors as possible mutation-proof, anti-hepatitis B & C agents

TIMOTHY M. BLOCK[1], ROBERT JORDAN[1], XUANYONG LU[1], ANAND MEHTA[1], DONALD PICKER[3], GARY JACOB[3], BARUCH S. BLUMBERG[4] and RAYMOND A. DWEK[2]

[1] *Department of Biochemistry and Molecular Pharmacology, Thomas Jefferson University College of Medicine, Philadelphia, Pa., 19107, USA*
[2] *University of Oxford, Oxford, OX1-3QU, UK*
[3] *Synergy Pharmaceuticals, Inc., Edison, NJ, 08837, USA*
[4] *Fox Chase Cancer Center, Philadelphia, Pa., 19101, USA*

Abstract

The morphogenesis of hepatitis B virus (HBV) and Bovine Viral Diarrhea Virus (BVDV) is more dependent upon the glucosidase step of glycoprocessing than are most host functions. Since BVDV is similar, with respect to its morphogenesis, to hepatitis C virus (HCV), it is speculated that inhibitors of glucosidases will have broad therapeutic value.

Introduction

It appears that inhibition of as little as 6% of cellular glycoprocessing, with either the glucosidase inhibitors nonyl or n-butyl DNJ (NN-DNJ, NB-DNJ), causes a 99% decrease in HBV gene product secretion. Under these conditions there is a negligible impact upon host glycoprotein secretion. Unlike the situation with other antiviral agents, the frequency of viruses that have gained resistance to these compounds may be low, or even zero. Indeed, NN-DNJ resistant BVDV and HBV could not be generated by either continuous passage in the presence of compound (for BVDV) or by site directed mutagenesis [for HBV, see 31]. Glucosidases mediate the first step of glycoprocessing, which is necessary for the proper folding and trafficking of some glycoproteins. We speculate that most, if not all, viruses that acquire their envelopes from intracellular membranes will be selectively sensitive to glucosidase inhibitors. Indeed, NN-DNJ has been shown to be effective in reducing the levels of enveloped woodchuck hepatitis virus *in vivo* [5]. The precise molecular reasons for the selective sensitivity of certain viruses to these inhibitors is discussed. The possibility of developing a class of well-tolerated antivirals to which resistance is rare has enormous implications for the future of therapy for chronic viral disease.

Frontiers in Viral Hepatitis Ed. by RF Schinazi, J-P Sommadossi and CM Rice. 301 — 314

The problem of HBV & HCV

Worldwide more than 400 million people are chronically infected with the hepatitis B and C viruses [HBV, HCV, see 1]. HBV and HCV are the etiological agents of a progressive liver disease in which 5-20% of those chronically infected may eventually develop life-limiting cirrhosis and hepatocellular carcinoma [22]. There is an immediate, desperate need for HCV therapeutics, and there is a significant need for effective HBV drugs which will complement nucleoside analogues.

Current therapeutic options

For both HBV and HCV, interferon alpha (an immune system modifying cytokine) has been shown to be effective in inducing patients to achieve "milestones" (not cures) in 5 to 30% of those treated [22]. At present, the only specific treatment for chronic hepatitis C is interferon alpha therapy, either on its own or in combination with the guanosine analogue ribavirin [22]. However, (a) parenteral administration is necessary, (b) the adverse side effects are use-limiting and (c) only half of the patients respond to treatment. Moreover, relapse in responder populations is common following cessation of therapy [22]. For HBV, the nucleoside analogue lamivudine is now available and is a highly effective anti-polymerase agent, achieving reductions of HBV viremia in almost all users [22].

However, there are problems associated with monotherapy in which the target of the compound is a virus-specified enzyme. As with HIV patients treated with AZT monotherapy, HBV patients treated with lamivudine alone acquire resistant mutants [6, 27]. For example, it is estimated that resistant mutants were present in as may as 34% of those treated with lamivudine, after two years [16, 27]. Given the problems associated with HIV monotherapy, many clinicians even wonder about the wisdom of monotherapy for HBV; if resistant mutants emerge, these patients will not even be eligible for liver transplantation — their final option. Although the pathogenecity of resistant mutants is unknown (and could be less than that of the wild type), the occurrence of mutants could seriously undermine and limit the usefulness of nucleoside therapy.

Role of glycoprocessing in host function

N-linked glycosylation of glycoproteins occurs via the action of oligosaccharide transferase, in the endoplasmic reticulim (ER). However, in the ER, mammalian cells begin to degrade (process) the 14-residue oligosaccharide immediately after its addition to the nascent, polypeptide backbone at specific amino acid sequences, called "sequons" (see Figure 1 [13]). This trimming reaction is temporally and spatially regulated, beginning with the removal of terminal and penultimate glucose residues by ER glucosidases I and II. After additional trimming, the glycoprotein is transferred to the Golgi complex, where the oligosaccharide is reconstructed into its characteristic glycoform. Although the enzymology of processing is well understood, the reason that

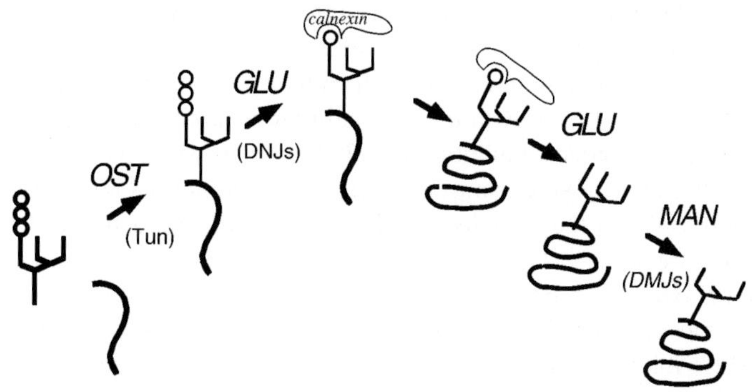

Figure 1. N-linked glycosylation and processing. The process of N-linked glycosylation is shown as the combination of the pitchfork-like oligosaccharide structure with the ribbon-like polypeptide (progressing from an unfolded to folded state) by the action of oligosaccharyltransferase (OST). This step is inhibited by tunicaymicin (Tun). Glucosidase enzymes (GLU) mediate removal of terminal glucose residues (shown as circles attached to the oligosaccharide). Calnexin (shown as a wrench) is thought to bind nascent polypeptides via monoglucose residues and mediate protein folding. Mannosidases (MAN) process the N-linked oligosaccharide further. GLU and MAN enzymes are inhibited by DNJs and DMJs, respectively.

the N-linked glycan is degraded soon after its transfer, only to be rebuilt in the Golgi had been an enigma [see 18].

The reasons for the tremendous cellular investment in *glycan processing* are even more surprising when considering that the process, in the ER, is nonessential (for tissue culture growth) [43]. Removal of the terminal glucose is apparently necessary for the transport of some, but not all, glycoproteins from the ER to the Golgi [28; 36; 34; 34a]. It has been proposed that the mono-glucosylated glycoprotein (the product of glucosidase) binds to cell chaperones such as calnexin [17]. Calnexin is hypothesized to help in protein folding and subsequent protein-protein interactions (oligomerization), and transport from the ER [18, 35]. Misfolded glycoprotein is either retained in the ER or continuously cycles between the ER and Golgi, possibly in association with with other cellular chaperones or transport proteins [12, 17].

Dependence of HBV and BVDV, and possibly HCV, to glucosidases

We have previously shown that the secretion of enveloped HBV DNA is sensitive to glucosidase inhibition. HBV is thought to bud by the rolling of its nucleocapsid into the ER or post-ER intracellular membranes [24]. Further mechanisms of glucosidase inhibitor action studies led us to propose that viruses that acquire their envelopes from intracellular membranes might be extremely sensitive, as a class, to glucosidase inhibitors. HCV and the Flaviviridae family, as a whole, are also thought to bud nucleocapsids through the ER or other internal membranes. Since HCV is difficult to grow in tissue culture, bovine viral diarrhea virus (BVDV) was used as its surrogate. BVDV is a flavivirus containing a positive stranded, infectious, 10 kb RNA genome that is translated into a 4,000-amino-acid polyprotein [23, 34]. Unlike HCV, however, methods for evaluation of its growth in tissue cultures are well defined.

Under conditions of modest inhibition of cellular glucosidases (which mediate a step in glycoprocessing), host glycoproteins are secreted at near normal levels (see Figure 2). However, nearly 100% of the secretion of HBV and bovine viral diarrhea virus (BVDV) is prevented (Figure 2).

Secretion of HBV and BVDV infectious virus is thus sensitive to glucosidase inhibitors. We have previously shown that HBV DNA accumulates within cells treated with glucosidase inhibitors such as NB-DNJ [31]. It was hypothesized that defective and not infectious forms of HBV were accumulating, transiently, within glucosidase-inhibited cells. This, however, could not be formally tested, since infectivity assays for HBV are difficult to perform.

The possibility that glucosidase inhibition caused an accumulation of infectious virus to be trapped within the cellular compartment was explored with BVDV. Briefly, BVDV-infected cells were left untreated or incubated with the glucosidase inhibitor, NB-DNJ. At three days after infection at an moi of less than one, the amount of infectious virus in the culture medium and within cell lysates was compared. As shown in Figure 3, in untreated cells, approximately two-thirds of the infectious virus remained cell associated, although a considerable titer was detectable in the medium. Cells treated with glucosidase inhibitors had nearly no detectable virus in either the cell medium or within the cellular compartment. These data suggest that glucosidase-inhibited cells do not accumulate infectious virus within the cellular compartment.

Glucosidase function is necessary for virus maturation

The glucosidases were shown to be the vulnerable step in glyco-processing by a series of pharmacological dissections. For example, inhibition of mannosidases with DMJ, which inhibits the glycoprocessing step immediately following glucose removal (see Figure 1), had no impact upon enveloped HBV or BVDV secretion (Figure 4).

Acylated DNJs

Previous studies have been performed with the simple imino sugar NB-DNJ (see Figure 5). Although it is orally active with excellent bio-availability and has been shown to be well tolerated in monkeys and humans [15], the high (millimolar) doses required to achieve an anti-HBV effect in tissue culture made the pursuit of more potent analogues desirable. Therefore, a survey of imino sugars with different biochemical structures and properties were tested for anti-HBV activity, with the hope of finding clues to structure-activity relationships that would provide a platform from which to develop a more realistic therapeutic compound.

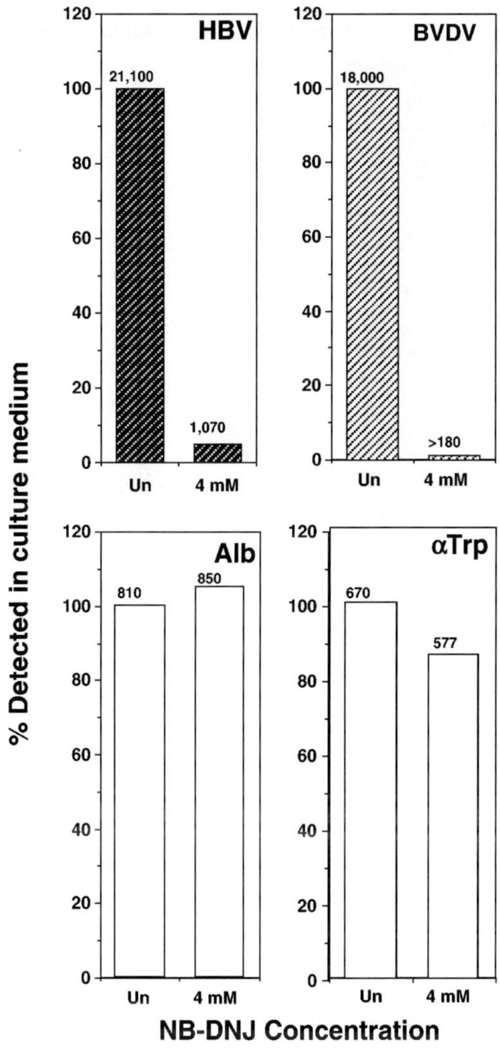

Figure 2. HBV and BVDV secretion is selectively sensitive to glucosidase inhibitors. The secretion of enveloped HBV and cellular polypeptides albumin (Alb, a nonglycosylated protein) and alpha 1 antitrypsin (αTrp, a glycosylated protein) from HepG 2.2.15 cells in the absence and presence of the glucosidase inhibitor NB-DNJ (4 mM) is shown. Briefly, after six days incubation of HepG 2.2.15 cells in the absence (UN) or presence (4 mM) of NB-DNJ, the amount of enveloped HBV, albumin and α1 antitrypsin secreted into the culture medium was determined. The value of the amount of HBV or polypeptide secreted in the absence of NB-DNJ is taken as 100%. HBV was measured by an immunoprecipitation (IP)-PCR. The intensity of the PCR product was detected by ethidium bromide staining, quantified by densitometry, with the raw OD value provided in the box. For polypeptide secretion, cells were labeled for 30 minutes with 35-S methionine. Three hours after labeling, culture medium was immunoprecipitated with specific antibody, followed by resolution through SDS PAGE. The bands specific for the polypeptide of interest were quantified by densitometry and raw values are presented in the box. Details of the assay can be found in Lu et al. (1996). Data presented here are from unpublished observations.

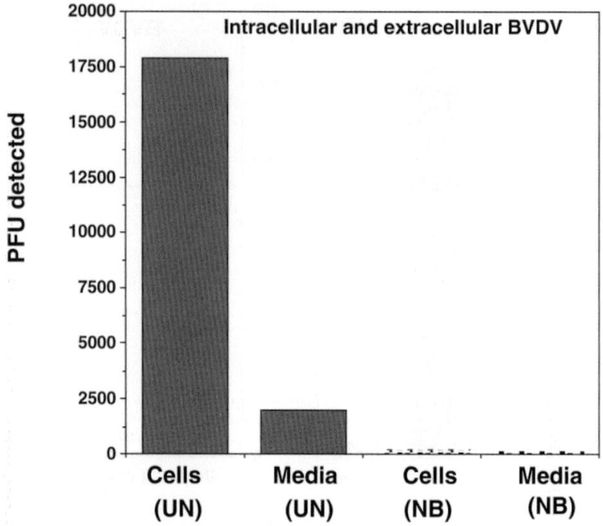

Figure 3. BVDV does not accumulate within the intracellular compartment of glucosidase-inhibited cells. BVDV-infected MDBK cells were grown in the absence (UN) or presence (NB) of 1 mg/ml (~4 mM) of NB-DNJ for three days. Media and cells were separated and the amount of virus (PFU) present was determined following freeze-thawing by standard methods. Infection was performed at a low (less than 1) multiplicity.

Each compound was tested for anti-HBV activity and cytotoxicity. A DNJ derivative possessing a 9 carbon alkyl side chain (called nonyl DNJ or NN-DNJ), shown in Figure 5, was selected for further study, since it possessed anti-HBV and anti-BVDV activity in the low micromolar range and could be easily produced [Dwek, unpublished]. The selectivity index of NN-DNJ was determined to be between 50 and 100, using a mitochondrial dehydrogenase (MTT) assay [21]. Curiously, NN-DNJ and NB-DNJ had a similar Ki for the glucosidase enzyme (Table 1), suggesting that the enhanced antiviral activity of NN-DNJ in cell-based assays was due to increased cellular association or uptake. This possibility was determined, in part, by analysis of tissue accumulation of radio-labeled compound in mice following oral administration, where NN-DNJ appeared to have an enhanced hepatotropism [47].

Treatment of chronic woodchuck hepatitis virus infection with NN-DNJ

With micromolar active glucosidase inhibitors, it was realistic to consider *in vivo* experiments. NN-DNJ was determined to be orally available and well tolerated in rodent studies, using in excess of 150 mg/kg (not shown). Therefore, the ability of NN-DNJ to reduce the levels of enveloped WHV DNA within the serum of chronically infected woodchucks was tested. The results were reported in Block et al. (1998). Briefly, 20 one-year-old

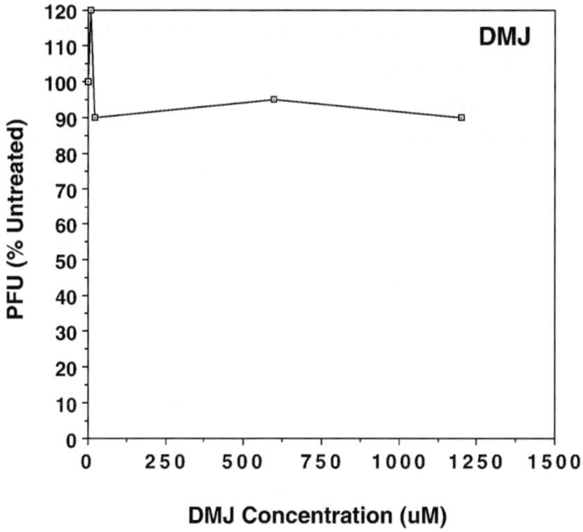

Figure 4. Inhibition of complex glycan formation with DMJ does not prevent HBV or BVDV secretion. MDBK cells were grown to confluence in six well plates and infected with 500 pfu of cp BVDV (NADL strain) per well for one hour at 37 degrees. The inoculum was then replaced with medium containing the indicated concentration of DMJ. After three days culture, medium supernatants were removed, and virus yields were determined by plaque assay. After three days the plaques resulting from this secondary infection were counted, and the results were expressed as percentage of the number of plaques resulting from infection with the inhibitor-free plaque assay supernatant (=100%). DMJ was used at concentrations of up to 1.5 mM, an inhibitor concentration sufficient to protect treated cells from killing by a complex-sugar binding lectin (ECA) (data not shown). Data and methods are as in Zitzmann et al. (1999).

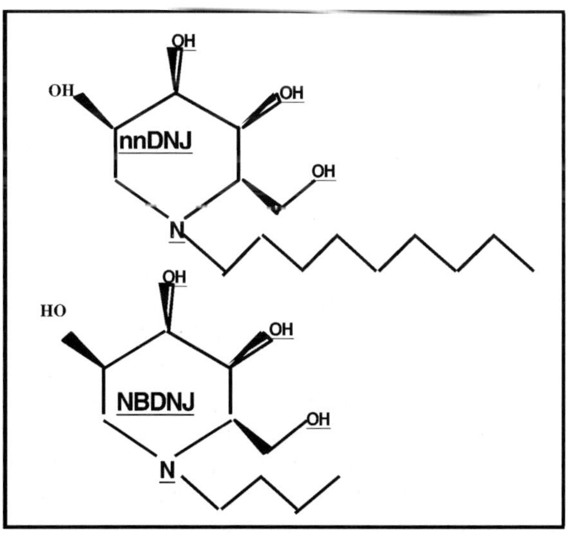

Figure 5. Structure of NN-DNJ and NB-DNJ. Chemical structures of the simple imino sugars nonyldeoxynojirimycin (NN-DNJ) and n-butyl deoxynojirimycin (NB-DNJ) are shown.

chronically infected woodchucks were divided into five treatment groups. Placebo or four different doses of NN-DNJ were administered orally, twice daily. All animals in all treatment groups thrived, showing no evidence of toxicity, using standard noninvasive means of evaluation (weight, liver function tests). The amount of total and enveloped WHV DNA in the serum was compared at zero and four weeks. Total DNA levels did not vary with dose group. However, the amount of enveloped WHV in woodchucks four weeks after treatment declined in a dose-dependent fashion (see Figure 6), with some animals lacking all detectable enveloped viral DNA.

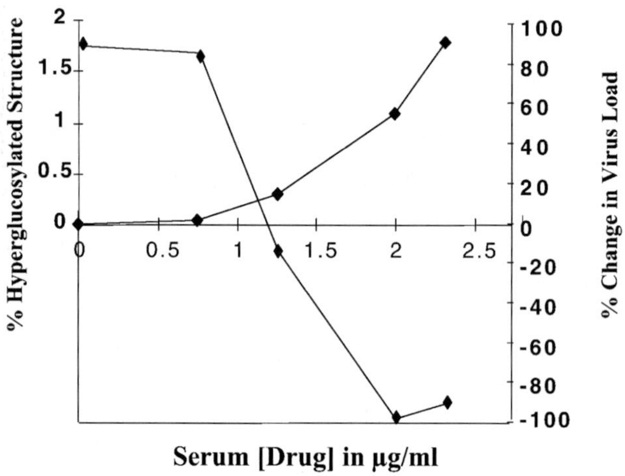

Figure 6. NN-DNJ-fed woodchucks experience a decline in enveloped WHV that correlates with unprocessed glycan. Woodchucks chronically infected with woodchuck hepatitis virus (WHV) were fed placebo or NN-DNJ by oral gavage. The amount of enveloped WHV in the serum was determined. The amount at four weeks after treatment is shown as a percentage of the amount prior to treatment (right Y-axis) and is plotted as a function of the amount of serum NN-DNJ (at four weeks after treatment), along with the amount of unprocessed glycan in the serum at four weeks of treatment. These methods and details are described in greater detail in Block et al., 1998.

The decline in enveloped viral DNA was shown to correlate with increasing amounts of serum NN-DNJ concentrations (see Figure 6 and Block et al., 1998). It was also of interest to determine if the decline in enveloped WHV DNA correlated with the extent to which the target enzyme, ER glucosidase, was inhibited. Since it was not possible to directly measure glucosidase enzyme activity in the treated animals, a surrogate marker for inhibition was developed. It was reasoned that the degree to which ER glucosidase was inhibited would be reflected in the accumulation of serum N-linked tri-glucosylated glycan. As shown in Figure 2, ER glucosidase mediates removal of terminal glucose residues from the nascent N-linked oligosaccharide. Therefore, inhibition of the enzyme would be expected to cause a buildup of tri-glucosylated structures. An HPLC assay to detect tri-glucosylated structures derived from serum glycoproteins was developed, and the results are summarized in Figure 6. Serum from animals fed placebo contained no detectable glc3man7 structures and did not experience any reductions in enveloped viral DNA. However, the amount of enveloped viral DNA in animals treated for four weeks with NN-DNJ decreased with increasing levels of glc3man7 structures. That is, there was a clear dose relationship between the level of glycoprocessing inhibition and antiviral impact. Moreover, as little as 1% net inhibition of glycoprocessing was associated with a maximum (2 logs) drop in viremia. This suggested that overall, small amounts of inhibition of glycoprocessing were sufficient to cause large drops in enveloped viral DNA levels.

This hypothesis was borne out by *in vitro* studies. The amount of enveloped HBV and hyperglucosylated N-linked glycan in the culture medium of 2.2.15 cells was measured as a function of NN-DNJ concentration. Figure 7 shows that the amount of hyperglucosylated glycan in the culture medium increases in an NN-DNJ-dose-dependent fashion, plateauing at about 3.3%. The reason that increased amounts of NN-DNJ do not result in increased amounts of hyperglucosylated structure is uncertain, but is likely due to the action of other cellular processing enzymes (such as the golgi endomannosidase), which can process most glycan structures independently of glucosidase. Significantly, as was seen *in vivo*, as little as 3% inhibition of total glycoprocessing was sufficient to cause a greater than 99% reduction in the secretion of enveloped HBV. The apparent ability of NN-DNJ to achieve the same antiviral activity as NB-DNJ under conditions where glycoprocessing was less inhibited could also mean that NN-DNJ possesses an antiviral activity that uses a mechansim in addition to glucosidase inhibition. This possibility is under investigation.

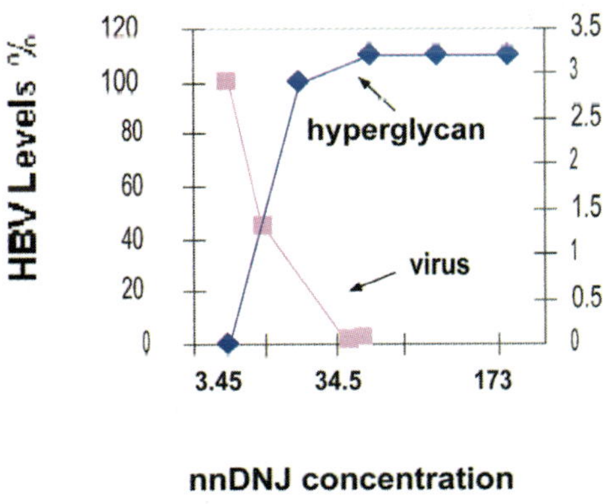

Figure 7. Correlation between inhibition of glycoprocessing and the NN-DNJ antiviral effect in tissue culture. After three days of incubation of HepG 2.2.15 cells, the indicated ug/ml concentration of either NN-DNJ culture medium was tested for the amount of enveloped HBV by immunoprecipitation (IP) PCR (as in Lu et al., 1995) or triglucosylated glycan, as in Block et al. (1998). The amount of HBV detected in untreated cells is considered to be 100%. Tri-glucosylated glycan (hyperglycan), derived by hydrazine release and fluor. labeling, from all secreted glycoproteins, was measured by normal phase HPLC (see Block et al., 1998) and accumulates when glucosidase is inhibited. It is considered to be proportional to the degree to which the enzyme has been inhibited.

Glucosidase-resistant mutants could not be isolated

Since HBV cannot be passed continuously in tissue culture, it has been unrealistic to determine if mutants resistant to glucosidase inhibitor could be spontaneously generated. However, BVDV is sensitive to glucosidase inhibitors and can be passaged continuously in tissue cultures. Therefore, the possibility that mutant BVDV resistant to NN-DNJ and NB-DNJ could emerge was tested by the serial passage of 1 x 10^5 PFU in the presence of various concentrations of inhibitor. At selected passages, the progeny were tested for the ability to grow in the absence and presence of a concentration of inhibitor known to reduce titers by 99%. Complete resistance is defined as equal titer formation in the absence or presence of inhibitor. Partial resistance was defined as the acquisition of a greater IC-90 (concentration of compound required to reduce titers by 90%) than was seen for wild type, parental virus.

As shown in Figure 8, after more than 20 passages, there is no evidence that resistant mutants of BVDV have emerged. In contrast, BVDV mutants resistant to a neutralizing monoclonal antibody appear within four passages (not shown).

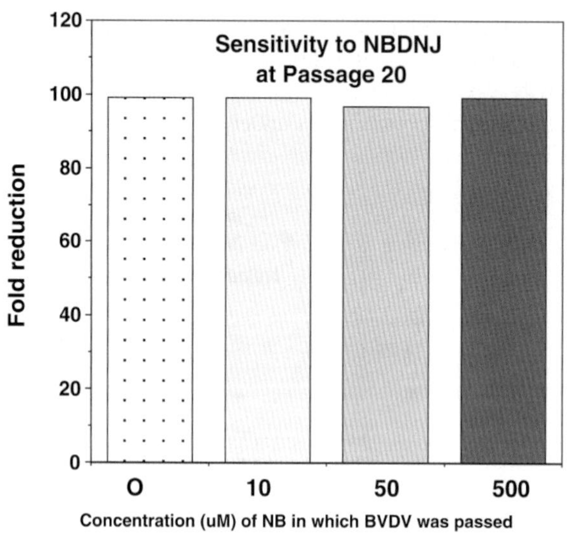

Figure 8. Sensitivity to NB-DNJ before and after passage of BVDV in the presence of various concentrations of compound. MDBK cells were infected with BVDV strain NADL at an moi of 0.01 in the presence of the indicated concentration of glucosidase inhibitor. After approximately 90% of the culture was judged, by analysis under light microscopy, to be "cytopathic", the culture was harvested and a "passage" was considered achieved. This cycle was repeated for 20 passages, after which the degree of sensitivity (fold reduction) of the continuously passaged virus to an amount of glucosidase inhibitor that decreases wild type, parental virus by 99%, was determined and is shown.

Conclusions

HBV and HCV are completely different viruses with strikingly similar natural histories of infection: both target the liver and cause chronic, probably immunopathological diseases [22]. Relevant to this discussion is the fact that their morphogenesis seems to be from the same intracellular organelles. Thus, although they are very different virologically, and drugs directed against HBV enzymes (such as lamivudine) are likely to be ineffective against HCV, we suggest that their shared intracellular morphogenesis profiles offer an exciting opportunity for intervention.

A growing body of evidence suggests that viruses that acquire their lipid envelopes and glycoproteins from intracellular membranes, such as the ER and Golgi, are extremely dependent upon the ER glucosidase. For example, we have observed that the secretion of HBV as well as production of BVDV, in tissue culture is prevented by glucosidase inhibitors [47]. BVDV is considered to be a good tissue culture surrogate of hepatitis C virus (HCV) [19]. Moreover, inhibition of HBV and BVDV was achieved under conditions in which little, if any, toxicity to the host was observed. HBV, HCV and BVDV are all believed to bud from the ER. Therefore, we hypothesize that viruses that bud from the ER can be selectively inhibited with glucosidase inhibitors. It is worthwhile mentioning that precise IC 50 determinations vary somewhat with culture conditions.

Clearly, certain classes of enveloped viruses are more sensitive to glucosidase mediated processing for their secretion than are most host functions. Moreover, mutant viruses refractory to the action of glucosidase inhibitors are rare. NN-DNJ is more potent than is NB-DNJ in the inhibition of HBV and BVDV secretion. This could be due in part to a preferential cellular uptake. It is also possible that NN-DNJ possesses antiviral mechanisms other than that of inhibiting glucosidases. This is being explored.

Targeting a host enzyme for a beneficial effect is, of course, not new and is the basis of many of the therapeutics in clinical use, from diabetes and cholesterol lowering medications to hypertension medications. However, it is less conventional to propose targeting a host enzyme for the treatment of a viral infection. The ultimate usefulness of these compounds as therapeutics will depend upon their safety profiles.

Acknowledgements

This manuscript and work was supported, in part, by an appropriation from The Commonwealth of Pennsylvania, The Hepatitis B Foundation, and Synergy Pharmaceuticals, Inc. Dr. Nicole Zitzmann (U. Oxford) is thanked for helpful comments and sharing unpublished results.

Table 1. Antiviral profiles of NB-DNJ and NN-DNJ:

Compound:	EC-50 (uM)	Ki (uM)	CC-50 (uM)
NB-DNJ	115	0.22	>5, 000
NN-DNJ	2.5	0.44	150

The amount of compound needed to inhibit 50% of the plaques produced by BVDV strain NADL in a single-step yield reduction assay (EC-50), 50% of rat liver glucosidase in a standard liquid enzyme assay, or kill 50% of the cells in culture, is shown. Data (for BVDV) are from R. Jordan (unpublished), with assay details as in Zitzmann et al., 1999. Data for glucosidase enzyme are from R. Dwek (U. Oxford, unpublished).

References

1. Alter, M. J. (1997) Epidemiology of hepatitis C. *Hepatology*. 26: Suppl. 1: 62S-65S.
2. Allen, M. I., M. Deslauriers, C. W. Andrews, et al. (1998) Identification and characterization of mutations in hepatitis B virus resistant to lamivudine. *Hepatology*. 27: 1670-77.
3. Beasley, R. P. (1988). The Hepatitis B virus. The major etiology of hepatocellular carcinoma. *Cancer*. 61: 1942-1956..
4. Block, T. M., Platt, F., Lu, X., Gerlich, W., Foster, G., Blumberg, B. S. and Dwek, R. A. (1994) Hepatitis B Virus secretion is inhibited by the imino sugar, N-butylnojirimycin *Proc. Natl. Acad. Sci. USA* 91, 2235-2239
5. Block, T. M., Lu, X., Mehta, A. S., Blumberg, B. S., Tennant, B., Ebling, M., Korba, B., Lansky, D. M., Jacob, G. S. and Dwek, R. A. (1998) Treatment of woodchucks chronically infected with woodchuck hepatitis virus with protein folding inhibitors. *Nature Medicine* 4, 610-614.
6. Chayuma, K., Y. Suzuki, Y., M. Kobayashi et al. (1998) Emergence and takeover of YMDD motif mutant hepaitis B virus during long term lamivudine therapy and re-takeover by wild type virus after cessation of therapy. *Hepatology* 27: 1711-1716.
7. Choukhi, A., Ung, S., Wychowski, C. and Dubuisson, J. (1998) Involvement of endoplasmic reticulum chaperones in the folding of hepatitis C virus glycoproteins. *Journal of Virology* 72, 3851-3858
8. Cullen, N. J., G. Moraleda, J. Sapatelli, C. Aldrich et al. (1998) The problems of resistance to antiviral drugs and immunotherapy in the woodchuck model of chronic hepatitis B virus. *IBC 4th International Conference on hepatitis*, (Book), Jan. 22/23, 1998, Wash., DC.
9. Datema, S. Olofsson, P. Romero. (1987), Inhibitors of protein glycosylation and glycoprotein processing in viral systems. *Pharmacol. Thera.* 33: 221-286
10. Donis, R. (1995) Molecular Biology of bovine virus diarrhea virus and its interactions with the host. *Vet. Clin. N. A.* 11: (3) 393-423.
11. Dubuisson, J. and Rice, C. M. (1996) Hepatitis c virus glycoprotein folding: disulfide bond formation and association with calnexin. *Journal of Virology* 70, 778-786
12. Dwek, R. A. (1995). Glycobiology: more functions for oligosaccharides. *Science*. 269: 1234-1235.
13. Elbein, A. D. (1991) Amino sugar compounds as antiviral and anti tumor agents, *Sem. Cell Biol.* 2; 309-317;
14. Ellgaard, L., Molinari, M. and Helenius, A. (1999) Setting the standards: Quality control in the secretory pathway. *Science* 286: 1882-1888.
15. Fischl, M, L. Resnick, R. Coombs, A. Kremer, J. Potage et al. (1994), The safety and efficacy of combination therapy N-butyl deoxynojirimycin (SC-48334) and Zidovudine in patients with HIV infection and 200-500 CD4 cells / mm3. *J. Acq. Imm.* Def. S., 7: 139-147
16. Fontanna, R. J. and A. S. F. Lok (1997) Combination Therapy for chronic hepatitis B. *Hepatology* 26: 234-237.
17. Hammand and Helenius, 1994, Quality control in the secretory pathway: retention of a misfolded

viral membrane glycoprotein involves cycling between the ER, Intermediate compartment and Golgi Apparatus, *Journal of Cell Biology*, 126: 41-52).

18. Helenius, A. (1994) How N linked oligosaccharides affect glycoprotein folding in the endoplasmic reticulum. *Mol. Biol. Cell.* 5: 253-265.
19. Henzler, H.-J., and Kaiser, K. (1998) Avoiding viral contamination in biotechnological and pharmaceutical processes. *Nat. Biotechnology.* 16: 1077-1079.
20. Herbert, D. N., B. Foellmer and A. Helenius (1995). Glucose trimming and reglucosylation determine glycoporein association with calnexin in the endoplasmic reticulum. *Cell.* 81: 425-433.
21. Heo, D. S., J. Park, K. Hata, et al. (1990) Evaluation of tetrazolium based semiautomatic colorimetric assay for measurement of human anti-tumor cytotoxicity. *Can Res.* 50: 3681-3690.
22. Hoofnagle, J. H. and Di Bisceglie, A. M. (1997). The treatment of chrnoic viral hepatitis. *New Engl. J. Med.* 336: 347-356.
23. Houghton, M., Han, J., Kuo, G., Choo, Q.-L., and Weiner, A. J. (1993) The relationship between HCV and the flaviviradae family. Pp 229-237. In *Viral Hepatitis, scientific basis and clinical management,* Zuckerman, A. J. and Thomas, H.C. Eds.) Churchill Livingston, London, UK
24. Huovila, A. P., A. Eder and S. Fuller (1992) Hepatitis B surface antigen assembles in a post ER, pre golgi compartment. *J. Cell Biol.* 118: 1305-1320.
25. Jansen. R. W., L. C. Johnson and D. R. Averett (1993) High capacity *in vitro* assessment of anti-hepatitis B virus compound selectivity by a virion specific polymerase chain reaction. *Antimicro Agent Chemo.* 37: 441-447.
26. Kim, P. S. and P. Arvin (1995) Calnexin and BiP as sequential molecular chaperones during thyroglobulin folding in the endoplasmic reticulum. *J. Cell Biol.* 128: 29-38.
27. Locarnini, S. and C. Birch (1999) Antiviral chemotherapy for chronic hepatitis B infection: lessons learned from treating HIV infected patients. *J. Hepatology* March, 536-547.
28. Lodish, H., A. Kong (1984). Glucose removal from N linked oligosacchairdes is required for efficient maturation of certain secretory glycoproteins from the rough endoplasmic reticulim to the Golgi compartment. *J. Cell. Biol.* 98: 1720-1729.
29. Lu, X., Mehta, A., Dwek, R., Butters, T. and Block, T. (1995) Evidence that N glycosylation is necessary for the secretion of hepatitis B virus *Virology* 213, 660-665
30. Lubas, W.A., Spiro, R.G. (1988). Evaluation of the role of rat liver golgi endo alpha mannosidase in processing N linked oligosaccharides. *J. Biol. Chem.* 263: 3990-3998.
31. Mehta, A., Lu, X., Block, T. M., Blumberg, B. S. and Dwek, R. A. (1997) Similar glycoproteins with drastically different sensities to glycosylation processing *Proc. Natl. Acad. Sci. USA* 94, 1822-1827
32. Mehta, A., Zitzmann, N., Rudd, P. M., Block, T. M. and Dwek, R. A. (1998) α-Glucosidase inhibitors as potential broad based antiviral agents. *FEBS Letters* 430, 17-22
33. Meunier, J., Fournillier, A., Choukhi, A., Cocquerel, L., Dubuisson, J., Wychowski, C. (1999) Analysis of the glycosylation sites of hepatitis C (HCV) glycoprotein E1 and the influence of E1 glycans on the formation of the HCV glycoprotein complex. *Journal of General Virology* 80, 887-896.
34. Miller, R. H. and Purcell, R. H. (1990) Hepatitis C virus shares amino acid sequence similarity with pestiviruses and flavi viruses as well as members of two plant virus sub groups. *Proc. Natl. Acad. Sci. USA* 87, 2057-2061

34a. Moore, S. E. and R. G. Spiro (1993) Inhibition of glucose trimming by castanospermine results in rapid degradation of unassembled major histocompatibility complex class I molecules. J. Biol. Chem. 268(6): 3809-3812.

35. Ou, W. J., P. H. Cameron, D. Y. Thomas and J. J. M. Bergeron (1993) Association of folding intermediates

of glycoproteins with calnexin. *Nature.* 364: 771-776.

36. Parent, B., T-K. Yeo and K. Olden (1986). Differential effects of 1-deoxynojirimycin on the intracellular transport of secretory glycoproteins in human hepatoma cells in culture. *Mol. Cell. Biochem.* 72: 21-33.
37. Patzer, E., Nakamura, G., Yaffe, A., Intracellular transport and secretion of hepatitis B surface antigen in mammalian cells. (1984), *J. Virol.* 51: 346-353
38. Patzer, E.J., Nakamura, G.R., Simonsen, G.C., Levinson, A.L., Brands, R.(1986), Intracellular packaging and assembly of hepatitis b surface antigen particles occurs in the endoplasmic reticulim. *J. Virol.* 58: 884-892
39. Platt F. G. Nieses, R. Dwek, T. Butters, (1994), NB-DNJ is a novel inhibitor of glycolipid biosynthesis, *J. Biol. Chem.* 269: 8362-8365
40. Rudd, P. M. and Dwek, R. A. (1997) Glycosylation: heterogeneity and the 3 dimensional structure of proteins. *Critical Reviews in Biochemistry and Molecular Biology* 32, 1-100
41. Sells, M. A., Chen, M. L. and Acs, G. (1987) Production of hepatitis b virus particles in Hep G2 cells transfected with cloned hepatitis b virus DNA. *Proc. Natl. Acad. Sci. USA* 84, 1005-9
42. Schang, L., M., J.Phillips, and P.A. Schaffer, (1998) Requirement of cellular cyclin-dependent kinases in herpes simplex virus replication and transcription. *Journal of Virology* 72, 5626-5637.
43. Stanley, P. (1984) Glycosylation mutants of animal cells. *Ann. Rev. Gen.* 18: 525-552.
44. Tennant, B., B. Baldwin, W. Hornbuckle, B. Korba, P. J. Cote and J. Gerin (1997) Animal models in the preclinical assessment of therapy for viral hepatitis. *Antiviral Thera.* 1 (Suppl) 4: 47-52.
45. Werr, M. and Prange, R. (1998) Role for calnexin and N-linked glycosylation in the assembly and secretion of hepatitis B virus middle envelope protein particles. *Journal of Virology* 72, 778-782
46. Wickner, S., Mauizi, M. R. and Gottesman (1999) Post translational quality control: folding, refolding and degrading proteins. *Science* 286: 1888-1893.
47. Zitzmann, N., A. Mehta, B. Blumberg, R. Dwek and T. M. Block (1999) Imino sugars inhibit the formation and secretion of BVDV, a pestivirus model of hepatitis C virus. *Proc. Natl. Acad. Sci.* 96: 11878-11882).

Nuclease resistant ribozymes directed against hepatitis C virus RNA plus and minus strand inhibit viral replication of a HCV/poliovirus chimera

L.M. BLATT, K.L JENSEN, L. BELLON, S.F. JAMISON, P.A. PAVCO and D.G. MACEJAK

Ribozyme Pharmaceuticals, Inc., 2950 Wilderness Place, Boulder, CO 80301

Abstract

Ribozymes are enzymatic RNA molecules that can be engineered to cleave specifically a target RNA sequence and are thus applicable to targeting viral RNA as a means to inhibit viral replication. We have chemically modified ribozymes to yield molecules that retain catalytic cleavage activity but are stabilized to nuclease degradation, and we have designed such ribozymes to target and cleave the highly conserved 5'-UTR of the HCV genome. This region of HCV RNA forms an internal ribosome entry site (IRES) that is required for efficient translation of the HCV polyprotein. Ribozymes targeting the HCV RNA plus strand as well as the minus strand were synthesized. To test the antiviral activity of the stabilized ribozymes, a plaque assay was implemented using an HCV/poliovirus (HCV/PV) chimera in which the HCV IRES directs translation of the poliovirus polypeptide. Treatment with ribozymes targeting the HCV RNA plus strand (sites 165, 195, 196, 282, 306, or 330) demonstrated significant inhibition of replication of the chimeric HCV/PV (>70-90%, $p < 0.01$). Likewise, treatment with ribozymes targeting the HCV RNA minus strand (sites -161, -170, -199, or -297) also resulted in a significant inhibition of replication of the chimeric HCV/PV (>70-90%, $p < 0.01$). To investigate potential effects of simultaneously targeting the plus and minus strands, dose-response curves of combination treatments were analyzed using the HCV/PV system. The combination studies demonstrated an additive effect of the ribozymes targeting the plus and minus HCV RNA strands that was linear over a dose range from 0-to-200 nM concentrations. A specific ribozyme mechanism of action was demonstrated by the lack of inhibitory effects on HCV/PV replication using either a scrambled binding arm attenuated control (SAC: tests for nonspecific activity of nucleotide content) or a binding arm attenuated control (BAC: tests for binding arm effects). These studies indicate that synthetic stabilized ribozymes directed against plus or minus strand HCV RNA demonstrate potent antiviral activity and have the potential to be effective therapeutic agents for the treatment of chronic hepatitis C.

Frontiers in Viral Hepatitis Ed. by RF Schinazi, J-P Sommadossi and CM Rice. 315 — 323

Hepatitis C virus (HCV) is an enveloped, plus-strand RNA virus of the genus Flaviviridae [1, 2]. HCV is an important pathogen worldwide, infecting over 150 million people [3]. Chronic infection with HCV can result in cirrhosis, liver failure and hepatocellular carcinoma [4, 5]. There is no vaccine for HCV, and current treatment with interferon and ribavirin is ineffective in a large percentage of patients [6, 7]. Interferon therapy is also associated with unpleasant side effects such as fever, diarrhea, lethargy and malaise [6, 7]. The poor growth of the virus in cell culture and the lack of an appropriate small animal model, however, have hampered development of new therapies.

We have circumvented this limitation by utilizing a chimeric poliovirus (PV) that contains the HCV RNA internal ribosome entry site (IRES) in place of the poliovirus IRES [8]. This chimeric HCV/PV replicates efficiently in cell culture and is dependent upon the HCV IRES. The IRES is required for translation of the viral polyprotein by a cap-independent mechanism [9, 10]. The 5' untranslated region (UTR) of HCV RNA that contributes to the IRES is highly conserved in sequence among HCV genotypes [11], and thus makes an excellent target for a ribozyme therapeutic.

Ribozymes are catalytic RNA molecules that can be designed to cleave a specific RNA sequence. We have designed a number of ribozymes to cleave specific sites in the HCV 5'UTR and its complementary minus-strand sequence. To determine if any of these sites are accessible to ribozyme cleavage during viral replication within the cellular milieu, we screened these ribozymes for the ability to inhibit replication of the HCV/PV chimera in cells in culture.

Materials and methods

Cells and virus

HeLa cells were maintained in DMEM (Gibco BRL, Grand Island, NY) supplemented with 5% fetal bovine serum. A cloned DNA copy of the HCV-PV chimeric virus was a gift of Dr. Eckard Wimmer (NYU, Stony Brook, NY). An RNA version was then generated by *in vitro* transcription and transfected into HeLa cells to produce infectious virus.

Ribozyme synthesis

Nuclease resistant ribozymes and control oligonucleotides containing 2'-*O*-methyl-nucleotides, 2'-deoxy-2'-*C*-allyl uridine, a 3'-inverted abasic cap, and phosphorothioate linkages were synthesized as described [12, 13]. Ribozymes targeting cleavage of the 5'UTR of HCV genotype 1b and controls were described previously [14]. Attenuated core controls have nucleotide changes in the core sequence that greatly diminish the ribozyme's cleavage activity. The attenuated controls either contain scrambled binding arms (referred to as SAC) or maintain binding arms (BAC) capable of binding to the mRNA target. Ribozymes targeting the minus strand have the catalytic core shown in Figure 1 and have seven nucleotide binding arms that allow base-pairing to the minus strand at the designated cleavage site.

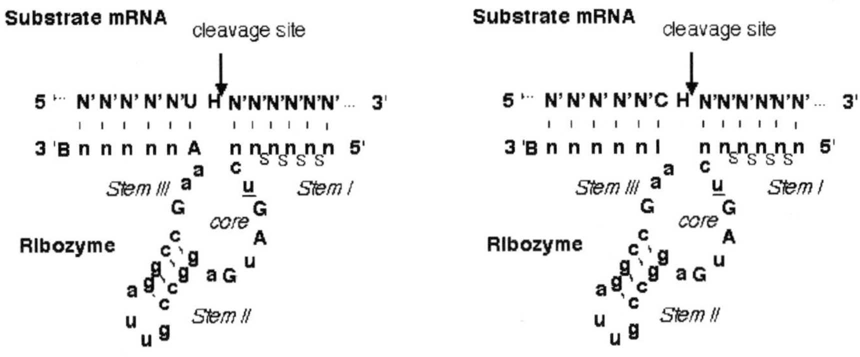

Figure 1. Ribozyme motifs. Ribozymes targeting UH (left panel) or CH (right panel) cleavage sites are shown base-paired to their target. Modifications are denoted as follows: upper case, ribonucleotide; lower case, 2'-*O*-methyl-nucleotide; s, phosphorothioate linkage; B, inverted 3'-3' deoxy-abasic; u̲, 2'-deoxy-2'-*C*-allyl-uridine; I, inosine; H = A, C, or U.

Ribozyme delivery

The use of lipid cytofectin, RPI.9778, was described previously [14]. HeLa cells were seeded in 96-well plates at a density of 9000-10,000 cells/well and incubated at 37°C under 5% CO_2 for 24 hours. Transfection of ribozyme or control oligonucleotides (200 nM) was achieved by mixing 10X ribozyme or control oligonucleotides (2000 nM) with 10X RPI.9778 (80 µg/ml) in DMEM (Gibco BRL) containing 5% fetal bovine serum (FBS) in U-bottom 96-well plates to make 5X complexes. Ribozyme/lipid complexes were allowed to incubate for 15 min at 37°C under 5% CO_2. Medium was aspirated from cells and replaced with 80 µl of DMEM (Gibco BRL) containing 5% FBS, followed by the addition of 20 µl of 5X complexes. Cells were incubated with complexes for 24 hours at 37°C under 5% CO_2. All experiments were repeated at least twice, and results reported were reproducible. After 24 hours, cells were lysed to release virus by three cycles of freeze/thaw. Virus was quantified by plaque assay. Viral yield is shown as mean plaque-forming units per ml (pfu/ml) + SEM. P values were determined by the Student's *t* test.

Plaque assay

Virus samples were diluted in serum-free DMEM (Gibco BRL) and 100 µl applied to Vero cell monolayers (~80% confluent) in 6-well plates for 30 minutes. Infected monolayers were overlaid with 3 ml 1.2% agar (Sigma) and incubated at 37°C under 5% CO_2. When plaques were visible (after two to three days) the overlay was removed, monolayers were stained with 1.2% crystal violet, and plaque-forming units were counted.

Results

We synthesized ribozymes targeting 15 UH (H = A, C, or U) sites in the HCV 5' UTR. These ribozymes contained chemical modifications to inhibit RNase digestion but retain cleavage activity of the ribozyme (Figure 1). In addition, we synthesized ribozymes targeting either UH or CH sites in the minus strand. The UH and CH ribozyme motifs are shown in Figure 1.

In order to examine the efficacy of ribozymes targeting the HCV 5'UTR in a replicating viral system, we employed an HCV/poliovirus (PV) chimera that contains the HCV IRES in place of the PV IRES [8]. This chimera replicates efficiently in HeLa cells, but is dependent upon the HCV IRES for translation. Cleavage of the HCV IRES could inhibit either translation and/or replication of full-length HCV/PV RNA. HeLa cells infected with HCV/PV were treated with various ribozymes targeting the HCV 5'UTR. After 24 hours, treated cells were lysed by three cycles of freeze/thaw to release virus, and infectious virus was quantified by plaque assay.

As shown in Figure 2A, treatment with ribozymes targeting the HCV RNA plus strand (sites 165, 195, 196, 282, 306, and 330) demonstrated significant inhibition of replication of the chimeric HCV-poliovirus (>70-90%, $p < 0.01$) compared to cells treated with a nonspecific control (SAC). In order to characterize the nature of inhibition due to the ribozyme molecule, ribozymes to two sites (195 and 330) were chosen for further study. A paired SAC was designed for each ribozyme. The SAC cannot bind to the target site due to the scrambled binding arm sequence, but contains the same base composition as the active ribozyme molecule. Treatment with ribozyme to site 195 significantly inhibited viral replication (Figure 2B) compared to paired SAC-treated cells, as we have previously reported [14]. In this experiment ribozyme to site 330 was not as efficacious as the site 195 ribozyme (Figure 2B). The paired SAC for site 330 did not inhibit viral replication and behaved similarly to the site 195 SAC (Figure 2B).

To confirm that a ribozyme catalytic mechanism was required for inhibition, we tested a binding competent, attenuated control (BAC) specific for site 195. The BAC retains the ability to bind to the same site as the ribozyme but contains two base changes in the catalytic core that greatly attenuate cleavage activity. As shown in Figure 2B, the BAC to site 195 did not inhibit HCV/PV replication, thus confirming that binding alone was not responsible for the inhibition observed.

We also screened ribozymes targeting a number of sites in the minus strand complementary to the 5'UTR (Figure 3). We assigned site numbering to the minus strand based on the plus strand. For example, ribozyme targeting site -96 cleaves the minus strand 3' of the nucleotide complementary to nucleotide 96 in the plus strand. In other words, site -97 is 97 nucleotides upstream from the 3' end of the minus strand. Cleavage of the minus strand would be expected to reduce RNA replicative intermediates and inhibit synthesis of nascent viral RNA plus strands. As shown in Figure 3, treatment with ribozymes targeting the HCV RNA minus strand at several UH sites (-161 or -297) and CH sites (-170 or -199) also resulted in a significant inhibition of HCV/PV replication (>70-90%, $p < 0.01$) compared to treatment with a general SAC. For comparison, treatment with ribozyme to site 195 of the plus strand is also shown.

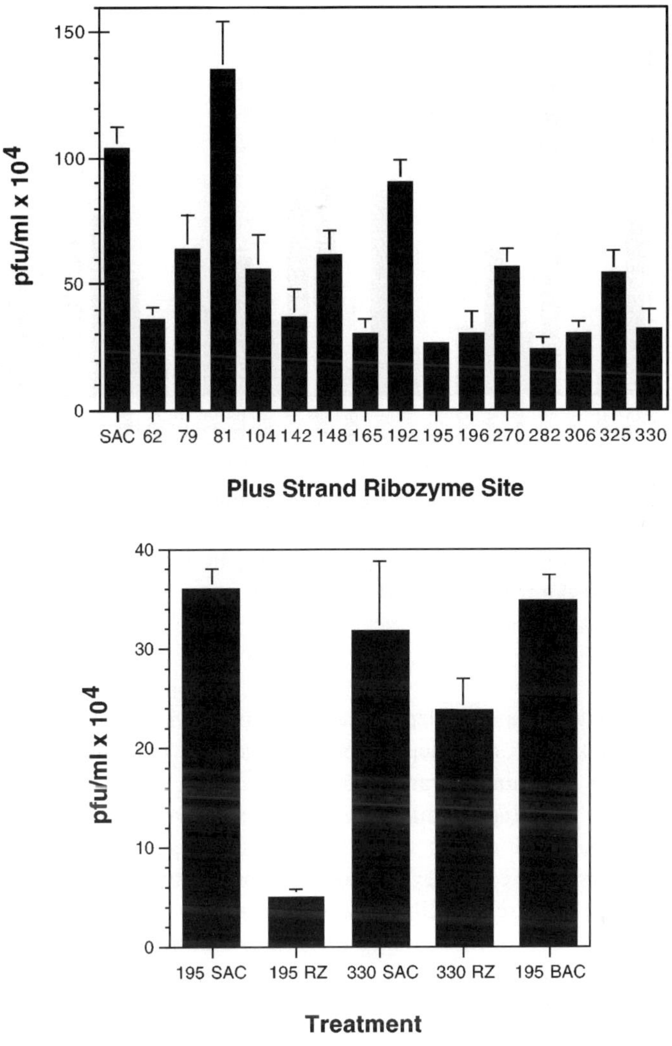

Figure 2. Inhibition of HCV/PV replication by ribozymes targeting HCV RNA plus strand. A) Ribozyme screen. B) Ribozyme inhibition is sequence dependent and requires the catalytic core. Plaque-forming units (pfu) ± SEM are shown from cells treated with ribozyme to the site as indicated. SAC, scrambled attenuated control. BAC, binding attenuated core control.

In order to demonstrate a dose-dependent inhibitory effect of a ribozyme targeting the plus or minus strand, we treated HCV/PV-infected cells with increasing doses of ribozyme targeting site +195 (Figure 4A). To maintain the same transfection conditions across the dose response, we mixed the active ribozyme with an SAC to achieve a total oligonucleotide concentration of 200 nM in order to keep the same total nucleic acid-to-lipid charge ratio in each transfection. Treatment with increasing doses of site

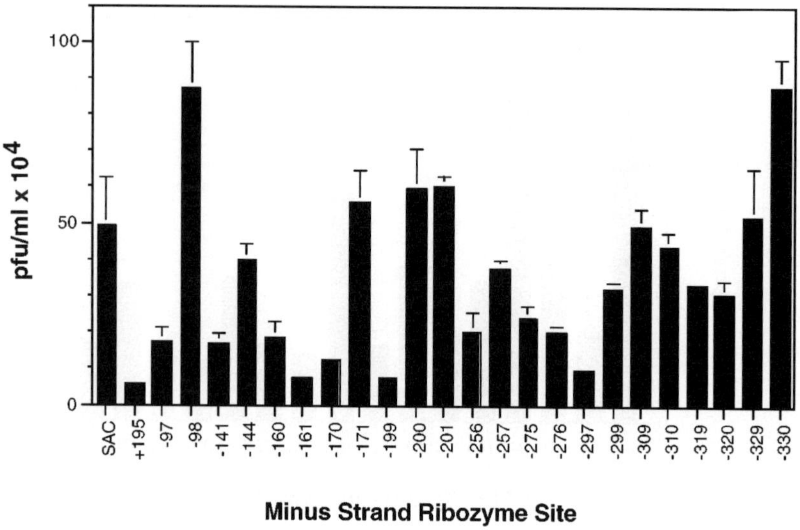

Figure 3. Inhibition of HCV/PV replication by ribozymes targeting HCV RNA minus strand. Plaque-forming units (pfu) ± SEM are shown from cells treated with ribozyme to the site as indicated. SAC, scrambled attenuated control. +195 targets plus strand.

+195 ribozyme resulted in a dose-dependent inhibition of viral replication (Figure 4A). We also observed similar dose-dependent inhibition in treatment with efficacious ribozymes targeting the minus strand. An example of a dose response with a less efficacious ribozyme targeting the minus (site -256) is shown in Figure 4B.

To investigate potential effects of simultaneously targeting the plus and minus strands, dose-response curves of several combination treatments were analyzed using the HCV/PV system (Figure 5). Ribozyme targeting site 195 of the plus strand was mixed at different doses with ribozyme targeting a site in the minus strand to maintain a total ribozyme dose of 200 nM. As a control, ribozyme to site 195 was mixed with ribozyme targeting site -330 of the minus strand, a ribozyme observed not to be efficacious when given alone (Figure 3). The dose response of this combination is similar to that of site 195 mixed with a paired SAC (Figure 4A). In this experiment, the other ribozymes targeting the minus strand significantly inhibit HCV/PV replication (>95%, $p < 0.01$) when given alone (0 nM site 195 ribozyme points in Figure 5), as does ribozyme to site 195 alone (200 nM dose in Figure 5). The transitional combinations of the ribozymes targeting the plus and minus HCV RNA strands appear to generate an intermediate effect over a dose range from 0-to-200 nM concentrations.

Discussion

Development of new therapies for patients with chronic HCV has been hampered by the poor growth of HCV in cell culture. This limitation could be circumvented by using

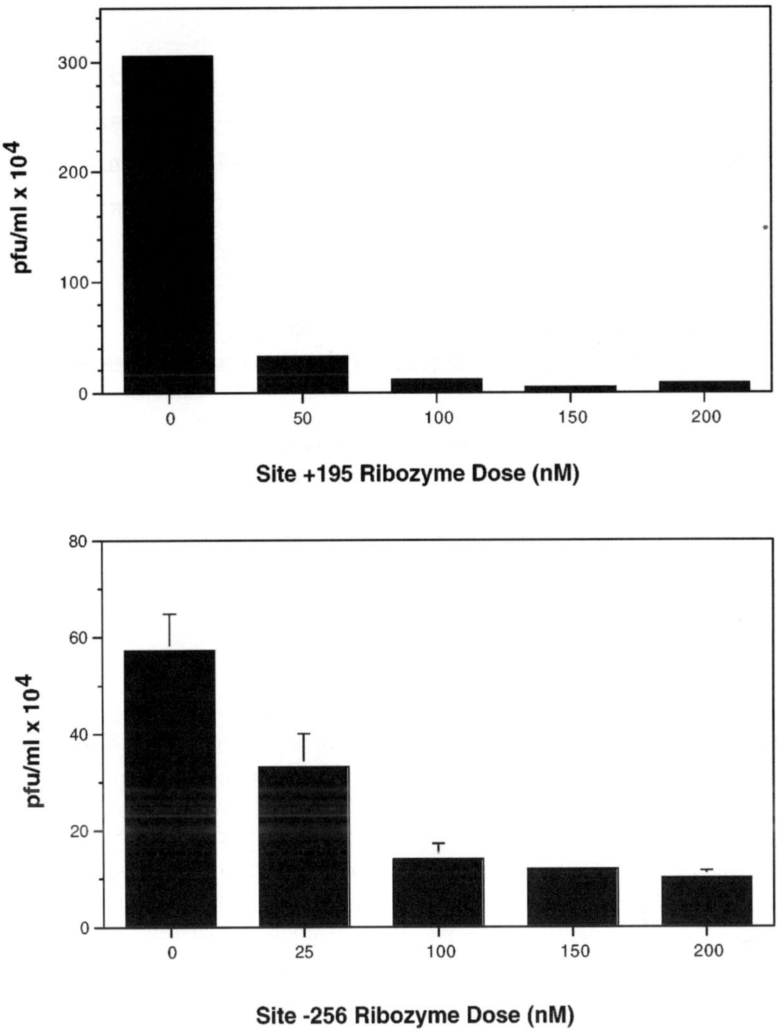

Figure 4. Ribozyme dose response. A) Ribozyme to site 195 of plus strand. B) Ribozyme to site -255 of minus strand. Plaque-forming units (pfu) ± SEM are shown from cells treated with the dose of ribozyme to the site as indicated. Active ribozyme was mixed with SAC to maintain a total dose of 200 nM.

a HCV/PV chimera that replicates efficiently in cell culture, but is dependent upon the HCV IRES [8]. Both HCV and PV are plus-strand RNA viruses that replicate in the cytoplasm of infected cells, and thus have analogous steps in their life cycles. The sequence of the HCV IRES is highly conserved among the various HCV genotypes [11], and therefore makes an excellent target for ribozyme therapy.

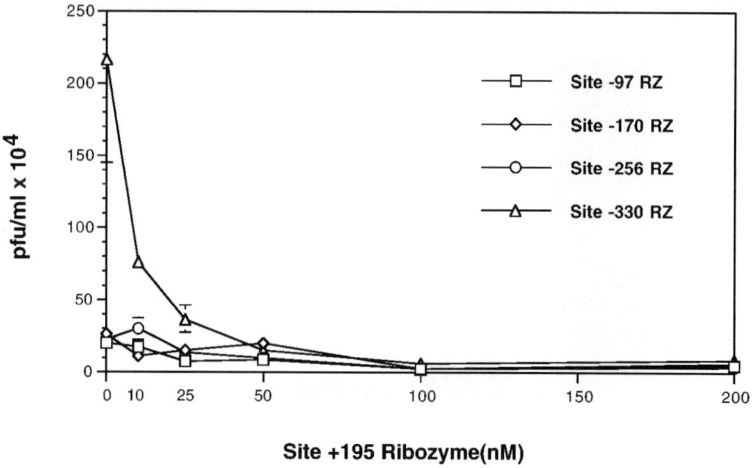

Figure 5. Combination treatment with ribozymes targeting plus and minus strand. Plaque-forming units (pfu) ± SEM are shown from cells treated with dose of ribozyme to site 195 of plus strand, as indicated. Ribozyme to site 195 was mixed with ribozymes to the minus strand, as shown, to maintain total dose of 200 nM.

Because there may be only a limited number of RNA sites accessible for targeting within cells due to RNA secondary structure or protein binding, we have screened ribozymes to a number of sites in the HCV 5'UTR and its complementary minus strand sequence. Treatment with ribozymes targeting sites 165, 195, 196, 282, 306, or 330 of the plus strand of HCV RNA or -161, -170, -199, and -297 of the complementary region in the minus strand significantly inhibited replication of the HCV/PV chimera. The level of inhibition for ribozymes targeting the plus or minus strand were similar, although the ribozyme targeting site 195 in the plus strand was consistently the most efficacious.

As previously reported [14] and shown in Figure 2B, the inhibition in viral replication by treatment with ribozyme to site 195 required a catalytic mechanism, since a catalytically attenuated ribozyme that maintained base-pairing did not inhibit viral replication. In addition, the inhibition due to treatment with ribozymes targeting the plus or minus strand was dose-dependent. Combination treatment with a ribozyme targeting the plus strand (site +195) and ribozymes targeting the minus strand appeared to give an intermediate level of inhibition. The potent antiviral activity of synthetic, stabilized ribozymes directed against the plus or minus strand of HCV RNA, as demonstrated here, support their potential to be effective therapeutic agents for the treatment of chronic hepatitis C.

Acknowledgements

We are grateful to Dr. Eckard Wimmer for supplying the HCV chimera, to Dr. Jim McSwiggen for bioinformatics and ribozyme design, and to Victor Mokler for synthesis of the ribozymes described.

References

1. Choo, Q.L., Kuo G., Weiner A.J., Overby L.R., Bradley D.W. and Houghton M. (1989). Isolation of a cDNA clone derived from a blood-borne non-A, non-B viral hepatitis genome. Science 244, 359-362.
2. Houghton, M., Weiner A., Han J., Kuo G. and Choo Q.-L. (1991). Molecular biology of the hepatitis C viruses: implications for diagnosis, development and control of viral diseases. Hepatology 14, 381-388.
3. Hoofnagle, J. (1997). Hepatitis C: The Clinical Spectrum of Disease. Hepatology 26, 15S-20S.
4. Tong, M.J., el-Farra N.S., Reikes A.R. and Co R.L. (1995). Clinical outcomes after transfusion-associated hepatitis C. New Engl. J. Med. 332, 1463-1466.
5. Sherlock, S. (1992). Viral hepatitis. Lancet 339, 802.
6. McHutchison, J.G., Gordon S.C., Schiff E.R., Shiffman M.L., Lee W.M., Rustgi V.K., Goodman Z.D., Ling M.H., Cort S. and Albrecht J.K. (1998). Interferon alpha-2b alone or in combination with ribavirin as initial treatment for chronic hepatitis C. New Engl. J. Med. 339, 1485-1492.
7. Poynard, T., Marcellin P., Lee S.S., Niedrau C., Minuk G.S., Ideo G., Bain V., Heathcote J., Zeuzem S., Trepo C. and Albrecht J. (1998). Randomized trial of interferon alpha2b plus ribavirin for 48 weeks or for 24 weeks versus interferon alpha2b plus placebo for 48 weeks for treatment of chronic infection with hepatitis C virus. Lancet 352, 1426-1432.
8. Lu, H.-H. and Wimmer E. (1996). Poliovirus chimeras replicating under the translational control of genetic elements of hepatitis C virus reveal unusual properties of the internal ribosomal entry site of hepatitis C virus. Proc. Natl. Acad. Sci. USA 93, 1412-1417.
9. Tsukiyama-Kohara, K., Iizuka N., Kohara M. and Nomoto A. (1992). Internal ribosome entry sites within hepatitis C virus RNA. J. Virol. 66, 1476-1483.
10. Wang, C., Sarnow P. and Siddiqui A. (1993). Translation of Human Hepatitis C Virus RNA in Cultured Cells is Mediated by an Internal Ribosome-Binding Mechanism. J. Virol. 67, 3338-3344.
11. Bukh, J., Purcell R.H. and Miller R.H. (1992). Sequence analysis of the 5' noncoding region of hepatitis C virus. Proc. Natl. Acad. Sci. USA 89, 4942-4946.
12. Beigelman, L., McSwiggen J.A., Draper K.G., Gonzalez C., Jensen K., Karpeisky A.M., Modak A.S., Matulic-Adamic J., DiRenzo A.B. and al. e. (1995). Chemical modification of hammerhead ribozymes. Catalytic activity and nuclease resistance. J. Biol. Chem. 270, 25702-25708.
13. Wincott, F., DiRenzo A., Shaffer C., Grimm S., Tracz D., Workman C., Sweedler D., Gonzalez C., Scaringe S. and Usman N. (1995). Synthesis, deprotection, analysis and purification of RNA and ribozymes. Nucleic Acids Res. 23, 2677-2684.
14. Macejak, D.G., Jensen K.L., Jamison S.F., Domenico K., Roberts E.C., Chaudhary N., von Carlowitz I., Bellon L., Tong M.J., Conrad A., Pavco P.A. and Blatt L.M. (2000). Inhibition of HCV RNA-dependent translation and replication of a chimeric HCV-poliovirus using synthetic stabilized ribozymes. Hepatology 769-776.

Mechanism of laser therapy of viral hepatitis

VICTOR OVSIANNIKOV

D. V. Efremov Scientific Research Institute of Electrophysical Apparatus, Saint Petersburg, Russia

The results of six-years' investigation in low-energy laser therapy for viral hepatitis are presented. A special infrared laser was used for this purpose. It was determined that laser therapy in combination with basic and detoxification therapies accelerated the recovery of patients and increased the quality of treatment. Different schemes for application of the laser were used for the treatment of patients with hepatitis B and hepatitis C virus. The safety of laser therapy was examined and, the mechanism of therapeutic effect was proposed based upon clinical observations and laboratory examinations. It was shown that the application of the laser action to the body led to activation (or stimulation) of adaptation reactions in the body: to normalization of peroxide oxidation of lipids, to normalization of immune system activity and, to activation of the blood production system. Laser therapy of viral hepatitis increases the quality of treatment, and there were no apparent relapses of diseases.

Introduction

Laser therapy of viral hepatitis has been used in St. Petersburg since 1993. It was proposed based on our clinical experience in laser treatment of some skin diseases [1] and some postoperative complications in oncology patients [2, 3], on investigation of laser activity on viruses in culture [4], on our theoretical notion about the mechanism of carcinogenesis [5-7] and interaction of laser radiation with tissue [1]. The parameters of laser radiation were determined from such observations as therapeutic effect, absence of negative side effects.

A special infrared laser with wavelength 890 nm was developed. It works in a periodic-pulse mode with an average power of 10-60 mW. It is easily transportable and can be operated by trained medical workers.

Method

The method of laser therapy for viral hepatitis involves the laser irradiation of blood in cubital veins, liver and thymus (breast-bone area) [8]. All laser actions are produced transcutaneously without any tissue heating. Calculations show that the temperature of

Frontiers in Viral Hepatitis Ed. by RF Schinazi, J-P Sommadossi and CM Rice. 325 — 331

tissue will not increase more than 1° C. The patients did not report feeling any heating during the period of laser treatment.

Investigations into the efficiency of laser therapy for viral hepatitis were conducted in the infectious clinics of two Medical Academies of St. Petersburg [9, 10]. The clinical observations (including general condition, intoxication, jaundice, hepatomegalia) and biochemical testing [including bilirubin levels (determined by Inderassik et al. method), choletelin (determined by Ilca method), β-lipoprotein (determined by Burstern and Samaill method), alaminotransferase (ALT) (determined by Reitman and Franckel method), Sublimate titer (determined by Greensted method), cell immunity of CD-cells (determined by Bach method)] were determined. Ultrasonic investigations of liver, gallbladder, pancreas and spleen were also conducted. The level of the anti-oxidation defense system was determined by measuring the concentration of thiol groups SH and SS in serum, by determining the ratio SH/SS, and by determining the intensity of free radical oxidation. The last was investigated by the method of inductance chemiluminescence of cells and serum.

Clinical efficiency of laser therapy

In the first stage of our investigations, we specified parameters of laser activity and checked the efficiency of laser therapy (conducted by T. Sologub and N. Pustasheva). In the second stage, the efficiency of laser treatment for different forms and stages of viral hepatitis as well as the cell or humoral mechanisms of the therapeutic effect of laser treatment were determined (conducted by N. Kuznetsov and O. Masterova).

Laser therapy was proposed to patients who had clear symptoms of hyperfermentemia, changes in biochemical indexes, presence of markers of viral hepatitis HBsAg, HBeAg, anti-HBV core antibody, anti-HCV, and absence of markers for hepatitis A virus (anti-HAVgGM) or hepatitis delta virus (anti-HDV).

Laser treatment was applied against a background of basic and detoxification therapies. In the first stage of investigation (64 patients: 21 women and 43 men; 56 patients with acute viral hepatitis B and C, six patients with chronic viral hepatitis C, two patients with chronic viral hepatitis B with cirrhosis), it was shown that laser therapy led to positive results in acute and chronic forms of disease, but was ineffective in patients with chronic viral hepatitis with cirrhosis [9].

Laser therapy was prescribed to patients after five to seven days in clinic. Most of these (75%) were in the main period of disease, and 25% were in the period of early convalescence (with persistent hyperfermentemia).

In the subsequent studies laser therapy was prescribed for all patients during the main period of disease. Identical groups of 20 patients (identical in sex, age, type of hepatitis) were used as control groups. They received the traditional treatment without any laser treatment. The course of laser therapy took five to ten days. All patients tolerated it very well, without any subjective (reported) complaints or objective complications.

The general clinical condition of patients improved after two to four days of laser therapy. Symptoms of skin intoxication, skin itch and pain in the right hypochondrium vanished, and dimensions of the liver decreased. The symptom of intoxication in laser patients vanished four to five days earlier than in patients in the control group, and their recovery was five to seven days earlier.

The laboratory examinations showed that positive changes of all biochemical indices took place after five courses of laser therapy (on average). Examples of improvement of the general condition of patients are shown in Table 1.

Table 1. Clinical observations in patients with acute viral hepatitis B

	Control group, days	Laser group, days
Duration of the symptom "General weakness"	13 ± 2	10 ± 1
Duration of the symptom "Lowering appetite"	13 ± 1	9 ± 1
Duration of jaundice	35 ± 2	29 ± 3
Duration of hepatomegalia period	38 ± 2	33 ± 3

The biochemical examinations of these patients at different stages of disease are shown in the Table 2.

Table 2. Biochemical examinations of patients with acute viral hepatitis B

	Bilirubin	μmole/l.h	ALT	Un/l	Thymol probe un	
Period of disease	Control group	Laser group	Control group	Laser group	Control group	Laser group
Main stage	239 ± 10	244 ± 10	1440 ± 20	1512.± 60	10 ± 1	10 ± 1
Jaundice period	143 ± 10	123 ± 10	840 ± 40	780 ± 30	9 ± 0.5	8.0 ± 0.5
Early convalescence	54 ± 5	36.4 ± 3.5	512 ± 36	504 ± 30	7 ± 1	7 ± 0.5
Convalescence	24 ± 2	17 ± 1	116 ± 24	112 ±13	7 ± 0.5	7 ± 05

All data from the biochemical examinations of patients from the laser group indicated a faster improvement than in the control group. The time to normalization of these parameters was shorter in the laser group.

The efficiency of laser therapy for patients with lingering forms of disease was investigated in the group of 50 patients with the acute form of viral hepatitis B (30 patients in the laser group and 20 patients in the control group). The bilirubin amount after the course of laser therapy was 17.2 ± 0.66 μmole/l.h in the laser group and 24 ± 2.4 μmole/l.h in the control group at the same time. The time to normalization was 52.5 ± 2.4 days in the laser group and 58.3 ± 2.4 days in the control group.

The investigation of thiol groups showed that concentration of the SH group in serum after the laser treatment increased 25%-30%, and the ratio of SH/SS concentrations increased from one up to four.

The investigation of the free radical oxidation processes by the method of inductance chemoluminescence of cells and serum led us to conclude that intensity of these processes in the blood of patients in the laser group was 30% less than in the control group. These results indicated an increased nonspecific resistance.

The investigation of immune status of patients was conducted in a group of 60 patients (30 — laser group and 30 — control group). After the course of laser therapy, CD-3 increased from 866 un. to 1238 un.; CD-4 increased from 546 un. to 781 un.

The laser treatment of patients with viral hepatitis C was carried out using different protocols in the two different clinics, resulting in different results. Patients in the first clinic (31 patients laser group and 20 patients control group) received the laser irradiation of liver, blood and thymus-breastbone. Laser treatment produced positive results in this group. Patients in the second clinic (20 patients laser group and 20 patients control group) received the laser irradiation of liver and blood in cubetal veins only. Laser therapy in this group led to apparent positive results, but the differences from the control patients were not statistically significant.

We know that the replication of HCV takes place in different organs, and this leads to damage in the different tissues. Therefore, the stimulation of the whole immune system is needed for the successful treatment of this disease. Irradiation of blood and liver is not enough for this purpose. The first protocol of laser treatment produced an improvement in the overall immune status of the patients and led to positive results in the treatment of HCV.

It is clear that the results of laser therapy depended on the stage of disease. We had the laser group of 48 patients: 20 patients with acute forms of hepatitis (eight — hepatitis B, 12 — hepatitis C) and 28 patients with chronic forms of hepatitis (nine — hepatitis B, 19 — hepatitis C). Statistically significant results (reduction of jaundice period and cytolytic period) were obtained in 83% of patients with acute hepatitis and in 68% of patients with chronic hepatitis.

The influence of laser treatment on the peroxide oxidation of lipids was investigated in a group of 150 patients with lingering forms of viral hepatitis B and C. For analysis purposes the patients were divided into two groups: the first with low indices of immune status (CD-3 — 866 ± 36 un., CD-4 — 546 ± 51 un., CD-8 — 308 ± 18 un.) before treatment, and the second with normal indices of immune status before treatment. Laser treatment led to increases in these indexes in the first group (CD-3 — 1238 ± 61 un., CD-4 — 781 ± 18 un., CD-8 — 501 ± 10 un.). In the second group these indices were lower at the beginning of treatment and increased to normal values in the period of early convalescence.

More than 300 patients with viral hepatitis have received laser treatment, and for most of them it gave positive results. We did not observe relapses of disease after laser therapy. All these results indicate that laser therapy can normalize a morphologic structure of live tissue and increase immune reactivity of the patient.

Mechanism of laser therapeutic action

For the purpose of discussion about the mechanism of laser therapeutic action, we take into account the results of laser treatment of HIV/AIDS patients [11-13].

There were several hypotheses about the primary action of low-energy laser radiation on a living tissue. They involved the effect of cell metabolism stimulation by activation of some cellular enzyme, conformation of intracellular fluid or biopolymers, activation of singlet oxygen, and temperature changes of cell membranes.

We suppose that laser radiation action on living cells can stimulate (normalize) the energy cycle of cells in cases in which they have been changed as a result of disease [1]. Some cellular molecules can receive the needed energy by means of absorption of laser radiation energy. If the cells have normal metabolic processes, the laser energy is dispersed in the tissue. The total laser energy is not enough for thermal action on tissue. This assumption can explain most of the phenomena of laser therapy. It helped us to calculate the parameters of laser radiation that were needed for irradiation of any patient area and permitted us to propose the appropriate protocol of laser treatment for the different stages and forms of viral hepatitis.

It is known that laser action on tissue can lead to increased microcirculation of blood in irradiated areas. The effect of increasing microcirculation can help to regenerate the damaged cells of the liver. At the same time, laser action on blood can lead to photo modification of the membranes of blood cells. It can lead to increased membrane permeability and to greater levels of biologically active substances in the blood stream, thereby affecting other organs, such as the adrenal gland.

Our analysis shows that by means of our special laser we could input enough laser energy for normalization of metabolism in blood, liver and bone marrow cells. This could lead to improved regeneration of liver cells, but only in the thin layer of liver.

Our investigation has shown that localized laser therapy could influence the immune and blood-production systems in patients [3]. During the laser irradiation of the thymus-breastbone, we could stimulate (normalize) the function of the thymus, which regulates many processes in the body. At the same time laser activity on the bone marrow cells could result in increasing the production of new, healthy blood cells, bone marrow being the source of new blood cells and the thymus being the site of lymphocyte maturation. We observed rapid positive changes in patients' blood and an improvement in their immune status.

Analysis of laser treatment of HIV/AIDS patients showed that normalization of blood components and immune status of patients takes place after a very short time — one course of laser therapy.

Investigation of the anti-oxidation defense system showed stimulation under laser therapy and normalization of the processes of peroxide oxidation of lipids. Perhaps this effect plays an important role in therapeutic efficacy of laser treatment. N. Kuznetsov and O. Masterova were the first who recognized this relationship.

We are not able to point out a single mechanism of therapeutic efficacy of laser treatment for viral hepatitis patients. Perhaps all the above-mentioned effects are present, and the real mechanism is as complex as the human organism itself. But now we can confirm that laser therapy can stimulate the defense mechanisms of the body, and that this leads to a shortening of the patient's recovery period, and to increasing the quality of life.

Innocuousness and safety of laser therapy

Laser therapy is a new and not widespread modality. Thus, questions of safety and tolerance are very important. We did not observe untoward effects or results from laser therapy in our protocols. The wavelength was chosen from the conditions of disposition of an object of irradiation. Visible radiation can be used for action at the skin's surface, or for superficial damage, but radiation near the infrared spectrum is more convenient for action under the skin, at the level of tissue or organs. Ultraviolet laser radiation cannot be recommended for therapy, because it can change the genetic properties of living cells [5]. Infrared laser radiation did not affect the genetic properties of cells, and using it is safe in this respect. Laser irradiation must produce therapeutic effects and should not heat tissue, so its power is limited from mW to $n \cdot 100$ mw. Some investigation has shown that at higher laser intensities, the suppression of cellular metabolism can occur.

Our research into laser effects on viruses *in vitro* has shown that virus infectivity remained unchanged under the low-energy laser radiation, if the initial virus activity was normal. Our practice of using laser treatment represents a new and different direction in the practice of medicine: infectious disease, surgery, oncology, neurology. Our results show that laser therapy does not lead to any negative side effects or any complications, provided the clinical application of lasers is made in conjunction with calculation of laser actions.

It ought to be mentioned that laser therapy methods can lead to negative results or to complications if used incorrectly. Therefore we are prepared to collaborate on international projects using laser treatment methods. We could visit foreign clinics for teaching and demonstrating laser treatment for such diseases as viral hepatitis or HIV.

Acknowledgments

The author acknowledges the Ministry of Atomic Energy of the Russian Federation for supporting his work.

References

1. Ovsiannikov VA and Krasavtseva LV. Application of Laser in the Practice of an Out-Patient Clinic. *Vestnik Khirurgii* V. 141, No. 7, p. 114-116, 1988.
2. Ovsiannikov VA, Barchuk AS, Gelfond ML. Quantum-Genetic Mechanism of Carcinogenesis and Laser Selective Action on Tumor. *Report of the XVI International Cancer Congress*, New-Delhi, India, 1994, Report Thesis v. 1, p.356.

3. Ovsiannikov VA. Analysis of the Low-Energy Laser Treatment of Some Cancer and Infectious Diseases. *Journal Clinical Laser Medicine & Surgery* V. 15, No. 1, p. 39-44, 1997.
4. Ovsiannikov VA and Shitikova GM. Laser Radiation Action on Viruses. *Perspective Directions of Laser Medicine* International Conference, Odessa, USSR, Report Thesis p. 361, 1992.
5. Ovsiannikov VA. Quantum-Genetic Theory of Carcinogenesis. Preprint NIIEFA K- 0646, Moscow, CNIIatominform, 1984.
6. Ovsiannikov VA. About Quantum-Genetic Theory of Carcinogenesis. Voprosy Oncologii V.32, No. 9, p. 72-74, 1986.
7. Ovsiannikov VA. About Possible Mechanism of Carcinogenesis and Laser Selective Action upon Metastases. Izvestiya Akad. Nauk USSR Ser. Phys. V. 52, No. 2, p. 312, 1988.
8. Ovsiannikov VA, Petrov IB, Pustashova NN, Sologub TV, Kuznetsov NI, Masterova OA. Laser Therapy of Viral Hepatitis. Laser & Technology V. 6, No. 3, p. 115-119, 1996.
9. Ovsiannikov VA, Kuznetsov NI, Masterova OA, Pustashova NN. Using laser treatment for viral hepatitis. — International Congress "Laser and Health - 99", Moscou, Russia, 1999. Report thesis p. 333.
10. Clinico-immunologic Substanationof Low-Energy Laser Radiation Using for Viral Hepatitis Treatment in Complex Therapies. Dissertation St Petersburg, 2000.
11. Ovsiannikov VA, Sizova NV, Maslov VP, Gnevasheva GI. The Treatment of HIV/AIDS Patients by Means of Laser Action. Report at XI Intern. Conference on AIDS, Vancouver, 1996, Report Thesis V. 2, p. 88.
12. Ovsiannikov VA, Sizova NV, Maslov VP, Gnevasheva GI. About Mechanism of Laser Treatment of HIV Patients. Report at IV Intern. Conference on AIDS, Manila, Philippines, 1997, Report Thesis p. 89.
13. Ovsiannikov VA, Sizova NV, Maslov VP, Rakhmanova AG. Efficiency of Laser Therapy for HIV-patients. — International Congress "Laser and Health - 99", Moscou, Russia, 1999. Report thesis p. 385.
14. Victor Ovsiannikov et al. Laser Therapy of Infectious Diseases: Results and Mechanism of therapeutic Action. -Proceeding of SPIE Vjlume 4606, Vol. 2, No. 35, p. 131 - 137.

DRUG DISCOVERY AND DEVELOPMENT: RESISTANCE AND THERAPEUTIC STRATEGIES IN HUMANS

Nomenclature for antiviral resistant human hepatitis B virus mutations in the polymerase region

LIEVEN J. STUYVER[1,2], STEPHEN A. LOCARNINI[3], ANNA LOK[4], DOUGLAS D. RICHMAN[5], WILLIAM F. CARMAN[6], JULES L. DIENSTAG[7], RAYMOND F. SCHINAZI[8] and THE HEP DART INTERNATIONAL COMMITTEE

[1] *Veterans Affairs Medical Center, Decatur, GA 30033, USA*
[2] *Pharmasset, Inc., Tucker, GA 30084, USA*
[3] *Victorian Infectious Diseases Reference Laboratory, North Melbourne, Victoria 3051, Australia*
[4] *University of Michigan Medical Center, Ann Arbor, MI 48109, USA*
[5] *San Diego Veterans Affairs Medical Center and University of California San Diego, La Jolla, CA 92093-00679, USA*
[6] *University of Glasgow, Division of Virology, Glasgow G11 5JR, Scotland*
[7] *Massachusetts General Hospital and the Department of Medicine, Harvard Medical School, Boston 02114, USA*
[8] *Department of Pediatrics, Emory University School of Medicine and Veterans Affairs Medical Center, Decatur, GA 30033, USA*

Abstract

There is currently no universally accepted numbering convention for the antiviral drug-related resistance mutations in the reverse transcriptase (rt) domain of the human HBV polymerase. The published inconsistencies have resulted from different HBV genotypes. A standardized numbering system for HBV polymerase is proposed. The new system is based on functional observations of HBV surface gene proteins (preS1, preS2, and HBsAg) and on the current convention used for HIV-1 polymerase proteins (protease, rt, and integrase), in which the amino acid numbering restarts at the first codon position of each domain. The HBV polymerase protein can be divided into four domains (terminal protein, spacer, rt, ribonuclease H), and each of these can be numbered separately. In this proposal, the HBV rt domain starts with the highly conserved EDWGPCDEHG motif, contains 344 amino acids, and the lamivudine-related resistance mutations are found at amino acid rtL180M (previously amino acid 528, 526, 515, or 525) and rtM204V/I (previously 552, 550, 539, or 549). The new consensus rt domain numbering system is genotype independent and allows investigators to number any previously and newly discovered antiviral-related amino acid change in a standardized manner.

Frontiers in Viral Hepatitis Ed. by RF Schinazi, J-P Sommadossi and CM Rice. 335 — 351

Introduction

An increasing number of treatment failures due to antiviral resistance have been recognized since the introduction of antiviral agents like lamivudine (3TC, Epivir) for the treatment of chronic hepatitis B virus infections [1-11]. In most cases amino acid variations in the reverse transcriptase (rt) domain of the HBV polymerase are apparent when compared with the pretreatment sequence [12, 13]. Confusion has resulted from the varying amino acid numbering systems used in the different published studies. At the *International Conference on Therapies for Viral Hepatitis*, held in Maui, December 12-16, 1999, it was decided to develop a uniform consensus numbering system for the rt domain of the HBV polymerase. In this manuscript, a guide is provided to the various numbering systems and their origin. In addition, a standardized system that is applicable to polymerases of all human HBV genotypes is proposed for adoption by the scientific community.

HBV genotypes

Inconsistencies in amino acid numbering of HBV polymerase result from the nature of the HBV genotypes. The family Hepadnaviridae contains two genera: the Orthohepadnaviruses (infecting humans, monkeys, apes, and rodents) and the Avihepadnaviruses (infecting birds). The type species for the family is HBV, a complex group of closely related viruses with narrow host specificity, namely hominoids. This complex group is characterized by a variety of genotypes, the definition of which is based on one of the following criteria: an inter-group divergence of 8% or more in the complete genome nucleotide sequence; or a 4.1% divergence or more of the surface gene [14, 15]. Consequently, HBV consists of at least seven different genotypes (A through G) [14, 16-20]. Additionally, another five HBV genotypes have been isolated from gibbons [21, 22], chimpanzees [23, 24], gorillas [25], and orangutans [26]. Until recently, these cases represented infected animals kept in zoos or research primate centers, but evidence is now available of HBV infections in wild-born animals [27]. Although cross-species transmission of hepadnaviruses among hominoids is possible [26], these ape viruses have never been detected in humans, so they have not been assigned a genotype number (Table 1).

Genotyping is currently performed by phylogenetic analysis [28], by fragment length polymorphisms [29, 30], by PCR [31, 32], or by using differential hybridization technologies [33]. Genotypes are distributed geographically. Genotype A is found worldwide; genotypes B and C are most predominant in Asia; genotype D is found in South Europe, the Americas, and Australia; genotype E is most commonly found in Africa; genotype F is found in native Americans and Polynesians; and genotype G is found in the US and Europe [33, 34].

Typical characteristics of prototype members of the different viral genotypes are shown in Table 1, which includes differences in the length of HBcAg and preS1 regions. Because the carboxyterminal portion of HBcAg and the complete ORF of the surface gene (preS1, preS2, and HBsAg) overlap with polymerase, these length

Table 1. Overview of the hominoid HBV genotypes including reference strains

Genotype	Genome nt	HBcAg aa	preS1 aa	preS2 aa	HBsAg aa	Surface antigen aa	Polymerase	Reference strain	Reference
A	3221	185	119	55	226	400	845	HBVADW2 (X02763	Valenzuela et al., 1980
B	3215	183	119	55	226	400	843	HPBADW1 (D00329)	Okamoto et al., 1986
C	3215	183	119	55	226	400	843	HBVADR4 (X01587)	Fujiyama et al., 1983
D	3182	183	108	55	226	389	832	HPBAYW (J02203)	Galibert et al., 1979
E	3212	183	118	55	226	399	842	BAS (X75657)	Norder et al., 1994
F	3215	183	119	55	226	400	843	FOU (X75658)	Norder et al., 1994
G	3248	195	108	55	226	399	842	FR1 (AF160501)	Stuyver et al. 2000
Gibbon 824 HBV	3182	183	108	55	226	389	832	gib824 (AJ131568)	Grethe, S et al., 2000
Gibbon HBV	3182	183	108	55	226	389	832	gib HBV (U46935)	Norder et al., 1996
Gorilla 97 HBV	3182	183	108	55	226	389	832	gor97 (AJ131567)	Grethe, S et al., 2000
Chimpanzee HBV	3182	183	108	55	226	389	832	LSH (D00220)	Vaudin et al., 1988
Orangutan HBV	NA	NA	108	55	226	389	NA	OHV (Y17559)	Warren, K.S. et al., 1999

NA: not available

polymorphisms affect the total length of the polymerase protein (Table 1). Although analysis of published sequences reveals many HBV strains with deletions [35, 36], these isolates are not seen as representative members of their genotype, but as variants that emerged during the course of a chronic infection.

In clinical settings, the genotype of the virus is usually unknown. Thus, the correct numbering of the amino acids in the rt domain is mostly speculative, and a source of considerable confusion.

The HBV polymerase gene: genome organization and comparison with other retroviral polymerases

During replication, a pregenomic RNA is produced which encodes for both HBcAg and polymerase [37, 38]. Polymerase is the second ORF on this mRNA and partially overlaps with the 3' end of the HBcAg cistron. In HIV-1, a comparable constraint exists, but polymerase translation occurs by ribosomal frameshifting [39, 40]. The precise mechanism for HBV polymerase translation is not known, although a leaky scanning mechanism [41, 42] or termination, backwards scanning and reinitiation [43] have been postulated.

Unlike HIV-1, the HBV polymerase is not proteolytically cleaved to mature, enzymatically active proteins, but consists of four domains [44]: a terminal protein (tp domain), which becomes covalently linked to negative-strand DNA during initiation of reverse transcription [45, 46]; a spacer domain, which is very tolerant to mutations and can be partially deleted without affecting polymerase activity [47-49]; the reverse transcriptase/polymerase (rt domain), which contains the conserved regions A through F, characteristic of RNA-dependent RNA polymerase (RdRP) and RNA-dependent DNA polymerase (RdDP) [50, 51]; and the RNAse H domain (rh domain) [52] (Figure 1). In contrast to HIV-1, the HBV polymerase does not contain an integrase domain.

In persistently infected patients, the daily HBV turnover is approximately 50 percent of the free virus population, with a total release of 10^{11} virus particles per day in the peripheral blood [53]. HBV rt lacks proofreading activity, resulting in high mutation frequencies of between 10^{-5} to 10^{-6} per site per year [54]. Consequently, there is an accumulation of multiple sequence variants (sequence evolution), some of which are selected during antiviral therapy. In addition, fluctuations in the intracellular [dTTP]/[dCTP] pools might give rise to a G to A hypermutation, which in some cases results in several Gs that are replaced by As throughout the entire genome [55, 56].

Numbering systems for HIV-1 polymerase and HBV surface gene

In HIV-1, the polymerase gene contains different domains, namely the protease domain, the rt domain, and the integrase domain. Amino acid numbering for each of these domains restarts at the first codon position of each domain.

For the HBV surface gene, amino acid numbering restarts at the first methionine of each of the subparts. The total length of the different gene products, preS1, preS2 and HBsAg, is provided in Table 1 and Figure 1; only the preS1 region has length polymorphisms. Consequently, the description of all functional parts in HBsAg (transmembrane regions, extracellular regions, major hydrophilic region, serological subtype determinants, antigenic variants) is identical for all genotypes. For example, the typical vaccine escape mutant is found at amino acid sG145R in all genotypes [57, 58].

A standardized nomenclature for HBV polymerase

The organization of the HBV polymerase is shown in Figure 1. The four domains are indicated, including the conserved regions A through E. In genotype A, the amino terminal part of tp has two additional amino acids (tpG17 and tpT18). This affects the ORF for HBcAg (cD153 and cR154), but not HBeAg (not shown), since this length polymorphism is located immediately carboxyterminal of the HBeAg processing site. None of the other human or ape HBV genotypes have this 2 amino acid insertion, but remarkably, there is a 5 amino acid insertion present at the same position in rodent hepadnaviruses (woodchuck hepatitis virus (WHV) [59], Arctic ground squirrel hepatitis virus (AGSHV) [60], and ground squirrel hepatitis virus (GSHV) [61]; not shown). Since the efficiency of the backwards scanning mechanism depends on the distance between the 3' end of the core ORF and initiation of the polymerase ORF [43] (143 nucleotides for genotype B – G, 149 for genotype A, 158 for rodent hepatitis viruses), these length polymorphisms might help control the translation of the polymerase protein from the pregenomic mRNA in a genotype dependent manner. The hydroxyl-group of the Y-residue needed for the protein-primed initiation of reverse transcription is indicated (Figure 1).

The amino-terminal part of preS1 is variable within genotypes (Table 1 and Figure 1). Because both the spacer domain and preS1 protein start at approximately the same nucleotide position, but in different reading frames, the length polymorphism is found in the amino-terminal part of the spacer domain. The spacer domain covers the complete preS1 domain, and most of the preS2 domain. The spacer domain is flexible and tolerates mutations and deletions [47-49]. It also explains, in part, the viability of non-genotype-specific preS1 variations found in many chronically infected patients [35, 62].

Unlike the currently used *separate functional domain numbering system* for the surface gene, a *continuous numbering system* has been used for the HBV polymerase. As a result, the numbering of the lamivudine-treatment related variants methionine (sensitive) to valine or isoleucine (resistant) in the YMDD motif (conserved region C in the HBV polymerase) is genotype dependent (Figure 1). Thus, for genotype A, it is M552V/I; for genotype B, C, and F, it is M550V/I; for genotype D, it is M539V/I; and for genotypes E and G, it is M549V/I.

Since the HBV polymerase is translated from one mRNA, independent initiation codons for the several domains (spacer, rt, and rh) are not present. There is no post-translational maturation by proteolytic cleavage, and therefore, cleavage sites cannot be determined. Border values between these domains are as yet not defined, although structural studies shed some light on this matter [44]. In the absence of experimental

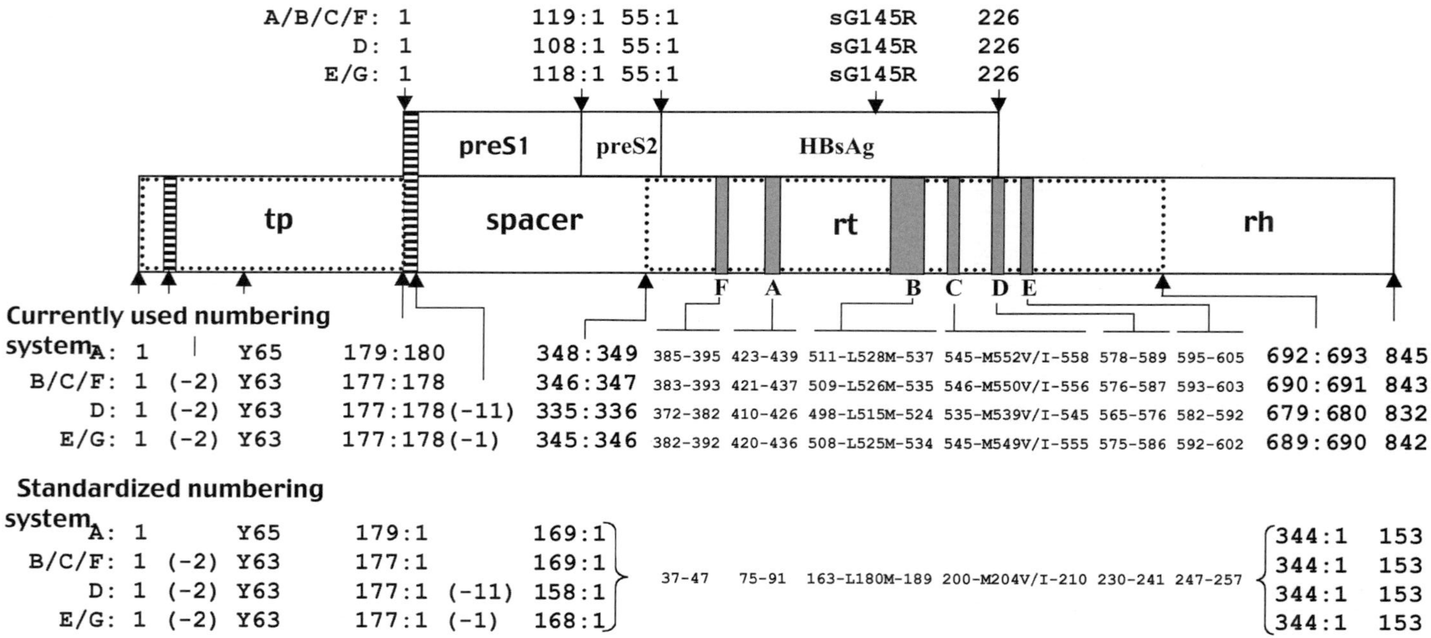

Figure 1. Organization of the HBV polymerase. The different domains of the HBV polymerase are indicated with a dotted line. Horizontally dashed boxes indicate the regions with genotype-related polymorphisms. The shaded boxes indicate the conserved regions of the rt domain of the HBV polymerase. The numbering is genotype related, and genotypes are indicated on the left. Amino acid numbering for the ape HBV strains is identical, as for human HBV genotype D.

evidence, a putative initiation site based on amino acid sequence alignments covering all genotypes (data not shown) is proposed, and indicated in Figure 1. In this proposal, the rt domain starts with the highly conserved 'EDWGPCDEHG...' motif, making the total length of the hominoid HBV rt domain 344 amino acids long. There is no rt length variability observed for the 12 HBV genotypes (Figure 1). In the woolly monkey hepatitis virus (WMHV) [63] and rodent hepatitis virus rt domains, there is length variability between conserved regions A and B, resulting in 346 and 342 amino acids for the respective rt domains (data not shown).

We propose that a *functional domain numbering* be adopted for the hominoid HBV polymerase. In this numbering system, tp domain and spacer domain numbering are genotype-dependent, but numbering of the rt and rh domains is genotype-independent. Consequently, the lamivudine-resistant amino acids are found at position rt180 (rtL180M in conserved region B; Figure 1) and, in the rtYMDD motif, at position rt204 (rtM204V/I in conserved region C; Figure 1) for all 12 genotypes. Note that possible tp and spacer mutants (if they emerge at all) will still be genotype-dependent, and that the rt domain numbering for the non-hominoid hepatitis viruses (WMHV, rodent hepadnaviruses, and Avihepadnaviruses) will be different (data not shown). To date, variability present in the rt of the non-human lentiviruses have not posed significant problems in drug-related amino acid numbering in clinically obtained HIV-1 strains.

Antiviral-resistance related amino acids in the rt conserved regions of HBV and HIV-1

Summaries of the drug-selected amino acid changes in the HBV rt domain have been published [12, 13]. From these papers and also from the published retroviral resistance table [64], it is clear that amino acid changes associated with rt inhibitors (nucleoside analogue and non-nucleoside inhibitors) are mostly present in the conserved regions A through E of the RdDP. In addition to these five regions, another conserved region, F, emerged after crystal structure analysis of the HCV RdRP [50]. This region F is also present in the HIV-1 rt (amino acids 68 to 78) and, based on sequence alignments, is also likely to be present in HBV (amino acids 37-47; Table 2). The positions of the reported drug-related mutations are shown in Table 2 [12, 13, 65]. There are no mutations reported for the HBV conserved region F, in contrast to HIV-1 where several AZT, DDI, DDC, and multi-drug resistance mutations are grouped together [64]. Adefovir dipovoxil (bis-POM-PMEA), a drug in clinical evaluations for HBV [66] and HIV-1[67], selects for a codon K70E mutation in HIV-1, but has not been linked to any domain F changes in HBV polymerase [68].

Huang et al. described the interaction between the HIV-1 rt enzyme and its substrate (rt•primer:template•dNTP complex) [69]. Several of the amino acids involved with these interactions are located in the conserved regions (Table 2). A remarkable homology is observed at those positions for HBV (standardized numbering) and HIV-1, respectively, at: rtR41 and R72; rtD45 and D76; rtD83 and D110; rtA87 and A114; rtG172 and G152; rtP177 and P157; rtY203M204D205D206 and Y183M184D185D186; and the "primer grip" motif rtM250G251 and M230G231. Additionally, interaction sites that were reported to be drug resistant in HIV-1 are found in sequences from untreated HBV patients (respectively for HBV (untreated) and HIV-1 (mutant): rtV43 and V74; rtF88 and F115; rtM171 and M151].

Consequences for HBsAg

Viral strains selected during antiviral treatment with resistant motifs in rt often show amino acid changes in the HBsAg ORF. For example, rtL180M would be responsible for changing the sS171W172 sequence of the HBsAg ORF into sL171W172, sS171X172 (with X a translational stop), or sP171W172 [70]. rtM204V can cause sI195W196 to change into either sM195W196, or sK195W196; and the rtM204I might result in sI195X196, sI195L196, sI195S196, or sT195L196 [70]. It is clear that the different nucleotide changes selected during lamivudine therapy might affect HBsAg differently. The importance of these HBsAg amino acid changes needs further investigation, since mutations in HBsAg could have a significant impact on immune recognition, replication capacity and virulence.

Consensus proposal for HBV polymerase nomenclature and viral load

For future antiviral studies with HBV, the HEP DART International Committee recommends the following:

1. HBV is highly mutable and replicates to high levels, resulting in a great genetic variation, both within an individual and among populations. Careful selection of the appropriate words to describe the nature of the observed changes is recommended. Some useful examples are listed below:
   Natural polymorphisms. Variations observed within an individual and between populations, as compared with the reference sequence. The sequences given in Table 1 might be used as reference.
   Variant. Sequence variations observed during therapy, as compared with the pre-therapy sequence obtained from the same patient. In some cases, these variants can confer drug resistance.
   Drug-resistant mutant. A sequence variant that is observed to emerge under a selective antiviral pressure, and that is confirmed to confer the phenotypic change in drug susceptibility assays. A less robust level of confirmation can be found in a statistically increased prevalence of this variant in treated *versus* untreated patients. Variants should only be claimed or proposed to be drug-resistant mutants if they qualify accordingly.
2. Resistance-related amino acids should be numbered with the standardized genotype-independent numbering system. Each mutation is preceded with the abbreviation of the protein name in lower case (rt, pt, rh, s, c, x; more details about this will be published by Lok et al.). This includes the lamivudine-associated amino acids at position rt180 (previously 528, 526, 515, and 525) and rt204 (previously 552, 550, 539, and 549); as well as the famciclovir-associated amino acids at position

Table 2. Genotype-dependent and independent amino acid numbering for the conserved regions of the HBV polymerase rt domain, and comparison with conserved regions in HIV-1 rt

Conserved region F

HBsAg aa numbering	29	30	31	32	33	34	35	36	37	38	39
HBsAg CONSENSUS aa sequence	P	Q	S	L	D	S	W	W	T	S	L
HBV pol genotype A aa numbering	385	386	387	388	389	390	391	392	393	394	395
HBV pol genotype B, C, and F aa numbering	383	384	385	386	387	388	389	390	391	392	393
HBV pol genotype D aa numbering	372	373	374	375	376	377	378	379	380	381	382
HBV pol genotype E and G aa numbering	382	383	384	385	386	387	388	389	390	391	392
HBV rt DOMAIN all genotypes aa numbering	37	38	39	40	41	42	43	44	45	46	47
HBV rt DOMAIN CONSENSUS aa sequence	T,S	T,A,E	E	S	R	L	V	V	D	F	S
HBV rt REPORTED DRUG RESISTANT aa											
HIV-1 rt aa numbering	68	69	70	71	72	73	74	75	76	77	78
HIV-1 rt CONSENSUS aa sequence	S	T	K	W	R	K	L	V	D	F	R
HIV-1 rt REPORTED DRUG RESISTANT aa		D,S +SS	E, N,R				V	T,I		L	

Conserved region A

HBsAg aa numbering	67	68	69	70	71	72	73	74	75	76	77	78	79	80	81	82	83
HBsAg CONSENSUS aa sequence	P	I,T	C	P	G	Y	R	W	M	C	L	R	R	F	I	I	F
HBV pol genotype A aa numbering	423	424	425	426	427	428	429	430	431	432	433	434	435	436	437	438	439
HBV pol genotype B, C, and F aa numbering	421	422	423	424	425	426	427	428	429	430	431	432	433	434	435	436	437
HBV pol genotype D aa numbering	410	411	412	413	414	415	416	417	418	419	420	421	422	423	424	425	426
HBV pol genotype E and G aa numbering	420	421	422	423	424	425	426	427	428	429	430	431	432	433	434	435	436
HBV rt DOMAIN all genotypes aa numbering	75	76	77	78	79	80	81	82	83	84	85	86	87	88	89	90	91
HBV rt DOMAIN CONSENSUS aa sequence	S	N	L	S	W	L	S	L	D	V	S	A	A	F	Y	H	L,I
HBV rt REPORTED DRUG RESISTANT aa	T	V,I	M														
HIV-1 rt aa numbering	102	103	104	105	106	107	108	109	110	111	112	113	114	115	116	117	118
HIV-1 rt CONSENSUS aa sequence	K	K	K	S	V	T	V	L	D	V	G	D	A	Y	F	S	V
HIV-1 rt REPORTED DRUG RESISTANT aa		N,Q, R,T			A,I,L		I							F	Y		

Table 2. Continued

Conserved region B

HBsAg aa numbering	155	156	157	158	159	160	161	162	163	164	165	166	167	168	169	170	171	172	173	174	175	176	177	178	179	180	181
HBsAg CONSENSUS aa sequence	S	W	A	F,LA,V,G	K,R	Y,F	L	W	E	W	A	S	V,A	R	F	S	W	L	S	L	L	V,A	P,Q	F	V	Q
HBV pol genotype A aa numbering	511	512	513	514	515	516	517	518	519	520	521	522	523	524	525	526	527	528	529	530	531	532	533	534	535	536	537
HBV pol genotype B, C, and F aa numbering	509	510	511	512	513	514	515	516	517	518	519	520	521	522	523	524	525	526	527	528	529	530	531	532	533	534	535
HBV pol genotype D aa numbering	498	499	500	501	502	503	504	505	506	507	508	509	510	511	512	513	514	515	516	517	518	519	520	521	522	523	524
HBV pol genotype E and G aa numbering	508	509	510	511	512	513	514	515	516	517	518	519	520	521	522	523	524	525	526	527	528	529	530	531	532	533	534
HBV rt DOMAIN all genotypes aa numbering	163	164	165	166	167	168	169	170	171	172	173	174	175	176	177	178	179	180	181	182	183	184	185	186	187	188	189
HBV rt DOMAIN CONSENSUS aa sequence	I,V	L,M	G	F	R	K	I	P	M	G	V,G	G	L	S	P	F	L	L	A	Q	F	T	S	A,S	I,L	C	S
HBV rt REPORTED DRUG RESISTANT aa	V			L							L				L			M				S					
HIV-1 rt aa numbering	143	144	145	146	147	148	149	150	151	152	153	154	155	156	157	158	159	160	161	162	163	164	165	166	167	168	169
HIV-1 rt CONSENSUS aa sequence	R	Y	Q	Y	N	V	L	P	Q	G	W	K	G	S	P	A	I	F	Q	S	S	M	T	K	I	L	E
HIV-1 rt REPORTED DRUG RESISTANT aa									M					A	S				L								

Conserved region C

HBsAg aa numbering	192	193	194	195	196	197	198	199	200	201	202
HBsAg CONSENSUS aa sequence	L	S,L	A,V	I	W	M	M,I	W	Y,F	W	G
HBV pol genotype A aa numbering	548	549	550	551	552	553	554	555	556	557	558
HBV pol genotype B, C, and F aa numbering	546	547	548	549	550	551	552	553	554	555	556
HBV pol genotype D aa numbering	535	536	537	538	539	540	541	542	543	544	545
HBV pol genotype E and G aa numbering	545	546	547	548	549	550	551	552	553	554	555
HBV rt DOMAIN all genotypes aa numbering	200	201	202	203	204	205	206	207	208	209	210
HBV rt DOMAIN CONSENSUS aa sequence	A	F	S	Y	M	D	D	V, L,M	V	L	G
HBV rt REPORTED DRUG RESISTANT aa	V				V,I			I			
HIV-1 rt aa numbering	180	181	182	183	184	185	186	187	188	189	190
HIV-1 rt CONSENSUS aa sequence	I	Y	Q	Y	M	D	D	L	Y	V	G
HIV-1 rt REPORTED DRUG RESISTANT aa		C,I			V,I,T				C	I	S

able 2. Continued

Conserved region D

HBsAg aa numbering	222	223	224	225	226							
HBsAg CONSENSUS aa sequence	L	W	V	Y,S	I							
HBV pol genotype A aa numbering	578	579	580	581	582	583	584	585	586	587	588	589
HBV pol genotype B, C, and F aa numbering	576	577	578	579	580	581	582	583	584	585	586	587
HBV pol genotype D aa numbering	565	566	567	568	569	570	571	572	573	574	575	576
HBV pol genotype E and G aa numbering	575	576	577	578	579	580	581	582	583	584	585	586
HBV rt DOMAIN all genotypes aa numbering	230	231	232	233	234	235	236	237	238	239	240	241
HBV rt DOMAIN CONSENSUS aa sequence	S	L,V	G	I	H	L	N	P,T	N,S, H,A	K	T	K
HBV rt REPORTED DRUG RESISTANT aa						I			S			
HIV-1 rt aa numbering	211	212	213	214	215	216	217	218	219	220	221	222
HIV-1 rt CONSENSUS aa sequence	R	W	G	L	T	T	P	D	K	K	H	Q
HIV-1 rt REPORTED DRUG RESISTANT aa	K				F,Y				Q,E			

Conserved region E.

HBV pol genotype A aa numbering	595	596	597	598	599	600	601	602	603	604	605
HBV pol genotype B, C, and F aa numbering	593	594	595	596	597	598	599	600	601	602	603
HBV pol genotype D aa numbering	582	583	584	585	586	587	588	589	590	591	592
HBV pol genotype E and G aa numbering	592	593	594	595	596	597	598	599	600	601	602
HBV rt DOMAIN all genotypes aa numbering	247	248	249	250	251	252	253	254	255	256	257
HBV rt DOMAIN CONSENSUS aa sequence	L	N H	F	M	G	Y	V,I	I	G	S,C	W,Y
HBV rt REPORTED DRUG RESISTANT aa		H					I				
HIV-1 rt aa numbering	227	228	229	230	231	232	233	234	235	236	237
HIV-1 rt CONSENSUS aa sequence	F	L	W	M	G	Y	E	L	H	P	D
HIV-1 rt REPORTED DRUG RESISTANT aa	L	R		——	——		V	I		L	

Legend to Table 2:

aa: amino acids
solid boxes: conserved amino acids through all RdRPs and RdDPs [Poch et al.,1989 #55]
dotted boxes: lamivudine-related resistant amino acids
—— HIV-1 rt interactions with template:primer
═══ HIV-1 rt interactions with nucleoside triphosphate
▬▬ HIV-1 rt interactions with primer:template and nucleoside triphosphate
...... Van der Waals interaction

rt173 (previously 521, 519, 508, and 518), rt180 (previously 528, 526, 515, and 525), and rt207 (previously 555, 553, 542, and 552). A guideline for using the standardized numbering system and for better understanding the drug-resistance mutations published in the past is shown in Table 2.

3. Amino acid changes related to antiviral resistance are indicated as follows: pretreatment (sensitive) amino acid – number – emerging (resistant) amino acid; for example rtM204V. The use of the term 'YMDD mutant' or 'YMDD variant' is strongly discouraged, because (a) only the methionine residue is prone to changes during antiviral treatment; (b) the V and I alleles may have different consequences; and (c) the effects on HBsAg should not be overlooked.
4. Different nucleotide changes in the rt domain might affect HBsAg differently. Therefore, the rt domain alterations should be mentioned both at the nucleotide and amino acid level, with indication of the consequences for the HBsAg ORF.
5. Some amino acids (Table 2: rtV163, rtS238, rtH248, and rtI253 in standardized numbering) have been reported in relation to an HBV-resistant profile. Since these motifs are also present in the consensus untreated sequence, it is recommended that the rt domain obtained during the course of a treatment schedule should always be compared with pretreatment sequences from the same individual. This will avoid misinterpretation between genotype-specific variability, strain variability, and drug-selected variants. It will also permit recognition of possible transmission of drug resistance (see definitions and comments above).
6. Viral load and changes in viral load should be expressed logarithmically (as log copies/ml). A log scale should be used for all graphs demonstrating viral load and activity of antiviral compounds in animal models and clinical studies.

Conclusion

This consensus document, which is adopted by the HEP DART International Committee, should provide a uniform method for numbering drug-related mutations in all HBV genotypes. This new numbering system will assume increasing importance as additional drugs become available to treat this disease. Data presented using this standardized format will provide consistency for numbering antiviral-related amino acid changes as they are discovered and enhance our understanding of drug resistance in HBV-infected individuals.

Acknowledgments

This work was previously published in Hepatology 2001;33:741-757. This work was supported in part by grants AI41980 (RFS), AI27670 (DDR), AI388858 (DDR), AI36214 (DDR) and grant AI29164 (DDR) from the National Institutes of Health and by the Research Center for AIDS and HIV Infection of the Atlanta and San Diego Veterans Affairs Medical Center.

Appendix

The HEP DART International Committee: Angeline Bartholomeusz, Australia; Adrian Di Bisceglie, USA; Robert A. de Man, the Netherlands; Geoffrey Dusheiko, UK; Phillip A. Furman, USA; Paolo La Colla, Italy; Ching-Lung Lai, Hong Kong; Johnson Y.N. Lau, USA; Michael P. Manns, Germany; Hubert GM Niesters, the Netherlands; Masao Omata, Japan; Suzane Kioko Ono-Nita, Brazil; Michael J. Otto, USA; Deenan Pillay, UK; Thierry Poynard, France; Jean-Pierre Sommadossi, USA; Daniel Shouval, Israel; Vincent Soriano, Spain; Howard Thomas, UK; Hans Will, Germany; and Fabien Zoulim, France.

References

1. Benhamou Y, Bochet M, Thibault V, Di Martino V, Caumes E, Bricaire F, Opolon P, et al. Long-term incidence of hepatitis B virus resistance to lamivudine in human immunodeficiency virus-infected patients. Hepatology 1999;30(5):1302-1306.
2. Dienstag JL, Schiff ER, Wright TL, Perrillo RP, Hann HW, Goodman Z, Crowther L, et al. Lamivudine as initial treatment for chronic hepatitis B in the United States. N Engl J Med 1999;341(17):1256-1263.
3. Hunt CM, McGill JM, Allen MI, Condreay LD. Clinical relevance of hepatitis B viral mutations. Hepatology 2000;31(5):1037-1044.
4. Kao JH, Chen PJ, Lai MY, Chen DS. Hepatitis B genotypes correlate with clinical outcomes in patients with chronic hepatitis B. Gastroenterology 2000;118(3):554-559.
5. Lai CL, Chien RN, Leung NW, Chang TT, Guan R, Tai DI, Ng KY, et al. A one-year trial of lamivudine for chronic hepatitis B. Asia Hepatitis Lamivudine Study Group [see comments]. N Engl J Med 1998;339(2):61-8.
6. Ling R, Mutimer D, Ahmed M, Boxall EH, Elias E, Dusheiko GM, Harrison TJ. Selection of mutations in the hepatitis B virus polymerase during therapy of transplant recipients with lamivudine. Hepatology 1996;24(3):711-713.
7. Mutimer D, Pillay D, Dragon E, Tang H, Ahmed M, O'Donnell K, Shaw J, et al. High pre-treatment serum hepatitis B virus titre predicts failure of lamivudine prophylaxis and graft re-infection after liver transplantation. J Hepatol 1999;30(4):715-721.
8. Ono-Nita SK, Kato N, Shiratori Y, Lan KH, Yoshida H, Carrilho FJ, Omata M. Susceptibility of lamivudine-resistant hepatitis B virus to other reverse transcriptase inhibitors. J Clin Invest 1999;103(12):1635-1640.
9. Perrillo R, Rakela J, Dienstag J, Levy G, Martin P, Wright T, Caldwell S, et al. Multicenter study of lamivudine therapy for hepatitis B after liver transplantation.Lamivudine Transplant Group. Hepatology 1999;29(5):1581-1586.
10. Pichoud C, Berby F, Stuyver L, Petit MA, Trepo C, Zoulim F. Persistence of viral replication after anti-HBe seroconversion during antiviral therapy for chronic hepatitis B. J Hepatol 2000;32(2):307-316.
11. Tillmann HL, Trautwein C, Bock T, Boker KH, Jackel E, Glowienka M, Oldhafer K, et al. Mutational pattern of hepatitis B virus on sequential therapy with famciclovir and lamivudine in patients with hepatitis B virus reinfection occurring under HBIg immunoglobulin after liver transplantation. Hepatology 1999;30(1):244-256.
12. Bartholomeusz A, Schinazi RF, Locarnini SA. Significance of mutations in the hepatitis B virus

polymerase selected by nucleoside analogues and implications for controlling chronic disease. Viral Hep Rev 1998;4(3):167-187.

13. Pillay D, Bartholomeusz A, Cane P, Mutimer D, Schinazi RF, Locarnini S. Mutations in the hepatitis B virus DNA polymerase associated with antiviral resistance. International Antiviral News 1998;6(9):167-169.
14. Norder H, Courouce AM, Magnius LO. Complete genomes, phylogenetic relatedness, and structural proteins of six strains of the hepatitis B virus, four of which represent two new genotypes. Virology 1994;198(2):489-503.
15. Okamoto H, Tsuda F, Sakugawa H, Sastrosoewignjo RI, Imai M, Miyakawa Y, Mayumi M. Typing hepatitis B virus by homology in nucleotide sequence: comparison of surface antigen subtypes. J Gen Virol 1988;69(10):2575-2583.
16. Fujiyama A, Miyanohara A, Nozaki C, Yoneyama T, Ohtomo N, Matsubara K. Cloning and structural analyses of hepatitis B virus DNAs, subtype adr. Nucleic Acids Res 1983;11(13):4601-4610.
17. Galibert F, Mandart E, Fitoussi F, Tiollais P, Charnay P. Nucleotide sequence of the hepatitis B virus genome (subtype ayw) cloned in E. coli. Nature 1979;281(5733):646-650.
18. Okamoto H, Imai M, Shimozaki M, Hoshi Y, Iizuka H, Gotanda T, Tsuda F, et al. Nucleotide sequence of a cloned hepatitis B virus genome, subtype ayr: comparison with genomes of the other three subtypes. J Gen Virol 1986;67(11):2305-2314.
19. Stuyver L, De Gendt S, Van Geyt C, Zoulim F, Fried M, Schinazi RF, Rossau R. A new genotype of hepatitis B virus: complete genome and phylogenetic relatedness. J Gen Virol 2000;81(1):67-74.
20. Valenzuela P, Quiroga M, Zalvidar J, Gray P, Rutter WJ. The nucleotide sequence of the hepatitis B viral genome and the identification of the major viral genes. New York: Academic Press; 1980.
21. Mimms LT, Solomon LR, Ebert JW, Fields H. Unique preS sequence in a gibbon-derived hepatitis B virus variant. Biochem Biophys Res Commun 1993;195(1):186-191.
22. Norder H, Ebert JW, Fields HA, Mushahwar IK, Magnius LO. Complete sequencing of a gibbon hepatitis B virus genome reveals a unique genotype distantly related to the chimpanzee hepatitis B virus. Virology 1996;218(1):214-223.
23. Vaudin M, Wolstenholme AJ, Tsiquaye KN, Zuckerman AJ, Harrison TJ. The complete nucleotide sequence of the genome of a hepatitis B virus isolated from a naturally infected chimpanzee. J Gen Virol 1988;69(6):1383-1389.
24. Zuckerman AJ, Thornton A, Howard CR, Tsiquaye KN, Jones DM, Brambell MR. Hepatitis B outbreak among chimpanzees at the London Zoo. Lancet 1978;8091(2):652-654.
25. Grethe S, Heckel JO, Rietschel W, Hufert FT. Molecular epidemiology of hepatitis B virus variants in non-human primates. J Virol 2000;74(11):5377-5381.
26. Warren KS, Heeney JL, Swan RA, Heriyanto, Verschoor EJ. A new group of hepadnaviruses naturally infecting orangutans (*Pongo pygmaeus*). J Virol 1999;73(9):7860-7865.
27. MacDonald DM, Holmes EC, Lewis JC, Simmonds P. Detection of hepatitis B virus infection in wild-born chimpanzees (Pan troglodytes verus): phylogenetic relationships with human and other primate genotypes. J Virol 2000;74(9):4253-4257.
28. Ohba K, Mizokami M, Ohno T, Suzuki K, Orito E, Lau JY, Ina Y, et al. Relationships between serotypes and genotypes of hepatitis B virus: genetic classification of HBV by use of surface genes. Virus Res 1995;39(1):25-34.
29. Mizokami M, Nakano T, Orito E, Tanaka Y, Sakugawa H, Mukaide M, Robertson BH. Hepatitis B virus genotype assignment using restriction fragment length polymorphism patterns. FEBS Lett 1999;450(1-2):66-71.

30. Li JS, Tong SP, Wen YM, Vitvitski L, Zhang Q, Trepo C. Hepatitis B virus genotype A rarely circulates as an HBe-minus mutant: possible contribution of a single nucleotide in the precore region. J Virol 1993;67(9):5402-5410.
31. Echevarria JE, Tenorio A, Courouce AM, Leon P, Echevarria JM. Polymerase chain reaction can resolve some undefined cases of hepatitis B virus antigenic subtyping. J Med Virol 1994;42(3):217-223.
32. Norder H, Hammas B, Magnius LO. Typing of hepatitis B virus genomes by a simplified polymerase chain reaction. J Med Virol 1990;31(3):215-221.
33. Van Geyt C, De Gendt S, Rombaut A, Wyseur A, Maertens G, Rossau R, Stuyver L. A line probe assay for hepatitis B virus genotypes. In: Schinazi RF, Sommadossi J-P, Thomas H, editors. Therapies for Viral Hepatitis. London: International Medical Press; 1998. p. 139-145.
34. Blitz L, Pujol FH, Swenson PD, Porto L, Atencio R, Araujo M, Costa L, et al. Antigenic diversity of hepatitis B virus strains of genotype F in Amerindians and other population groups from Venezuela. J Clin Microbiol 1998;36(3):648-651.
35. Gerken G, Kremsdorf D, Capel F, Petit MA, Dauguet C, Manns MP, Meyer zum Buschenfelde KH, et al. Hepatitis B defective virus with rearrangements in the preS gene during chronic HBV infection. Virology 1991;183(2):555-565.
36. Pollicino T, Campo S, Raimondo G. PreS and core gene heterogeneity in hepatitis B virus (HBV) genomes isolated from patients with long-lasting HBV chronic infection. Virology 1995;208(2):672-677.
37. Nassal M, Schaller H. Hepatitis B virus replication--an update. J Viral Hepat 1996;3(5):217-226.
38. Nassal M. Hepatitis B virus replication: novel roles for virus-host interactions. Intervirology 1999;42(2-3):100-116.
39. Bebenek K, Roberts JD, Kunkel TA. The effects of dNTP pool imbalances on frameshift fidelity during DNA replication. J Biol Chem 1992;267(6):3589-2596.
40. Reil H, Kollmus H, Weidle UH, Hauser H. A heptanucleotide sequence mediates ribosomal frameshifting in mammalian cells. J Virol 1993;67(9):5579-5584.
41. Lin CG, Lo SJ. Evidence for involvement of a ribosomal leaky scanning mechanism in the translation of the hepatitis B virus pol gene from the viral pregenome RNA. Virology 1992;188(1):342-352.
42. Fouillot N, Tlouzeau S, Rossignol JM, Jean-Jean O. Translation of the hepatitis B virus P gene by ribosomal scanning as an alternative to internal initiation. J Virol 1993;67(8):4886-4895.
43. Hwang WL, Su TS. Translational regulation of hepatitis B virus polymerase gene by termination-reinitiation of an upstream minicistron in a length-dependent manner. J Gen Virol 1998;79(9):2181-2189.
44. Lanford RE, Kim YH, Lee H, Notvall L, Beames B. Mapping of the hepatitis B virus reverse transcriptase TP and RT domains by transcomplementation for nucleotide priming and by protein protein interaction. J Virol 1999;73(3):1885-1893.
45. Weber M, Bronsema V, Bartos H, Bosserhoff A, Bartenschlager R, Schaller H. Hepadnavirus P protein utilizes a tyrosine residue in the TP domain to prime reverse transcription. J Virol 1994;68(5):2994-2999.
46. Zoulim F, Seeger C. Reverse transcription in hepatitis B viruses is primed by a tyrosine residue of the polymerase. J Virol 1994;68(1):6-13.
47. Radziwill G, Tucker W, Schaller H. Mutational analysis of the hepatitis B virus P gene product: domain structure and RNase H activity. J Virol 1990;64(2):613-620.
48. Kim Y, Hong YB, Jung G. Hepatitis B virus: DNA polymerase activity of deletion mutants. Biochem Mol Biol Int 1999;47(2):301-308.
49. Li JS, Fourel I, Jaquet C, Trepo C. Decreased replication capacity of a duck hepatitis B virus mutant with altered distal pre-S region. Virus Res 1991;20(1):11-21.

50. Lesburg CA, Cable MB, Ferrari E, Hong Z, Mannarino AF, Weber PC. Crystal structure of the RNA-dependent RNA polymerase from hepatitis C virus reveals a fully encircled active site. Nat Struct Biol 1999;6(10):937-943.
51. Poch O, Sauvaget I, Delarue M, Tordo N. Identification of four conserved motifs among the RNA-dependent polymerase encoding elements. EMBO J 1989;8(12):3867-3874.
52. Wei X, Peterson DL. Expression, purification, and characterization of an active RNase H domain of the hepatitis B viral polymerase. J Biol Chem 1996;271(51):32617-32622.
53. Nowak MA, Bonhoeffer S, Hill AM, Boehme R, Thomas HC, McDade H. Viral dynamics in hepatitis B virus infection. Proc Natl Acad Sci U S A 1996;93(9):4398-4402.
54. Orito E, Mizokami M, Ina Y, Moriyama EN, Kameshima N, Yamamoto M, Gojobori T. Host-independent evolution and a genetic classification of the hepadnavirus family based on nucleotide sequences. Proc Natl Acad Sci U S A. 1989;86(18):7059-7062.
55. Gunther S, Sommer G, Plikat U, Iwanska A, Wain-Hobson S, Will H, Meyerhans A. Naturally occurring hepatitis B virus genomes bearing the hallmarks of retroviral G-->A hypermutation. Virology 1997;235(1):104-108.
56. Vartanian JP, Meyerhans A, Sala M, Wain-Hobson S. G-->A hypermutation of the human immunodeficiency virus type 1 genome: evidence for dCTP pool imbalance during reverse transcription. Proc Natl Acad Sci U S A 1994;91(8):3092-3096.
57. Carman WF, Zanetti AR, Karayiannis P, Waters J, Manzillo G, Tanzi E, Zuckerman AJ, et al. Vaccine-induced escape mutant of hepatitis B virus. Lancet 1990;336(8711):325-329.
58. Waters JA, Kennedy M, Voet P, Hauser P, Petre J, Carman W, Thomas HC. Loss of the common "A" determinant of hepatitis B surface antigen by a vaccine-induced escape mutant. J Clin Invest 1992;90(6):2543-2547.
59. Galibert F, Chen TN, Mandart E. Nucleotide sequence of a cloned woodchuck hepatitis virus genome: comparison with the hepatitis B virus sequence. J Virol 1982;41(1):51-65.
60. Testut P, Renard CA, Terradillos O, Vitvitski-Trepo L, Tekaia F, Degott C, Blake J, et al. A new hepadnavirus endemic in arctic ground squirrels in Alaska. J Virol 1996;70(7):4210-4219.
61. Seeger C, Ganem D, Varmus HE. Nucleotide sequence of an infectious molecularly cloned genome of ground squirrel hepatitis virus. J Virol 1984;51(2):367-375.
62. Nakajima E, Minami M, Ochiya T, Kagawa K, Okanoue T. PreS1 deleted variants of hepatitis B virus in patients with chronic hepatitis. J Hepatol 1994;20(3):329-335.
63. Lanford RE, Chavez D, Brasky KM, Burns RBr, Rico-Hesse R. Isolation of a hepadnavirus from the woolly monkey, a New World primate. Proc Natl Acad Sci USA 1998;95(10):5757-5761.
64. Schinazi RF, Larder BA, Mellors JW. Mutations in retroviral genes associated with drug resistance: 1999-2000 update. International Antiviral News 1999;7(4):46-69.
65. Hussain M, Lok AS. Mutations in the hepatitis B virus polymerase gene associated with antiviral treatment for hepatitis B. J Viral Hepat 1999;6(3):183-194.
66. Gilson RJ, Chopra KB, Newell AM, Murray-Lyon IM, Nelson MR, Rice SJ, Tedder RS, et al. A placebo-controlled phase I/II study of adefovir dipivoxil in patients with chronic hepatitis B virus infection. J Viral Hepat 1999;6(5):387-395.
67. Kahn J, Lagakos S, Wulfsohn M, Cherng D, Miller M, Cherrington J, Hardy D, et al. Efficacy and safety of adefovir dipivoxil with antiretroviral therapy: a randomized controlled trial. JAMA 1999;282(24):2305-2315.
68. Xiong X, Yang H, Westland CE, Zou R, Gibbs CS. *In vitro* evaluation of hepatitis B virus polymerase mutations associated with famciclovir resistance. Hepatology 2000;31(1):219-224.

69. Huang H, Chopra R, Verdine GL, Harrison SC. Structure of a covalently trapped catalytic complex of HIV-1 reverse transcriptase: implications for drug resistance. Science 1998;282(5394):1669-1675.
70. Stuyver L, Van Geyt C, De Gendt S, Van Reybroeck G, Zoulim F, Leroux-Roels G, Rossau R. A line probe assay for monitoring drug-resistance in HBV-infected patients during antiviral therapy. J Clin Microbiol 2000;38(702-707):702-707.

Complex genotypic changes during failure of HBV nucleoside analogue therapy

DEENAN PILLAY[1], DAVID MUTIMER[2], NIGEL BURROUGHS[3], DAVID COOPER[4] and PATRICIA CANE[1]

[1] *PHLS Antiviral Susceptibility Reference Unit, Division of Immunity and Infection, University of Birmingham Medical School, UK*
[2] *Liver and Hepatobiliary Unit, University Hospital NHS Trust (Queen Elizabeth Hospital), Birmingham, UK*
[3] *University of Warwick, Coventry, UK*
[4] *National Centre in HIV Epidemiology and Clinical Research, University of New South Wales, Darlinghurst, New South Wales, Australia*

Introduction

A range of nucleoside analogues have activity against hepatitis B virus (HBV), including lamivudine, famciclovir and entecavir. In addition, adefovir is a potent nucleotide analogue inhibitor of this virus. Controlled studies of lamivudine in chronic HBV infection and its prophylaxis against re-infection in liver transplantation have demonstrated its clinical efficacy. However, there is a risk of emergence of lamivudine resistance, with an estimated incidence of at least 14% per year in treated immunocompetent patients [5]. Variations in the incidence of resistance and clinical impact of resistance are also apparent between patient groups.

This review focuses on our clinical experience of HBV antiviral drugs and the HBV genotypic correlates of success and failure. Infection in three groups of treated patients will be considered: a) liver transplant recipients given HBV to prevent re infection; b) chronic HBV infected patients; and c) HBV/human immunodeficiency virus-1 co-infected patients. Through ongoing clinical studies, we explore the virological nature of drug resistance, the apparent clinical properties of resistant viruses, and finally, the potential cross-resistance profiles of these viruses in a clinical setting.

Virological relapse in lamivudine-treated patients, defined by a rising HBV viral load, is commonly associated with mutations in the HBV polymerase gene, specifically within the highly conserved YMDD motif (M550I or M550V) [9]. This is analogous to HIV resistance to lamivudine, which is caused by mutations within the same motif. Initially, the number of mutations observed within the HBV polymerase associated with resistance was limited, with M550V but not M550I being associated with L526M. These have been termed Type 1 (M550V, L526M) or Type II (M550I) mutations [1]. In contrast, famciclovir resistance was described as being associated

Frontiers in Viral Hepatitis Ed. by RF Schinazi, J-P Sommadossi and CM Rice. 353 — 364

with V519L and L526M. Based on the crystallographic model of HIV reverse transcriptase, conserved domains A-E of HBV polymerase have been described (A: 421-436; B: 505-528; C: 546-557; D: 575-590; E: 592-600), whereby A, C and D may participate in nucleoside triphosphate binding and catalysis, and domains B and E may be involved in template and primer positioning. In this model, penciclovir and lamivudine resistance mutations can be ascribed to different enzyme domains (B domain, and B and C domains, respectively) (Pillay et al., 1998).

The emergence of resistance is limited by genetic constraints related to loss of replicative capacity. It has been difficult to assess the fitness of resistant genotypes emerging in clinical practice, owing to the absence of a routine cell culture system for HBV. Transfection experiments suggest that the characteristic YMDD mutations, as well as others associated with lamivudine and famciclovir resistance, are variably associated with reduced replication and polymerase activity [8]. A further constraint on genetic variability is that the open reading frame (ORF) encoding the surface antigen overlaps that of the polymerase. Thus, resistance mutations may alter HBsAg amino acid sequence, possibly leading to alterations in their potential cell binding domains [3]. The precise impact of drug resistance mutations on HBsAg function remains to be determined, although it is essential that the implications of HBV drug resistance mutations for surface antigen structure are documented when characterising these polymerase changes.

Another variable in the published series of HBV drug failure is the form in which HBV DNA levels are expressed. Firstly, assays of variable sensitivity have been utilised, and secondly, results have been expressed either on a linear or logarithmic scale. It is apparent that sensitive assays are required in order to appreciate the dynamics and early detection of viral rebound on therapy. Further, given the huge amount of viral replication and production, it is advisable that these results are expressed in a log scale. We recommend against using the well-established hybridisation assay for quantitation of HBV DNA due to its lack of sensitivity, poor dynamic range and its expression of results in an inappropriate form (pg/ml rather than viral DNA copies/ml).

Transplantation

The nature of HBV drug resistance was explored by studying HBV viral load rebound in five transplant recipients, four of whom received lamivudine pre- and post-transplantation and one of whom received lamivudine prophylaxis shortly following transplantation. Detailed viral load measurements and HBV polymerase cloning and sequencing were undertaken in order to explore the precise characteristics of the rebound viruses. Resistant virus from all patients showed either the Type I or II changes involving the M550 codon. However, more detailed analysis identified the complexity of these apparently straightforward changes.

The viral load changes and timing of treatment for one patient (Patient A) is illustrated in Figure 1. In addition, the allied population sequencing results are documented in Table 1. Drug resistance was associated with L526M and M550V relative to the pretreatment sequence. The latter change led to an HBsAg change of I195M, with an

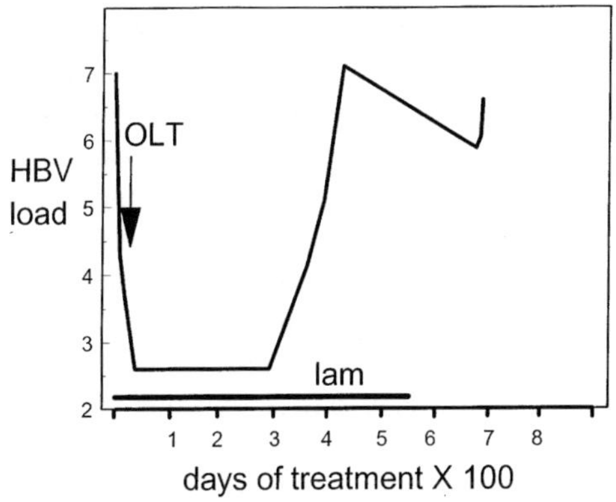

Figure 1. HBV viral load changes in Patient A

Table 1. Changes in HBV sequence relative to pretreatment for Patient A (pol amino acids 483-583, HBsAg amino acids 129-226)

Days from start of treatment	pol 526	pol 538 sAg184	pol 550 sAg 195	pol 553 sAg 198
0	TTG (L)	CGT (R) V	ATG (M) I	GTG (V) M
412	ATG (M)	CGT/C (R) V/A	GTG (V) M	GTG (V) M
474	ATG (M)	CGT/C (R) V/A	GTG (V) M	GTG (V) M
592	ATG (M)	CGT/C (R) V/A	GTG (V) M	GTG (V) M
655	A/TTG (M/L)	CGT/C (R) V/A	G/ATG/C (M/V/I*) I/M	G/TTG (V/L) M/I

* several possible combinations: see Table 2.

apparent mixture of nucleotides at polymerase codon 538 (CGT/C) that were silent in the polymerase reading frame, but leading to a mixture of V and A at HBsAg position 184. Within three months of cessation of lamivudine treatment, but not at 27 days post-cessation, there was a change in the HBV population, with new mixes detected at codons 526, 550 and 553 and with possible mixtures elsewhere. It was therefore decided to examine this population more closely by sequencing of multiple clones. Fourteen clones from day 655 samples were sequenced, and the amino acids changes are identified in Table 2. It can be seen that there was no emergence of virus wild type at position 550, but this position was now a mixture of ATC (I) and GTG (V). All clones showing M550V also had L526M, but one of four clones which had M550I also had L526M. Other changes in a minority of clones which had not been detected by the population sequencing were also observed. In total, of only 14 clones sequenced, there appeared to be nine different genome populations represented. The relative fitness (or indeed, viability) of these variants is unknown, but our failure to detect wild type virus indicates that reversion does not invariably occur in the absence of drug pressure. It is likely that the apparent reversion observed in some patients represents an outgrowth of preexisting wild type virus that has persisted during drug treatment. In the transplant scenario, this preexisting population would be that which infected the new liver following transplantation. This is likely to be a far narrower range of species than the pre-existing population in an individual infected for many years with chronic infection; thus, virus evolution following transplantation may differ from that in chronic infection, and this deserves further study.

Table 2. Deduced polymerase amino acid changes relative to pretreatment samples seen in clones derived from day 655 sample of Patient A

Polymerase codon									
Clone:	494	508	526	542	550	553	555	561	575
1	Y-F		L-M		M-V				L-M
2			L-M		M-V				
3			L-M		M-V				L-M
4			L-M		M-V				L-M
5					M-I*	V-L			
6					M-I	V-L		Q-R	
7			L-M		M-V				L-M
8			L-M	P-L	M-V				
9			L-M		M-V				
10					M-I	V-L			
11		I-L	L-M		M-V				L-M
12			L-M		M-V		L-S		
13			L-M		M-V				
14			L-M		M-I	V-L			

* All I550 are encoded by ATC

A different pattern was observed for a second patient (Patient B) who started on lamivudine 116 days prior to transplantation. Resurgence of replication occurred 242 days following treatment (126 days after transplant), and this patient was subsequently unsuccessfully treated with famciclovir and ganciclovir (Figure 2). Emergence of virus on lamivudine was associated with the polymerase mutations L526M, M550V and S565A (Table 3). This virus did not respond to subsequent famciclovir therapy for 110 days, but the majority species remained the same, indicating that selective pressure was

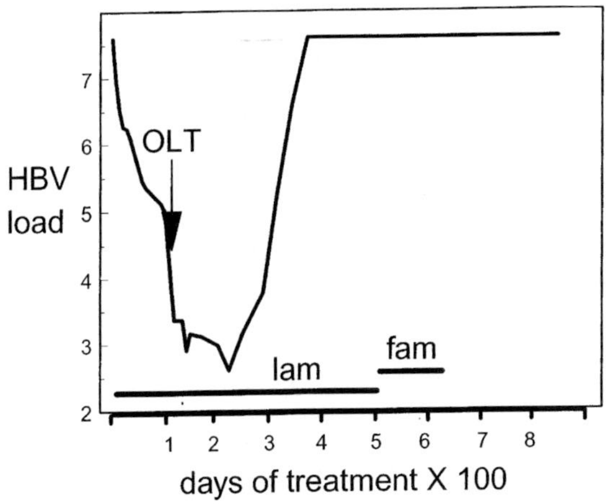

Figure 2. HBV viral load changes in Patient B.

maintained by this drug. Apparently complete reversion back to wild type polymerase at codons 526, 550 and 565 occurred within 148 days of stopping famciclovir, but the revertant virus also showed F567Y and L491M changes. This again suggests that this genome represented outgrowth of a minority archive species within the re-infected liver.

In order to explore the potential predictors of emergence of drug resistance post-transplantation, we prospectively studied ten consecutive patients receiving lamivudine prophylaxis and progressing to transplant. Resistance developed in five of these patients eight to 15 months post-transplant (Table 4). Emergence of resistance was predicted by the HBV viral load prior to initiation of lamivudine pre-transplantation ($>10 \times 10^6$ c/ml). By contrast, the nadir of viral load achieved following initiation of lamivudine pre-transplant did not appear associated with emergence of resistance. These observations are consistent with the pre-existence of minority species of HBV which have reduced susceptibility to lamivudine. The absolute frequency of these species will be higher in patients in whom steady state viral load is high, and this determines the likelihood that these species will remain present at the time of transplant, despite a very significant reduction in viral load by lamivudine. It is therefore more likely that these species will re-infect the liver following transplantation.

There has also been speculation that lamivudine-resistant HBV species have reduced pathogenicity and/or replicative capacity. This has important implications for clinical practice. For instance, should lamivudine be continued as monotherapy despite emergence of drug resistance, should lamivudine be stopped, or should alternative therapies be initiated? During prospective monitoring of transplant recipients receiving lamivudine prophylaxis, four patients were identified with graft re-infection associated with lamivudine-resistant virus. All patients develop liver failure with onset of liver dysfunction associated with the emergence of genotypic resistance, thus suggesting that the proposed virological attenuation consequent on drug resistance may not manifest as such *in vivo*, particularly in the post-transplant immunocompromised patient [6].

Table 3. Changes in HBV sequence relative to pretreatment for Patient B (pol amino acids 483-583, HBsAg amino acids 129-226)

Days from start of treatment	pol 491	pol 494 sAg 140		pol 526	pol 550 sAg 195		pol 565 sAg 210		pol 567 sAg 213		pol 570 sAg 216	
-72	CTG (L)	TAC (Y)	T	CTG (L)	ATG (M)	I	TCC (S)	S	TTT (F)	L	GTG (V)	Stop*
56	CTG (L)	TAC (Y)	T	CTG (L)	ATG (M)	I	TCC (S)	S	TTT (F)	L	GTG (V)	Stop*
130	CTG (L)	TAT (Y)	I	CTG (L)	ATG (M)	I	TCC (S)	S	TTT (F)	L	GTT (V)	L
305	CTG (L)	TAC (Y)	T	ATG (M)	GTG (V)	M	GCC (A)	R	TTT (F)	L	GTT (V)	L
361	CTG (L)	TAC (Y)	T	ATG (M)	GTG (V)	M	GCC (A)	R	TTT (F)	L	GTT (V)	L
511	CTG (L)	TAC (Y)	T	ATG (M)	GTG (V)	M	GCC (A)	R	TTT (F)	L	GTT (V)	L
620	CTG (L)	TAC (Y)	T	ATG (M)	GTG (V)	M	GCC (A)	R	TTT (F)	L	GTT (V)	L
679	CTG (L)	TAC (Y)	T	ATG (M)	GTG (V)	M	GCC (A)	R	TTT (F)	L	GTT (V)	L
748	CTG (L)	TAC (Y)	T	ATG (M)	GTG (V)	M	GCC (A)	R	TTT (F)	L	GTT (V)	L
790	ATG (M)	TAC (Y)	T	CTG (L)	ATG (M)	I	TCC (S)	S	TAT (Y)	I	GTT (V)	L
818	ATG (M)	TAC (Y)	T	CTG (L)	ATG (M)	I	TCC (S)	S	TAT (Y)	I	GTT (V)	L
827	ATG (M)	TAC (Y)	T	CTG (L)	ATG (M)	I	TCC (S)	S	TAT (Y)	I	GTT (V)	L

*C Terminal 11 amino acids of HBsAg missing

Table 4. Outcome of 10 HBV infected patients treated with lamivudine as prophylaxis prior to liver transplantation

Patient	Pre-lamivudine DNA titre (genomic copies/ml serum)	Duration of treatment before transplantation (days)	Pre-transplant DNA titre (genomic copies/ml serum)	Post-transplant follow-up (days)	Outcome
1	>40 million	61	1,129	610	alive/mutant infection
2	>40 million	113	2,280	704	dead/mutant infection
3	>40 million	36	354,500	480	alive/mutant infection
4	11,569,640	56	14,360	856	alive/mutant infection
5	10,018,160	58	<400	505	dead/mutant infection
6	3,004,280	52	4,960	1,125	alive PCR-negative
7	2,859,480	55	4,800	1,557	alive PCR-negative
8	5,960	170	<400	1,077	alive PCR-negative
9	1,840	93	<400	851	alive PCR-negative
10	<400	150	<400	1,117	alive PCR-negative

Chronic infection

As discussed above, the traditional view of HBV drug resistance mutations is that virus variants with M550V also show the L526M change, but that the latter is not observed in association with M550I. Since it is believed that the L526M represents an important change associated with famciclovir resistance, we have tested the hypothesis that the Group II lamivudine-resistant variants (M550I) retain sensitivity to famciclovir *in vivo*. Five chronically infected patients with lamivudine-resistant HBV were identified with the M550I mutation (lacking L526M), and famciclovir was added to existing lamivudine therapy in these individuals. We reasoned that continuing lamivudine treatment would maintain a selective pressure for the M550I mutation already existing. Strikingly, no patients treated with combination therapy had a decline in HBV viral load $>1\log_{10}$. We also noted a continual evolution of the virus over greater than three-months follow-up of double therapy, whereby all but one patient had a detectable population of L526M, with the presence of M550I in three of these four cases. The classical Group 1 variant (L526M, M550V) appeared as the majority population in only one patient (Table 5).

Sequencing of multiple clones from each of three patients failing lamivudine monotherapy demonstrated the pre-existence of these L526M/M550I species as minority populations prior to addition of famciclovir.

Table 5. Sequential treatment of chronic HBV: HBV polymerase changes associated with clinical lamivudine and famciclovir resistance

Polymerase amino acid positions		519	526	550
Pretreatment genotype (all patients)		V	L	M
Patient 1	— LAM failure	V	L	I
	— LAM + FAM failure	V	L/M	I
Patient 2	— LAM failure	L	L	I
	— LAM + FAM failure	L	L/M	I
Patient 3	— LAM failure	V	L	I
	— LAM + FAM failure	V	L	I
Patient 4	— LAM failure	V	L/M	I
	— LAM + FAM failure	V	L/M	I
Patient 5	— LAM failure	L	L/M	I/V
	— LAM + FAM failure	L	M	V

Genotypic changes were identified by population sequencing. 13. LAM = lamivudine; FAM = famciclovir; I = isoleucine

These data strongly support the hypothesis that the emergence of HBV drug resistancein chronic infection is associated with a large range of viral variants, albeit as minority populations [7]. This is significant in that rapid emergence of resistance to second-line therapy may occur, dependent on the precise genotypes represented within the quasispecies. Further, this reinforces the view, widely accepted within HIV clinical research circles, that sequential therapy for HBV infection is likely to be suboptimal compared to potent first-line combination therapy.

A number of differences have been observed between the emergence of lamivudine resistance in transplant recipients compared to those patients with chronic infection. We therefore undertook detailed mathematical analysis of the dynamics of emergence of resistance in our transplant and chronic infection cohort of patients. Three patients with post-transplant emergence of drug resistance and six chronic HBV carriers with resistance were studied. Using Markov Chain Monte Carlo methods, we identified that the virus dynamics between these two sets of patients were significantly different. Firstly, lamivudine-resistant mutants grew faster in transplant patients compared to chronic carriers. Secondly, the mutant emerged significantly earlier in transplant patients (average 374 days relative to start of therapy) compared to non-transplant patients (average 570 days of therapy). These observations may be due to immunosuppressive therapy in transplant recipients or an increase in the number of susceptible cells at transplant [2]. Thus, the availability of an uninfected liver allows a higher rate of growth following re-infection compared to the chronic infected states in which the continual infection of hepatocytes from newly produced virus is dependent on the turnover of infected hepatocytes and generation of new uninfected cells.

The application of mathematical models to emergence of HBV drug resistance, as has been established for HIV, is important in order to inform the appropriate use of antiviral drugs in these different clinical settings.

HBV/HIV-1 co-infection

Co-infection with HIV-1 and HBV is not uncommon. The natural history of HBV infection is modified within this scenario. Higher HBV viral loads and a higher rate of HBV reactivation are observed in comparison with HIV-1-uninfected individuals. Furthermore, an exacerbation of HBV hepatitis has been observed in co-infected individuals treated with HAART, presumably reflecting the immunopathological basis of HBV-induced liver disease. It is therefore important to develop strategies for control of HBV replication in HIV infected patients. A number of case reports and small studies of co-infected individuals have demonstrated an anti-HBV effect of lamivudine in this context. More recently a large retrospective study of co-infected patients enrolled within the CAESAR Study has been reported. This was a randomised double-blind, placebo controlled trial of lamivudine (at a dose of 150 mg twice a day) or lamivudine plus loviride (a non-nucleoside reverse transcriptase inhibitor subsequently withdrawn from use) added to zidovudine-containing regimens for patients with advanced HIV infection. At 52 weeks of study, HBV DNA was reduced by a median of 2 $\log_{10}$ c/ml in the lamivudine arm, compared with no reduction in the placebo-treated patients. A trend towards lower alanine transferase (ALT) levels and delayed progression of HIV disease were also observed in the lamivudine arms [4]. Since this represented a unique data set for co-infected patients, we explored the emergence of HBV drug resistance in this cohort.

Of the 97 co-infected individuals receiving lamivudine in this study, approximately 40% had high HBV viral load measurements at weeks 44 to 52 of study (>10,000 c/ml). Genotypic analysis of HBV from 13 of these 20 patients was undertaken, which demonstrated key lamivudine-resistance mutations in five patients by the final time point. This translates into a one-year incidence of resistance of approximately 14%, comparable to data from non-HIV infected patients. Thus, in this cohort, eight patients with high HBV DNA levels after 52 weeks of lamivudine had wild type HBV polymerase sequence. We then compared changes in ALT levels over the course of treatment between those failing with or without genotypic drug resistance. Of interest, those with mutations within HBV polymerase had a mean fall in ALT from baseline of 52 μ/l, compared to a mean rise of 12 μ/l in those without emergence of drug resistance, despite similar baseline liver function (Table 6). This observation supports the theory that HBV polymerase mutants may be replication defective, as demonstrated *in vitro*. Nevertheless, we identified one patient with genotypic HBV resistance who developed a transient hepatitis flare, as has previously been observed following withdrawal of

Table 6. Virological data for 13 HBV/HIV-1 co-infected patients treated for 52 weeks with lamivudine. The data are separated between those with mutant hepatitis B virus (HBV) polymerase and those with wild type. HBV polymerase and HIV reverse transcriptase (RT) endpoints refer to relevant resistant-associated mutations within the respective genes. All sequences were confirmed as wild type at baseline, at the relevant positions.

	HBV DNA (copies/ml)					HIV RNA (copies/ml)			
Patient No.	Baseline	Nadir + (if appropriate)	Endpoint	HBV Polymerase Endpoint	Change in ALT (IU/L)	Baseline	Final	Change in CD_4 Cell Count (x 10^6/L)	HIV RT Endpoint
1	>$4x10^7$	$7.1x10^4$	$1.6x10^5$	w/t	+39	$6.0x10^4$	$3.3x10^4$	-45	M184I
2	>$4x10^7$	-	$2.3x10^5$	w/t	+67	$5.2x10^4$	$3.9x10^4$	+47	M184V
3	>$4x10^7$	$1.9x10^6$	>$4x10^7$	w/t	+7	$9.9x10^2$	$1.6x10^3$	+25	M184V
4	inh	-	$1.0x10^4$	w/t	+40	$1.5x10^5$	$1.0x10^5$	+69	M184V
5	inh	-	$1.6x10^5$	w/t	+7	$2.2x10^4$	$5.5x10^3$	+107	M184V
6	>$4x10^7$	$7.6x10^3$	$4.0x10^4$	w/t	-21	$2.1x10^5$	$2.7x10^4$	-37	M184V
7	>$4x10^7$	-	$1.8x10^5$	w/t	-50	$6.8x10^4$	$4.1x10^4$	+2	M184V
8	>$4x10^7$	$1.1x10^5$	$4.7x10^5$	w/t	+8	$1.1x10^4$	$5.6x10^3$	+56	M184V
9	>$4x10^7$	$3.2x10^4$	$9.0x10^6$	M550V; L526M	-68	$7.9x10^3$	$5.0x10^2$	-10	nd
10	>$4x10^7$	$1.6x10^4$	$4.5x10^5$	M550V; L526M	-96	$3.6x10^4$	$5.5x10^3$	+29	M184V
11	>$4x10^7$	$2.1x10^5$	$4.7x10^5$	M550M/V;L526M/L	-32	$2.8x10^4$	$3.1x10^3$	+87	M184V
12	$1.1x10^6$	$9.3x10^3$	$1.2x10^6$	M550I	+475	$2.7x10^4$	$8.2x10^2$	+28	nd
13	$6.2x10^6$	-	$4.6x10^5$	M550V; L526M	-14	$2.6x10^4$	<$4x10^2$	+65	nd

+ for those patients with a demonstrable HBV viral load rebound during the period of study, the nadir viral-load value reached is given.

ALT, alanine transferase; w/t, wild type; M, methionine; V, valine; I, isoleucine; L, leucine; nd, HIV RT sequencing not done due to insufficient HIV viral load; inh, inhibiting sample in HBV quantitative polymerase chain reaction assay

lamivudine therapy for HBV. A further conclusion from this analysis is that for a significant proportion of lamivudine-treated patients, poor suppression of HBV (>10,000 c/ml) is not necessarily associated with drug resistance, but more probably with inadequate potency of a monotherapy regimen against the background of an extremely high viral replication rate.

Lamivudine is commonly prescribed for HIV infection, and it is very likely that a large number of co-infected patients have therefore received this drug. Our results suggest that the clinical and virological benefit of HBV lamivudine monotherapy in such patients should be balanced against a potential for emergence of drug resistance.

Conclusion

In summary, we have explored the emergence of HBV drug resistance against lamivudine in a range of patient groups. Differences in the dynamics of emergence of resistance between transplant and non-transplant patients have been identified through detailed virological monitoring, and genotypic analysis of HBV polymerase has demonstrated the quasispecies nature of this virus. Therefore, it is likely that monotherapy drug pressure selects for a wide range of viral species, the presence of which may compromise subsequent nucleoside analogue therapy.

It is essential that new strategies for therapy of HBV are based on highly potent combination regimens, thereby reducing the risk of emergence of drug resistance.

References

1. Allen, M.I., Deslauriers, M., Andrews, C.W., et al., 1998. Identification and characterisation of mutations in hepatitis B virus resistant to lamivudine. Hepatology 27, 1670-1677.
2. Burroughs, N.J., Pillay, D., Mutimer, D., 1999. Significance testing of clinical data using virus dynamics models with a Markov chain Monte Carlo method: application to emergence of lamivudine-resistant hepatitis B virus. Proc. R. Soc. Lond. B. 266, 59-2366.
3. Cane, P.A., Mutimer, D., Ratcliffe, D., et al., 1999. Analysis of Hepatitis B virus quasispecies changes during emergence and reversion of lamivudine resistance in liver transplantation. Antivir. Ther. 4(1), 7-14.
4. Dore, G.J., Cooper, D.A., Barrett, C., et al., 1999. Dual efficacy of lamivudine on human immunodeficiency virus/hepatitis B virus coinfected patients from a randomised, controlled study (CAESAR). J. Infect. Dis. 180, 607-613.
5. Lai, C.L., Chien R.N., Leung N.W., et al., 1998. A one year trial of lamivudine for chronic hepatitis B. Asia hepatitis lamivudine study group, NEJM 339(2) 61-68.
6. Mutimer, D., Pillay, D., Shields, P., et al., 2000. Outcome of lamivudine resistant Hepatitis B virus infection in the liver transplant recipient. Gut 46, 107-113.
7. Mutimer, D., Pillay, D., Cook, P., et al., 2000. Selection of multi-resistant hepatitis B virus during sequential nucleoside analogue therapy. J. Infect. Dis. 181(2), 713-716.
8. Ono-Nita, S.K., Kato, N., Shiratori, Y., et al., 1999. Susceptibility of lamivudine-resistant hepatitis B virus to other reverse transcriptase inhibitors. J. Clin. Invest. 103, 1635-1640.

9. Pillay, D., Bartholomeusz, A., Cane, P., et al., 1998. Mutations in the hepatitis B DNA polymerase associated with antiviral resistance. Int. Antiviral News 6, 167-169.

Lamivudine for chronic hepatitis B: Efficacy, safety, resistance, and current treatment issues

NATHANIEL A. BROWN

Idenix Pharmaceuticals, Inc., 125 CambridgePark Drive, Cambridge, MA 02476 USA

Introduction

Lamivudine (β-L-2',3'-dideoxy-3'-thiacytidine) is an orally bioavailable L-cytidine analog which inhibits human immunodeficiency virus (HIV) and hepatitis B virus (HBV) replication *in vitro* at nanomolar concentrations. In recent years, lamivudine tablet formulations have been subjected to extensive clinical investigations in both HIV- and HBV-infected patients, leading to regulatory approvals for HIV infection (as part of combination therapies) from 1995 onward, and regulatory approvals for chronic hepatitis B (as a monotherapy) from 1998 onward. Currently, lamivudine is regulatory-approved for use in the treatment of patients with chronic hepatitis B in over 50 countries worldwide.

The antiviral, pharmacologic, and human pharmacokinetic properties of lamivudine have been reviewed elsewhere [1]. This review focuses on the cumulative Phase II and III data from the worldwide clinical trial program for lamivudine in patients with chronic hepatitis B. As the first of a new generation of orally-bioavailable HBV therapeutics, the accumulated clinical data for lamivudine provide insights on what the future may hold for monotherapy and combination therapy with additional HBV antiviral agents. This review summarizes existing scientific and clinical data, primarily from GlaxoWellcome-sponsored clinical trials of lamivudine. This data review is not intended as prescribing information for treating hepatitis B patients; in this regard, clinicians should consult regulatory-approved product labels for lamivudine in their respective countries.

Phase II clinical trial results

The primary efficacy endpoint assessed in the Phase II dose-ranging trials of lamivudine in hepatitis B patients was reduction of serum HBV DNA levels, reflecting suppression of HBV replication. This endpoint was chosen because reductions in HBV DNA levels had previously been shown to be associated with improvements in HBV-associated liver inflammation, and possibly with HBeAg loss and seroconversion (i.e., gain of detectable anti-HBe). The results of Phase II dose-ranging trials indicated that lamivudine treatment

Frontiers in Viral Hepatitis Ed. by RF Schinazi, J-P Sommadossi and CM Rice. 365 — 381

of patients with chronic hepatitis B consistently afforded marked reductions in serum HBV DNA levels, with maximal reductions at daily doses of 100 mg and above [2-5]. In the Phase II trials, estimates of lamivudine's anti-HBV effect were artificially lowered by two methodologic limitations: (a) the studies utilized a conventional solution hybridization assay used in earlier interferon trials, which could not detect HBV DNA reductions to levels below approximately 10^6 genomes/ml; and (b) for data-analysis purposes, HBV DNA data from the Phase II trials were log-transformed, and 'negative' values were arbitrarily assigned a positive value of one-half of the lower limit of detection of the solution hybridization assay (typically 0.8 pg/ml, one-half of 1.6 pg/ml). The latter analytic convention truncated the observed HBV DNA reductions in the Phase II trials at this lower boundary of analysis (0.8 pg/ml), artificially limiting the observed HBV DNA reductions to about two $\log_{10}$ in most patients.

To address these methodologic limitations of the Phase II virologic data, sera from a Phase IIb trial of extended lamivudine treatment were reexamined by sensitive quantitative PCR methods (Roche Monitor™ assay) [6]. The PCR results from this trial indicated that the 23 patients experienced a median reduction in serum HBV DNA levels of 5.1 $\log_{10}$ during the first six months of treatment [6]. In individual patients, treatment-related reductions in serum HBV DNA levels ranged from 2.7 to 7.4 $\log_{10}$. Thus, all patients in this Phase IIb trial experienced a >99% reduction in circulating HBV DNA with lamivudine treatment, and the typical viral load reduction was >10,000-fold.

Phase III clinical trial results

Four controlled phase III trials were conducted internationally in HBeAg-positive adult patients with chronic hepatitis B: a placebo-controlled, Asian multicenter study in treatment-naïve patients; a placebo-controlled, U.S. multicenter study in treatment-naïve patients; an active comparator study (lamivudine vs. interferon vs. a 24-week combination regimen) conducted in Europe, Canada, and several other locales, where patients were also treatment-naïve; and an international study (placebo vs. lamivudine vs. a 24-week combination regimen) involving patients who previously failed to respond to alpha-interferon. The results of these Phase III clinical trials, investigating primarily one-year treatment periods, have recently been published or reported in abstract form [7-10]. These four Phase III trials afforded primary (intent-to-treat) efficacy analyses for 958 patients treated with any of the following: placebo, lamivudine monotherapy, interferon alpha-2b monotherapy, or a 24-week combination regimen of lamivudine plus interferon.

The results of the four Phase III trials indicated that lamivudine treatment consistently led to reduced hepatic necroinflammatory activity, reduced progression of hepatic fibrosis (in treatment-naïve patients), enhanced HBeAg loss and seroconversion, and normalization of serum ALT levels [6-9]. These four efficacy endpoints were prospectively defined in the Phase III protocols. The results of the Phase III trials are summarized in further detail below, before the review of results in patients with HBeAg-negative CHB and other patient groups.

Changes in hepatic necroinflammatory activity and fibrosis

Clinical outcomes in viral hepatitis patients are ultimately associated with the extent of progression of necroinflammatory damage in the liver. Chronic necroinflammatory activity, related to ongoing HBV or HCV replication, is ultimately responsible for end-stage cirrhosis and may be an important tumor-promoting stimulus for hepatocellular carcinoma. Hence, in trials of antiviral agents for viral hepatitis, it is important to assess treatment effects on liver inflammation and fibrosis.

As in hepatitis C trials with interferon, histologic responses were measured in the lamivudine trials as 2-point-or-greater reductions in the Knodell histologic activity index, i.e., the Knodell HAI score [11, 12]. The Phase III protocols required documentation of histologic features of chronic viral hepatitis in pretreatment liver biopsies, and the availability of histologic slides from pretreatment and follow-up liver biopsies (the latter at Week 52 visits). For the Phase III histologic assessments, biopsy slide evaluations were performed by independent expert hepatopathologists. Slide readings were blinded with regard to patient identification, treatment assignment, date, and sequence (i.e., baseline vs. follow-up) [7-10]. Confirmatory histologic assessments included separate slide 'ranking' evaluations, in which paired biopsy slides (baseline and follow-up) from each patient were evaluated by the hepatopathologists for global severity of histologic features, separately for necroinflammatory and fibrosis features. In these 'ranking' analyses, the pathologists were blinded to patient identifiers, treatment, date, and sequence of the biopsy slides (baseline vs. follow-up). The pathologists knew only that the two slides before them for the 'ranking' comparison were from the same patient. The task was to rank one slide as 'worse' or both slides as the 'same' (for necroinflammatory features, then separately for fibrosis features).

Across the Phase III trials, 17-26% of patients, distributed proportionately across the randomized treatment groups, lacked paired evaluable liver biopsies. In the intent-to-treat analyses featured in most lamivudine publications, patients for whom two evaluable biopsies were not available were counted as histologic non-responders, thus conservatively controlling against bias in any missing data, but potentially leading to underestimates of histologic treatment effects.

As summarized in Figure 1, in the three placebo-controlled Phase III trials, histologic responses were consistently more frequent in lamivudine recipients than in placebo-treated patients ($P < 0.01$ for each trial) [7, 8, 10]. In the active-comparator trial, histologic responses were more common with lamivudine, but the difference compared to interferon was not statistically significant [8]. For unclear reasons, in this study histologic response was proportionally lowest in the combination treatment group [8]. In each trial, the results of the separate slide 'ranking' analyses confirmed the significant lamivudine treatment effect observed with Knodell HAI scoring. Also, subanalyses of the HAI component scores confirmed a significant treatment effect (2-point or greater reductions) in the sum of the first three components of the Knodell score, a sum which is usually termed the "necroinflammatory" HAI score.

Another histologic endpoint prospectively incorporated into the lamivudine trials was analysis of progression of fibrosis, defined as the appearance of worsening in a patient's follow-up (Week 52) biopsy compared to the same patient's baseline biopsy,

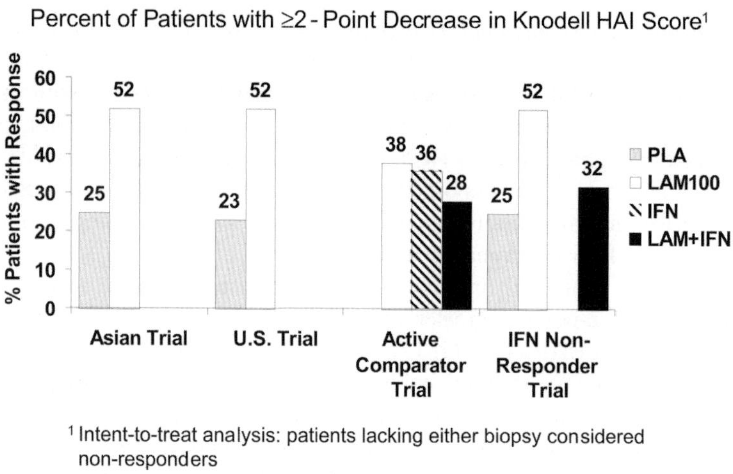

Figure 1. Effect of treatment on liver histology.

in the blinded slide-ranking evaluations. As shown in Figure 2, fibrosis progression in patients was significantly less common with lamivudine treatment, in the multicenter Asian and U.S. trials which enrolled previously untreated (i.e., interferon-naïve) patients ($P < 0.01$ in comparison to placebo, in both trials). In contrast, the difference in fibrosis progression in the trial involving interferon non-responders did not reach statistical significance (4% for lamivudine vs. 7% for placebo), perhaps because patients in this trial already had advanced histologic disease at baseline (19% with cirrhosis, many others with grade 3 fibrosis). In the active comparator trial, as shown in Figure 2, fibrosis progression was observed in 17% of lamivudine patients, 30% of interferon patients, and 32% of patients in the combination therapy group ($p = 0.051$ for the lamivudine vs. interferon comparison) [10].

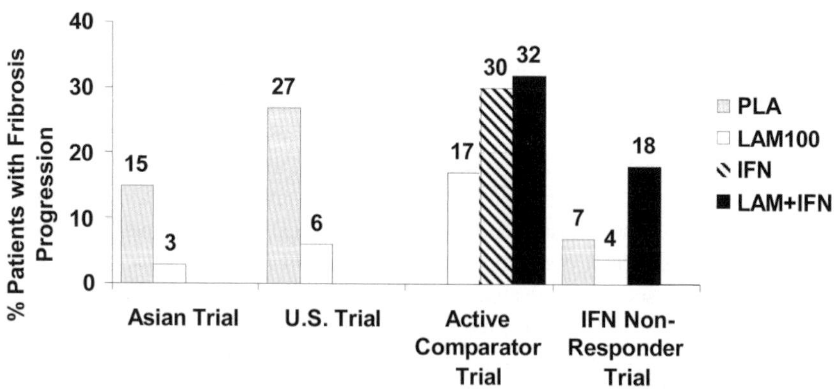

Figure 2. Effect of treatment on fibrosis progression.

In contrast to fibrosis progression, improvement in fibrosis was not a pre-defined, statistically-evaluated endpoint in the lamivudine trial program. Hence the apparent improvement in preexisting fibrosis, evident for many patients in the Phase III trials, deserves further evaluation in future studies. Finally, although progression to cirrhosis was expected to be a relatively rare event in the one-year Phase III trials, an exploratory analysis of the Phase III histologic results revealed that, overall, 1.8% of lamivudine-treated patients progressed to cirrhosis during the one-year Phase III trial periods, compared to 7.1% of placebo-treated patients ($p = 0.04$) [13].

HBeAg and HBsAg loss and seroconversion

Histologic improvements correlate with suppression of HBV replication, i.e., with serum HBV DNA reductions, regardless of whether HBeAg or HBsAg seroconversion are observed [14]. However, HBeAg loss and seroconversion (HBeAg loss with gain of anti-HBe) are associated with multilog reductions in serum HBV DNA levels, reflecting a patient's transition to a generally durable state of markedly reduced HBV replication; and this state of reduced HBV replication is usually associated with histologic improvement, except in patients with preexisting advanced cirrhosis [14-16). The long-term histologic improvements associated with HBeAg loss/seroconversion appear to explain the observation that HBeAg responses are usually a good predictor of improved long-term clinical outcomes, i.e., improved survival and reduced incidence of cirrhosis-related liver failure [15, 16]. Therefore, observations regarding HBeAg responses (loss or seroconversion) are important for two reasons. First, HBeAg response provides a potential opportunity to discontinue nucleoside antiviral therapy (while continuing to observe the patient). And second, HBeAg response in a pre-cirrhotic patient provides some assurance, albeit preliminary, of the probability of an improved longer-term clinical outcome.

In the Phase III trials in treatment-naïve Asian and Western patients, lamivudine-treated patients showed significantly enhanced rates of HBeAg response (loss and seroconversion) compared to placebo recipients. HBeAg loss rates at Week 52, for the various treatment regimens in the four Phase III trials, are illustrated in Figure 3. Three-component HBeAg seroconversion (loss of detectable HBeAg, loss of detectable HBV DNA, and gain of detectable anti-HBe) was the featured analysis for HBeAg responses in the Phase III trial program, although simple HBeAg loss and 2-component HBeAg seroconversion (loss of HBeAg with gain of anti-HBe) were also significantly enhanced with lamivudine [7, 8].

In the the active comparator trial, HBeAg loss (22% and 22%) and seroconversion (18% and 19%) were similar at one year for lamivudine and interferon, and proportionally somewhat better at one year with the combination regimen (lamivudine+interferon), as illustrated in Figure 3 [9]. The increment in HBeAg seroconversion with the combination regimen was not statistically significant in the primary (intent-to-treat) data analysis, but did achieve significance in two secondary efficacy-subset analyses. Therefore the issue as to whether the combination of lamivudine plus interferon will result in enhanced HBeAg seroconversion rates needs further prospective study. Furthermore, in this study it was notable that other efficacy endpoints (e.g., ALT nor-

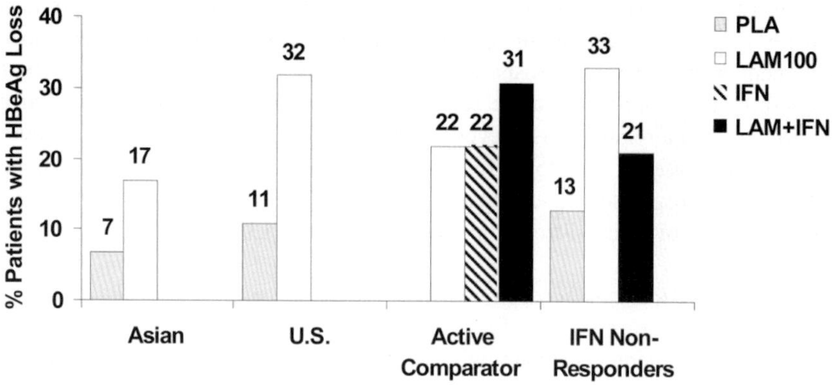

Figure 3. Effect of treatment on HBeAg loss.

malization) and safety considerations favored lamivudine monotherapy over interferon monotherapy and the combination regimen.

In the international trial with interferon non-responders, sustained HBV DNA response and ALT normalization were significantly better for lamivudine recipients, and 3-component HBeAg seroconversion was proportionally best for the lamivudine group, but was not statistcally superior to placebo (18% vs 13%, p = ns), in part due to the high seroconversion rate in the placebo group in this trial [10]. In a secondary analysis of data from this trial, HBeAg loss was significantly better with lamivudine (33% vs. 13% for placebo, $p < 0.04$), and data from the follow-up period indicated that patients with HBeAg loss alone had responses that appeared equally durable post-treatment, compared to patients with 2- or 3-component HBeAg seroconversion [10]. As shown in Figure 3, in this study HBeAg loss with lamivudine monotherapy was proportionally better than results achieved with the combination regimen (21%). In this regard, it is important to note that this study exclusively enrolled interferon non-responders, in contrast to the active-comparator trial described above, which enrolled interferon-naïve patients.

The 3-component HBeAg seroconversion endpoint prospectively defined in the lamivudine trials differs from the HBeAg loss endpoint used in most interferon trials [17]. HBeAg loss is more frequent than 3-component seroconversion, although most patients with HBeAg loss also exhibit undetectable serum HBV DNA (in hybridization assays), and most eventually develop detectable anti-HBe. This difference in the featured HBeAg response endpoint can give rise to confusion when comparing results across lamivudine and previous interferon trials [18]. In the placebo-controlled Western trials, i.e., the U.S. multicenter and international interferon non-responder trials, HBeAg loss was observed in 32-33% of lamivudine patients at Week 52, similar to the 20-40% HBeAg loss rates reported for interferon [14, 17].

Exploratory regression analyses of combined data from the Phase III lamivudine trials indicates that, with lamivudine treatment (as for interferon), HBeAg loss and seroconversion are proportional to pretreatment ALT levels, presumably signifying better treatment-related clearance of HBV replication in patients with ongoing immune responses to HBV infection [14, 19]. The combined Phase III data indicate that, for each baseline ALT level, the frequency of HBeAg responses to lamivudine at one year is at least as high as that for interferon treatment [19]. In contrast to several reported analyses of interferon data, in multivariate regression analyses of the Phase III lamivudine data, pretreatment HBV DNA level did not reach statistical significance as a predictor of HBeAg responsiveness to lamivudine [19].

There are increasing data that, with extension of lamivudine therapy past one year, HBeAg loss and seroconversion can be cumulative [20-23]. To date, the only substantial longer-term data are from a multicenter follow-on study conducted in Asia, in which 58 patients have had a continuous assignment to lamivudine treatment (100 mg/day). As shown in Figure 4, annual data updates on this continuous-treatment Asian cohort indicate an encouraging pattern of cumulative HBeAg loss and seroconversion during up to four years of lamivudine treatment to date, especially in patients with elevated ALTs pretreatment [20-23]. At four years, cumulative HBeAg loss was greater than 60% for patients with any elevated level of ALT pretreatment, and more than 70% for patients with pretreatment ALT levels greater than twofold above normal [23].

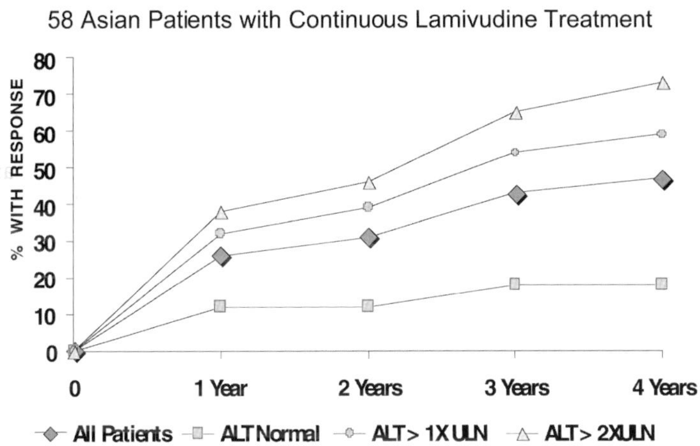

Figure 4. HBeAg loss over four years by pretreatment ALT level.

For patients who experienced HBeAg loss and/or HBeAg seroconversion in the Western Phase III studies, such responses have generally been durable after discontinuation of lamivudine treatment, with posttreatment data now extending to two years or more [8, 10, 24-26]. Similar to observations on HBeAg seroconversion, it appears likely that HBsAg seroconversion will be cumulative over time in HBeAg responders. In a recent update of data from a posttreatment follow-up study, 9 of 43 (21%) previous HBeAg responders to lamivudine had achieved durable HBsAg seroconversions (undetectable serum HBsAg and detectable anti-HBs) [26]. Thus, in immunocompetent hepatitis B patients with compensated liver disease treated for a year or more with lamivudine, when HBeAg loss or seroconversion occurs (as documented on two or more successive clinic visits) appears to be a reasonable time to discontinue treatment, although clinical follow-up should continue routinely [8, 25].

HBV DNA reductions and ALT normalization

Virologic response and ALT normalization were prospectively-defined secondary efficacy endpoints in the lamivudine Phase III trials. The Phase III results indicated that, as in the Phase II trials, lamivudine treatment consistently resulted in marked reductions in serum HBV DNA levels, with median values remaining undetectable for lamivudine-treated patients at the end of the one-year Phase III treatment periods [7-10]. Overall, in the Phase III trials about 30% of patients had detectable serum HBV DNA (in the solution hybridization assay) at the end of one year of treatment, although the quantitative HBV DNA values in such patients were typically substantially below their pretreatment levels.

As might be expected in light of the treatment-related reductions in hepatic necroinflammatory activity described above, serum ALT levels were consistently improved with lamivudine treatment, with patients typically achieving normal ALT levels within four to12 months after the start of lamivudine treatment in the Phase III trials [7-10]. As noted above, in the active comparator trial, serum ALT normalization was significantly better at one year for lamivudine, compared to either interferon or the 24-week combination regimen [9, 27].

Phase III safety observations

In the Phase III trials, the safety profile of lamivudine was consistently similar to placebo during the one-year treatment periods, with regard to both clinical adverse events and laboratory abnormalities [7-10, 28]. Posttreatment, more grade 3-4 ALT elevations were observed in patients discontinued from lamivudine, compared to placebo, but clinically severe posttreatment adverse events were rare (<1% of patients), and the incidence of such severe events was not different for patients discontinuing lamivudine or placebo [8-10, 28]. Despite these assurances from the controlled data, in patients who have not HBeAg-seroconverted prior to the discontinuation of lamivudine treatment, it is likely that replication-active hepatitis B will return, and it is recommended that patients who are discontinued from treatment should be periodically monitored for evidence of return of disease activity (clinically, and for HBV serologic markers and serum liver function tests).

One report indicated that severe disease flares, including hepatic decompensation, can occasionally be seen in patients with disease breakthroughs on long-term lamivudine therapy, associated with the emergence of lamivudine-resistant, YMDD-mutant HBV (see below) [29]. None of the patients died, and the disease flare was associated with potentially beneficial HBeAg seroconversion in eight of 12 patients, including durable HBeAg seroconversions and disease remissions in the three patients with transient hepatic decompensation [29]. Due to these observations, further analyses of combined Phase II-IV lamivudine data were undertaken, leading to observations that:

(a) liver-related severe adverse events were significantly more common in placebo-treated patients compared to lamivudine recipients; and (b) liver-related serious adverse events were rare (<1% per year) and were about equally common in patients with PCR-detectable YMDD-mutant HBV vs. residual wild-type HBV [30].

Drug-resistant HBV mutants: Impact on response

Many reports now support the notion that mutations affecting the methionine codon in the conserved YMDD motif in the HBV polymerase/reverse transcriptase are the primary mutations for HBV resistance to lamivudine *in vitro* [31-36]. These mutations result in a variant HBV polymerase, with either valine or isoleucine substituted for the methionine residue in the YMDD motif, which is located within the catalytic domain of the polymerase. With other examples of antiviral resistance (e.g., HIV and herpesviruses), the emergence of viral strains with reduced antiviral susceptibility is not automatically associated with complete loss of clinical response, in contrast to assumptions from clinical experiences with microbial resistance during acute bacterial infections. In patients with chronic viral infections, this potential dissociation between viral resistance *in vitro* and clinical response *in vivo* occurs principally for two reasons: (a) viral strains with mutations associated with reduced drug susceptibility tend to exhibit reduced replication competence, because the primary resistance mutations structurally affect viral gene products that are critical for replication (e.g., polymerases); and (b) chronic immune responses contribute to an ongoing virus-host equilibrium. Such previous lessons in anitviral resistance appear fully applicable to the clinical resistance considerations for lamivudine in hepatitis B patients, as discussed below.

Early reports indicated that the development of YMDD-mutant HBV, detected by PCR amplification of HBV DNA from patient sera, is associated with variably diminished virologic and clinical responses to lamivudine [31-33]. Hence, in the four Phase III trials, the incidence and clinical significance of YMDD-variant HBV were studied systematically by PCR amplification of HBV DNA from all available patient sera at Week 52 (and selected other timepoints), regardless of the patients' clinical and virologic status. With this approach, YMDD-mutant HBV were detectable after one year of therapy in 14-32% of lamivudine-treated patients in the individual Phase III trials, with a higher incidence in the Western studies (27-32%) compared to the Asian study (14-16%) [7-10]. In the Asian follow-on treatment study, the incidence of detectable YMDD mutants has been cumulative, with YMDD mutants detectable by PCR methods in 42% of patients at year two, 53% at year three, and 70% at year four [20-23].

While some patients with YMDD mutants in the clinical trials maintained undetectable HBV DNA levels (in conventional assays) and normal ALT levels, most such patients exhibited a variably diminished therapeutic response. In each study, patients with YMDD-mutant HBV were found to have reduced HBeAg loss/seroconversion compared to lamivudine-treated patients with wild-type HBV [7-10]. Also, patients with YMDD mutants were less likely to show sustained ALT normalization and sustained non-detectable HBV DNA [7-10, 20-23]. However, patients with YMDD mutants tended to maintain improved median HBV DNA levels, ALT levels, and histologic scores, compared to their pretreatment values and compared to placebo-treated patients [7-10, 20-23, 37].

At the time of emergence of YMDD-mutant HBV, a proportion of patients will experience return of elevated serum ALT levels, often associated with return of serum HBV DNA to levels $>10^6$ genomes/ml. However, these elevated ALT and HBV DNA levels most often subside, or partially subside, over the subsequent two to eight months, after which patients tend to maintain improved or partially improved ALT and HBV DNA levels. For the subgroup of patients who do not maintain at least partial efficacy responses on long-term lamivudine therapy — e.g., patients whose serum ALT and HBV DNA levels return toward pretreatment values, or who exhibit clinical or histologic evidence of disease progression — discontinuation of therapy, or addition of other therapeutic agents should be considered.

In the overall Phase III data, patients who developed YMDD mutants tended to have higher pretreatment HBV DNA levels compared to patients who lacked detectable YMDD mutants. After one year of treatment, HBV DNA in patients with YMDD mutants remained substantially reduced (median HBV DNA at one year = 22 pg/ml compared to 138 pg/ml at pretreatment baseline); but these results were not as good as those for patients without YMDD variants (median HBV DNA at one year = undetectable by hybridization) [37]. The two-, three-, and four-year results from the Asian follow-on treatment study indicated that patients who developed YMDD mutants typically continued to maintain substantially reduced HBV DNA levels on continued lamivudine, and median ALT levels remained improved by 50% or more in the same group [20, 21, 23]. Cumulatively one third (13/39) of these Asian patients with YMDD-mutant HBV had HBeAg seroconverted with up to four years of treatment [23].

The observation that HBV DNA levels tend to remain improved with lamivudine treatment for prolonged periods in patients with lamivudine-resistant HBV variants indicates a potentially interesting and important contrast between HBV resistance and HIV resistance — i.e., a potentially slower and less frequent development of viral variants with "compensatory mutations" during HBV infection compared to HIV infection. HIV patients, after the development of YMDD-altered (codon 184-mutant) HIV variants, tend to exhibit initially depressed HIV RNA levels, but are likely to show a relatively early return or partial return of HIV RNA toward pretreatment levels, in association with the emergence of viral subpopulations with compensatory mutations restoring, or partially restoring, the replication competence lost with the YMDD-associated (codon 184) primary resistance mutation. Late secondary mutations involving HBV polymerase mutations outside the YMDD motif, possibly compensatory in their replication effects, have been reported in occasional hepatitis B patients on prolonged lamivudine therapy [38]. However, in the overall lamivudine clinical trial experience to date, these mutations appear to be unusual, at least in the first four years of lamivudine treatment. The clinical significance of YMDD-mutant and other lamivudine-resistant HBV variants, with regard to diminution of clinical efficacy, remains to be elucidated through additional studies.

De novo combination therapy remains strongly preferable in HIV patients due to the high mutability of HIV and the irreversible loss of memory CD4 lymphocytes with virologic breakthrough. The slower emergence of virologic resistance, and the regenerative capacity of the liver (associated with substantially slower deterioration in target organ function in HBV patients) together support investigation of clinical strategies of monotherapy and sequential combination regimens, as well as *de novo* combination regimens, in patients with chronic hepatitis B. *De novo* combination treatment strategies may be particularly desirable in subgroups of hepatitis B patients for whom the medical risks of virologic breakthrough are high – e.g., patients with advanced cirrhosis or immunodebilitated organ transplant recipients.

Clinical results for other patient groups

Aside from patients with clinically compensated, HBeAg-seropositive chronic hepatitis B, several other patient groups comprise important components of the worldwide disease burden associated with chronic HBV infection — e.g., patients with HBeAg-negative chronic hepatitis B due to pre-core mutant HBV, patients with decompensated cirrhosis, endstage patients requiring liver transplantation, and children with active chronic hepatitis B. Current results for each of these patient subgroups are summarized briefly below, with references for further details as needed.

Over the past fifteen years, HBeAg-seronegative chronic hepatitis B, due to so-called pre-core mutant HBV, has been reported with increasing frequency, especially in the countries of the Mediterranean littoral and in Southeast Asia. For patients with HBeAg-seronegative hepatitis B, the trials of lamivudine treatment include one large controlled study conducted in southern Europe, and several investigator-initiated studies. In the large controlled trial, 125 patients with HBeAg-negative chronic hepatitis B were randomized to lamivudine (100 mg/day) or matching placebo for six months [39]. After six months, patients with detectable HBV DNA were to be withdrawn from treatment, but kept in the study for further observation, while patients with undetectable HBV DNA were to continue treatment to month 12 followed by an additional six months of observation. The study results indicated that the combined efficacy response of clearance of detectable serum HBV DNA (using the Chiron bDNA assay) and normalization of serum ALT levels was achieved at six months by 63% of lamivudine recipients, but only 6% of placebo recipients ($p < 0.001$) [39]. At 12 months, lamivudine recipients showed significant improvements in liver histology compared to baseline. However, data from the six-month posttreatment follow-up period indicated that only 30% of lamivudine recipients maintained undetectable HBV DNA off-treatment, and fewer still (17%) maintained normal ALT levels posttreatment [40]. Thus, as had previously been observed for interferon, most lamivudine-treated patients experienced return of active disease after discontinuation of one year of therapy. Current studies in this patient group are directed toward exploration of longer treatment periods and elucidation of efficacy parameters that might be useful in predicting durable posttreatment responses.

In the liver transplant setting, lamivudine has been studied as a treatment for post-transplant recurrences of hepatitis B and as a prophylactic agent for reducing post-transplant recurrences through pre- and post-transplant suppression of HBV replication [41-44]. While efficacy for both uses has been reported from open-label studies, the issue of antiviral resistance appears especially important in such patients, who tend to have high levels of HBV replication (with steroids and immunsuppression), and who are often debilitated, immunosuppresssed, and lacking in hepatic 'reserve' due to cirrhosis or rapidly progressive HBV infection. Patients in these clinical settings appear to generally experience initial treatment benefit, and post-transplant recurrences appear partially reduced by lamivudine treatment in historical comparisons [41-43]. However, patients in these settings sometimes develop return of severe or fatal disease due to loss of virologic control, whether with wild-type HBV or YMDD-mutant HBV [41-43]. For prevention of post-transplant HBV recurrences, the combination of lamivudine with hepatitis B immune globulin (HBIg) prophylaxis has been reported to offer substantially improved efficacy [44]. Of concern, some lamivudine-treated transplant recipients, after previous treatment with HBIg (and, in some cases, famciclovir) have had recurrences of HBV viremia and rapid disease progression associated with evolution of HBV mutants displaying both YMDD mutations and HBIg-associated polymerase mutations [45, 46], However, other post-transplant patients with YMDD mutants from the same clinical study site have not exhibited rapid disease progression [46]. Complex polypharmacy is often utilized in the organ transplant setting, and the potential for unique HBV mutational patterns in this setting, affecting HBV antiviral susceptibility and replication competence, remains subject to further study.

Ongoing and future studies

Ongoing sponsored lamivudine trials include: (a) Asian and Western follow-up trials of extended lamivudine treatment (i.e., treatment for up to five years, in non-seroconverted patients from the Phase III trials); (b) an international trial in children with chronic hepatitis B; (c) a multicenter, clinical-endpoints trial in Asia, investigating delay in hepatic decompensation in biopsy-documented HBV cirrhotics; and (d) several investigator-initiated studies. Further studies in patients with pre-core mutant HBV infection and patients with HIV/HBV co-infection are anticipated. Additionally, several trials investigating lamivudine in conjunction with other agents are underway or in late planning stages. Collaborative studies involving lamivudine and adefovir will address add-on therapy for patients with YMDD-mutant HBV and return of elevated ALTs, as well as *de novo* combination therapy in treatment-naïve patients with chronic hepatitis B. Collaborative studies of lamivudine plus pegylated interferons will be initiating shortly. As other new anti-HBV agents reach phase II-III clinical development, it is likely that collaborative explorations of various sequential and *de novo* combination treatment regimens will be undertaken by clinical investigators and by pharmaceutical sponsors. A key question at this juncture is whether combinations of orally-bioavailable nucleoside analogs will enhance HBeAg response rates observed with lamivudine alone, or whether treatment regimens employing adjunctive immunomodulatory therapies will be needed to achieve this goal.

Current treatment issues

The most important issue for clinicians trying to reduce the global disease burden associated with chronic HBV infection is the current worldwide lack of clinical recognition of HBsAg carriers, and identification of carriers with active liver disease, most of whom are asymptomatic. With interferon and lamivudine widely available, many patients with chronic hepatitis B can now be clinically managed, and an appreciable fraction can achieve durable treatment responses. Unfortunately, in most countries more than 80-90% of HBsAg carriers are currently unrecognized. Perhaps because little could be done for hepatitis B patients until recently, very few countries have attempted broad screening programs to detect and clinically evaluate HBsAg carriers. Under the present circumstances in both Asian and Western countries, many HBsAg carriers with long-standing subclinical hepatitis will continue to develop advanced cirrhosis and decompensated liver disease by the time of initial clinical recognition,

Non-response to interferon and treatment breakthrough on lamivudine are important issues, and a significant proportion of hepatitis B patients will need additional therapeutic options for successful long-term management of their disease. Nonetheless, substantial therapeutic progress has been made in the past 10-15 years with these two agents, and further progress is likely to be afforded with the availability of additional agents currently under investigation. It appears likely that chronic hepatitis B will be clinically manageable, if not curable, in most patients within the next seven to 10 years. Such imminent therapeutic progress provides a strong stimulus for immediate attention to public campaigns directed toward increased disease awareness and HBV screening, globally. These efforts can go hand-in-hand with expansion of universal HBV vaccination efforts worldwide, to achieve long-term control of the massive burden of death and disease caused by chronic HBV infection.

Conclusions

For non-decompensated, non-immunosuppressed patients with chronic hepatitis B, the accumulating data for lamivudine support a clinical strategy of treating patients with HBV-replicative chronic hepatitis B until HBeAg loss or seroconversion is observed, followed by clinical observation for future signs of return of HBV replication and hepatitis disease activity. Longitudinal follow-on study results to date suggest continuing viral load reductions, ALT improvements, and histologic imrpovements in patients who do not achieve HBeAg responses in the first year of treatment. The Asian trial data indicate that a majority of hepatitis B patients with elevated ALTs may achieve HBeAg seroconversion with up to four years of lamivudine treatment [23]. The development of YMDD-mutant HBV is common with prolonged lamivudine therapy (about 70% of patients at four years), and is associated with variably diminished therapeutic efficacy; but most patients with YMDD mutants continue to experience improved ALT and HBV DNA levels compared to their pretreatment values, and some have achieved durable HBeAg seroconversions. New clinical studies with lamivudine will focus on add-on therapies for patients with virologic breakthrough and return of liver disease (e.g., elevated ALTs), and investigations of *de novo* combination regimens in therapy-naïve patients.

Acknowledgements

This data summary was provided on behalf of the many clinical collaborators, consultants, and Glaxo Wellcome staff involved in the sponsored clinical trial program investigating lamivudine for the treatment of hepatitis B worldwide. Special gratitude is owed to the principal investigators of the Phase III trials (Dr. C-L Lai, Dr. J. Dienstag, Dr. S. Schalm, Dr E. Schiff, Dr. N. Tassopoulos), to several clinical consultants (Dr. R. Perrillo, Dr. D. L. Tyrrell, Dr. A. Lok, Dr. J. Heathcote, Dr. M. Rizzetto, W. Maddrey), and to project colleagues at Glaxo Wellcome (Dr. D.F. Gray, Dr. J. Dent, M. Woessner, Dr. L. Condreay, L. Crowther, S. Gardner, Dr. M. Atkins, J. Barber, Dr. R. Davis, M. Sullivan, P. McPhillips, Dr. A. Moorat, Dr. C. Hunt, and Dr. M. Rubin).

References

1. Jarvis B and Faulds D. Lamivudine: a review of its therapeutic potential in chronic hepatitis B. *Drugs* 1999; 58(1): 101-141
2. Tyrrell DLJ, Mitchell MC, de Man RA, Schalm SW, Main J, Thomas HC, Fevery J, Nevens F, Beranek P and Vicary C. Phase II trial of lamivudine for chronic hepatitis B. *Hepatology* 1993; 18 (No. 4, Pt 2): 112A
3. Dienstag JL, Perrillo RP, Schiff ER, Bartholomew M, Vicary C, and Rubin M. A preliminary trial of lamivudine for chronic hepatitis B infection. *New England Journal of Medicine* 1995;333:1657-1661
4. Lai CL, Ching CK, Tung A, Li E, Young J, Hill A, Wong BC, Dent J, and Wu PC. Lamivudine is effective in suppressing hepatitis B virus DNA in Chinese hepatitis B surface antigen carriers: a placebo-controlled trial. *Hepatology* 1997; 25: 241-244
5. Nevens F, Main J, Honkoop P, Tyrrell DL, Barber J, Sullivan MT, Fevery J, De Man RA, and Thomas HC. Lamivudine therapy for chronic hepatitis B: a six-month randomized dose-ranging study. *Gastroenterology* 1997;113:1258-1263
6. Gauthier J, Bourne EJ, Lutz MW, Crowther LM, Dienstag JL, Brown N, and Condreay L. Quantitation of hepatitis B viremia and emergence of YMDD variants in patients with chronic hepatitis B treated with lamivudine. *Journal of Infectious Diseases* 1999; 180:1757-1762
7. Lai CL, Chien RN, Leung NWY, Chang T, Guan R, Tai D, Ng K, Wu PC, Dent J, Barber J, Stephenson S, and Gray F. A one-year trial of lamivudine for chronic hepatitis B. *New England Journal of Medicine* 1998;339:61-68
8. Dienstag JL, Schiff ER, Wright TL, Perillo RP, Han HWL, Goodman Z, Crowther L, Condreay L, Woessner M, Rubin M and Brown NA. Lamivudine as initial treatment for chronic hepatitis B in patients from the United States. *New England Journal of Medicine* 1999; 341:1256-1263
9. Schalm SW, Heathcote J, Cianciara J, Sherman M, Willems B, Dhillon A, Moorat A, Barber J and Gray DF. Lamivudine and alpha-interferon combination treatment of patients with chronic hepatitis B: a randomised trial. *Gut* 2000; 46: 562-568
10. Schiff E, Karayalcin S, Grimm I, Perrillo R, Dienstag J, Husa P, Schalm S, Crowther L, Sullivan M,

Woessner M, McPhillips P, Brown N and the International Lamivudine Investigator Group. A placebo controlled study of lamivudine and interferon alpha-2b in patients with chronic hepatitis B who previously failed interferon therapy. *Hepatology* 1998; 28 (No. 4, Pt 2): 388A

11. Farrell GC, Bacon BR, and Goldin RD for the Clinical Advisory Group for the Hepatitis C Comparative Study. Lymphoblastoid interferon alfa-n1 improves the long-term response to a 6-month course of treatment in chronic hepatitis C compared with recombinant interferon alpha-2b: results of an international randomized controlled trial.. *Hepatology*. 1998; 27: 1121-1127.
12. Lindsay KL. Therapy of hepatitis C: overview. *Hepatology* 1997; 26 (Suppl.1): 71S-77S
13. Goodman Z, Dhillon AP, Wu PC, Gray F, Atkins M, Stevenson C, Barber J, Brown N, Crowther L and Woessner M. Lamivudine treatment reduces progression to cirrhosis in patients with chronic hepatitis B. *Journal of Hepatology* 1999; 30 (Suppl 1): 59
14. Perrillo RP, Schiff ER, Davis GL, Bodenheimer HC Jr, Lindsay K, Payne J, Dienstag JL, O'Brien C, Tamburro C, Jacobsen IM, Sampliner R, Feit D, Lefkowitch J, Kuhns M, Meschievitz C, Sanghvi B, Albrecht J and Gibas A. A randomized, controlled trial of interferon alpha-2b alone and after prednisone withdrawal for the treatment of chronic hepatitis B. *New England Journal of Medicine* 1990; 323: 295-301
15. Niederau C, Heintges T, Lange S, Goldmann G, Niederau CM, Mohr L and Haussinger D. Long-term follow-up of HBeAg-positive patients treated with interferon alpha for chronic hepatitis B. *New England Journal of Medicine* 1996; 334:1422-1427
16. Lau DTY, Everhart J, Kleiner DE, Park Y, Vergalla J, Schmid P and Hoofnagle JH. Long-term follow-up of patients with chronic hepatitis B treated with interferon alfa. *Gastroenterology* 1997; 113: 1660-1667
17. Wong DKH, Cheung AM, O'Rourke K, Naylor CD, Detsky AS and Heathcote J. Effect of alpha-interferon treatment in patients with hepatitis B e antigen-positive chronic hepatitis B. *Annals of Internal Medicine* 1993; 119: 312-323
18. Omata M. Treatment of chronic hepatitis B infection (editorial). *New England. Journal of Medicine* 1998; 339: 114-115.
19. Perrillo RP, Schalm SW, Schiff ER, Brown N, Woessner M and Sullivan M. Predictors of HBeAg seroconversion in chronic hepatitis B patients treated with lamivudine. *Hepatology* 1999; 30: 317A
20. Leung NWY, Lai CL, Chang TT, Guan R, Lee CM, Ng KY, Wu PC, Dent JC, Edmundsen S and Liaw YF. Three year lamivudine therapy in chronic HBV. *Journal of Hepatology* 1999; 30: 59
21. Liaw YF, Leung NYW, Chang TT, Guan R, Tai DI, Ng KY, Chien RN, Dent J, Roman L, Edmundsen S and Lai CL for the Asia Hepatitis Lamivudine Study Group. Effects of extended lamivudine therapy in Asian patients with chronic hepatitis B. *Gastroenterology* 2000; 119: 172-180
22. Lok ASF. Lamivudine therapy for chronic hepatitis B: is longer duration of treatment better? (editorial) *Gastroenterology* 2000; 119: 263-266
23. Chang TT, Lai CL, Liaw YF, Guan R, Lim SG, Lee CM, Ng KY, Leung NWY, Nicholls GJ, Pearce MA and Dent JC. Incremental increases in HBeAg seroconversion and continued ALT normalization in Asian chronic HBV (CHB) patients treated with lamivudine for four years. *Antiviral Therapy* 2000; 5 (Suppl. 1): 44 (abstract 077).
24. Schiff E, Cianciara J, Kowdley K, Norkrans G, Perillo R, Tong M, Crowther L, Wakeford J, Woessner M, Stevenson C and Brown N. Durability of HBeAg seroconversion after lamivudine monotherapy in controlled phase II and III trials. *Hepatology* 1998; 28 (No. 4, Pt 2): 163A.
25. Dienstag JL, Schiff ER, Mitchell M, Casey DE, Gitlin N, Lissoos T, Gelb LD, Condreay L, Crowther L, Rubin M and Brown N. Extended lamivudine retreatment for chronic hepatitis B: maintenance of viral

suppression after discontinuation of therapy. *Hepatology* 1999; 30: 1082-1087

26. Schiff E, Cianciara J, Karayalcin S, Kowdley K, Woessner, M, McMullen, S, Pearce M and Brown N. Durable HBeAg and HBsAg seroconversions after lamivudine for chronic hepatitis B. *Journal of Hepatology* 2000; 32 (Suppl. No. 2): 99
27. Heathcote J, Schalm SW, Cianciara J, Farrell G, Feinman V, Sherman M, Dhillon AP, Moorat AE, and Gray DF. Lamivudine and Intron A combination treatment in patients with chronic hepatitis B infection. *Journal of Hepatology* 1998; 28: 43
28. Leung N, Dienstag J, Schiff E, Sullivan M, Atkins M, Grice R, Woessner M, Brown N, Hunt CM. Clinical safety profile of lamivudine treatment in a large cohort of hepatitis B patients. *Hepatology* 1998; 28 (No. 4, Pt 2):587A
29. Liaw Y-F, Chien R-N, Tsai S-L, Chu C-M. Acute exacerbation and hepatitis B virus clearance after emergence of YMDD motif mutations during lamivudine therapy. *Hepatology* 1999; 30: 567-572
30. Leung NWY, Lai CL, Dienstag J, Schiff E, Heathcote J, Atkins M, Marr C, Woessner M, Maddrey WC. Long-term safety of lamivudine in patients with chronic hepatitis B. *Abstracts of the N.I.H. Workshop on the Management of Hepatitis B: 2000*, p. 92 (poster 3.5)
31. Tipples GA, Ma MM, Fischer KP, Bain VG, Kneteman NM and Tyrrell DLJ. Mutation in HBV RNA-dependent DNA polymerase confers resistance to lamivudine *in vivo*. *Hepatology* 1996; 24: 714-717
32. Ling R, Mutimer D, Ahmed M, Boxall HE, Elias E, Dusheiko GM and Harrison TJ. Selection of mutations in the hepatitis B virus polymerase during therapy of transplant recipients with lamivudine. *Hepatology* 1996; 24: 711-713
33. Bartholomew MM, Jansen RW, Jeffers LJ, Reddy KR, Johnson LC, Bunzendahl H, Condreay LC, Tzakis AG, Schiff E and Brown N. Hepatitis-B-virus resistance to lamivudine given for recurrent infection after orthotopic liver transplantation. *Lancet.* 1997; 349: 20-22
34. Chayama K, Suzuki Y, Kobayashi M, Kobayashi M, Tsubota A, Hashimoto M, Miyano Y, Koike H, Kobayashi M, Koida I, Arase Y, Saitoh S, Murashima N, Ikeda K and Kumada H. Emergence and takeover of YMDD motif mutant hepatitis B virus during long-term lamivudine therapy and re-takeover by wild type after cessation of therapy. *Hepatology* 1998; 27: 1711-1716
35. Melegari M, Scaglioni PP and Wands JR. Hepatitis B virus mutants associated with 3TC and famciclovir administration are replication defective. *Hepatology* 1998; 27: 628-633
36. Allen MI, Deslauriers M, Andrews CW, Tipples GA, Walters KA, Tyrrell DLJ, Brown N for the Lamivudine Clinical Investigation Group and Condreay LD. Identification and characterization of mutations in hepatitis B virus resistant to lamivudine. *Hepatology* 1998; 27:1670-1677
37. Atkins M, Hunt CM, Brown N, Gray F, Sanathanan L, Woessner M, Lai CL, Dusheiko G, Dienstag J, Wright T, Barnard J, Bourne E and Condreay L. Clinical significance of YMDD mutant hepatitis B virus (HBV) in a large cohort of lamivudine-treated hepatitis B patients. *Hepatology* 1998; 28 (No. 4, Pt 2):319A
38. Yeh CT, Chien RN, Chu CM and Liaw YF. Clearance of the original hepatitis B virus YMDD-motif mutants with emergence of distinct lamivudine-resistant mutants during prolonged lamivudine therapy. *Hepatology* 2000; 31: 1318-1326
39. Tassopoulos NC, Volpes R, Pastore G, Heathcote J, Buti M, Goldin R, Hawley S, Barber J, Condreay L, Gray DF, and the Lamivudine Pre-Core Mutant Study Group. Efficacy of lamivudine in patients with hepatitis B e antigen-negative/hepatitis B virus DNA-positive (precore mutant) chronic hepatitis B. *Hepatology* 1999; 29: 889-896
40. Tassopoulos NC, Volpes R, Pastore G, Heathcote J, Buti M, Gray DF, Barber J and Hawley S.

Post-lamivudine follow-up of patients with HBeAg negative chronic hepatitis B. *Journal of Hepatology* 1999; 30 (Suppl. No. 1): 117

41. Perrillo R, Rakela J, Dienstag J, Levy G, Martin P, Wright T, Caldwell S, Schiff E, Gish R, Villeneuve JP, Farr G, Anschuetz G, Crowther L, Brown N, and the Lamivudine Transplant Group. Multicenter study of lamivudine therapy for hepatitis B after liver transplantation. *Hepatology* 1999; 29: 1581-1586
42. Grellier L, Mutimer D, Ahmed M, Brown D, Burroughs AK, Rolles K, McMaster P, Beranek P, Kennedy F, Kibbler H, McPhillips P, Elias E and Dusheiko G. Lamivudine prophylaxis against reinfection in liver transplantation for hepatitis B cirrhosis. *Lancet* 1996; 348: 1212-15
43. Perrillo RP, Schiff ER, Dienstag JL, Gish R, Dickson R, Adams P, Brown N, Gardner S, and Anschuetz G. Lamivudine for prevention of recurrent hepatitis B after liver transplantation: final results of a U.S./Canadian multicenter trial. *Hepatology* 1999; 30 (No. 4, Pt 2): 222A.
44. Markowitz JS, Martin P, Conrad AJ, Markmann JF, Seu P, Yersiz H, Goss JA, Schmidt P, Pakrasi A, Artinian L, Murray N, Imagawa DK, Holt C, Goldstein L, Stribling R and Busuttil RW. Prophylaxis against hepatitis B recurrence following liver transplantation using combination lamivudine and hepatitis B immune globulin. *Hepatology* 1998; 28: 585-589
45. Tillman HL, Trautwein C, Bock T, Boker KHW, Jackel E, Glowienka M, Oldhafer K, Bruns I, Gauthier J, Condreay LD, Raab HR and Manns MP. Mutational pattern of hepatitis B virus on sequential therapy with famciclovir and lamivudine in patients with hepatitis B virus reinfection occurring under HBIg immunoglobulin after liver transplantation. *Hepatology* 1999; 30: 244-256
46. Tillmann HL, Bock TC, Locarnini SA, Torresi J, Jaeckel E, Rosenau J, Finger A, Boeker KH, Klempnauer J, Manns MP and Trautwein C. Risk factors for selection of YMDD mutants, their consequences in liver transplant recipients, ranging from sudden onset of liver failure to no disease. *Hepatology* 2000; 32 (No. 4, Pt 2): 376A

Clinical experience and follow-up with lamivudine in the Asian population

CHING-LUNG LAI and MAN-FUNG YUEN

Division of Hepatology, Department of Medicine, Queen Mary Hospital, The University of Hong Kong, Hong Kong

Introduction

To date, there are only two therapeutic agents, interferon and lamivudine, that have been generally approved by regional authorities for the treatment of chronic hepatitis B virus (HBV) infection. Lamivudine, unlike interferon-α, has equal efficacy for both Chinese and Caucasian patients with chronic HBV infection and negligible adverse effects.

Lamivudine is the (-) enantiomer of the deoxycytidine analogue 2'-deoxy-3'-thiacytidine. It acts mainly by suppressing the replication of HBV. However, it also has some indirect immunomodulatory effect.

Lamivudine exhibits two modes of viral suppression [1]. First, the active metabolite lamivudine 5'-triphosphate mimics deoxycytidine triphosphate and is incorporated into newly synthesized HBV DNA to cause chain termination. Second, lamivudine 5'-triphosphate demonstrates competitive inhibition of both the viral DNA-dependent DNA polymerase and the RNA-dependent DNA polymerase activity (i.e., reverse transcriptase activity). There are four possible sites of action for lamivudine (Figure 1) [2]. The most obvious site is at the step of reverse transcription of the pre-genomic mRNA into the nascent minus-strand DNA (Figure 1, pathway 1). This has been proven by *in vitro* assays. The second site of action interrupts the formation of plus-strand DNA from the nascent minus-strand DNA, which is dependent on viral DNA polymerase activity (Figure 1, pathway 2). This inhibition has also been demonstrated by *in vitro* assays. Lamivudine may also exert its effect by inhibiting the completion of double-stranded DNA, thereby interrupting cccDNA formation. This will inhibit the amplification and replenishment of this intranuclear store of cccDNA (Figure 1, pathway 3) and the formation of cccDNA during the initial infection (Figure 1, pathway 4). These sites of action, though difficult to prove, are highly likely.

T-cell hyporesponsiveness to HBV antigens is well documented in patients with chronic HBV infection and may represent a critical pathogenic determinant of viral persistence. The mechanism is not known, but may be related to the high viral or antigen load typically observed in these patients.

Boni, et al. have used the reduction of viral and antigen load by lamivudine as an experimental model to investigate the importance of these two factors in the immune response to HBV infection [3]. Twelve patients with hepatitis B e antigen-positive (HBeAg-positive) chronic, active hepatitis received lamivudine 100 mg daily for 12

Frontiers in Viral Hepatitis Ed. by RF Schinazi, J-P Sommadossi and CM Rice. 383 — 390

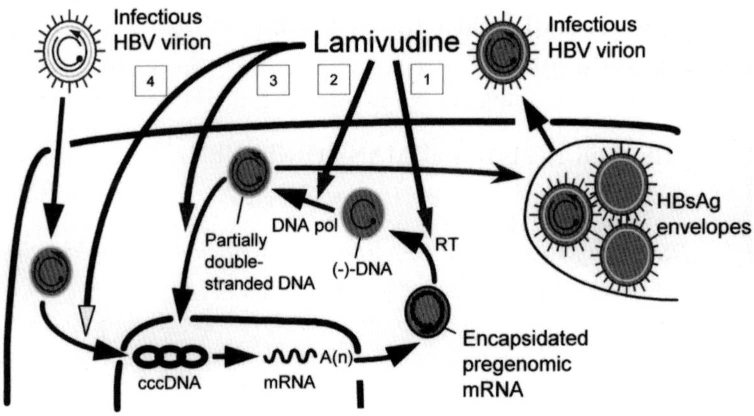

Figure 1. The four possible sites of action of lamivudine in the replicative cycle of the hepatitis B virus (HBV = hepatitis B virus, cccDNA = covalently closed circular DNA, mRNA = messenger RNA, RT = reverse transcriptase, (-)-DNA = minus-strand DNA, DNA pol = DNA polymerase, HBsAg = hepatitis B surface antigen) (Diagram adapted from: Lai CL, MF Yuen. Profound suppression of hepatitis B virus replication with lamivudine. J Med Virol 2000;61:367-373)

months and were then followed up for six months. The T-cell response to HBcAg and HBeAg before treatment initiation was low, but with lamivudine therapy the responses to both antigens showed a rapid and significant increase that persisted throughout the treatment period. After seven to14 days of lamivudine therapy, significant and sustained enhancement of the proliferative CD4-mediated response to HBeAg and HBcAg was noted in 10 patients (83%). These patients also showed an increased frequency of HBeAg-specific T cells and enhanced responses to mitogens and recall antigens, such as phytohaemagglutinin, tetanus toxoid and mouse anti-human CD3 monoclonal antibody. A temporal association was noted between recovery of T-cell reactivity to viral antigens and a reduction in viraemia. The enhanced proliferative responses to HBV proteins and the increased frequencies of circulating HBeAg-reactive T cells were generally preceded by, or temporally associated with, a decline in serum HBV DNA. An enhancement of CD8-positive CTL frequency and reactivity was also observed. These findings indicate that lamivudine therapy overcomes T-cell hyporeactivity. This effect is probably related to a reduction in the level of viraemia.

Experience of lamivudine in Asian patients with HBV infection

Treatment of chronic HBV infection

A multicenter, one-year trial of lamivudine involving 358 Chinese patients with chronic HBV infection showed that lamivudine reduced hepatitis activity (in 54%, 49% and 25% of patients on lamivudine 100 mg daily, lamivudine 25 mg daily and placebo, respectively), decreased progression of fibrosis (which occurred in 3%, 6% and 15% for the same respective drugs), increased HBeAg seroconversion (in 16%, 13% and 4%, respectively) and improved normalization of alanine aminotransferase (ALT) (in 72%, 65%, 24%, respectively) [4]. All the percentages for lamivudine 100 mg daily were significantly better than those for the patients on placebo. However, 15% of patients after one year of either dosage of lamivudine developed mutation in the tyrosine, methionine, aspartate and aspartate (YMDD) motif of the catalytic domain of the HBV DNA polymerase (see below).

For the patients who do not achieve HBeAg seroconversion in the first year, lamivudine will have to be given for a longer period. There are three questions concerning the long-term use of lamivudine. Firstly, will the improvement in HBeAg seroconversion and histology continue with longer periods of lamivudine treatment? Secondly, is lamivudine-induced HBeAg seroconversion stable and sustained when lamivudine is stopped? Thirdly, what are the long-term implications of YMDD-variant HBV?

In the Asian study mentioned above, a proportion of the patients were randomized to continue receiving the same dosage of lamivudine at the end of the first and second year. After the third year, all the patients were offered open-label lamivudine 100 mg daily for two more years. In all, 58 out of the 358 patients received lamivudine 100 mg daily continuously for three years; 44 of these 58 went on to receive a fourth year of lamivudine 100 mg daily. In these 58 patients, the rate of HBeAg seroconversion was 22%, 29%, 40% and 47% at the end of the first, second, third and fourth years respectively. It is well documented that elevated pretreatment ALT level is a major determinant for HBeAg seroconversion [5]. The HBeAg seroconversion rates for the patients with elevated pretreatment ALT and for those with pretreatment ALT of greater than twice above the upper limit of normal are shown in Figure 2. At the end of four years of continuous lamivudine, 73% of patients with pretreatment ALT levels greater than twice the upper limit of normal had HBeAg seroconversion. In the Asian population, there is thus a cumulative increase in HBeAg seroconversion with continuous lamivudine therapy, especially in patients with elevated ALT levels.

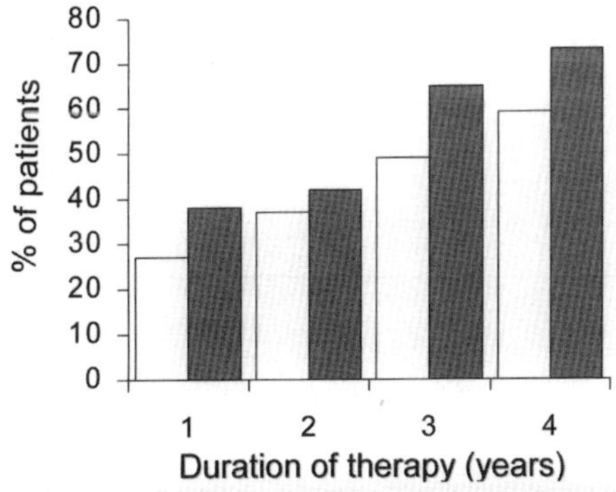

Figure 2. The percentage of patients with elevated pretreatment alanine transaminase levels achieving HBeAg seroconversion on four years of continuous lamivudine therapy. The blank bars represent the patients with alanine transaminase levels above the upper limit of normal at baseline. The shaded bars represent the patients with alanine transaminase levels greater than twice the upper limit of normal at baseline.

In 26 patients who were taken off lamivudine after HBeAg seroconversion, out of the original 358 patients, 21 (81%) remained positive for antibody against HBeAg (anti-HBe) with a median follow-up period of over 12 months. The stability of HBeAg seroconversion is comparable to that observed in Caucasians who are taken off lamivudine after HBeAg seroconversion. In Asian patients with chronic hepatitis B, seroreversion to HBeAg after spontaneous HBeAg seroconversion is relatively common. In a study by Lok and her colleagues, ten out of 31 Chinese patients with spontaneous HBeAg seroconversion had reversion back to HBeAg-positivity, usually within six months [6]. Spontaneous HBeAg seroconversion was only stable in 21/31 (68%) of Chinese patients. Lamivudine-induced HBeAg seroconversion is therefore at least as stable as (probably more stable than) spontaneous HBeAg seroconversion in Chinese patients with chronic hepatitis B infection.

Eighty-one of the 358 patients had a third liver biopsy at the end of the third year (Table 1). In the 38 patients who did not develop the YMDD-variant HBV, 63.2% had continued histologic improvement, and only 13.2% had histologic deterioration. (Histologic improvement, and deterioration are defined as a change in the histologic activity index score of two points or more.)

Table 1. The improvement or worsening in histology in 81 patients on three years of continuous lamivudine therapy with biopsies at baseline and at the end of the third year. Improvement or worsening in histology is defined as a change in the total histologic activity index (HAI) score by two points or more.

	Improved n (%)	*No change* n (%)	*Worsened* n (%)
Non-YMDD (38 pts)	24 (63.2)	9 (23.7)	5 (13.2)
YMDD (43 pts)	21 (48.8)	12 (27.9)	10 (23.3)
YMDD > 2 yr (7 pts)	4 (57.1)	2 (28.6)	1 (14.3)
YMDD 1-2 yr (17 pts)	8 (47.1)	4 (23.5)	5 (29.4)
YMDD < 1 yr (19 pts)	9 (47.4)	6 (31.6)	4 (21.1)

YMDD-variant hepatitis B virus

The major site of mutation of HBV associated with lamivudine therapy is the tyrosine methionine asparate aspartate amino acid (YMDD) motif. The YMDD motif is a highly conserved motif in the catalytic domain of the reverse transcriptase (RT)/DNA polymerase and is shared by all hepadnaviruses as well as retroviruses. The variants are characterized by the mutation of the methionine (codon 552) to either valine or isoleucine (YMDD to YVDD or YIDD). There is often a contributing mutation in the "B domain" of the RT where the leucine (codon 528) is mutated to methionine. Other sites of mutation are less commonly found and of doubtful clinical significance.

The amino acid changes of the YMDD motif, YVDD and YIDD, also result in changes in the amino acid in sequence of HBsAg in positions 195 and 196 respectively. Since the immunodominant protective epitope (the "a" determinant from amino acid position 124 to 147) of the surface antigen is situated away from these mutations, it is unlikely that the YMDD-variant HBV would affect the immune response.

In the wild type HBV, the YMDD motif is in a region with high affinity for nucleotides, hence facilitating the formation of the nascent minus strand of the HBV DNA (Figure 3). Lamivudine has an affinity for the RT domain of the virus, probably because it binds at a pocket formed partly by the methionine in position 552. At the presumed binding site of lamivudine, the side chain of the methionine in position 552 is in van der Waal contact with lamivudine, with a distance of approximately 3Å [7]. The presence of lamivudine will suppress the formation of minus-strand HBV DNA by chain termination and competitive inhibition of the RT activity. With the mutation of methionine in the YMDD motif to isoleucine or valine (YMDD to YIDD or YVDD), the length of the amino acid side chain gets shorter. Allen, et al. postulates that this increases the size of the binding pocket, thereby attenuating the affinity of lamivudine for the RT domain. Lamivudine therefore has little or no inhibitory effect on the replication of the YMDD-variant HBV.

However, with the alteration in the configuration of the YMDD region when the methionine in position 552 is mutated, the interaction between nucleotides and the active catalytic site of the RT is also affected, so that viral replication of the YMDD-variant HBV is less competent than that of the wild type HBV.

The marked impairment in replication competence of HBV bearing the YI/VDD mutations has been demonstrated in transiently transfected the untreated HCC cell lines, and in HEK 293 human embryo kidney-derived cell lines (latter cell lines requiring deoxynucleotide depletion with hydroxyurea treatment) [8].

In the 58 Chinese patients on continuous lamivudine therapy for over three years, the incidence of YMDD-variant HBV at the end of the first, second, third and fourth years of lamivudine was 16%, 38%, 56% and 67%, respectively. Despite the emergence of YMDD-variant HBV, the median HBV DNA level was significantly lower than the pretreatment HBV DNA level. The median ALT level rose with the development of the variants, but remained below the pretreatment level. The lower HBV DNA levels suggest the YMDD-variant HBV is, less replication-competent than the wild-type HBV, and the lower ALT levels suggest that the YMDD-variant HBV causes less aggressive disease than the wild-type HBV.

Among the 81 Chinese patients who had a liver biopsy at the end of the third year, 43 patients had YMDD-variant HBV. Forty-nine% of these patients still had improvement of liver histology; only 23% of patients had worsening of liver histology (Table 1). The proportion of patients with improvement in histology was similar, irrespective of whether the patients had the YMDD variants for less than one year, for one to two years, or for over two years.

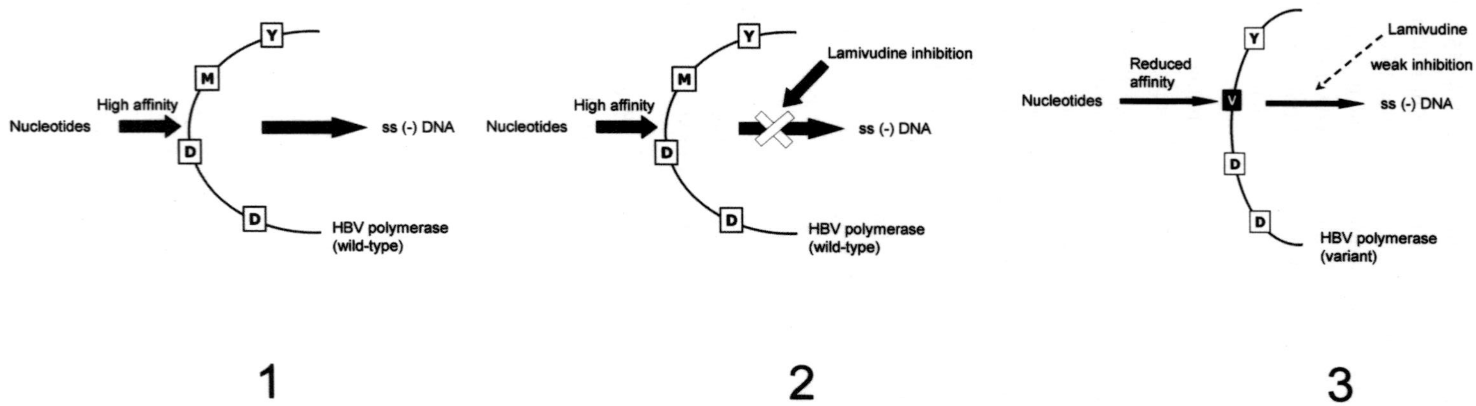

Figure 3. Diagrammatic representation of the effect on lamivudine binding and nucleotide affinity with the mutation of the YMDD motif in the hepatitis B virus DNA polymerase/reverse transcriptase domain. (Y = tyrosine, M = methionine, D = aspartate, V = valine, ss(-)DNA = single-stranded negative hepatitis B virus DNA.) (1) shows the high affinity of the YMDD motif for nucleotides, facilitating the formation of the single-stranded negative hepatitis B virus DNA. (2) shows the effect of the close contact of lamivudine with the side chain of the methionine in the YMDD motif. (3) shows the increase in the size of the binding pocket with mutation of methionine to valine in the YMDD motif, and the effect of such a mutation on the lamivudine binding to the motif and on the affinity for nucleotides.

Lamivudine in liver transplantation in Asian patients

In the Caucasian population, lamivudine monotherapy has been used successfully in both the prevention [9] and the treatment [10] of recurrence of hepatitis B after liver transplantation.

The Liver Transplant Team (University Departments of Medicine and of Surgery), Queen Mary Hospital, Hong Kong, had been using lamivudine as a single agent for the prevention of recurrence of hepatitis B as well as for *de novo* hepatitis B after liver transplantation since 1995. Patients with end-stage hepatitis B cirrhosis were given lamivudine 100 mg daily at least one month before transplantation. For patients presenting with acute fulminant hepatitis B or *de novo* hepatitis B after liver transplantation, lamivudine 100 mg daily was given as soon as possible.

Up to April 2000, there were 54 liver transplant patients requiring lamivudine: 47 with end-stage hepatitis B cirrhosis (36% HBeAg positive and 64% anti-HBe positive at the time of transplantation), three with acute fulminant hepatitis B and four with *de novo* hepatitis B after liver transplantation. Five patients died soon after the transplantation; six died later from unrelated causes, one patient with *de novo* hepatitis B died of fibrosing cholestatic hepatitis within two weeks of acquiring the hepatitis B infection.

The 42 surviving patients had a median follow-up of 24 months (range four to 56 months). Thirty patients lost the hepatitis B surface antigen (HBsAg) after the transplantation, the majority within two months of the operation. Of these 30 patients, eight subsequently developed antibody against HBsAg (anti-HBs). In ten patients who were still positive for HBsAg, nine became anti-HBe positive, and only one patient was still positive for HBeAg. The two remaining patients developed the YMDD-variant HBV at 14 and 18 months after the liver transplantation. The first patient required a second liver transplantation, the explanted liver showing fibrosing cholestatic hepatitis. Both patients received adefovir dipivoxil, which successfully suppressed the YMDD variants.

An incidence of 4.8% for the development of YMDD variants with a median follow-up of 24 months is low compared to the incidence in the post-transplant patients in the Caucasian series and to the incidence in Chinese patients with asymptomatic hepatitis B infection. The reason for the low incidence of YMDD variants in the Chinese post-transplant patients is not known, but may be related to the low level of viral replication in Chinese patients requiring transplantation, in whom the HBV infection would have lingered on for several decades.

Conclusions

Long-term lamivudine monotherapy in the Chinese patients with chronic HBV infection results in incremental increases in HBeAg seroconversion, especially in patients with elevated ALT levels. There is also continued improvement in histology in the majority of patients. HBeAg seroconversion is stable after discontinuation of lamivudine. However, the incidence of YMDD-variant HBV also increases with the long-term use of lamivudine. But, in spite of the development of the YMDD-variant HBV, the HBV

DNA and ALT levels in the majority of patients remain below the pretreatment levels, indicating that the YMDD-variant HBV is probably less replication competent and less aggressive than the wild type HBV. Up to 49% of patients with the YMDD-variant still show histologic improvement.

Lamivudine monotherapy is also useful in preventing the recurrence of hepatitis B infection and in treating *de novo* hepatitis B infection after liver transplantation in Chinese patients. The incidence of YMDD-variant HBV is low in these patients.

The future for the treatment of chronic hepatitis B infection probably lies in combination therapy. But whether lamivudine should be combined with an immunomodulator such as interferon or therapeutic vaccines, or with other nucleoside analogues remains to be determined.

Reference:

1. Johnson MA, Moore KHP, Yuen GJ, Bye A, Palses GE. Clinical pharmacokinetics of lamivudine. Clinical Pharmacokinetics 1999;26(1):41-66.
2. Lai CL, MF Yuen. Profound suppression of hepatitis B virus replication with lamivudine. J Med Virol 2000;61:367-373.
3. Boni C, Bertoletti A, Penna A, Cavalli A, Pilli M, Urbani S, Scognamiglio P, Boehme R, Panebianco R, Fiaccadori F, Ferrari C. Lamivudine treatment can restore T cell responsiveness in chronic hepatitis B. J Clin Invest 1998;102:968-75.
4. Lai CL, Chien RN, Leung NWY, Chang TT, Guan R, Tai DI, et al. A one-year trial of lamivudine for chronic hepatitis B. N Engl J Med 1998;339(2):61-8.
5. Chien RN, Liaw YF, Atkins M, The Asian Hepatitis Lamivudine Trial Group. Pretherapy alanine transaminase level as a determinant for hepatitis B e antigen seroconversion during lamivudine therapy in patients with chronic hepatitis B. Hepatology 1999;30:770-4.
6. Lok ASF, Lai CL, Wu PC, Leung EKY, Lam TS. Spontaneous hepatitis B e antigen to antibody seroconversion and reversion in Chinese patients with chronic hepatitis B virus infection. Gastroenterology 1987;92:1839-43.
7. Allen MI, Deslauriers M, Andrew CW, Tipples GA, Walters KA, Tyrell DLJ, Brown N, Condreay L. Identification and characterization of mutations in hepatitis B virus resistant to lamivudine. Hepatology 1998;27:1670-7.
8. Melegari M, Scaglioni PP, Wands JR. Hepatitis B virus mutants associated with 3TC and famciclovir administration are replication defective. Hepatology 1998;27:628-33.
9. Grellier L, Mutimer D, Ahmed M, Brown D, Burroughs AK, Rolles K, McMaster P, Beranek P, Kennedy F, Kibbler H, McPhillips P, Elias E, Dusheiko G. Lamivudine prophylaxis against reinfection in liver transplantation for hepatitis-B cirrhosis. Lancet 1996;348:1212-5.
10. Perrillo R, Rakela J, Dienstag J, Levy G, Martin P, Wright T, Caldwell S, Schiff E, Gish R, Villeneuve JP, Farr G, Anschuetz G, Crowther L, Brown N, the Lamivudine Transplant Group. Multicenter study of lamivudine therapy for hepatitis B after liver transplantation. Hepatology 1999;29:1581-6.

Impaired response to 5 mU/day interferon treatment in African-Americans with chronic hepatitis C

ALESSANDRA COLANTONI,
NICOLA DE MARIA and DAVID H. VAN THIEL

*Division of Gastroenterology and Hepatology,
Loyola University Medical Center, Building 114, Room 48,
2160 South 1st Ave, Maywood, IL 60153, USA*

Abstract

In the USA, the prevalence of hepatitis C virus (HCV) infection is higher among African-Americans than among Caucasians. The aim of this study was to determine the response rate to interferon (IFN) treatment for chronic HCV infection in these two racial groups.

Thirty-one African-Americans and 62 Caucasians with chronic hepatitis C were studied. The patients were matched for age, gender, severity of liver disease, and viral genotype. They were treated with IFN (5 mU/day) for 12 months. The following endpoints were chosen to evaluate the response rate to IFN treatment: *on-therapy*, after six months of IFN; and *end-of-therapy*, at the end of the 12 months of treatment. African-Americans had a significantly reduced response to IFN as compared to Caucasians at all endpoints. No differences in pretreatment serum ALT, HCV-RNA, iron and ferritin levels or hepatic iron contents between the two groups were found. Our results indicate that African-Americans have a reduced response to high-dose IFN treatment as compared to Caucasians. Both environmental and genetic factors may be implicated in this impaired ability to clear HCV infection.

Introduction

Interferon-alpha (IFN) is an effective treatment for hepatitis C virus (HCV) infection. A sustained response to IFN in chronic hepatitis C is achieved in 15% to 20% of cases when IFN is used alone, and in 30 to 40% when Ribavirin is added to IFN [1]. Both virus and host-related factors have been associated with an elevated likelihood of response to anti-viral treatment in patients infected with HCV [3]. These factors include younger age, absence of cirrhosis, etc. A recent study suggested that African-Americans may have an impaired response to IFN treatment as compared to Caucasians [6]. The prevalence of HCV infection is higher among African-Americans than it is in Caucasians [4]. Thus, it is likely that a higher number of individuals from this racial

Frontiers in Viral Hepatitis Ed. by RF Schinazi, J-P Sommadossi and CM Rice. 391 — 398

group will seek medical care for HCV-related liver disease and will develop, in a medium- to long-term future, complications related to HCV chronic infection.

The aim of the present study was to examine the response to high-dose IFN treatment (5 mU/day) in a case control study comparing African-American and Caucasian individuals with chronic hepatitis C.

Materials and methods

Patients

The present study is a retrospective, case-control study wherein the response rate to IFN for chronic HCV infection was evaluated in African-Americans (study group) and compared to Caucasians (control group). The patient population consisted of consecutive African-American subjects seen at the West Penn Hospital in Pittsburgh, PA, and at the Loyola University Medical Center in Maywood, IL, for HCV-related chronic hepatitis between January 1995 and October 1998. They were treated with IFN 5 mU/day for 12 months. All African-Americans were American citizens born in the United States. Two Caucasian subjects for each African-American, seen during the same time frame at both centers, were used as controls. Before starting the treatment, all subjects had an evaluation consisting of blood cell count, indicators of liver injury, such as AST, ALT, alkaline phosphatase, γ-GTP, total bilirubin, a quantitation of serum HCV-RNA, the analysis HCV genotype, a panel of hepatitis B markers (HBsAg, anti-HBs, anti-HBc) and serum HBV-DNA, a panel of autoantibodies titers (anti-mitochondrial, anti-nuclear, anti-smooth muscle, anti-microsomal and anti-LKM-1), serum iron and ferritin levels, total iron binding capacity and calculated transferrin saturation. A pretreatment liver biopsy for histology, HCV-RNA and HBV-DNA determination was obtained for each patient. Each patient was also evaluated for history of alcohol abuse (defined as use of more than 40 mg alcohol/day for at least six months) or intravenous drug abuse. The criteria for inclusion in the study were: serum anti-HCV and HCV-RNA positivity; age between 18 and 75 years; absence of confounding factors, such as active hepatitis B, autoimmune markers, active alcohol abuse, metabolic disorders, or human immunodeficiency virus positivity; WBC count below $2,000 \times 10^3/mm^3$; platelets count below 50,000/μl; no history of ascites, bleeding varices, or hepatic encephalopathy.

Thirty-one African-Americans were included in the study and were matched in terms of age, gender ratio, cirrhosis index, modified Knodell score and viral genotype with a control group of 62 Caucasians (Table 1). The selection of the control group was based solely on the presence of matching entry criteria. No differences in the pretreatment serum ALT levels, iron and ferritin levels, or hepatic iron content between the two groups were found.

Liver morphology

Two observers read all liver biopsies and scored them using a modified Knodell score, wherein each of the four parameters assessed (periportal necrosis, intralobular necrosis,

Table 1. Characteristics of the study and control groups

	African-Americans (n = 31)	Caucasians (n = 62)
Age (years)	53.5 ± 1.6	52.1 ± 1.2
Male/Female	15/16	30/32
Weight (lbs)		
Male	215.3 ± 14.1	245 ± 21.4
Female	160.8 ± 12.0	152 ± 13.0
Cirrhosis/Non-cirrhosis	9/22	18/44
History of:		
ETOH	43%	38%
IVDU	39%	36%
Diabetes	10%	5%
Genotype:		
1a	36%	36%
1b	56%	54%
Others	8%	10%
Knodell score	8.0 ± 0.4	8.0 ± 0.6
periportal necrosis	1.9 ± 0.2	1.7 ± 0.2
lobular inflammation	1.5 ± 0.1	1.6 ± 0.2
portal inflammation	2.4 ± 0.1	2.5 ± 0.2
fibrosis	2.2 ± 0.2	2.5 ± 0.3
ALT	87.9 ± 15.4	101.4 ± 10.6
HCV-RNA	53.6 ± 8.8	87.7 ± 16.3
Iron - serum	112.5 ± 11.7	115.5 ± 7.7
Ferritin		
Male	458 ± 91.6	735.3 ± 260.8
Female	169.1 ± 35.3	248.8 ± 49.4
Iron - liver		
Male	999.6 ± 131.0	754.5 ± 136.1
Female	522.0 ± 104.1	379.6 ± 41.6

ETOH: alcohol abuse; IVDU: intravenous drug use

portal inflammation, and fibrosis) was scored from 0 (normal) to 4 (worse case) [7]. A score of 2 or less indicates normal liver morphology; scores of 3-6 are considered as mild chronic hepatitis; scores of 7-11 as moderate hepatitis; scores of 12-16 are considered as severe hepatitis with cirrhosis.

IFN treatment protocol

IFN was administered at a dose of 5 mU/day subcutaneously for 12 months. The patients were monitored utilizing routine blood cell counts, ALT, AST, alkaline phosphatase, γ-GTP and total bilirubin levels. Serum HCV-RNA was assessed monthly. The response to IFN treatment is defined as ALT normalization and HCV-RNA disappearance from the serum. The response to IFN was evaluated "on therapy" (after six months of treatment) and at the "end of therapy" (at the end of the 12 months of treatment). IFN administration was discontinued in those individuals who, at the end of a 12-month course of treatment, were persistently HCV-RNA negative in their serum with at least three consecutive monthly negative results. Those individuals who still had HCV-RNA detectable in their serum at the end of the 12 months of IFN administration were considered for other forms of treatment.

Quantitative PCR for HCV-RNA

HCV-RNA quantification was performed at the Central Blood Bank of Pittsburgh utilizing reverse transcriptase-polymerase chain reaction (rt-PCR). RNA was extracted from serum or frozen hepatic tissue using RNAzol B (Biotech Lab, Houston, TX). Complementary DNA was synthesized from the RNA using Moloney murine leukemia virus reverse transcriptase (Gibco BRL, Long Island, NY) and the downstream primer HCV 102 (nucleotide 276-244 of the 5' nontranslated region). Primers HCV 101 (nucleotide 26-49) and HCV 102 were then used to amplify the entire complimentary DNA preparation. The amplified product was detected by liquid hybridization with probe HCV 104 (nucleotide 157-188) followed by polyacrylamide gel electrophoresis and autoradiography. All samples were assayed in duplicate and were only reported as positive or negative when the duplicate agreed. Duplicates that did not agree were reported as indeterminate. Several negative controls were included with each run, none of which was ever positive.

Measurement of HBV-DNA

HBV-DNA levels were measured in serum and liver samples. Liver tissue was homogenized with zirconium beads and a beadbeater in phosphate-buffered saline. DNA was extracted using the QIAamp blood kits (Qiagen, Chatsworth, CA). PCR was performed with 10 pmoles each of primers HBV 201 (nt 455-474) and HBV 202 (nt 713-694) corresponding to the HBsAg sequence, as reported by Ono et al. [8], in 2.5 mM $MgCl_2$, 4 mM dNTP, 1 unit Taq enzyme and Taq buffer. Cycling conditions consisted of 94°C (30"), 50°C (15") and 30°C (30"), with a final extension for seven min at 72°C. Amplified product was detected by liquid hybridization with probe HBV 203 (nt 599-628), followed by polyacrylamide gel electrophoresis and autoradiography. All samples were assayed in duplicate and reported as positive or negative only when duplicates agreed. Results were deemed interpretable only when the 600 copy/ml control was read as positive and all negative controls were negative. All PCR reactions were performed in the presence of uracil-N-glycosylase to prevent amplicon contamination [9]. To verify that negative results were not due to the absence of DNA or to amplification inhibition, amplification of a fragment of the human factor V gene was performed on liver samples.

Human research approval

All of the subjects enrolled in this study gave an informed written consent before each procedure as well as before starting IFN treatment. The study conforms to the ethical guidelines of the 1975 Declaration of Helsinki.

Statistical analysis

The results are expressed as mean values ± SEM. The univariate analysis was made by Student's T test or by Yates' corrected chi-square test. A p-value less than 0.05 was considered to be significant.

Results

The treatment was tolerated well by all patients. The reported side effects consisted of fever, muscle pain and a flu-like syndrome shortly after IFN administration.

The response rate to high-dose IFN treatment at the two endpoints is reported in Table 2. Twenty-nine of the 31 African-Americans and 59 of the 62 Caucasians reached the second endpoint and completed the treatment course. In two cirrhotic individuals, one African-American and one Caucasian, IFN was suspended before the end of the treatment due to the deterioration of mental status and sepsis, respectively. Two patients, one African-American and one Caucasian, were lost to follow-up before the completion of the treatment course. One Caucasian patient underwent liver transplantation after six months of IFN therapy.

Table 2. Response rates to IFN treatment in the study and control groups

	On-therapy			End-of-therapy			Break-through
	all subjects	CAH	cirrhotics	all subjects	CAH	cirrhotics	all subjects
All subjects	45/93 (48%)	36/66 (55%)	9/27 (33%)	34/88 (39%)	30/65 (46%)	4/23 (17%)	10/43 (23%)
African-Americans	8/31[1] (26%)	7/22[1] (32%)	1/9 (11%)	3/29[2] (10%)	3/21[2] (14%)	0/8 (0%)	5/8[3] (63%)
Caucasians	37/62[1] (60%)	29/44[1] (66%)	8/18 (44%)	31/59[2] (53%)	27/44[2] (61%)	4/15 (27%)	5/35[3] (14%)

CAH: chronic hepatitis without cirrhosis

[1] = $p < 0.01$

[2] = $p < 0.0004$

[3] = $p < 0.004$

The African-American group presented a significantly reduced response rate at both endpoints as compared to the Caucasian group. In particular, after six months of therapy, only eight African-American subjects were HCV-RNA negative and had normalized their serum transaminase levels as compared to 37 Caucasians ($p < 0.01$). The difference between groups at the second endpoint was even more evident: only 10% of African-Americans were still HCV-RNA negative at the end of a 12-month course of IFN treatment, while 53% of Caucasians were HCV-RNA negative and showed normal ALT levels ($p < 0.0003$).

The difference between the two racial groups was still evident, even considering only individuals with chronic hepatitis without cirrhosis ($p < 0.0003$). By comparing the "end-of-therapy" response rates to those at the intermediate "on-therapy" endpoint, it appears that African-Americans had a higher virus "breakthrough" rate than did the Caucasian group (63% versus 14%, respectively, $p < 0.004$).

Discussion

In the present study, a reduced response rate to IFN therapy in African-Americans with chronic hepatitis C is demonstrated. At the end of IFN treatment, only 10% of African-American individuals had a biochemical and virological response to the therapy as compared to 53% of the individuals in the Caucasian group. African-American patients showed both an impaired response at the "on-therapy" endpoint as compared to the Caucasians (26% versus 60%, respectively, $p < 0.01$), and a higher viral "breakthrough" rate, having five out of eight individuals returning HCV-RNA positive after a temporary HCV-RNA negativity (63%) as compared to 14% Caucasian individuals.

The reason for the impaired response to IFN treatment among African-Americans chronically infected with HCV is not readily apparent. Both socioeconomic and genetic factors could be responsible for this observation. A simple factor that might play a prominent role is that a difference in compliance with therapy may exist for the two groups studied. However, the strict monitoring of the patients in the present study with a follow-up schedule requiring frequent interactions between patients and investigators make this an unlikely possibility.

In a large epidemiological study on mortality and morbidity among races in the USA, it has been shown that, even after adjusting the statistics for group income in order to avoid any potential economic bias, African-Americans still have a higher mortality and morbidity rate for most causes of illness and death as compared to Caucasians [12]. This finding indicates that either some behavioral or environmental factor of the African-American population is unfavorable as compared to Caucasians, or that a genetic factor is involved. Among the environmental factors that potentially influence the response to IFN treatment, diet needs to be considered. Chronic hepatitis C is thought to be a disease process in which free radicals are produced and oxidative stress plays a pathogenic role [13, 4]. Anti-oxidant compounds such as vitamins have been reported to have a protective effect on the course of chronic viral hepatitis and may enhance the response to IFN [15]. Therefore, differences in the amount of vegetables consumed daily by the different racial groups may need to be taken into consideration and may affect the response rate to various anti-viral treatments of chronic hepatitis C.

Another factor that may be considered as potentially responsible for the higher mortality and morbidity rates among African-American males is greater serum levels of testosterone as compared to Caucasians [16]. Higher testosterone levels may increase the risk of developing cardiovascular diseases, hypertension, and prostate cancer. The effect of sex hormones on the course of viral hepatitis is not known, although regardless of race, females do better than males when exposed to viral hepatitis. Intriguingly, in the present study, the "on-therapy" response rate of males as compared to females was reduced and close to statistical significance in the African-American group, but not in the Caucasian group. This difference, however, canceled out at the "end-of-therapy" endpoint.

It is of some interest that African-Americans have a higher death rate from cancer than Caucasians, even when statistics are equilibrated for all recognizable socioeconomic and biomedical factors known to affect outcome [12, 17-20]. This finding, combined with the known increased prevalence of certain autoimmune disorders (such as SLE) among African-Americans, suggests the possibility of an aberrant or somehow altered immune response in African-Americans that may contribute to a reduced ability to clear a HCV infection [25].

In conclusion, the data reported document an impaired response in African-Americans with chronic hepatitis C treated with IFN. Further studies are needed to identify and establish a role for environmental or genetic factors that might determine this difference in response as compared to Caucasians.

References

1. Carithers RL Jr, Emerson SS. Therapy of hepatitis C: meta-analysis of interferon alpha-2b trials. *Hepatology* 1997; 26 (Suppl 1): 83S-88S.
2. McHutchison JG, Gordon SC, Schiff ER, et al. Interferon alpha-2b alone or in combination with ribavirin as initial treatment for chronic hepatitis C. Hepatitis Interventional Therapy Group. *N Engl J Med* 1998; 339: 1485-92.
3. Davis GL, Lau JY. Factors predictive of a beneficial response to therapy of hepatitis C. *Hepatology* 1997; 26: 122S-127S.
4. Murphy EL, Bryzman S, Williams AE, et al. Demographic determinants of hepatitis C virus seroprevalence among blood donors. *JAMA* 1996; 275: 995-1000.
5. Kelen GD, Green GB, Purcell RH, et al. Hepatitis B and hepatitis C in emergency department patients. *N Engl J Med* 1992; 326: 1399-404.
6. Reddy R, Hoofnagle JH, Tong MJ, et al. Low rates of response to Interferon in African-Americans with chronic hepatitis C. *Hepatology* 1998; 28 (Suppl): 497A.
7. Knodell RG, Ishak KG, Black WC, Chen TS, Craig R, Kaplowitz N, et al. Formulation and application of a numerical scoring system for assessing histological activity in asymptomatic chronic active hepatitis. *Hepatology* 1981; 1: 431-5.
8. Ono Y, Onda H, Sasada R, Igarashi K, Sugino Y, Nishioka K. The complete nucleotide sequences of the cloned hepatitis B virus DNA: subtype adr and adw. *Nucleic Acids Res* 1983; 11: 1747-57.

9. Longo MC, Berninger MS, Hartley JL. Use of uracil DNA glycosylase to control carry-over contamination in polymerase chain reactions. *Gene* 1990; 93: 125-8.
10. Cacciola I, Pollicino T, Squadrito G, Cerenzia G, Orlando ME, Raimondo G. Occult hepatitis B virus infection in patients with chronic hepatitis C liver disease. *N Engl J Med* 1999; 341: 22-6.
11. De Maria N, Friedlander L, Colantoni A, Leandro G, Van Thiel DH. prior inactive HBV infection impairs the response to high dose Interferon treatment for chronic hepatitis C. *J Hepatol* 1999; 30 (Suppl 1): 246.
12. Davey Smith G, Neaton JD, Wentworth D, Stamler R, Stamler J. Mortality differences between black and white men in the USA: contribution of income and other risk factors among men screened for the MRFIT. MRFIT Research Group. Multiple Risk Factor Intervention Trial. *Lancet* 1998; 351: 934-9.
13. De Maria N, Colantoni A, Fagiuoli S, et al. Association between reactive oxygen species and disease activity in chronic hepatitis C. *Free Radic Biol Med* 1996; 21:291-5.
14. Farinati F, Cardin R, De Maria N, et al. Iron storage, lipid peroxidation and glutathione turnover in chronic anti-HCV positive hepatitis. *J Hepatol* 1995; 22: 449-56.
15. Andreone P, Gramenzi A, Bernardi M. Vitamin E for chronic hepatitis B. *Ann Intern Med* 1998; 128: 156-7.
16. Ellis L, Nyborg H. Racial/ethnic variations in male testosterone levels: a probable contributor to group differences in health. *Steroids* 1992; 57: 72-5.
17. Franzini L, Williams AF, Franklin J, Singletary SE, Theriault RL. Effects of race and socioeconomic status on survival of 1, 332 black, Hispanic, and white women with breast cancer. *Ann Surg Oncol* 1997; 4: 111-8.
18. Zaki A, Natarajan N, Mettlin CJ. Early and late survival in Hodgkin disease among whites and blacks living in the United States. *Cancer* 1993; 72: 602-6.
19. Troisi RJ, Freedman AN, Devesa SS. Incidence of colorectal carcinoma in the U.S.: an update of trends by gender, race, age, subsite, and stage, 1975-1994. *Cancer* 1999; 85: 1670-6.
20. Robbins AS, Whittemore AS, Van Den Eeden SK. Race, prostate cancer survival, and membership in a large health maintenance organization. *J Natl Cancer Inst* 1998; 90: 986-90.

Novel combined approaches to hepatitis C therapies

MARKUS CORNBERG and MICHAEL P. MANNS

Dept. Gastroenterology and Hepatology, Medizinische Hochschule Hannover, Hannover, Germany

Hepatitis C virus infection is the main hepatitis health problem in developed countries. Acute hepatitis C infection takes a chronic course in 50-80% of patients. Up to one to two percent of the population are chronically infected. Chronic hepatitis C is one of the leading causes of cirrhosis and end-stage liver cirrhosis, thus effective therapies are required. For many years interferon alpha has been the standard treatment of choice for patients with chronic hepatitis C infection. However, interferon alpha monotherapy is successful (i.e., leads to a sustained virological response) in only 10-15% of patients. Therefore, several antiviral adjuncts with immunomodulatory or anti-inflammatory properties have been tested to improve response rates. Most of them did not show additional benefit. Only the combination of interferon alpha and ribavirin could significantly enhance sustained virological response to 40%. More recently, several new antiviral agents have been explored to further improve response rates, and of these, amantadine, thymosin alpha-1, maxamine and mycophenolate mofetil are the most promising adjuncts. Modification of the interferon dosing schedule with induction-dosing and daily interferon regimens is another strategy to improve response rates. New interferons with either advanced biological activity, such as consensus interferon, or longer half-life and more favourable pharmacokinetics, such as pegylated interferons, may be more effective and improve response rates. Ongoing trials with the combination of pegylated interferons and ribavirin claim sustained response rates of about 50% with an acceptable safety profile. In the near future new treatment modalities will be available to directly suppress the hepatitis C virus. Helicase, protease and the RNA polymerase are potential targets for effective new drugs to suppress HCV replication.

Introduction

Treatment of chronic hepatitis C virus (HCV) infection has markedly improved since the introduction of combination therapy with interferon alpha (IFN) and ribavirin. The standard combination therapy (3x3 MU IFN tiw + 1,000/1,200 mg ribavirin daily) enhanced the sustained virological response to 40%, compared to only 15% using IFN monotherapy. Treatment response depends on HCV genotype and baseline levels of HCV-RNA [1, 2]. For patients who have relapsed following interferon monotherapy, about 50% can achieve sustained response when retreated with IFN and ribavirin [3].

Frontiers in Viral Hepatitis Ed. by RF Schinazi, J-P Sommadossi and CM Rice. 399 — 411

Therefore, combination therapy was approved by the FDA in 1998 and has become the standard treatment for naïve and relapse patients. However, patients with the most prevalent genotype 1 and high viral loads still have an unfavourable outcome. Almost three-fourths of these patients will not eliminate the virus with IFN and ribavirin. Also, patients who did not respond to an earlier IFN monotherapy showed a disappointing response to a standard combination therapy. A metaanalysis of 23 trials showed that combination therapy leads to sustained virological response in only 7.4% of patients [4]. Therefore, combination therapy is not recommended as a regular therapy for nonresponder patients. New treatment strategies have to be evaluated to achieve higher response rates in nonresponders and patients with unfavourable baseline characteristics, such as genotype 1, high viral load, advanced fibrosis or cirrhosis. Options to improve sustained response rates include modified regimes such as induction dosing or daily dosing, new therapeutic agents in combination with interferon alpha, and the use of new interferons.

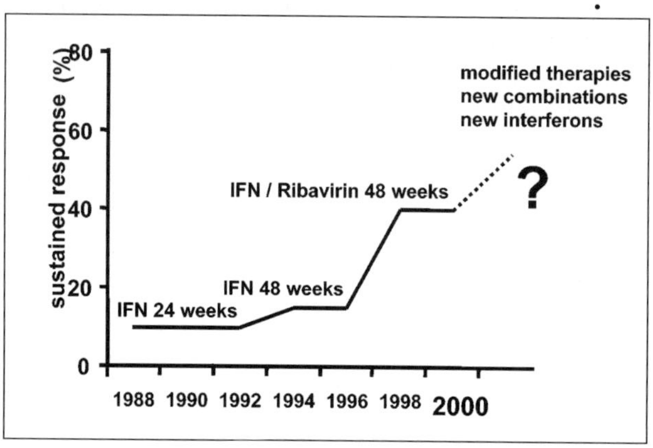

Figure 1. Development of HCV therapies. Between 1992 and 1994 the standard regimen of interferon alpha 3 MU tiw was increased from six months to 12 months in Europe. Thereafter, sustained virological response rates could be achieved in almost 20% of naïve patients. With the combination of ribavirin and interferon alpha, treatment efficacy could be improved markedly. New therapeutic modalities may further increase sustained response rates.

Modified therapies

An early virological response is important for a sustained response to antiviral treatment in hepatitis C. Zeuzem, et al. have demonstrated that all patients with a sustained virological response had an initial decline in HCV-RNA levels in serum of more than 3 logs within the first four weeks of treatment [5]. Viral kinetic studies gave evidence for an increased antiviral effect of higher dosages of interferon alpha (induction-dosing) and daily versus thrice-weekly IFN treatment schedules. Many groups have assessed the impact of interferon-alpha dose and regimen (tiw versus daily) on HCV kinetics [6, 7]. In these studies it was shown that there was a significant and more rapid reduction of HCV-RNA levels among patients who were treated by daily dosing schedules.

Van Vlierberghe, et al. have determined the efficacy of an eight-week daily-dosing induction period versus a tiw induction regimen of interferon alpha-2b in 317 naïve patients, in a controlled, multicenter randomized trial. Daily induction treatment resulted in an increased earlier response rate at week four (48.6% of patients HCV-RNA negative versus 30.8% of patients HCV-RNA negative) and week eight (66.5% of patients HCV-RNA negative versus 47.1% of patients HCV-RNA negative) [8]. These data suggest that daily administration of interferon could result in a higher rate of early viral clearance and perhaps in higher sustained response rates. On the basis of these data, a multicentre controlled trial of induction therapy with high-dose daily interferon alpha-2b and ribavirin in 625 patients with chronic hepatitis C was initiated [9]. 308 patients were treated with 1,000 or 1,200 mg ribavirin plus 10 MU IFN alpha-2b daily for two weeks, followed by 5 MU daily for six weeks, 3 MU daily for 16 weeks, and 3 MU tiw for 24 weeks. 317 patients were treated with the standard therapy regimen of 3 MU IFN alpha-2b tiw and 1,000 or 1,200 mg ribavirin. As expected, viral clearance occurred more rapidly in the induction group, and after eight weeks of treatment, HCV-RNA clearance was higher in patients treated with the daily induction-dosing regimen (44% vs. 32%). However, the daily induction regimen did not result in a significant improvement of viral response, either at the end of treatment or 12 weeks following completion of therapy. By the end of treatment, HCV-RNA was no longer detectable in 68% of patients in the induction group compared to 61% of standard therapy patients. Twelve-week follow-up response rates were 49% and 45%, respectively [9]. Thus, these data suggest that daily dosing should be continued throughout the six to 12 months of treatment.

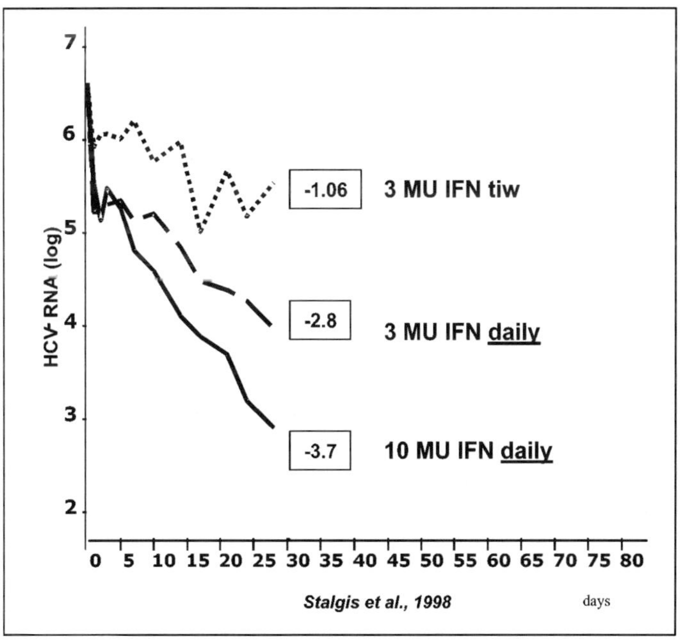

Figure 2. Viral kinetics. Daily dosing of interferon alpha leads to a more rapid HCV-RNA reduction than tiw schedules [6]

New drugs in combination with interferon alpha

Recent clinical trials have focused on supplemental drugs, such as ribavirin, that may enhance the efficacy of interferon alpha therapy. A large number of possible adjuncts have been evaluated, including ursodeoycholic acid, nonsteroidal anti-inflammatory agents, mycophenolate mofetil, thymosin alpha-1, maxamine, and amantadine. Most clinical trials have given disappointing results. Although some of these drugs may have an additional therapeutic effect, at present, none has been demonstrated to be superior to the combination therapy of interferon alpha and ribavirin.

Amantadine

Amantadine is a chiral tricyclic amine that has been demonstrated to inhibit specifically the replication of influenza A virus. Although an antiviral effect of amantadine on HCV-replication was not demonstrated, several preliminary reports gave hints of a possible benefit when used for treatment of hepatitis C [10-13]. Other studies did not show an advantage of dual therapy with IFN and amantadine in IFN nonresponders and naïve patients [14-16]. Although Zeuzem, et al. did not observe an additional benefit of the combination therapy with IFN and amantadine compared to IFN monotherapy in 119 naïve patients, combination with amantadine showed a trend to reduce IFN-related side effects such as fatigue and lethargy [16].

Triple therapy

Pilot studies promised more effective response rates with the combination therapy of interferon alpha, ribavirin and amantadine in nonresponder patients [12, 13]. Our own data confirm these preliminary results. The aim of our study was to evaluate a regimen of IFN induction therapy plus ribavirin, and IFN induction therapy with ribavirin and amantadine or placebo in 26 IFN-nonresponder patients [17]. IFN-alpha 2b was given at a high dose during the induction period: 10 MU qd for two weeks, 5 MU qd for two weeks, 3 MU qd for eight weeks, followed by 3 MU every other day for another nine months. 1,000-1,200 mg ribavirin and 200 mg amantadine or placebo were given orally qd. Overall initial virological response was 65%. There was a trend towards earlier viral clearance in group A (amantadine) at days 14-60. After 90 days of therapy (end of daily dosing) at a high rate (eight patients (31%)), viral breakthrough was observed. However, in group B (placebo) a viral breakthrough was seen more frequently (six patients (50%) vs. two patients (14%) in group A). Overall sustained response was 30%. In group A sustained response was 43% vs. 17% in group B. Evaluation of viral kinetics showed that patients with rapid HCV clearance were more likely to achieve sustained response [17]. This confirms data from previous studies [5, 7, 18].

Thymosin alpha-1

Thymosin alpha-1 (TA1) is a synthetic, immunomodulatory 28-amino-acid peptide that has been demonstrated to increase the activity of natural killer cells and maturate

Table 1. Combination of amantadine with interferon alpha. While some reports seemed to be promising, many studies do not reveal an additional benefit in the treatment of chronic hepatitis C.

Study	Patients	Regimen	Response (R)
[11]	180 naïve	A) 6 MU IFN alpha-2a tiw	Initial biochemical R
		B) 6 MU IFN alpha-2a tiw	A) 31%
		+ 200 mg amantadine qd	B) 63.8%
[13]	60 nonresponder	A) 5 MU IFN tiw	Sustained virological R
		+ 800-1.000 mg ribavirin	A) 5%
		B) 5 MU IFN tiw	B) 48%
		+ 800-1.000 mg ribavirin qd	
		+ 200 mg amantadine qd	
[15]	30 naïve	A) 4, 5 MU IFN alpha-2a tiw	Sustained virological R
		B) 4, 5 MU IFN alpha-2a tiw	A) 20%
		+ 200 mg amantadine qd	B) 21, 4%
[14]	29 nonresponder	A) 3 MU IFN alpha-2a tiw	Sustained virological R
		+ 1,000 mg ribavirin qd	A) 15%
		B) 3 MU IFN alpha-2a tiw	B) 0%
		+ 200 mg amantadine qd	
[16]	119 naïve	A) 6 MU IFN alpha-2a tiw 24 weeks	Sustained virological R
		3 MU IFN alpha-2a tiw 24 weeks	A) 10%
		+ 200 mg amantadine qd	
		B) 6 MU IFN alpha-2a tiw 24 weeks	B) 22%
		3 MU IFN alpha-2a tiw 24 weeks	
		+ 200 mg placebo qd	

$CD4^+$ T helper cells. TA1 appears to stimulate native interferons and cytokines such as interleukin 2 [19].

In terms of viral hepatitis, there is evidence that TA1 may be effective in the treatment of hepatitis B [20, 21]. To evaluate a possible effect in the treatment of chronic hepatitis C, Sherman and his group initiated a randomized, placebo-controlled trial testing a combination of interferon alpha-2b and thymosin alpha-1 in 109 naïve HCV-positive patients. Thirty-five patients received 1.6 mg of TA1 subcutaneously twice weekly and 3MU IFN tiw, 37 patients received placebo and 3 MU IFN tiw, and 37 patients received placebo for both agents. All patients were treated for 26 weeks. Virological end-of-treatment response was observed in 37.1% of patients treated with IFN and TA1, 18.9% of patients treated with IFN and placebo, and in 2.7% of the control patients. Cumulative, sustained biochemical responses were 14.2% and 8.1% in the IFN/TA1 and IFN groups, respectively. Moreover, histological improvement (more than 2 points decrease in the HAI score) was observed more frequently in the combination arm than in the comparison groups. Unfortunately, the study design was not able to demonstrate true sustained response rates, because relapsers were removed from the follow-up and retreated with other regimens [22]. In summary, combination therapy with TA1 and interferon appears to have an additional therapeutic effect, but large trials are warranted to confirm this suggestion. However, immunomodulator drugs such as TA1 may be promising adjuncts for common and future HCV treatment modalities, since immunopathogenesis of HCV has been linked to impaired NK and TH_1-T cell responses.

Mycophenolate mofetil

Mycophenolate mofetil (MMF), a morpholinoethyl ester of mycophenolic acid (MPA), is currently used as an immunosuppressive agent. After oral administration, MMF is hydrolysed to MPA, the active compound, which is a potent inhibitor of inosine monophosphate dehydrogenase (IMPDH) such as ribavirin. It has been demonstrated that MMF is more effective than ribavirin or 5-ethynyl-1-β-D-ribofuranosylimidazole-4-carboxamide (EICAR) to inhibit the IMPDH [23]. IMPDH catalyses a key step in purine nucleotide biosynthesis. Therefore inhibition of IMPDH results in a depletion of the intracellular GTP and dGTP pools. Lack of guanosine nucleotides may lead to a reduction of *de novo* synthesis of viral RNA and DNA. MPA has been shown to inhibit the replication of a number of viruses, including arena viruses (Junin and Tacaribe), yellow fever virus, reovirus-1, parainfluenza-3 virus, Coxsackie B4 virus, Epstein-Barr virus and human immunodeficiency virus. Also, an effect of MPA on HBV replication in primary human hepatocyte cultures was observed [24]. Eight of 11 HCV-positive patients who received MMF after liver transplantation showed a decline in HCV-RNA levels and a normalisation of ALT levels [25]. Our results in the treatment of 44 interferon nonresponder patients with IFN alpha-2a and MMF (one week 6 MU IFN tiw and 500 mg MMF, one week 6 MU IFN tiw and 1000 mg MMF, 22 weeks 6 MU IFN tiw and 2000 mg MMF) were disappointing. This pilot study was discontinued because of inefficacy (own unpublished results).

Data on other potent IMPDH inhibitors such as VX-497 and VX-148 are awaited.

Maxamine

Maxamine (histamine dihydrochloride) specifically inhibits the release of reactive oxygen metabolites from phagocytic cells in the liver by blocking histamine receptors, and thus may protect immune cells, including CD4 lymphocytes and natural killer (NK) cells from free radical-induced apoptosis. This also allows increased effectiveness of naturally occurring or added cytokines, including IL-2 and interferon alpha. Therefore, combination of maxamine might allow reduction of treatment dose of these cytokines which would also decrease toxicity and side effects. Thus a phase II multicentre trial of maxamine and interferon alpha-2b was initiated to evaluate the effective dose of maxamine with standard IFN in 129 naïve patients with chronic hepatitis C [26]. All patients received 3 MU IFN tiw and 3, 5, 6 or 10 mg maxamine subcutaneously per week for 48 weeks. Initial virological response rates after 24 weeks of therapy ranged from 57-69% across the four arms, while ALT was normalised in 44-73%, respectively. Side effects of maxamine were transient flush, temporary headache, tachycardia, and hypotension. This first result suggests that maxamine may improve the efficacy of IFN therapy, thus maxamine might be an alternative adjunct in place of ribavirin. However, sustained response rates have to be awaited and larger trials are needed to confirm this preliminary data.

New interferons

Interferon alpha was the first approved drug for the treatment of hepatitis C virus infection. But the efficacy of standard interferon alpha is low and sustained viral clearance is reached in only 15% of patients [1, 2]. Although ribavirin has doubled response rates compared to IFN monotherapy, the therapeutic situation is still unsatisfactory. An alternative approach to improve the response rates in patients with chronic hepatitis C is to modify the interferon regimen in combination therapy. New interferons with enhanced biological or pharmacodynamic potency may increase response rates.

Consensus interferon (CIFN)

Consensus interferon is a novel bioengineered "consensus" molecule, composed of the most frequently observed amino acid at each position of the alpha interferons. CIFN shares an 89%, 30% and 60% homology with IFN-α, IFN-β and IFN-ω. CIFN has a tenfold increased affinity to the type-1 IFN-receptor compared to IFN alpha-2a or IFN alpha-2b. Compared to the mass base, CIFN displays five to 10 times greater biological activity than other type-1 interferons [27-29]. Moreover, CIFN induces peak mRNA levels of IFN-induced genes at lower concentrations than IFN-α 2b [30].

Despite the increased antiviral efficacy *in vitro*, there was no significant difference in the viral response rates between CIFN (9 μg tiw) and IFN-α 2b (tiw) in patients. However, patients infected with HCV genotype 1 showed a faster and more pronounced decline in serum HCV-RNA concentrations with CIFN treatment compared to IFN-α 2b therapy. In addition, patients infected with HCV genotype 1 treated with CIFN had undetectable HCV-RNA at a greater percentage than patients in the IFN-α 2b group at the end of treatment (24% vs. 15%) and after the follow up (8% vs. 4%) [31]. Also patients who did not respond to a previous IFN therapy seem to benefit from a second therapy with CIFN to some degree.

A multicenter, open-label, phase III study was conducted in 337 patients with chronic hepatitis C virus (HCV) infection who had either not responded to a previous interferon therapy or had relapsed after discontinuation of therapy with consensus interferon or interferon alpha-2b [32]. Patients were treated with a higher dose of consensus interferon (15 μg three times a week for 24 or 48 weeks). For relapsers, the sustained HCV-RNA response rate was 58% (48 weeks) and 28% (24 weeks), respectively. Sustained HCV-RNA response rate among previous nonresponders was low, but no lower than the rate of combination therapy with standard IFN and ribavirin (13% after 48 weeks). These data demonstrate that re-treatment with consensus interferon is effective in IFN relapse patients, but does not markedly improve viral clearance rates in nonresponders [32]. Data on combination with ribavirin are still not available. Our preliminary data on combination with consensus interferon and ribavirin suggest a possible improvement of response rates in nonresponders (unpublished results).

Amino acid position	1	2	3	4	5	6	7
IFN α a	gly	asn	gly	phe	leu	lys	asn
IFN α b	thr	gly	val	phe	his	lys	asn
IFN α d	trp	asn	leu	asn	leu	glu	leu
IFN α f	trp	phe	gly	gly	leu	lys	leu
IFN α g	trp	asn	gly	asn	his	glu	his
IFN α j	gln	gly	val	phe	leu	lys	asn
Consensus	trp	asn	gly	phe	leu	lys	asn

Figure 3. Consensus interferon is a composition of the most frequently observed amino acid at each position of the IFNs-a

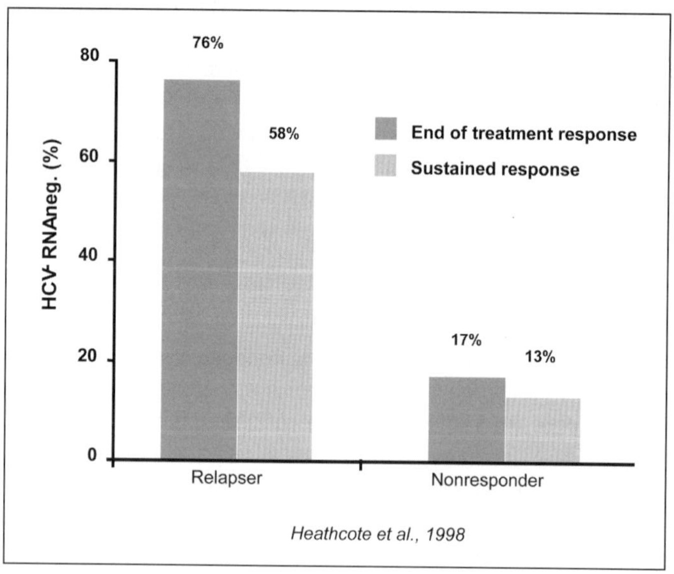

Figure 4. CIFN therapy (15 μg tiw, 48 weeks) in relapse patients and nonresponder patients [32].

Pegylated interferon alpha (PegIFN)

Polyethylene glycol (PEG) is a small molecule that can be polymerised into long chains and attached to proteins. Two pegylated IFNs are now undergoing clinical trials. PegIFN alpha-2a is a modified IFN alpha-2a by the covalent attachment of a branched 4,000 Dalton methoxy polyethylene glycol moiety. PegIFN alpha-2b consists of IFN alpha-2b attached to a single 12,000 Dalton PEG molecule. PegIFN alpha-2a and PegIFN alpha-2b have a decreased systemic clearance rate and a prolonged plasma half-life (approx tenfold compared to standard IFNs), which allow once weekly dosing. The two PegIFNs appear to have different characteristics. Half-lives are slightly different and metabolism and elimination rates differ. PegIFN alpha-2a is predominantly metabolised in the liver, whereas PegIFN alpha-2b elimination is predominantly renal. Due to these properties, comparison of both PegIFNs is difficult. The first clinical trials demonstrated that monotherapy with PegIFN alpha-2a or PegIFN alpha-2b improved sustained response rates compared to standard interferons. PegIFN alpha-2a *(PEGASYS)* was compared with a standard IFN alpha-2a regimen (6 MU IFN tiw 12 weeks, 3 MU IFN tiw 36 weeks) in 531 naïve patients with chronic hepatitis C. This trial demonstrated a promising 39% response rate in patients treated with PegIFN versus 19% in the standard IFN group [33]. Previous dose-finding studies indicated that the optimum dose for PegIFN alpha-2a is 180 μg per week. In a dose-finding study comparing PegIFN alpha-2b *(PegIntron)* with standard IFN alpha-2b, patients were randomized to receive IFN (3 MU IFN tiw) or 0.5, 1.0, or 1.5 μg/kg of PegIFN alpha-2b. The results demonstrated that PegIFN alpha-2b is significantly more effective (twofold) at higher dosages (1.0 and 1.5 μg/kg) compared to conventional IFN [34]. Even in patients with liver cirrhosis, 29% of patients had a sustained virological response with a 180 μg PegIFN alpha-2a regimen for 48 weeks [35]. The first clinical trials with the combination of PegIFN and ribavirin showed significantly higher initial response rates compared to the standard therapy with IFN and ribavirin, and thus it is predicted to have higher sustained response rates [36, 37, 38]. No additional side effects were observed, and the application only once weekly may improve compliance of patients. According to these promising results, combination of PegIFN and ribavirin may become standard treatment in naïve patients and especially in patients with unfavourable baseline characteristics.

Summary

Chronic hepatitis C virus is a worldwide health burden that leads to liver cirrhosis in a significant number of patients and enhances the risk for developing a liver carcinoma. The current standard therapy (3 MU IFN thrice weekly and ribavirin) leads to a sustained virological response in 40% of patients. Molecular modification of interferons improved pharmacodynamic and biological properties. Clinical trials with new interferons showed that consensus interferon may improve response rates in unsuccessfully pretreated patients and patients with HCV-genotype 1. Treatment with PegIFN will double response rates achieved with standard IFN monotherapy. Studies on these new interferons in combination with ribavirin are ongoing, and first results are promising.

Table 2. Pegylated interferon alpha (PegIFN) treatment is more effective than standard interferon alpha dosing regimens:

Study	Regimen	Patients	Initial response	Sustained response
[33]	PegIFN alpha-2a (180 μg oiw for 48 weeks)	267	66% (48 weeks)	39%
	IFN alpha-2a (6 MU tiw 12 weeks, 6 MU tiw 36 weeks)	264	27%	19%
[34]	IFN alpha-2b (3 MU tiw 48 weeks)	303		12%
	PegIFN alpha-2b (0,5 μg/kg oiw for 48 weeks)	315		18%
	PegIFN alpha-2b (1,0 μg/kg oiw for 48 weeks)	297	41%	25%
	PegIFN alpha-2b (1,5 μg/kg oiw for 48 weeks)	304		23%
[35]	PegIFN alpha-2a in patients with cirrhosis (180 μg oiw for 48 weeks)	87	43%	29%
[36]	IFN alpha-2b plus ribavirin (3 MU tiw + 1.000/1.200 mg for 48 weeks)	504	55%	47%
	PegIFN alpha-2b plus ribavirin (1.5 μg oiw 4 weeks, 0.5 μg oiw 44 weeks + 1.000/1.200 mg for 48 weeks)	514	56%	47%
	PegIFN alpha-2b plus ribavirin (1.5 μg oiw + 800 mg for 48 weeks)	517	64%	54%
[37]	PegIFN alpha-2a plus ribavirin (180 μg oiw + 1.000/1.200 mg for 48 weeks)	20	80% (24 weeks)	50%
[38]	PegIFN alpha-2a plus ribavirin (180 μg oiw + 1.000/1.200 mg for 48 weeks)	453	69%	56%
	PegIFN alpha-2a plus placebo (180 μg oiw + 1.000/1.200 mg for 48 weeks)	224	59%	30%
	IFN alpha-2b plus ribavirin (180 μg oiw + 1.000/1.200 mg for 48 weeks)	444	52% (48 weeks)	45%

Modification of interferon alpha dose or timing and combinations with complementary therapeutic agents such as amantadine may increase efficacy in special groups, such as nonresponders. For these groups an individually tailored treatment regimen may be favourable.

Future antiviral drugs may comprise molecules that directly inhibit HCV protein function and interfere with viral replication. NS3/4A serine protease, RNA helicase, and RNA-dependent RNA polymerase may be potential targets for new drugs. Furthermore, antisense oligonucleotides or ribozymes may become new treatment options to inhibit HCV replication.

References

1. Poynard T, Marcellin P, Lee SS, Niederau C, Minuk GS, Ideo G et al. Randomised trial of interferon alpha2b plus ribavirin for 48 weeks or for 24 weeks versus interferon alpha2b plus placebo for 48 weeks for treatment of chronic infection with hepatitis C virus. International Hepatitis Interventional Therapy Group (IHIT). *Lancet* 1998; 352:1426-1432.
2. McHutchison JG, Gordon SC, Schiff ER, Shiffman ML, Lee WM, Rustgi VK et al. Interferon alpha-2b alone or in combination with ribavirin as initial treatment for chronic hepatitis C. Hepatitis Interventional Therapy Group. *N Engl J Med* 1998; 339:1485-1492.
3. Davis GL, Esteban-Mur R, Rustgi V, Hoefs J, Gordon SC, Trepo C et al. Interferon alpha-2b alone or in combination with ribavirin for the treatment of relapse of chronic hepatitis C. International Hepatitis Interventional Therapy Group. *N Engl J Med* 1998; 339:1493-1499.
4. Wedemeyer H, Jackel E, Wedemeyer J, Frank H, Schuler A, Trautwein C et al. [Is combination therapy of chronic hepatitis C with interferon alpha and ribavirin in primary interferon nonresponders indicated?--An analysis of personal experiences and review of the literature]. *Z Gastroenterol* 1998; 36:819-827.
5. Zeuzem S, Lee JH, Franke A, Ruster B, Prummer O, Herrmann G et al. Quantification of the initial decline of serum hepatitis C virus RNA and response to interferon alfa. *Hepatology* 1998; 27:1149-1156.
6. Stalgis C, McHutchison J, Bekkering F, Perelson AS. Prediction of early viral clearance with daily IFN+Rib using a mathematical model. *Hepatology* 1998; 28:398A.
7. Neumann AU, Lam NP, Dahari H, Gretch DR, Wiley TE, Layden TJ et al. Hepatitis C viral dynamics in vivo and the antiviral efficacy of interferon-alpha therapy. *Science* 1998; 282:103-107.
8. Van Vlierberghe H, Leroux-Roels G, Burgeois N, Nevens F, Colle I, Henrion J et al. Daily induction treatment with α 2b interferon in naive chronic hepatitis C patients results in a higher early response. A controlled multicenter randomized trial. *Hepatology* 1999; 30:631A.
9. Carithers RL, Jr., Zeuzem S, Manns MP, McHutchison JG, Perrillo RP, Bailey R. et al. Multicenter, randomized, controlled trial comparing high dose daily induction interferon plus ribavirin versus standard interferon alpha-2b plus ribavirin. *Hepatology* 2000; 32:317A.
10. Smith JP. Treatment of chronic hepatitis C with amantadine. *Dig Dis Sci* 1997; 42:1681-1687.
11. Mangia A, Cascavilla I, Villani MR, Andriulli A. Amantadine HCl + IFN improves response in naive pts: Interim evaluation of a controlled study. *Hepatology* 1999; 30:436A.
12. Brillanti S, Foli M, Di Tomaso M, Gramantieri L, Masci C, Bolondi L. Pilot study of triple antiviral therapy for chronic hepatitis C in interferon alpha non-responders. *Ital J Gastroenterol Hepatol 1999*; 31:130-134.
13. Brillanti S, Levantesi F, Masi L, Foli M, Bolondi L. Triple antiviral therapy as a new option for patients with interferon nonresponsive chronic hepatitis C. *Hepatology* 2000; 32:630-634.
14. Khalili M, Denham C, Perrillo R. Interferon and ribavirin versus interferon and amantadine in interferon nonresponders with chronic hepatitis C. *Am J Gastroenterol* 2000; 95:1284-1289.
15. Yang SS, Tu TC, Wu CH. Combination of interferon alfa-2a and amantadine does not improve the efficacy of interferon therapy in patients with chronic hepatitis C. *Hepatology* 1999; 30:369A.

16. Zeuzem S, Teuber G, Naumann U, Berg T, Raedle J, Hartmann S et al. Randomized, double-blind, placebo-controlled trial of interferon alfa2a with and without amantadine as initial treatment for chronic hepatitis C. *Hepatology* 2000; 32:835-841.
17. Cornberg M., Jaeckel E, Schuler A, Koerbel J.N., Wedemeyer H, Mansuroglu T. et al. Treatment of chronic hepatitis C in nonresponder patients with high daily induction dosing of interferon alpha-2b, ribavirin and amantadine/placebo. *Hepatology* 2000; 32:351A.
18. Zeuzem S. Clinical implications of hepatitis C viral kinetics. *J Hepatol* 1999; 31:61-64.
19. Low TL, Goldstein AL. Thymosins: structure, function and therapeutic applications. *Thymus* 1984; 6:27-42.
20. Mutchnick MG, Appelman HD, Chung HT, Aragona E, Gupta TP, Cummings GD et al. Thymosin treatment of chronic hepatitis B: a placebo-controlled pilot trial. *Hepatology* 1991; 14:409-415.
21. Andreone P, Cursaro C, Gramenzi A, Zavagliz C, Rezakovic I, Altomare E et al. A randomized controlled trial of thymosin-alpha1 versus interferon alfa treatment in patients with hepatitis B e antigen antibody--and hepatitis B virus DNA--positive chronic hepatitis B. *Hepatology* 1996; 24:774-777.
22. Sherman KE, Sjogren M, Creager RL, Damiano MA, Freeman S, Lewey S et al. Combination therapy with thymosin alpha1 and interferon for the treatment of chronic hepatitis C infection: a randomized, placebo- controlled double-blind trial. *Hepatology* 1998; 27:1128-1135.
23. Gong ZJ, De Meyer S, Clarysse C, Van Pelt JF, Coopmans T, Neyts J et al. Differential anti-HBV activity *in vitro* of three potent inhibitors of inosine monophosphate dehydrogenase: mycophenolic acid (MPA), 5-ethynyl-1-β-D-ribofuranosylimidazole-4-carboxamide (EICAR) and ribavirin. *Hepatology* 1998; 28:586A.
24. Gong ZJ, De Meyer S, Clarysse C, Verslype C, Neyts J, De Clercq E et al. Mycophenolic acid, an immunosuppressive agent, inhibits HBV replication *in vitro*. *J Viral Hepat* 1999; 6:229-236.
25. Platz KP, Mueller AR, Willimski C, Mansoorian B, Berg T, Neuhaus R et al. Indication for mycophenolate mofetil therapy in hepatitis C patients undergoing liver transplantation. *Transplant Proc* 1998; 30:2232-2233.
26. Yoav L., Nevens F, Hyle S., Gehlsen K.R. A phase II dosing regimen study of histamine dihydrochloride (Maxamine) and interferon alpha-2b (IFN-A-2B) as initial therapy for hepatitis C: 24-week interim report. *Hepatology* 2000; 32:443A.
27. Blatt LM, Davis JM, Klein SB, Taylor MW. The biologic activity and molecular characterization of a novel synthetic interferon-alpha species, consensus interferon. *J Interferon Cytokine Res* 1996; 16:489-499.
28. Hu CJ, Ozes ON, Klein SB, Blatt LM, Taylor MW. Comparison of the *in vitro* host range of recombinant met-interferon- con1, interferon alpha-2b, and interferon-beta. *J Interferon Cytokine Res* 1995; 15:231-234.
29. Ozes ON, Reiter Z, Klein S, Blatt LM, Taylor MW. A comparison of interferon-Con1 with natural recombinant interferons- alpha: antiviral, antiproliferative, and natural killer-inducing activities. *J Interferon Res* 1992; 12:55-59.
30. Klein SB, Blatt LM, Taylor MW. Consensus interferon induces peak mRNA accumulation at lower concentrations than interferon-alpha 2a. *J Interferon Res* 1993; 13:341-347.
31. Tong MJ, Reddy KR, Lee WM, Pockros PJ, Hoefs JC, Keeffe EB et al. Treatment of chronic hepatitis C with consensus interferon: a multicenter, randomized, controlled trial. Consensus Interferon Study Group. *Hepatology* 1997; 26:747-754.
32. Heathcote EJ, Keeffe EB, Lee SS, Feinman SV, Tong MJ, Reddy KR et al. Re-treatment of chronic hepatitis C with consensus interferon. *Hepatology* 1998; 27:1136-1143.

33. Zeuzem S, Feinman SV, Rasenack J, Heathcote EJ, Lai MY, Gane E et al. Evaluation of the safety and efficacy of once-weekly PEG/INTERFERON alfa-2a (PEGASYS^{TM}) for chronic hepatitis C. A multinational, randomized study. *J.Hepatol.* 2000; 32:29.
34. Trepo C, Lindsay K, Niederau C, Shiffman M, Gordon S, Hoefs J et al. Pegylated interferon alpha-2b (PEG-INTRON) monotherapy is superior to interferon alpha-2b (INTRON A) for the treatment of chronic hepatitis C. *J.Hepatol.* 2000; 32:29.
35. Heathcote EJ, Shiffman ML, Cooksley G, Dusheiko GM, Lee SS, Balart L et al. Multinational evaluation of the efficacy and safety of once-weekly peginterferon α-2a (PEG-IFN) in patients with chronic hepatitis C (CHC) with compensated cirrhosis. *Hepatology* 1999; 30:621A.
36. Manns MP, McHutchison JG, Gordon SC, Rustgi VK, Shiffman M, Reindollar R et al. Peginterferon alpha-2b plus ribavirin compared to interferon alpha-2b plus ribavirin for the treatment of chronic hepatitis C: a randomized trial. *Lancet* 2001; 358(9286):958-965.
37. Fried MW, Shiffman M, Reddy R, Smith C, Marino G, Goncalez JR et al. Pegylated (40kDa) Interferon Alpha-2a (PEGASYS) in Combination With Ribavirin: Efficacy And Safety Results From a Phase III, Randomized, Actively Controlled, Multicenter Study. *Gastroenterology* 2001; 120.Suppl. A-55.

Consensus + pegylated interferon

JENNY HEATHCOTE

University of Toronto

Introduction

Worldwide, chronic viral hepatitis due to infection with either hepatitis B or hepatitis C is responsible for the majority of chronic liver disease. Chronic infection is associated with an increased risk of hepatocellular carcinoma, the prevalence of which is particularly high in areas of the world where chronic viral hepatitis B and C are common. The rate of hepatocellular carcinoma appears to be increasing even in areas where the prevalence of hepatitis B and C are low, simply because the overall number of infected persons (especially with hepatitis C) has increased over the last few decades [1, 2]. Hence it is of great importance that improved therapies for these chronic viral infections of the liver be developed.

Interferon therapy for hepatitis C

Interferons have been the mainstay of treatment for chronic hepatitis B and C. Alpha interferons interrupt viral uptake, replication and clearance via several mechanisms. However, their overall therapeutic benefit has been somewhat disappointing.

Consensus interferon

Consensus interferon was developed by scanning alpha interferon subtypes and then assigning the most frequently observed amino acid at each position to form a novel "consensus" molecule [3]. Thus a DNA coding sequence was synthesized based on this derived consensus sequence, and the molecule was cloned in a recombinant E. coli expression system. The *in vitro* antiviral activity of this recombinant consensus interferon (CIFN) has been compared to two other commonly used recombinant alpha interferons; namely, interferon alpha 2a and interferon alpha-2b. In different cell expression systems using both HeLa and ME-180 cells infected with vesicular stomatitis virus or herpes simplex virus-1, the activity of CIFN appears to be 1-2 logs greater than the other two alpha-recombinant interferons [4].

Frontiers in Viral Hepatitis Ed. by RF Schinazi, J-P Sommadossi and CM Rice. 413 — 423

Therapeutic trials of CIFN

A large study was designed to compare two doses of CIFN (3 & 9 mcg) with the standard dose (at that time) of interferon alpha-2b (three million units). Both drugs were to be given by subcutaneous injection three times a week (ttw) for six months. Seven hundred and four patients were randomized to this study. Standard virological (HCV RNA) and biochemical (serum ALT) markers of response were monitored during treatment and for six months after cessation of therapy. Responses were defined as end-of-treatment and end-of-observation response, the latter being at 24 weeks following cessation of therapy. Serum HCV RNA was detected using a quantitative, multicycle RT-PCR method (NGI, Culver City, CA) with a lower limit of detectability of 100 copies/ml.

This study demonstrated that CIFN at 9 mcg ttw had an efficacy rate that was no different from interferon alpha-2b (3 million units ttw) given for six months. Sustained biochemical response (SBR) was 20% for both, and the sustained virological response (SVR) was 12% for those randomized to CIFN 9 mcg and 11% in those randomized to 3 million units of interferon alpha-2b [5] (Table 1). Subgroup analysis showed that CIFN was significantly more effective than interferon alpha-2b in patients who had a high viral load (>4.8 $\times$ 10^6 copies per ml). A sustained virological response was observed in none of the 61 patients with high titre HCV RNA-randomized IFN alpha 2b, whereas 7.5% of those patients randomized to CIFN 9 mcg dose had a sustained virological response (Figure 1). The 3 mcg dose of CIFN was found to be ineffective. The rate of sustained virological response was found to be similar regardless of severity of liver disease present, i.e., a 10% SR-24 virological in those with cirrhosis and/or heavy fibrosis, and 12% virological SR in those patients who had little or no fibrosis at baseline [6] (Table 2).

During the conduct of this study it was recognized that six months of treatment with interferon was less effective than 12 months for chronic hepatitis C. Hence a second phase of the study was designed, whereby those subjects who at the end of the six month observation period following initial therapy were found either to have not responded, or to have had a virological and/or biochemical relapse following cessation of therapy, were offered re-treatment with a higher dose of CIFN (15 mcg ttw). Patients were randomized to receive re-treatment for either six or 12 months. Three hundred and thirty seven patients agreed to enter this second phase (Figure 2). The criteria for successful therapy were the same as those used in the initial trial. The re-treatment response rate to treatment did not depend on the type of IFN prescribed previously. The sustained virological response (SVR) rates in patients who were prior nonresponders was 13% in those who received 48 weeks of therapy and 5% in those re-treated for only six months. The sustained virological response in patients who were prior responders but who subsequently relapsed was higher: 58% in those given 48 weeks of re-treatment and 28% in those given only 24 weeks of re-treatment [7] (Table 3). Not all patients who had had a virological response to six months of therapy and who then relapsed following the first phase of this trial had a sustained virological response to re-treatment: 25% appeared to be resistant to re-treatment.

As in the initial phase of this study, successful outcome of re-treatment was dependent on viral genotype and initial baseline HCV-RNA titre. In genotype 3 patients

Table 1. ALT and HCV RNA responses

	ETR		SR-24 wk	
	CIFN 9 μg (n = 232)	IFN-α2b (n = 240)	CIFN 9 μg (n = 232)	IFN-α2b (n = 240)
ALT normal	42%	37%	20%	20%
HCV RNA undetectable	35%	27%	12%	11%

Tong et al., Hepatology 1997;26(3):747-754

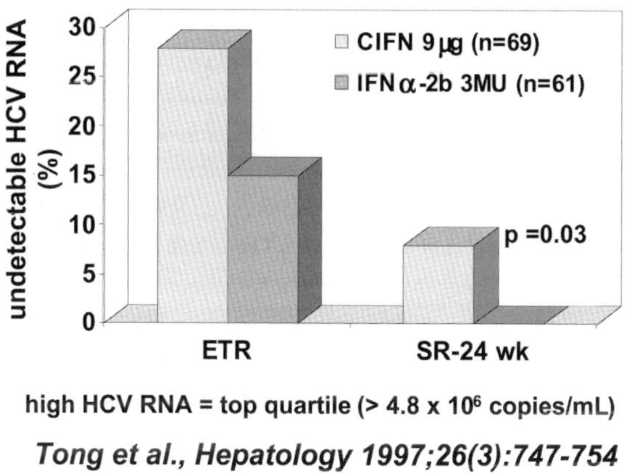

Figure 1. HCV RNA response in patients with high HCV RNA levels.

Table 2. ALT and HCV RNA response for cirrhotics / fibrotics vs. non-fibrotics

		ETR SR		24 wk	
		ALT	HCV RNA	ALT	HCV RNA
non-fibrotics	(n = 137)	49%*	39%	23%	12%
cirrhotics/fibrotics	(n = 62)	31%	27%	15%	10%

* $p < 0.05$ compared with cirrhotics and fibrotics.

Everson et al., Hepatology 1999;30:271-276

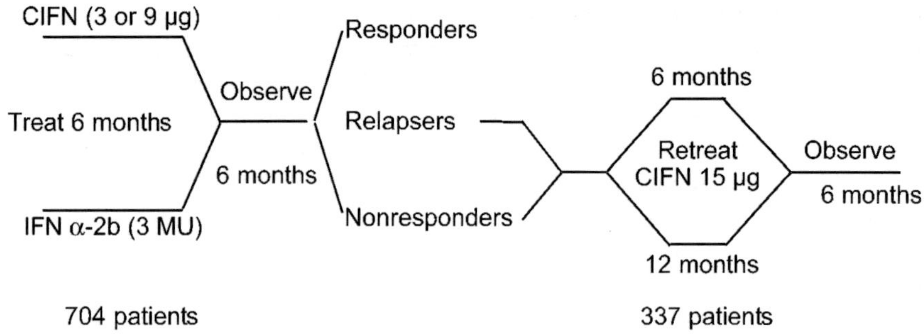

Figure 2. Phase 3 CIFN study retreatment.

Table 3. HCV RNA response after retreatment with CIFN 15 µg

	All Patients		Prior Non Responders		Prior Responders	
	24 wks (n = 107)	48 wks (n = 102)	24 wks (n = 75)	48 wks (n = 80)	24 wks (n = 32)	48 wks (n = 33)
End of treatment	35%	36%	19%	17%	72%	76%
End of observation	12%	27%*	5%	13%	28%	58%**

* $p = 0.008$ (24 vs 48 wks)
** $p = 0.024$ (24 vs 48 wks)
Heathcote et al., Hepatology 1998;27:1136

(n = 30) who received 48 weeks of re-treatment, those who were prior nonresponders had a 25% SVR and the prior relapsers an 88% SVR. Whereas in those with genotype 1 infections (n = 150), the prior nonresponders had a 12% SVR and the prior relapsers a 44% SVR (Table 4). The sustained response rate was significantly higher in those who had a baseline viral load of $<2 \times 10^6$, compared to those whose baseline viral load was higher than this (Table 5).

Breakthroughs

Throughout the re-treatment trial, monthly serum samples were taken for measurement of HCV RNA. Among 467 patients who, following initial treatment, were classified as being nonresponders (HCV RNA detectable at the end of treatment), some had in fact had undetectable HCV RNA during the course of therapy, but had subsequently broken through. These "breakthroughs" represented 28% of the so-called nonresponder population (86/312). Patients who were found to have viral breakthroughs during

Table 4. HCV RNA response to retreatment for prior HCV RNA nonresponders and prior HCV RNA relapsers

	prior NR				prior relapsers			
	ETR		SR		ETR		SR	
	24 wk	48 wk	24 wk	48 wk	24 wk	48 wk	24 wk	48 wk
genotype 1								
n = 150	11%	15%	3%	12%	64%	75%	35%	44%
genotype 2								
n = 23	57%	50%	0%	25%	75%	63%	25%	50%
genotype 3								
n = 30	60%	0%	40%	25%	77%	88%	15%	88%

Excluding 3 μg CIFN.
Heathcote et al., Hepatology 1998;27:1136

Table 5. HCV RNA response to retreatment in genotype 1 patients based on viral concentration for prior HCV RNA nonresponders and prior HCV RNA relapsers

Baseline HCV RNA in 9223	prior NR				prior relapsers			
	ETR		SR		ETR		SR	
	24 wk	48 wk	24 wk	48 wk	24 wk	48 wk	24 wk	48 wk
$< 2 \times 10^6$								
n = 18	0%	67%	0%	50%	75%	67%	75%	67%
$> 2 \times 10^6$	13%	10%	4%	8%	60%	77%	20%	38%

Heathcote et al., Hepatology 1998;27:1136

initial IFN therapy differed from those without breakthroughs, in that the latter had higher baseline viral loads (3.7×10^6 compared to 2.5×10^6), and they also had a higher prevalence of genotype 1 infections (85% versus 67%). No association with the development of antibodies to interferon could be found to explain the development of breakthroughs. There was no significant difference in either baseline histology or the percentage of those who required dose reduction during treatment, according to whether or not a "breakthrough" took place [8] (Table 6). When the response to re-treatment in nonresponders was analyzed according to whether or not a breakthrough in HCV RNA had occurred, the re-treatment SVR in those who were found to have had a

Table 6. Baseline characteristics of patients with viral breakthroughs

	all NR n = 312	NR with breakthroughs n = 86	NR without breakthroughs n = 226
baseline median HCV	3.3×10^6	2.5×10^6	3.7×10^6 *
% genotype 1	88%	67%	85%**
baseline median HAI	7.0	7.0	7.0
% with dose reduction	14%	17%	12%

* p = 0.011
** p = 0.001
Heathcote et al., Hepatology 1999;30:562-566

breakthrough was higher (28%) than in those re-treated patients who had not had a prior breakthrough (8%) (Table 7).

HCV RNA response by race

Initial response to interferon therapy in patients with hepatitis C was analyzed according to race, and it was observed that the 40 African-Americans included in the study had significantly lower ETR and SVR (5% and 3%, respectively), when compared to the responses seen in the 380 Caucasian subjects (33% and 12%, respectively). This was independent of type of interferon received (Table 8) [9]. Further analysis of sera according to different racial groups showed that African Americans had a significantly higher rate of genotype 1 infections and somewhat higher baseline viral loads although the latter were not significantly different from that found in Caucasians. Initial baseline histology was no different. Hence the reason for this poorer response rate in African-Americans appears to be related to the prevalence of genotype 1, although other as yet unknown factors may also play a role (Table 9).

Safety data

The number of serious adverse events which were reported following treatment with either CIFN or interferon alpha-2b were similar when compared head-to-head. In the second re-treatment trial of relapsers and nonresponders, where larger doses of CIFN were used, the number of serious adverse events, despite the larger dose and the longer treatment period, were no different. But one third of patients on the 15 mcg dose required dose reductions, (this had only been necessary in 12-16% of patients during the initial study involving lower doses). Dropouts due to adverse events were 7% in the first study and 4% in those randomized to CIFN 15 mcg for 24 weeks, and 10% in those who were randomized to 48 weeks in the re-treatment study (Table 10).

Table 7. Response to re-treatment in patients with HCV RNA breakthroughs

	all HCV RNA NR n = 68	NR with breakthroughs n = 18	NR without breakthroughs n = 50
Re-treatment sustained HCV RNA response	13%	28%*	8%
Re-treatment sustained ALT response	18%	39%**	10%

Retreatment for 12 months with 15 μg CIFN

* $p = 0.102$

** $p = 0.014$

Heathcote et al., Hepatology 1999;30:562-566

Table 8. HCV RNA responses by race — interferon therapy CHC

	end of treatment	sustained response
Caucasian (380)	33%*	12%**
African-Americans (40)	5%*	3%**
Hispanics (40)	28%	10%
Asians (10)	40%	30%

* $p = 0.04$

** $p = 0.07$

Reddy et al., Hepatology 1999;30:787-793

Table 9. Ethnic differences in response to IFN for CHC baseline parameters by race

Feature	Caucasians (n = 380)	African-Americans (n = 40)	Hispanic Whites (n = 40)	Asian-Americans (n = 10)
median HCV RNA level	3.0×10^6	3.6×10^6	1.9×10^6	1.4×10^6
genotype 1	66%*	88%*	69%	40%
cirrhosis	12%	5%	20%	10%

all groups comparable in age, gender and HAI score

* $p < 0.004$

Reddy et al., Hepatology 1999;30:787-793

Table 10. Safety data

	Initial treatment		Re-treatment	
	CIFN (9 μg)	IFN α-2b (3MU)	CIFN 24wk (15 μg)	CIFN 48 wk (15 μg)
Dropouts due to adverse events	7%	7%	4%	10%
Serious adverse events	8%	8%	4%	7%
Dose reductions	16%	12%	33%	36%

How can the efficacy of interferon be improved?

The overall sustained response rate following interferon monotherapy ranges between 10 and 20%, depending on the duration and probably the dose of therapy. It is now recognized that if interferon is combined with the nucleoside analogue, ribavirin, an increased sustained response rate is observed, accomplished chiefly by a reduction in the relapse rate [10, 11]. Unfortunately, treatment with this combination therapy is associated with an increased rate of side effects (21% withdrawal rate when patients are asked to take 48 weeks of therapy).

Interferon therapy has an immediate antiviral effect, but when it is given intermittently, i.e., three times a week (ttw), viral rebound occurs within 48 hours, (prior to the next injection) [12] (Figure 3). The efficacy of standard interferons is limited by the trough in antiviral activity between doses. Thus the rationale for IFN pegylation was generated (Table 11). With its high molecular weight (40 kDa), polyethylene glycol attached in a branched manner at a single site induces a slower sustained absorption rate and a much reduced renal clearance. Thus detectable serum IFN levels are reduced over the course of the week in treated patients [13]. Clearance of the PEG (40 kaD) IFN alpha 2a is chiefly via the liver.

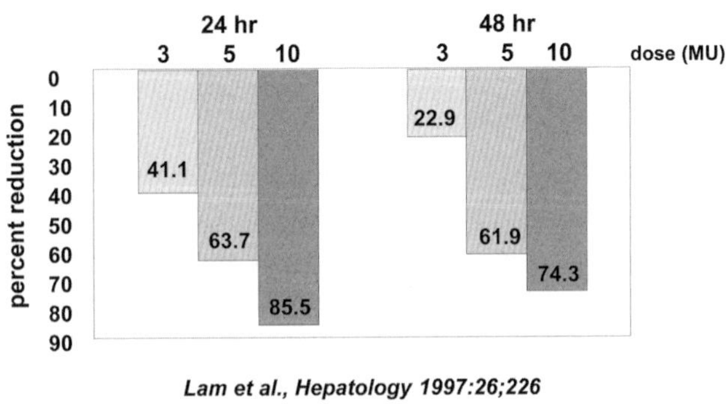

Figure 3. Reduction in HCV RNA following single dose of interferon alpha.

Table 11. Variables in pegylated protein characteristics

- PEG molecular weight and branching
  - Branched, high-molecular-weight PEGs provide sustained absorption and produce greater ↓ in renal clearance
- Type of bond between PEG and protein
  - Some bonds are stronger than others
  - Strength of bond determines durability of PEG protein

Katre, Adv Drug Delivery Rev. 1993;10:91-114.

Table 12. Summary of pharmacokinetic parameters in healthy subjects

PK Parameter [a]	40kDa PEG-IFN α2a 180 μg sc (n = 10)	IFN α2a 3 MIU sc (n = 34)
MAT [b] (h)	59 ± 24	2.6 ± 1.8
T max (h)	78 ±27	10 ±3
C max (ng/mL or U/mL)	14.2 ± 2.5	13.4 ± 3.7
t 1/2 (h)	77 ± 45	9 ± 6
CI/F (mL/h)	82 ± 38	11836 ± 3238
% absorbed	61	80

[a] mean ± SD except for MAT, which is mean ± SE

[b] MAT — mean absorption time; time required for 50% to be absorbed

IFN data from Xu et al., Hepatology 1998;28(Suppl):702A

IFN α2a which was 11836±

Pharmacokinetic parameters of PEG 40kDa IFN alpha 2a in healthy subjects

The pharmacokinetics of PEG 40kDa IFN alpha 2a, 180 mcg sc, have been compared to that of IFN alpha 2a, 3 million units sc, given to healthy subjects. The percent of IFN absorption with pegylated IFN was 61% compared to 80% with IFN alpha 2a. The T_{max} (hr) is significantly higher with PEG (40kDa) IFN alpha 2a, 78 ± 27 (hr) compared to 10 ± 3 (hr) with standard IFN alpha 2a. The $t_{1/2}$ (h) following injection with PEG 40k Da IFN alpha 2a was 77 ± 45 (hr) compared to 9 ± 6 (hr) when standard IFN therapy is given. The renal clearance of PEG 40 ka Da IFN alpha 2a was 82 ± 32 ml/hr, markedly less than that for standard IFN alfa 2a, 11,836 ± 3,238 mls per hr. This improvement in PK profile of PEG 40k IFN alpha 2a may be a key to enhancing IFN efficacy in the treatment of chronic hepatitis C, and possibly hepatitis B.

Summary

These studies describe major advances in interferon therapy for patients with chronic viral hepatitis. Long-acting PEG 40kDa IFN alpha 2a has now been shown to be more efficacious than standard, short-acting interferon monotherapy given on an intermittent basis. It remains unknown whether the side-effect profile will be different. The standard interferons described vary in their antiviral activity, CIFN being more effective than IFN alpha 2b in patients with hepatitis C who have a viral load $>4.8 \times 10^6$ copies/ml. In the future, the treatment of patients chronically infected with viral hepatitis should be tailored to specific viral and host-derived pretreatment variables.

References

1. Taylor-Robinson S, Foster G, Arora S, Hargreaves S & Thomas HC. Increase in primary liver cancer in the UK, 1979-94. Lancet 1997;350:1143.
2. El-Serag HB, Mason A. Rising incidence of hepatocellular carcinoma in the United States. N. Eng J Med 1999;340:745-750.
3. Blatt LM, Davis JM, Klein SB & Taylor MW. The biologic activity and molecular characteristics of a novel synthetic interferon alpha series, consensus interferon. J. Interferon Cytokine Res. 1996;16:489-499.
4. Ozes ON, Reiter ZVI, Klein S, Blatt LM & Taylor MW. A comparison of interferon con-1 with natural recombinant interferonsα: antiviral antiproliferative and natural killer-inducing activities. J Interferon 1992;12:55-59.
5. Tong M, Reddy R, Lee W, Pockros PJ, Hoefs JC, Keefe E, Hollinger FB et al. Treatment of chronic hepatitis C with consensus interferon: a multicenter, randomized, controlled trial. Hepatology 1997;26:747-754.
6. Everson G, Jensen DM, Craig JR, Van Leeuwen D, Bain V, Ehrinpreis M, Albert D et al. Efficacy of Interferon treatment for patients with chronic hepatitis C: comparison of response in cirrhotics, fibrotics or nonfibrotics. Hepatology 1999;30:271-276.
7. Heathcote J, Keefe E, Lee S, Feinman SV, Tong M, Reddy KR, Albert DG et al. Re-treatment of chronic hepatitis C with consensus Interferon. Hepatology 1998;27:1136-1143.
8. Heathcote E, James S, Mullen K, Hauser SC, Rosenblate H, Albert D and the Consensus Interferon study group. Chronic hepatitis C virus patients with breakthroughs during Interferon treatment can successfully be retreated with Consensus Interferon. Hepatology 1999;30:562-566.
9. Reddy K, Hoofnagle J, Tong M, Lee M, et al. Racial differences in responses to therapy with interferon in chronic hepatitis C. Hepatology 1999;30:787-793.
10. Poynard T, Marcellin P, Lee S. et al. Randomised trial of interferon alpha-2b plus ribavirin for 48 weeks or for 24 weeks versus interferon alpha-2b plus placebo for 48 weeks for treatment of chronic infection with hepatitis C virus. Lancet 1998;352:1426-1432.

11. McHutchison J, Gordon S, Schiff E. et al. Interferon alpha-2b alone or in combination with ribavirin as initial treatment for chronic hepatitis C. The New England Journal of Medicine 1198;339:1485-1492.
12. Lam NP, Neumann AU, Gretch DR, Wiley TE, Perelson AS et al. Dose independent acute clearance of hepatitis C genotype 1 virus with Interferon alfa. Hepatology 1997;26:226-231.
13. Heathcote EJ, Pockros PJ, Fried MW, Bain MA and DePamphilis J. The pharmacokinetics of pegylated 40k Interferon alfa 2a (PEG/IFN) in chronic hepatitis C (CHC) patients with cirrhosis. Gastroenterology 1999;116:G3190N Abstract.
14. Xu et al. Single dose, safety/tolerability and pharmacokinetic/pharmacodynamics (PK/PD) following administration of ascending subcutaneous doses of pegylated-interferon (PEG-IFN) and interferon α-2a (IFN α-2a) to healthy subjects. Hepatology 1998;28:702A.
15. Heathcote EJ, Shiffman M, Cooksley G, Dusheiko G, Lee S et al. Peginterferon alfa-2a in patients with chronic hepatitis C and cirrhosis. New Eng J Med 2000;343:1673-1680.
16. Zeuzem S, Feinman V, Rasenack J, Heathcote J, Lai MY et al. Peginterferon alfa-2a in patients with chronic hepatitis C. New Eng J Med 2000;343:1666-1672.

Impact of interferon alpha-2b and of combination with ribavirin on progression of liver fibrosis in patients with chronic hepatitis C

THIERRY POYNARD[1], JOHN MCHUTCHISON[2], GARY L. DAVIS[3], RAFAEL ESTEBAN-MUR[4], ZACHARY GOODMAN[5], PIERRE BEDOSSA[6] and JANICE ALBRECHT[7]

[1] *Service d'Hépato-Gastroentérologie Groupe Hospitalier Pitié-Salpêtrière, 47 Boulevard de l'Hôpital 75651 PARIS Cedex 13, France*
[2] *Scripps Clinic and Research Foundation, Division of Gastroenterology/Hepatology (203N), 10666 N Torrey Pines Road, La Jolla, CA 92037, USA*
[3] *Section of Hepatobiliary Diseases, P.O. Box 100214, University of Florida, Gainesville, FL 32610-0214, USA*
[4] *Servei de Medicine Interna-Hepatologia, Valle Hebron Hospital, 119, 08035, Barcelona, Spain*
[5] *Department of Hepatic and Gastrointestinal Pathology, Armed Forces Institute of Pathology, Washington, DC 20306-6000, USA*
[6] *Service d'Anatomie Pathologique, Hôpital de Bicètre, 94275 Kremlin Bicêtre, France*
[7] *Janice Albrecht, Schering-Plough Research Institute, Kenilworth, NJ, USA*

Summary

The hypothesis that treatment with a combination of interferon alpha-2b (IFN) and ribavirin (R) can alter the rate of progression of liver fibrosis was examined among 1,972 chronic hepatitis C patients. A sustained virological response was obtained in 44% with IFN-R vs 15% with IFN, and in 0% of controls. In responders, the annual rate of fibrosis decreased by 189% compared to controls, and septal fibrosis disappeared in 56%. In nonresponders, the rate of fibrosis decreased by 66% and progression to septal fibrosis was observed in only 15%. These results, not apparent in individual trials, demonstrated that IFN-R dramatically reduces the rate of fibrosis progression.

Frontiers in Viral Hepatitis Ed. by RF Schinazi, J-P Sommadossi and CM Rice. 425 — 439

Introduction

Current understanding of HCV infection has been advanced by the concept of liver fibrosis progression [1]. HCV can be lethal usually only when it leads to cirrhosis, the last stage of liver fibrosis. Therefore, an accurate estimate of fibrosis progression represents an important surrogate endpoint for evaluation of the vulnerability of any given patient for these potential complications, and for assessment of any treatment's impact on natural history. Of major interest is the fact that approved treatments in chronic hepatitis C — interferon [2-5] and, recently, the combination of interferon alpha-2b and ribavirin [6-9] — have not only antiviral, but also anti-fibrotic and immunomodulatory effects [10-12]. Thus, these treatments have the potential to affect the fibrosis progression in patients regardless of the virologic response.

Limitations on any estimate of fibrosis include (i) the difficulty in obtaining paired liver biopsies, (ii) the necessity for large numbers of patients to achieve statistical power, and (iii) the heterogeneity of fibrosis assessments. Even in randomized trials less than 50% of patients undergo a second liver biopsy after the end of treatment [5]. Because the time elapsed between biopsies is relatively short (usually between 12 to 24 months), the number of events (transition from one stage to another) is rare. Therefore, comparisons of fibrosis progression rates require a large sample size to observe significant differences. Metanalysis is considered as a possible method of increasing the power of comparisons, but unfortunately the overall number of patients with paired biopsies in published trials is small, and many trials used invalidated or inappropriate fibrosis scoring systems [13-14].

Because of these limitations, the actual impact of HCV treatment on the liver fibrosis progression rate in patients with chronic hepatitis C, regardless of virological response, is unknown. We have published elsewhere a specific study on the progression of liver fibrosis [9] observed in two randomized trials of the combination of interferon alpha-2b and ribavirin. We want to present here the results from a larger database of patients with paired liver biopsies.

Patient database

The individual data from five randomized trials [12] and from a single center cohort [1] have been gathered with permission of the principal investigators. The randomized trials included: an 18-month, IFN multicenter French trial [4], an International [7] and US [8] multicenter trial of ribavirin-interferon in naïve patients, and US [9] and International [9] multicenter trials of ribavirin-interferon in relapsers. The single-center cohort (DOSVIRC) represents all the patients with hepatitis C followed in the Hepato-Gastroenterology Department of the Pitié-Salpêtrière hospital, retrospectively before 1993 and prospectively thereafter. Patients with biopsy and serological confirmation of chronic hepatitis C were included if they had both pre- and posttreatment liver biopsies which were available for interpretation by the METAVIR scoring system for fibrosis stage and activity grade. Patients were excluded if they did not have paired biopsies, were co-infected with HBV or HIV, or had other forms of liver disease. In all trials a signed informed consent was obtained, after the nature and possible consequences of the studies were explained.

A database consisting of all studies was created containing the following information: gender, age at first biopsy, age at infection, presumed mode of infection (parenteral, usually IV drug use, transfusion, other or unknown), consumption of alcohol (none, less than 50 g per day, 50 g or more per day), type of treatment (IFN-R, IFN, control), duration of treatment (six, 12, or more than 12 months), METAVIR fibrosis stage and activity grade at first and second biopsy, time elapsed between the two biopsies in months, ALT response (normalization) at three months, ALT response at the end of treatment, ALT response at the end of follow-up (six months after the end of treatment), quantification of virus before treatment, at three months, at the end of treatment, at the end of follow-up (six months after the end of treatment), and viral genotype [1, 2, 3, 4, 5, 6]. Virological response was defined as no detectable quantity in the serum (that is, less than 100 copies per ml).

Liver biopsies were fixed, paraffin-embedded and stained with at least hematoxylin eosin safran and Masson's trichrome or picrosirius red for collagen. For each liver biopsy, a stage of fibrosis and a grade of activity was established, according to the following criteria. Fibrosis was staged on a scale of 0 to 4: F0 = no fibrosis, F1 = portal fibrosis without septa, F2 = few septa, F3 = numerous septa without cirrhosis and F4 = cirrhosis. Reproducibility of results between pathologists using this method has been established [14-15]. The grading of activity, or the intensity of the necroinflammation, was scored as follows: A0 = no histological activity, A1 = mild activity, A2 = moderate activity, and A3 = severe activity. One of three pathologists (Pierre Bedossa, Zacharie Goodman, Frederic Charlotte) reviewed the biopsies without any information concerning the clinical, biological or treatment characteristics. Biopsies of insufficient size to allow for valid assessment of the extent of fibrosis were discarded.

For four trials [7-9] serum HCV-RNA levels were determined in a single, central laboratory (NGI, Los Angeles, CA) using a quantitative reverse transcription multicycle polymerase chain reaction assay with a lower limit of detection of 100 copies/ml [16] and HCV genotyping was done using the INNO-LiPA HCV (Innogenetics, Zwijnaarde, Belgium) second-generation assay [17]. For the two other trials, quantification of serum HCV RNA used the bDNA method (Chiron 2.0, Emeryville, CA), the qualitative PCR AMPLICOR (Roche, Basel, Switzerland) performed in a single laboratory (CNRS 1484), and HCV genotyping used COP-PCR [18]. Equivalence between the two quantitative assessments has been validated [4, 16], as well as the two genotyping methods [19]. Characteristics of the 1,972 patients included are given in Table 1.

Assessment of fibrosis progression

The assessment of fibrosis progression over time was evaluated as previously described [1, 5]. The "observed" (direct) fibrosis progression rate was defined as the ratio between the difference in fibrosis stage, expressed in METAVIR units, between two biopsies and the interval between the two biopsies in years. For example, for a patient with fibrosis stage 2 at the first biopsy and stage 3 at the second biopsy, performed two years later,

Table 1. Characteristics of 1,972 patients included

Characteristic	Number of patients and means
Type of trial (Ref)	**N = 1972**
DOSVIRC cohort	287
IFN 18 months	176
IFN-Ribavirin naive US	670
IFN-Ribavirin naive international	562
IFN-Ribavirin relapser US	125
IFN-Ribavirin relapser international	152
Treatment received	N = 1972
Control	102
IFN 6 months	506
IFN 12 months or more	518
IFN + Ribavirin 6 months	522
IFN + Ribavirin 12 months	324
Age	N = 1972
Mean (years)	44.3
95% CI	43.8-44.8
Gender	N = 1972
Male (%)	1245 (63%)
Female (%)	727 (37%)
Source of infection	N = 1972
Transfusion	604 (31%)
Intravenous drug use	732 (37%)
Other or Unknown source	636 (32%)
Duration of infection	N = 1564 Missing for 408
Mean years	16.5
95% CI	16.0-16.9
Duration between biopsies (month 95% CI)	N = 1962 19.7 (19.1-20.2)
METAVIR fibrosis stage	N = 1972
No fibrosis (F0)	43 (2%)
Portal fibrosis (F1)	1279 (65%)
Few septa (F2)	331 (17%)
Many septa (F3)	204 (10%)
Cirrhosis (F4)	115 (6%)
METAVIR activity grade	N = 1972
None (A0)	51 (2%)
Mild (A1)	586 (30%)
Moderate (A2)	749 (38%)
Severe (A3)	586 (30%)
Genotype determination	N = 1770 Missing for 202
1	1143 (64%)
1a	456

Table 1. Continued

Characteristic	Number of patients and means
1b	543
1	144
2	237 (13%)
3	331 (19%)
4	47 (3%)
5	8 (0.5%)
6	4 (0.5%)
Initial serum HCV RNA assessment	N = 1694 Missing for 278
Median (copies/ml)	3.800.000
95% CI	3.600.000-4.000.000

the fibrosis progression rate was 0.500 fibrosis units per year. The advantage of this assessment is that the duration is known exactly. The limitations are that the duration between biopsies is rather short (mean = 20 months) in comparison to the mean time transition between fibrosis stages (seven years) [3], and there is a risk of sampling and interpretation errors for both biopsies. Therefore, we also used an "estimated" (indirect) fibrosis progression rate per year that was defined as the ratio between the fibrosis stage in METAVIR units and the estimated duration of infection in years. In this model it is assumed that the patient has no liver fibrosis on the day of infection (stage F0) and that the fibrosis progression is constant. For example, for a patient with fibrosis stage 2 and an eight-year duration of infection, the fibrosis progression rate was 0.250 fibrosis unit per year. The advantages of this assessment are the longer duration (mean = 16 years), and there is no variability at infection, if the assumption of F0 is correct. The limitations are that the duration of infection was unknown in 408 patients out of 1,972 (21%), and even when known, it remains an estimate (i.e., it is assumed that the first transfusion or the first IV drug injection was the true date of infection). It is also possible that some patients may have already had fibrosis (e.g., due to alcohol) the day of infection. For a given patient the impact of treatment on the spontaneous fibrosis progression rates was expressed as the difference between the observed rate (between the two biopsies performed before and after treatment) and the estimated rate before treatment. The relative impact was expressed as the ratio between this difference and the estimated rate before. The progression of fibrosis outside the portal tract with constitution of bridging or septa (F2) has been considered as the first critical threshold for significant or progressive disease due to HCV; the second critical threshold was the occurrence of an extensive fibrosis (F3 or F4), since these patients risk clinical complications. We have therefore compared the percentages of patients worsening, improving or not changing with respect to these fibrosis stages.

In order to take into account the factors associated with the natural progression of liver fibrosis, we performed a multivariate analysis. In non-treated patients we had previously observed [1] that the stage of fibrosis on the day of biopsy was dependent on the duration of infection (time-risk factor) and on three host-risk factors: sex, age at infection, and consumption of alcohol. Two variables were considered as estimates of time-related risk factors: the age at biopsy and the estimated duration of infection, defined as the period between the presumed date of infection and the date of biopsy. We had not previously identified virus factors as independent risk factors for liver fibrosis progression before treatment, but this could have been related to a lack of power, as genotypes and viral levels were available in only 376 and 173 patients, respectively, in the first model [1]. Therefore, we performed a new analysis in 1,139 treatment-naïve patients with complete data, to check if genotype and quantity of serum HCV RNA were associated with spontaneous liver fibrosis progression. Robust and logistic regression analyses were used. The explained variable was the fibrosis progression rate per year. Several models were constructed: the core model included age at biopsy, sex, genotype 2, 3 or neither, and RNA quantity (in $\log_{10}$). There was no association between genotype or viral load whichever analysis was used (details not shown). The mean, estimated fibrosis progression rate was 0.161 METAVIR units per year in patients with genotype 2 or 3 versus 0.150 in other genotypes (ns). In patients with a viral load greater than 3.5 million copies per ml, the rate was 0.150, the same as seen in patients with a viral load equal to or lower than 3.5 million copies per ml.

Estimation of treatment impact

Methods

The next step was the estimation of treatment impact in treated patients. We hypothesized that treatment: (i) results in an *absolute* regression of fibrosis stage in patients with a sustained virological response during treatment and thereafter, (ii) results in a *relative* reduction of the fibrosis progression in virological nonresponders during the treatment period, in comparison to spontaneous progression with an unknown restart of progression thereafter.

To determine the sustained virological response according to treatment, we used univariate and multivariate analyses and metanalyses. A sustained virological response (<100 copies/ml) was obtained in 44% by IFN-R (366/839) vs 15% by IFN (106/732; $p < 0.0001$), and in none of 102 controls ($p < 0.0001$ versus both treated groups). The sustained virological response could not been assessed in 299 patients, because no serum specimen was available. Because these results were obtained in different trials, sensitivity analyses were performed to take into account the randomization process, the treatment duration, risk factors and the previous history of treatment. For taking into account the randomization process and treatment duration, metanalyses of individual data were performed for patients included in four randomized trials comparing IFN-R to IFN, for 48 weeks, for 24 weeks, for treatment-naïve patients, and for patients who had relapsed after a previous unsustained response to interferon. The methodology of metanalysis was fully respected, as all the treatments, study designs and endpoints were identical in these four randomized trials. In the trial comparing IFN-R for 48 weeks, IFN alone for 48 weeks and IFN-R for 24 weeks, this last arm was excluded as there was no randomized IFN alone for 24 weeks group with which to compare. All analyses were performed by Peto et al. and Der Simonian methods. A total of 1,287 patients were analyzed. A sustained virological response was obtained in 5% of patients treated with IFN for 24 weeks, 17% treated with IFN for 48 weeks, 42% treated with IFN-R for 24 weeks and 47% treated with IFN-R for 48 weeks. All the differences were highly significant in favor of the combination IFN-R: the mean increase in sustained virological response for IFN-R was 34% (95% CI: 27-46%; chi-square = 57; $p < 0.001$), from a mean of 11% with IFN to 45% with IFN-R. The mean difference was higher in relapsers (50%; 95% CI 41-59%) than in treatment-naïve patients (29%; 95% CI 24-34%). Inside these subgroups there was no heterogeneity. To determine the impact of treatment adjusted for risk factors, we then performed several multivariate analyses which all showed consistent results. In robust and logistic regression analyses, six factors were independently associated with sustained response: ribavirin combination ($p < 0.0001$), genotype 2 and 3 ($p < 0.0001$), low viral load (<3.5 million copies/ml) ($p < 0.0001$), age at biopsy (<40 years) ($p = 0.0003$), female sex ($p = 0.01$) and absence of septal fibrosis ($p = 0.02$). Squared correlations were, respectively, 0.25 and 0.33. In patients with less than three response factors, there was a very significant advantage for the 48-week regimen; 35% sustained response (65/187; 95% CI 28-42%) versus 21% for the 24-week combination regimen (47/225; 95%CI 15-26%; $p = 0.002$). These findings permit consolidation (larger sample size without heterogeneity) into what has been observed in individual trials [12]: a very significant improvement in sustained virological response with combination IFN-R and, for patients with few response factors, an increase in response by extending the duration of therapy to 48 weeks.

Impact in responders

The next step was to estimate, in the group of sustained responders, the impact of treatment on fibrosis progression. For this purpose we compared, in 382 responders with known duration of infection, the fibrosis progression rate observed after treatment between the two biopsies, versus the progression rate estimated before treatment, and also versus the progression observed in two control groups: an historical control (84 patients without treatment, with two biopsies and a known duration of infection) and a simulated control group of 382 patients with the characteristics of the responders. The simulated control group was obtained by calculating the expected fibrosis progression rate according to a regression function. For this purpose we used another database of 1,157 patients never treated and with a known duration of infection [3]. By logistic regression the expected fibrosis progression rate per year was = 0.058 - (0.0035 × duration of infection in years) + (0.0037 × age at infection in years) + (0.021 × sex (0 if female, 1 if male)) + (0.028 × alcohol consumption (0 if less than 50 g per day, 1 if 50 g or more)). The mean estimate was lower in the present population of 1,564 patients (0.111) than in the 1,157 previous ones (0.252). This was not surprising, as patients included in the present database were younger, histologically less severe and never declared an alcohol consumption greater than 50 gr of alcohol. In comparison to the estimated fibrosis progression rate, the simulated estimate was very conservative and precluded the risk of false-positive conclusions. Using these estimates, there was a dramatic decrease of the fibrosis progression rates among the sustained responders, from 0.177 METAVIR fibrosis unit per year before treatment to -0.157 after, a 189% relative decrease ($p < 0.0001$), and from 0.107 for the simulated rate, a 247% relative decrease ($p < 0.0001$) (Table 2). The graphical representation of the treatment impact is given in Figure 1. Panel A illustrates the comparison to estimated progression before treatment, and Panel B illustrates the simulated progression. This impact was proportional to the initial fibrosis stage, with -0.012 in patients without septal fibrosis (F0 or F1) and -0.695 in patients with septal fibrosis (F2-F4). This means in terms of fibrosis regression that if the rate is constant, a patient with grade F2 at the beginning of treatment should regress to F1 in a mean of 1/0.695 = 1.4 years (95% CI

Table 2. Mean fibrosis progression rate per year for 1361 patients with an estimated duration of infection and RNA sustained response assessment. All differences versus controls, historical or simulated, were highly significant ($p < 0.001$). Fibrosis progression rates of simulated controls stratified by treatment groups were identical (107 to 114 10^{-3} fibrosis METAVIR unit per year) to those not stratified (data not shown).

Treatment and response	Mean fibrosis progression rate in F-METAVIR 10^{-3} units-per-year mean (95% CI) *(number of patients)*						Significance	
	Estimated before first biopsy			Observed between biopsies			Observed vs ctrl	Observed vs before
Historical Controls	**210**	**(165_256)**	**(n = 86)**	**267**	**(162_323)**	**(n = 86)**		**ns**
All treated	156	(141-171)	(n = 1275)	-12	(-48_23)	(n = 1275)	0.0001	0.0001
Simulated controls	*111*	*(111_111)*	*(n = 1275)*	*111*	*(111_111)*	*(n = 1275)*		
Sustained								
Responders	177	(147_206)	(n = 382)	-157	(-211_-103)	(n = 382)	0.0001	0.0001
Simulated controls	*108*	*(108_108)*	*(n = 382)*	*108*	*(108_108)*	*(n = 382)*		
Nonresponders	147	(129_165)	(n = 893)	50	(5_94)	(n = 893)	0.0001	0.0001
Simulated controls	*113*	*(112_113)*	*(n = 893)*	*113*	*(112_113)*	*(n = 893)*		
IFN alone	199	(170_227)	(n = 573)	33	(-26_91)	(n = 573)	0.0001	0.0001
Sustained								
Responders	321	(209_433)	(n = 77)	-156	(-258_-53)	(n = 77)	0.01	0.0001
Nonresponders	152	(127_177)	(n = 496)	62	(-3_127)	(n = 496)	0.0001	0.01
IFN-Ribavirin	140	(123-157)	(n = 702)	-49	(-93_-5)	(n = 702)	0.0001	0.0001
Sustained								
Responders	140	(117_163)	(n = 305)	-157	(-221_-94)	(n = 305)	0.01	0.0001
Nonresponders	141	(116_165)	(n = 397)	34	(-25_93)	(n = 397)	0.0001	0.001

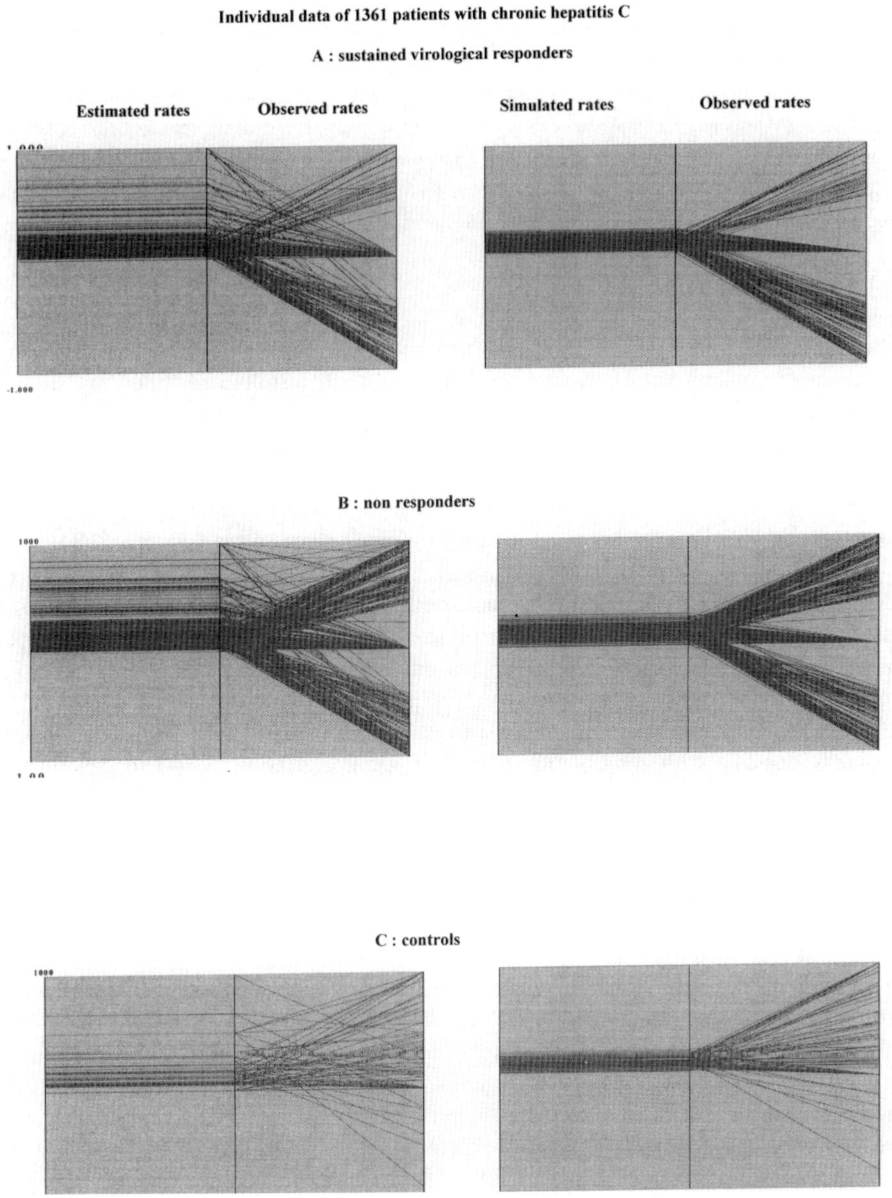

Figure 1. Fibrosis progression rate per year in F METAVIR units before and after treatment. Each individual data set from 1,361 patients with two biopsies and a presumed date of infection is represented by a line. The left panels have two parts. The first shows the estimated fibrosis progression rate per year, from the initial infection to the first liver biopsy (horizontal lines in the left part of the panel); this is calculated by dividing the fibrosis stage (fibrosis METAVIR unit) at the first biopsy by the duration of infection in years. The vertical axis represents the range rate from -1.000 to +1.000 fibrosis-METAVIR units per year. The second part shows the variation from this estimated fibrosis progression rate to the observed fibrosis rate between the first and the second biopsies (transversal lines in the right part of the panel). If there is no change, the second part of the line is horizontal.

Figure 1 (continued) If the fibrosis rate increases the line goes up; if the fibrosis rate decreases the line goes down. The right panels are based on the same principle, but the first part (horizontal line) shows the simulated fibrosis rate. This rate is calculated by a regression function. Panels A, B and C show the fibrosis progression rate of sustained responders, nonresponders and controls, respectively. This dynamic representation of fibrosis progression illustrates graphically that there was a much greater reduction in progression rates in treated patients, both responders and nonresponders, than in controls. It also illustrates the heterogeneity of these progression rates with a 3-modal distribution after treatment.

from 1.1 to 1.9 years). The hypothesis of a continual fibrosis decrease in virological sustained responders has been confirmed by long-term histological follow-up studies [6, 20, 21].

Because of the limitations of the fibrosis progression estimates, we determined more pragmatically the treatment impact according to the stage of liver fibrosis (Table 3). All the comparisons between sustained responders and controls were highly significant, whatever the initial stage. Among patients with many septa (stage F3), 6% (2/34; 95% CI 1-20%) progressed to cirrhosis (F4) vs 60% (6/10; 95% CI 26-88%; $p = 0.0007$) in controls. This is a very important clinical result because mortality occurs for the most part only in cirrhotic patients, and so far no study has demonstrated such a clear impact on the incidence of cirrhosis. According to our findings, in 58 patients with stage F3 treated by IFN-R combination, a sustained response was obtained in 38% (22/58; 95% CI: 26-52%). Therefore, in $0.38 \times (1-0.06) = 36\%$ of patients with extensive fibrosis, it is now possible with combination therapy to eradicate the virus and to prevent the occurrence of cirrhosis.

We next determined the impact of treatment on histological inflammatory activity. Improvement of at least one METAVIR grade was observed in 81% (381/472; 95% CI 77-84%) of sustained responders versus 14% (14/102; 95% CI 8-22%) of controls ($p < 0.0001$). Among sustained responders initially with A2 or A3, 87% (308/356; 95% CI 83-90%) returned to A0 or A1 after treatment. This result is very impressive, because in contrast to the very sensitive Knodell Histological Activity Index (ranging from 0 to 20), a difference in one METAVIR activity grade (ranging from 0 to 3) represents a 30% improvement of necro-inflammatory features.

Finally, for sustained responder patients, we tried to identify predictive factors of fibrosis improvement. No variable (in multivariate analysis; data not shown) was predictive of the fibrosis regression, except initial fibrosis stage, the higher stage showing more improvement. In particular, there was no difference in rates between IFN-R combination, IFN alone or the initial activity grade. These findings lead to the conclusion that, whatever the treatment used, when a sustained virological response is obtained, activity and fibrosis improve dramatically in a short follow-up, and even in the advanced stages. In individual trials this impact on fibrosis progression had been missed.

Table 3. Evolution of fibrosis after treatment among nonresponders and sustained responders, according to their initial stages. Whatever the initial stages, comparisons between sustained responders and controls or between nonresponders and controls were highly significant ($p < 0.001$). Among patients with at least a few septa at the first biopsy (F2 or more), septal fibrosis disappeared in 56% (95% CI 46-66%) of sustained responders versus 9% (95% CI 3-22%) of controls ($p < 0.0001$). Among patients without septal fibrosis at the first biopsy (F0 or F1), only 7% of sustained responders progressed to septal fibrosis or beyond versus 48% of controls ($p < 0.0001$).

3A. Evolution of fibrosis in patients with minimal fibrosis at first biopsy before treatment (none = F0 or portal fibrosis = F1)

Fibrosis stage	**Patients with no (F0) or portal (F1) fibrosis at first biopsy**					
At second biopsy	**Controls**		**Nonresponders**		**Sustained Responders**	
No (F0) or portal (F1)	30	(52%)	665	(85%)	346	(93%)
Few septa (F2)	22	(38%)	88	(11%)	23	(6%)
Many septa (F3) or cirrhosis (F4)	6	(10%)	33	(4%)	2	(1%)
Total	58	(100%)	786	(100%)	371	(100%)

3B. Evolution of fibrosis in patients with moderate fibrosis at first biopsy before treatment (few septa = F2)

Fibrosis stage at second biopsy	**Patients with few septa (F2) at first biopsy**					
	Controls		**Nonresponders**		**Sustained Responders**	
No (F0) or portal (F1)	4	(12%)	65	(44%)	36	(69%)
Few septa (F2)	11	(32%)	40	(27%)	7	(14%)
Many septa (F3) or cirrhosis (F4)	19	(56%)	43	(29%)	9	(17%)
Total	34	(100%)	148	(100%)	52	(100%)

3C. Evolution of fibrosis in patients with extensive fibrosis at first biopsy before treatment (Many septa = F3 or cirrhosis = F4)

Fibrosis stage at second biopsy	**Patients with many septa (F3) or cirrhosis (F4) at first biopsy**					
	Controls		**Nonresponders**		**Sustained Responders**	
No (F0) or portal (F1)	0	(0%)	31	(19%)	21	(43%)
Few septa (F2)	2	(20%)	24	(14%)	15	(31%)
Many septa (F3) or cirrhosis (F4)	8	(80%)	110	(67%)	13	(26%)
Total	10	(100%)	165	(100%)	49	(100%)

Impact in nonresponders

The next step was to assess if IFN-R treatment has an impact on the fibrosis progression rate among nonresponders, in comparison to rates before treatment and in comparison to untreated controls. For this purpose we used the same estimates as in sustained responders, the fibrosis progression rate per year and the evolution of fibrosis stage. The striking conclusion was that, although the impact was weaker than in sustained responders, IFN-R in nonresponders slowed the natural fibrosis progression observed before treatment, and in comparison to historical or simulated controls. There was a very significant decrease in the fibrosis progression rates, from 0.147 METAVIR fibrosis units per year before treatment to 0.050 after, which represents a 66% relative decrease ($p < 0.0001$), and from 0.113 in simulated controls, a 46% relative decrease ($p < 0.0001$) (Table 2). However, this effect was very heterogeneous, with a non-normal distribution, in contrast to what was observed in responders. In order to explain this heterogeneity, we compared the characteristics of these 893 nonresponders according to their fibrosis response: improvement (n = 126), stabilization (n = 596) and worsening (n = 171). Whatever the univariate or multivariate methods used (logistic, robust regression, discriminant analyses), few factors were identified. In these nonresponders the fibrosis response was highly associated with the initial stage of fibrosis. In patients without septal fibrosis (F0 or F1), the mean fibrosis progression rate was 0.141. Among patients with at least septal fibrosis, the mean fibrosis progression rate after treatment was -0.197 per year. The only other factor independently associated with fibrosis response was age. Patients with worsening fibrosis were older (73% more than 40 years) in comparison to patients who improved (33% more than 40 years; $p < 0.001$).

Next we determined the treatment impact in nonresponders according to the stage of liver fibrosis (Table 3). All the comparisons between nonresponders and controls were highly significant, whatever the initial stage. Among patients without septal fibrosis, only 15% (121/786; 95% CI 13-18%) of nonresponder patients progressed to septal fibrosis, compared to 48% (28/58; 95% CI 35-62) of controls ($p < 0.0001$). Among patients with at least septal fibrosis, septal fibrosis disappeared in 31% (96/313; 95% CI 26-36%) of nonresponders, compared to 9% (4/44; 95%CI 3-22%) of untreated controls ($p < 0.0001$). These findings argue against the concept of stopping treatment in patients without virological response. From our results, if the treatment impact is constant, and if the treatment is not interrupted, a patient with grade F2 at the beginning, when treated with IFN-R, should regress to F1 in a mean of 1/0.197 = 5.1 years (95% CI from 3.0 to 15.6 years). Among patients with extensive fibrosis (stage F3), 36% (95%CI 26-47%) progressed to cirrhosis (F4) vs 60% (95% CI 26-88%; $p = 0.09$) in controls. In terms of activity features, there was also a very significant impact of treatment, with improvement of at least one METAVIR grade in 33% (358/1099; 95% CI 30-35%) of nonresponders versus 14% (14/102; 95% CI 8-22%) of controls ($p < 0.0001$).

Impact of interferon-ribavirin independent of virological response

Lastly, we wanted to explore whether IFN-R combination compared to IFN alone had a greater impact on histological endpoints, independently of the sustained virological response. For this purpose we performed metanalyses of histological endpoints by combining individual data from the four randomized trials comparing IFN-R to IFN. The overall metanalysis without stratification on the virological response showed that there were 21% (95% CI 16-26%; p = 0.02) more patients who reduced inflammatory activity (by at least one METAVIR grade) in the IFN-R group (58%) in comparison to IFN alone (37%); there were also 4% (95% CI 1-8%; p = 0.04) fewer patients who worsened their fibrosis stage in the IFN-R group (15%) in comparison to IFN alone (19%). The stratified analysis showed that IFN-R combination was more effective than IFN alone in reducing hepatic inflammation, independent of the virological response. IFN-R increased by 6% (95% CI 1-12%, chi-square = 5, p = 0.02, heterogeneity test not significant) the percentage of patients who reduced inflammatory activity (by at least one METAVIR grade). Interestingly, this additional effect of IFN-R versus IFN alone was no different among sustained responders (8%; from 74 to 82%) than nonresponders (6%; from 31 to 37%). Therefore, if most of the reduced inflammatory activity effect was accounted for by sustained virological response, there is a remaining component which resulted from independent and unknown mechanisms. This phenomenon has already been observed with IFN alone (in randomized trials versus control, there are more patients with inflammatory activity improvement than with virological response) and is even greater with the IFN-R combination. No significant differences were observed in favor of IFN-R combination versus IFN alone for the fibrosis effect in responders or in nonresponders.

Conclusion

In summary, in our population of patients, these results have demonstrated that IFN-R combination treatment slows the rate of progression of liver fibrosis, and therefore has an impact on the natural history of chronic hepatitis C. With this combination a virological sustained response was obtained in 47% of patients. In these responders, moderate and severe activity disappeared in 86% of patients, and septal fibrosis disappeared in 56% of those in whom it was present before therapy. Among the nonresponders, treatment reduced the rate of fibrosis progression by 66% compared to controls and reduced the likelihood of developing septal fibrosis by 79% (69%-15%/69%) for those in whom it was not present before therapy.

We conclude that IFN-R has the potential to reduce the morbidity and mortality of chronic hepatitis C in sustained virological responders and to allow for stabilization of nonresponders awaiting new generations of drugs.

Acknowledgement

Supported by research grants from Schering Plough Research Institute, Kenilworth, NJ, USA, by Direction de la Recherche Clinique Assistance Publique Hôpitaux de Paris, Syndicat National Français de l'Industrie Pharmaceutique and by Association pour la Recherche contre le Cancer, Paris, France.

References

1. Poynard T, Bedossa P, Opolon P, for the OBSVIRC, METAVIR, CLINIVIR and DOSVIRC groups. Natural history of liver fibrosis progression in patients with chronic hepatitis C. Lancet 1997;349:825-32.
2. Poynard T, Leroy V, Cohard M, Thevenot T, Mathurin P, Opolon P, Zarski JP. Meta-analysis of interferon randomized trials in the treatment of viral hepatitis: Effects of dose and duration. Hepatology 1996;24:778-89.
3. Camma C, Giunta M, Linea C, Pagliaro L. The effect of interferon in chronic hepatitis C: a quantitative evaluation of histology by meta-analysis. J Hepatol 1997;26:1187-99.
4. Poynard T, Bedossa P, Chevalier M, Mathurin P, Lemonier C, Trepo C, Couzigou P, Payen JL, Sajus M, Costa JM, Vidaud M, Chaput JC, and the multicentre study group. A comparison fo three interferon alpha-2b regimens for the long-term treatment of chronic non-A, non-B hepatitis. New Engl J Med 1995;332:1457-62.
5. Sobesky R, Mathurin P, Charlotte F, Moussalli J, Olivi M, Vidaud M, Ratziu V, Opolon P, Poynard T. Modeling the impact of interferon alfa treatment on liver fibrosis progression in chronic hepatitis C: a dynamic view. Gastroenterology 1999;116:378-386.
6. Shiratori Y, Imazeki F, Moriyama M, Yano M, Arakawa Y, Yokosuka O, Kuroki T, Nishiguchi S, Sata M, Yamada G, Fujiyama S, Yoshida H, Omata M. Histologic improvement of fibrosis in patients with hepatitis C who have sustained response to interferon therapy. Ann Intern Med. 2000;132:517-24.
7. Poynard T, Marcellin P, Lee SS, Niederau K, Minuk GS, Ideo G, Bain V, Heathcote J, Zeuzem S, Trepo C, Albrecht J. Randomised trial of interferon alpha2b plus ribavirin for 48 weeks or for 24 weeks versus interferon alpha2b plus placebo for 48 weeks for treatment of chronic infection with hepatitis C virus. Lancet 1998;352:1426-32.
8. Mc Hutshison J, Gordon S, Schiff E, Shiffman ML, Lee WM, Rustgi VK, Goodman ZD, Ling MH, Cort S, Albrecht J. Interferon alpha-2b alone or in combination with ribavirin as initial treatment for chronic hepatitis C. N Engl J Med 1998;339:1485-92.
9. Davis G, Esteban-Mur R, Rustgi V, Hoefs J, Gordon SC, Trepo C, Shiffman ML, Zeuzem S, Craxi A, Ling MH, Albrecht J. Interferon alpha-2b alone or in combination with ribavirin for the treatment of relapse of chronic hepatitis C. N Engl J Med 1998;339:1493-9.
10. Poynard T, McHutchison J, Davis GL, Esteban-Mur R, Goodman Z, Bedossa P, Albrecht J. Impact of interferon alpha-2b and ribavirin on progression of liver fibrosis in patients with chronic hepatitis C. Hepatology in press
11. Patterson JL, Fernandez-Larson R. Molecular action of ribavirin. Rev Infect Dis 1990;12:1332-46.
12. Pilette C, Fort J, Riflet H, Cales P. Anti-fibrotic effects of interferons. Mechanisms and therapeutic prospects. Gastroenterol Clin Biol 1997;21:466-71.
13. Ning Q, Brown D, Parodo J et al. Ribavirin inhibits viral-induced macrophage production of TNF, IL-1,

the procoagulant fg12 prothrombinase and preserves Th1 cytokine production but inhibits Th2 cytokine response. J Immunol 1998;160:3487-93.

14. The METAVIR cooperative group. Inter- and intra-observer variation in the assessment of liver biopsy of chronic hepatitis C. Hepatology 1994;20;1:15-20.
15. Bedossa P, Poynard T for the French METAVIR group. An algorithm for the grading of activity in chronic hepatitis C. Hepatology 1996;24:289-93.
16. Tong MJ, Hwang SJ, Lefkowitz et al. Correlation of serum HCV RNA and alanine aminotransferase levels in chronic hepatitis C patients during treatment with ribavirin treatment with ribavirin. J Gastroenterol Hepatol 1994;9:587-91.
17. Stuyver L, Rossau R, Wyseur A et al. Typing of hepatitis C virus isolates and characterisation of new subtypes using a line probe assay. J Gen Virol 1993;74:1093-102.
18. Sajus M, Olivi M, Videau M et al. analysis of genotypes by a fluorescent competitive oligonucleotide priming PCR (COP PCR):AASLD Chicago 1994. Hepatology 1994;20:244a. abstract.
19. Stuyver L, Rossau R, Wyseur A et al. Typing of hepatitis C virus isolates and characterisation of new subtypes using a line probe assay. J Gen Virol 1993;74:1093-102.
20. Shindo M, Di Bisceglie AM, Hoofnagle JH. Long-term follow-up of patients with chronic hepatitis C treated with α-interferon. Hepatology 1992;15:1013-6.
21. Marcellin P; Boyer N; Gervais A et al. Long-term histologic improvement and loss of detectable intrahepatic HCV RNA in patients with chronic hepatitis C and sustained response to interferon-alpha therapy. Ann Intern Med 1997;127:875-81.

Decorin expression in chronic hepatitis C; effect of interferon alpha treatment

ILONA KOVALSZKY[1], KATALIN JÁRMAY[2], JÓZSEF DUDÁS[1] and ZSUZSA SCHAFF [3]

[1] *First Institute of Pathology and Experimental Cancer Research, Semmelweis University, Budapest, Hungary*
[2] *First Department of Internal Medicine, Albert Szent-Györgyi Medical University, Szeged, Hungary*
[3] *Second Department of Pathology, Semmelweis University, Budapest, Hungary*

Hepatitis C virus (HCV) is the most common infection causing chronic hepatitis [1, 2, 3]. The chronic necroinflammatory process exerted against HCV-infected hepatocytes activates the mononuclear-macrophage system. This activation results in the increased production of cytokines and growth factors. With increased levels of TNF-α and its receptors, IL-1β, IL-2, IL-6, IL-8, IFN-γ, TGF-β1, intercellular and vascular adhesion molecules are reported to mediate and maintain the chronic inflammation [4-8]. Apoptosis of hepatocytes by TNF-α and Fas-Fas ligand interaction-mediated death signals lead to loss of liver parenchyma [9]. However, these molecules, besides participating in the inflammatory process, also activate the synthesis of extracellular matrix proteins [10, 11, 12]. Thus, fibrous remodelling of the liver is a characteristic feature of chronic hepatitis.

Hepatic stellate cells (HSC) and myofibroblasts are the major cell populations responsible for production of extracellular matrix in the liver. TGF-α, PDGF, IGF, and IL-1β promote proliferation of HSCs, while TGF-β1 and IL-6 stimulate their matrix protein synthesis [13]. TNF-α — the level of which is characteristically high in chronic hepatitis C (CHC) — inhibits the proliferation and apoptosis of HSCs as well as the synthesis of certain matrix proteins [14-16]

Liver fibrogenesis and wound healing have several common features [17]. However, it also seems that the cytokine-induced proteoglycan synthetic response of HSCs differs significantly from that of the fibroblasts.

This is also true for decorin, which is a small leucine-rich extracellular matrix (ECM) proteoglycan. Both TNF-α and TGF-β1 downregulate decorin synthesis of fibroblasts [16]. In contrast, HSCs and myofibroblasts respond to TGFβ–1 activation by increased decorin synthesis [11].

Decorin has been proven to regulate extracellular matrix assembly. This molecule has been reported to bind and neutralize TGFβ-1 [18], and to effect the maturation of collagen fibers. In experimental models, decorin has given protection against glomerulosclerosis [19, 20] and glial scarring [21]. Considering the overall regulatory effect of decorin on

Frontiers in Viral Hepatitis Ed. by RF Schinazi, J-P Sommadossi and CM Rice. 441 — 449

fibrogenesis, we surmised a similar potential in hepatitis C-induced liver fibrosis. Therefore, we studied the changes of decorin expression in CHC samples. Besides untreated samples, changes in decorin expression after IFN-α treatment were also analysed.

Materials and methods

Twenty-eight percutaneous needle biopsies and five surgical liver specimens were studied from HCV-positive patients. Twenty patients were enrolled in an IFN-α trial. Half of them received 3 MIU IFN-α-2b (Intron-A, Schering-Plough) three times a week for six months, the other half for twelve months. The therapeutic response was evaluated by fine needle biopsies taken before the end and six months after the end of treatment.

Detection of decorin

Deparaffinized, rehydrated sections were boiled in a microwave oven in 0.01 M citrate buffer at pH 4.0 for 2x5 minutes [22], and digested with 0.01% trypsin for 10 minutes at room temperature. Endogenous peroxidase was inhibited, and nonspecific binding sites were masked by nonimmune goat serum diluted in 5% albumin. Antiserum against decorin was applied in 1:3000 dilution at 37°C for 90 minutes. Biotin-labelled antirabbit goat serum was used in 1:200 dilution, and ABC reaction was carried out. At the last step of ABC, biotinylated tyramin diluted 1:125 in 0.03% H_2O_2 was added, and the sections were incubated for 10 minutes [23]. Subsequently, a second round of ABC reaction was carried out. 3-3' diaminobenzidine tetrahydrochloride 0.05 mg/ml in 0.0003% H_2O_2 was used as a chromogen. The sections were then counterstained with hematoxylin. For controls, the primary antibody was replaced by nonimmune rabbit serum.

Evaluation of liver specimens

The guidelines of Desmet et al. [24] were followed to determine histological grading and staging. For the scoring of decorin, a semiquantitative scoring system based on the publication of Chevallier et al. [25] was used. Four parameters were graded from 0-3: the immunopositivity in the *periportal (zone 3)* and *perisinusoidal (zone 2)* areas, around *central veins (zone 1)* as well as the *expression unrelated to these anatomical structures* (i.e. presence of porto-portal or veno-portal bridging reactions, positivity around individual hepatocytes or hepatocyte islands). To make the results comparable to staging, the final scores were divided by 3; thus the maximum score was 4.

Isolation of RNA, Northern blot and RT-PCR

Total RNA was isolated by the method of Chirgwin et al. [26]. Ten μg of total RNA were size-selected by agarose gel electrophoresis and transferred onto Hybond membrane (Amersham, USA). Filters were hybridized with specific cDNA probes labelled with ($\alpha^{32}P$) dCTP by using a random priming kit. Hybridization was performed at 65°C in Quick-hyb solution (Stratagene, USA) for two hours. After post-hybridization washes with 2x and 0.1x SSC, 0.1% SDS filters were exposed to Kodak X-Omat films at -70°C. GAPDH of the same filter was used as an internal standard.

Results

Expression of decorin in normal liver and at various stages of CHC

Normal human livers contain very low amounts of decorin. The antibody localizes the proteoglycan in the sparse connective tissue of the portal triad, around the central vein and the fibrous capsule of the liver (Figure 1).

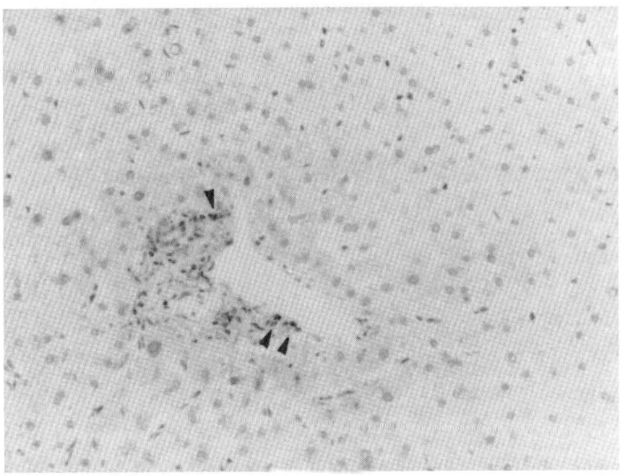

Figure 1. Decorin immunostaining in normal liver. Hardly detectable spot-like reaction was seen in the connective tissue of portal triad. Original magnification × 200.

Decorin proved to be a very sensitive detector of chronic hepatitis. Minimal lesions were characterized by the increase of periportal decorin depositions, which occurred as spot-like reactions in the connective tissue among the lymphocytes (Figure 2a). The periportal deposition became more and more dominant in moderate lesions (Figure 2b). Together with the disruption of the limiting plate, decorin invaded towards the perisinusoidal region (Figure 3). In the severe lesions, strong and widespread deposition in all four regions was observable (Figure 3, 4). Bridging reaction was found between the central veins and portal area or in porto-portal localization. An early indication of this alteration was a stronger perisinusoidal positivity orienting towards a certain direction, as if guiding the proliferating matrix cells and matrix protein deposition (Figure 5).

In cirrhotic samples, decorin was typically found in the fibrotic septa either in its spot-like or collagen-bound fiber-like form (Figure 6), at which time the perisinusoidal reaction became weaker.

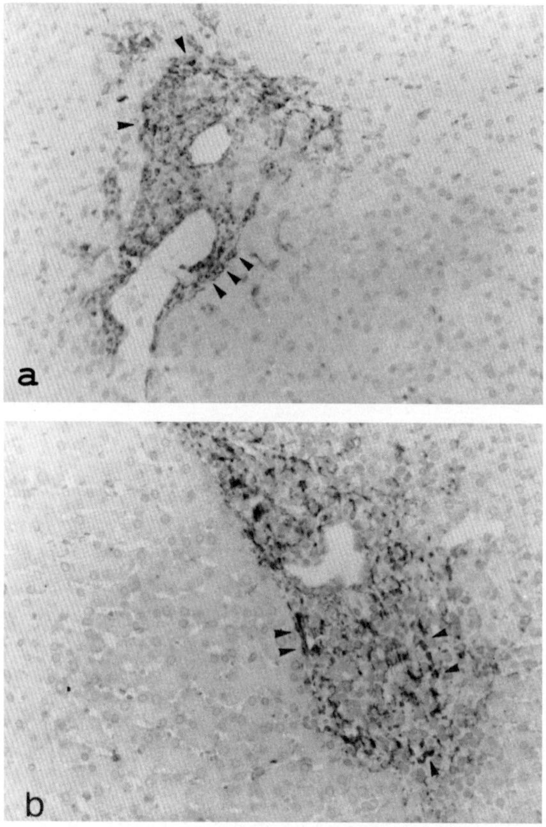

Figure 2. Minimal (a) and mild (b) lesions. Increasing amounts of inflammatory cells occurred in the portal area, among which scattered spot-like reactions could be observed. Original magnification × 200.

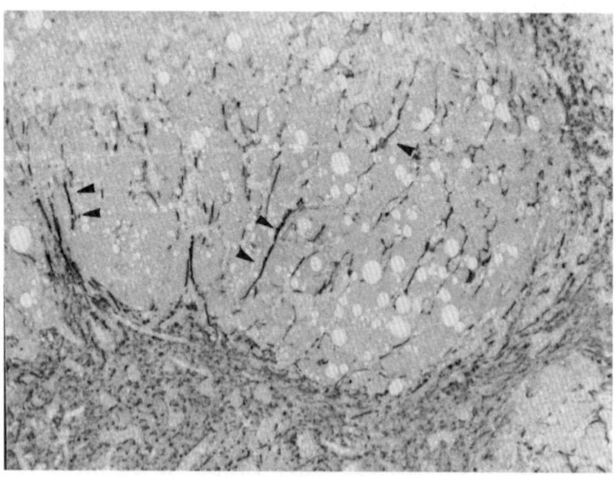

Figure 3. Severe lesion. Wide portal area with proliferating bile ducts, surrounded by decorin positivity. The limiting plate is destroyed, decorin reaction occurred along the sinusoids. The hepatocytes show fatty degeneration. Original magnification × 200.

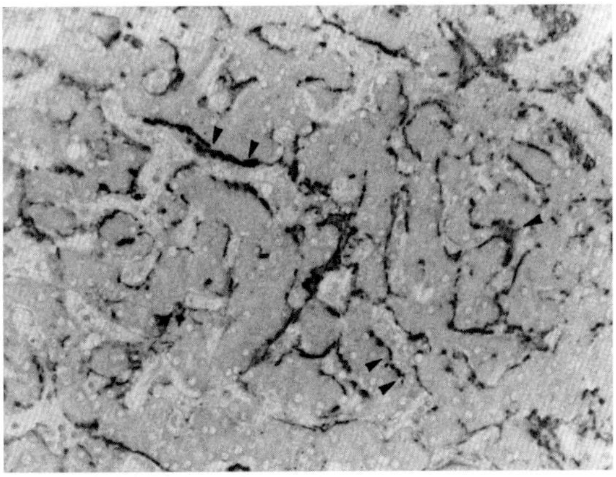

Figure 4. Severe CHC. Strong perisinusoidal decorin deposition can be observed. Original magnification × 400.

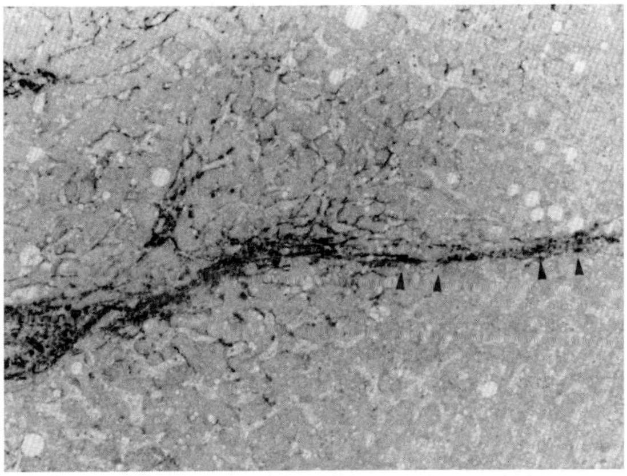

Figure 5. Bridging fibrosis. Decorin deposition is seen spreading from a portal tract toward the central vein. Original magnification × 200.

Similarly to TGF-β1, the expression and deposition of decorin paralleled the grade of inflammation.

The increased production of decorin was regulated at the mRNA level. Decorin transcript was abundant in HCV cirrhosis. This upregulation went parallel with that of the TGF β-1 mRNA steady-state level (Figure 7). Decorin became dominant among the liver proteoglycans. Western blot indicated that the glycanation pattern of the molecule became more heterogeneous, manifesting in a wide smeary band.

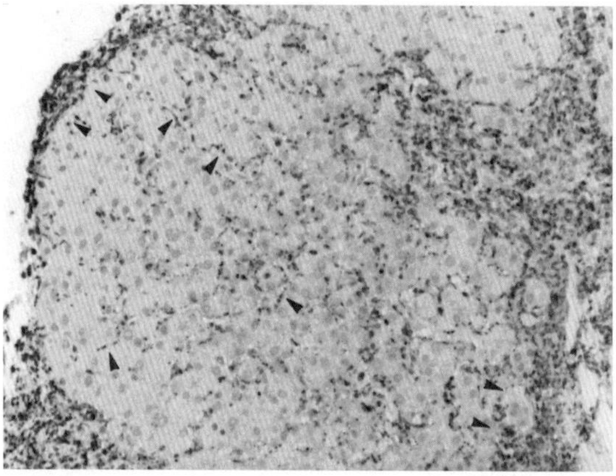

Figure 6. Active liver cirrhosis. Regenerative nodule surrounded by mononuclear cell-infiltrated septum. Strong decorin positivity can be seen in the fibrous septum. Spot-like reaction is shown along the sinusoids. Original magnification × 200.

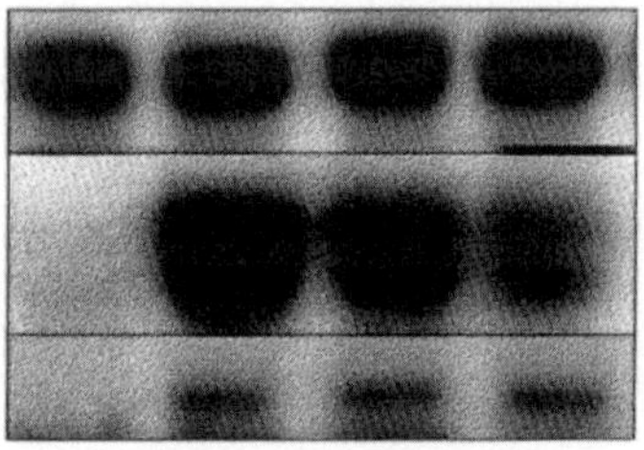

Figure 7. Northern hybridization of normal, acutely damaged and severe CHC liver specimens. No expression of TGF-beta 1 and decorin was detectable in the normal liver. Strong upregulation occurred in damaged liver specimens. GAPDH: internal standard for hybridization. 1: normal liver, 2: acute liver injury, 3, 4: chronic hepatitis C.

Decorin expression after IFN-α therapy

The therapy was administered for six months and one year, respectively. Indication of improvement of the inflammatory process could already be found after six months, but one year was necessary to obtain convincing signs of the effect. IFN-α treatment resulted in a significant decrease in decorin expression, analyzed in all zones together ($p < 0.03$). Investigating the zones separately, significant changes were detectable in the perivenular region (zone 1) as well as in the portal tract (zone 3) ($p < 0.05$). The decrease in the perisinusoidal region (zone 2) was not found to be of significant value. IFN-α treatment could not inhibit the progression of liver fibrosis.

Discussion

Chronic liver injuries regularly cause liver fibrosis and cirrhosis. These alterations develop as a consequence of imbalance of extracellular matrix synthesis and degradation [27]. The activation of matrix production starts in the early phase of the disease [28].

Our observations indicated that decorin deposition was one of the earliest signs of fibrogenesis activaton, which went parallel with the inflammatory activity [29]. Little is known about the transcriptional and translational regulation of decorin in the liver. In contrast to other tissues, TGF-β1 upregulates the expression on the mRNA level [11], while the effect of TNF-α and IL-1β is not known.

It is a further question whether the HCV virus itself affected the expression of decorin. We observed a distinct glycanation pattern of decorin isolated from CHC specimens. In other aspects, cirrhosis and fibrosis of various origins did not differ from each other. This means that the inflammation, rather than the virus itself, induces decorin deposition.

Interferon alpha treatment for one year effectively inhibited the decorin deposition, especially in the portal and perivenular regions, which are the main sites of the inflammatory process [30]. Interestingly, these were the regions where TGF-β1 co-localized with decorin. This raises the possibility that INF-α acts via a TGF-β mediated route. In fibroblasts IFN-α downregulates TGF-β1 production on the transcriptional level [31].

It is important to stress that cases with a low histological activity index were more prone to improvement, with decorin expression regressing to an even lower histological grade.

Decorin has been reported to be capable of inhibiting the biological activity of TGF-β1, especially in terms of matrix production [18, 19, 20, 21]. Considering the decorin functions described so far, this molecule may be more important in the pathobiology of CHC than has been predicted [32]. This potential, however, remains to be assessed. At this stage of our knowledge, decorin has proved to be a useful marker for both early fibrogenesis and the therapeutic response to IFN-α, helping to better assess the actual pathological grade and stage of chronic hepatitis.

Acknowledgement

This work was supported by the National Science Foundation (OTKA) grant T 029017; T 023579; AKP 98-78 3, 2; FKFP 0305/1999.

References

1. Trepo C, Pradat P. Hepatitis C virus infection in Western Europe. *J. Hepatol.,* 1999;31: Suppl 1:80-83.
2. Hoofnagle JH, Hepatitis C. The clinical spectrum of disease. *Hepatology* 1997:26: Suppl 1 15-20.
3. Seeff LB, Natural history of hepatitis C. *Hepatology* 1997.Suppl 1 21-58.
4. Grungreiff K, Reinhold D, Ansorge S. Serum concentration of sIL-2R, IL-6, TGF-beta1, neopterin, and

zinc ion chronic hepatitis C patients treated with interferon-alpha. *Cytokine* 1999;11:1076-80.

5. Huang YS, Hwang SJ, Chan CY, Wu JC, Chao Y, Chang FY, Lee SD. Serum levels of cytokines in hepatitis C-related liver disease: a longitudinal study. *Chung Hua I Hsueh Tsa Chih* 1999;62:327-33.
6. Itoh Y, Okanue T, Ohnishi N, Sakamato N, Nishioji K, Nakagawa Y, Minam M, Murakami Y, Kashima K. *Am. J. Gastroenterol.*, 1999; 94:1332-40.
7. Kaplanski G, Farnarier C, Payan MJ, Bongrand P, Durand JM. Increased levels of soluble adhesion molecules in the serum of patients with hepatitis C. Correlation with citokine concentrations and liver inflammation and fibrosis. *Dig.Dis.Sci.* 1997;42:2277-84
8. Napoli J, Bishop GA, McGuiness PH, Painter DM, McCaughan GW. Progressive liver injury in chronic hepatitis C infection correlates with increased intrahepatic expression of Th1-associated cytokines. *Hepatology* 1996;24:759-65.
9. Hayashi N, Mita E. Fas system and apoptosis in vial hepatitis. *J. Gastroenterol. Hepatol.,* 1997;12:S223-26.
10. Roulot D, Sevcsik AM, Coste T, Strosberg AD, Marullo S. Role of transforming growth factor beta type II receptor in hepatic fibrosis in rats. *Hepatology* 1999;29:1730-38.
11. Gressner AM, Krull N, Bachem MG. Regulation of proteoglycan expression in fibrotic liver and cultured fat-storing cells. *Pathol. Res.Pract.* 1994; 190: 864-82.
12. Hsu JY, Hsu MY, Sorger T, Herlyn M, Levine EM. Heparin/endothelial cell growth supplement regulates matrix gene expression and prolongs life span of vascular smooth muscle cells through modulation of interleukine-1. *In vitro Cell Dev. Biol. Anim.* 1999;35:647-54.
13. Tsukamoto H. Cytokine regulation of hepatic stellate cells in liver fibrosis. *Alcohol Clin. Exp.Res.* 1999; 23:911-16.
14. Saile B, Matthes N, Knittel T, Ramadori G. Transforming growth factor beta and tumor necrosis factor alpha inhibit both apoptosis and proliferation of activated rat hepatic stellate cells. *Hepatology* 1999; 30: 196-202.
15. Tufvesson E, Westergren-Thorsson G. Alteration of proteoglycan synthesis in human lung fibroblasts induced by interleukine-1 beta and tumor necrosis factor-alpha. *J. Cell Biochem.* 2000;77:198-309.
16. Mauviel A, Santra M, Chen YQ, Uitto J, Iozzo RV. Transcriptional regulation of decorin gene expression. Induction by quiescence and repression by tumor necrosis factor-alpha. *J. Biol. Chem.* 1995; 270:11692-700.
17. Li D, Friedman SL. Liver fibrogenesis and the role of hepatic stellate cells: new insights and prospects for therapy. *J. Gastroenterol. Hepatol.* 1999.14:618-33.
18. Yamaguchi Y, Mann DM, Rouslahti E. Negative regulation of transforming growth facto-b by the proteoglycan decorin. *Nature* 1990;346:281-84
19. Border WA, Noble NA, Yamamoto T, Harper JR, Yamaguchi Y, Pierschbacher MD, Rouslahti E. Natural inhibitor of transforming growth factor-b protects against scarring in experimental kidney disease. *Nature* 1992;360:361-64.
20. Isaka Y, Brees DK, Ikegaya K, Kaneda Y, Imai E, Noble NA, Border WA, Gene therapy by skeletal muscle expression of decorin prevents fibrotic disease in rat kidney. *Nat. Med.* 1996;2: 418-23.
21. Loga A, Baird A, Berry M. Decorin attenuates gliotic scar formation in the rat cerebral hemisphere. *Exp. Neurol.* 1999;159:504-10.
22. Shi SR, Key ME, Kalra KL. Antigen retrieval in formalin-fixed, paraffin embedded tissues: An enhancement method for immunohistochemical staining based on microwave oven heating of tissue sections. *J. Histochem.* 1991:39:741-48.
23. Adams JC. Biotin amplification of biotin and horseradish peroxidase signals in histochemical stains.

J Histochem Cytochem 40:1457-1463. 1992.

24. Desmet VJ, Gerber M, Hoofnagle JH, Manns M, Scheuer PJ. Classification of chronic hepatitis: diagnosis, grading and staging. *Hepatology* 19:1513-1520. 1994.
25. Chevallier M, Guerret S, Chossegross P, Gerard F, Grimaud J-A. A histological semiquantitative scoring system for evaluation of hepatic fibrosis in needle liver biopsy specimens: Comparison with morphometric studies. *Hepatology* 20:349-355. 1994.
26. Chirgwin JM, Przybyla AE, McDonnald RJ, Rutter WJ, Isolation of biologically active ribonucleic acid from sources enriched in ribonuclease. *Biochemistry* 18:5294-5300. 1979.
27. Alcoado R, Arthur MJP, Iredale JP. Pathogenesis of liver fibrosis. *Clin. Sci.* 1997;92:103-12.
28. Nakatsukasa H, Nagy P, Evarts RP, Hsia C-C, Marsden E, Thorgeirrson SS. Cellular distribution of transforming growth factor-β1 and procollagen types I, III, and IV transcript in carbon tetrachloride-induced rat liver fibrosis. *J. Clin. Invest.* 1990;85:1833-1843.
29. Gallai M, Kovalszky I, Knittel T, Neubauer K, Armbrust T, Ramadori G. Expression of extracellular matrix proteoglycans perlecfan and decorin in carbon-tetrachloride-injured rat liver and isolated liver cells. *Amer. J. Pathol.* 1996;148:1463-71.
30. Tredget EE, Wang R, Shen Q, Scott PG, Ghahary A. Transforming growth factor-beta mRNS and protein in hypertrophic scar tissues and fibroblasts> antagonism by IFN-alpha and IFN gamma in vitro and in vivo. *J. Interferon cytokine* 2000;20:143-51
31. Jarmay K, Gallai M, Karacsony G, Ozsvar Zs, Schaff Zs, Lonovics J, Kovalszky I. Decorin and actin expression and distribution in patients with chronic hepatitis C following interferon alpha-2b treatment. *J. Hepatol.* 2000:32:993-1002.
32. Iozzo RV. The biology of the small leucine-rich proteoglycans. *J. Biol. Chem.*1999;274:18843-18846.

Preclinical and clinical development of the anti-HIV, anti-HBV oxathiolane nucleoside analog emtricitabine

GEORGE R. PAINTER[1], LAURENCE T. RIMSKY, PHILLIP A. FURMAN[1], DENNIS C. LIOTTA[2] RAYMOND F. SCHINAZI[2] and JOSEPH B. QUINN

[1] *Triangle Pharmaceuticals, 4611 University Dr., Durham, NC 27717-0530, USA*
[2] *Emory University School of Medicine/VA Medical Center, Decatur, GA 30033, USA*

Introduction

Acquired immunodeficiency syndrome (AIDS) was first described in the United States in 1981, with the unexplained appearance of Kaposi's sarcoma, *Pneumocystis carinii* pneumonia and other opportunistic infections in previously healthy homosexual males [1]. Affected individuals became susceptible to opportunistic infections and specific immune deficiency resulting from the depletion of $CD4^+$ lymphocytes. Intensive investigation revealed the etiologic agent of AIDS to be a lymphotropic retrovirus, the human immunodeficiency virus (HIV) [2, 3]. Today, three classes of drugs are available to treat patients infected with HIV: the nucleoside reverse transcriptase inhibitors (NRTI), the nonnucleoside reverse transcriptase inhibitors (NNRTI), and the protease inhibitors (PI). The currently accepted standard of care for HIV infection involves the use of three drug combination regimens [4]. The use of combination therapy has profoundly reduced the morbidity and mortality associated with HIV infection. However, the approved anti-HIV drugs and the combination(s) of these drugs have significant limitations including toxicity, the selection of drug-resistant variants, pharmacokinetic interactions with other agents and poor adherence due to complex dosing regimens. These limitations have necessitated the continued search for anti-HIV agents with an improved clinical profile.

Hepatitis B virus (HBV) also constitutes a major worldwide health threat. In addition to the morbidity associated with acute clinical infection, chronic liver disease, cirrhosis, hepatitis delta virus infection and primary hepatocellular carcinoma are recognized sequelae [5]. The reservoir for HBV includes an estimated worldwide population of 300 million carriers. Approximately 25% of chronic carriers will die from primary hepatocellular carcinoma or cirrhosis of the liver. At present there are only two approved therapies for the treatment of HBV infection, α-interferon and lamivudine. The limited efficacy of α-interferon and the emergence of lamivudine-resistant HBV variants have made it clear that additional therapies are needed for the treatment of acute and chronic

Frontiers in Viral Hepatitis Ed. by RF Schinazi, J-P Sommadossi and CM Rice. 451 — 484

HBV infection. These new therapies will include combination regimens analogous to those used to treat HIV infections.

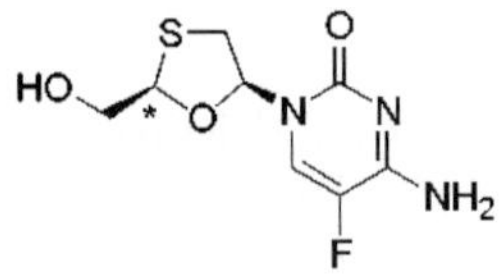

Figure 1. Structure of emtricitabine (524W91, FTC) [6]. The oxathiolane ring, which is an analog of a 2',3'-dideoxyribose ring, has the L configuration at what corresponds to the 4' position (*). This is in contrast to naturally occurring nucleosides, which have a D configuration at this position.

The 2',3'-dideoxynucleoside analog (2R,5S)-5-fluoro-1-[2-(hydroxymethyl)-1,3-oxathiolan-5-yl]cytosine (Figure 1) is a potent and selective inhibitor of HIV and HBV replication *in vitro* and *in vivo*. Clinical studies have demonstrated the drug to be very effective in suppressing both HIV and HBV in infected patients. In this report we will present an overview of the preclinical and clinical studies conducted to date on emtricitabine and when possible critique differences between emtricitabine and other nucleoside analogs currently approved for the treatment of HIV and HBV disease. Particular attention will be paid to comparing the antiviral activity of emtricitabine to that of lamivudine and differentiating the activities of the two compounds based on the introduction of fluorine into the C-5 position of emtricitabine.

In vitro antiviral activity

The antiviral activity of emtricitabine has been shown to be specific for HIV-1, HIV-2, and HBV. No activity has been observed at concentrations up to 100 µM against HSV-1, HSV-2, HCMV, VZV, coronavirus, yellow fever virus, respiratory syncytial virus, rotavirus, influenza virus, or rhinovirus [7].

Anti-HIV activity

The ability of emtricitabine to inhibit replication of HIV-1 and HIV-2 in cell culture has been studied extensively using various human T-lymphoid cell lines (MT-2, MT-4, CEM and HT4-6C), and PMBCs infected with laboratory-adapted strains of HIV-1 (III_B, LAI or LAV) and HIV-2 (ZY, ROD2). The results are summarized in Table 1. A comparison of the *in vitro* potency of emtricitabine to that of the other nucleoside analogues currently used to treat HIV is difficult owing to the wide variety of cell types, virus strains and assay conditions used by the numerous investigators who have determined EC_{50} values for these compounds. However, if EC_{50} data derived from PBMCs infected with the LAI, LAV or III_B strain of HIV-1 are used as the basis of comparison, emtricitabine and the nucleoside analogues currently approved for human use can be divided into three potency groups. The most potent group includes emtricitabine and AZT, with EC_{50} value ranges of 0.001 to 0.01 μM and 0.001 to 0.058 μM, respectively. The second potency group includes d4T, 3TC and ddC, with EC_{50} value ranges of 0.04 to 0.09 μM, 0.04 to 0.53 μM, and 0.01 to 0.23 μM, respectively. The least potent group includes ddI and abacavir, with EC_{50} value ranges of 0.46 to 19 μM, and 3.7 μM, respectively.

Table 1. Inhibitory effect of emtricitabine on the replication of laboratory strains of HIV-1 and HIV-2

Virus (strain)	Cell Type	EC_{50} (μM)
HIV-1 (IIIB)	CEM	0.1[a,b]
	MT-4	0.5[a,b]
	PBMC	0.01[b]
HIV-1 (LAV)	CEM	0.009[a]
	HT4-6C	0.02[a]
	PBMC	0.009[b], 0.001[d]
HIV-1 (LAI)	CEM	0.04[c]
	MT-2 PBMC	0.62[c], 0.001[e]
	PBMC	0.03[c]
HIV-2 (2ZY)	MT4	1.5[a]
	CEM	0.1[a]
HIV-2 (ROD2)	PBMC	0.007[b]

a. [8]
b. [7]
c. Personal Communication, K. Borroto-Esoda, Triangle Pharmaceuticals
d. [9]
e. [10]

Several investigators have compared the anti-HIV activity of emtricitabine with that of lamivudine in the same assay, thereby eliminating any ambiguities introduced by an interassay comparison. The results are summarized in Table 2. Although different laboratory strains of virus, different cell types and different assay methods were used by the investigators in these studies, emtricitabine consistently showed greater activity than lamivudine with the activity advantage ranging from three- to 11-fold.

Table 2. Comparison of the anti-HIV activity of emtricitabine (FTC) with lamivudine (3TC) using various laboratory strains of HIV-1

		EC_{50} (μM)		
HIV subtype	Cell Line	FTC	3TC	Sensitivity Ratio[d]
LAI[a]	PBMC	0.018	0.19	11
IIIB[b]	PBMC	0.01	0.07	7
IIIB[b]	MT4	0.5	3.2	6
LAI[a]	MT2	0.3	1.6	5
HXB2[c]	MT4	0.09	0.24	3
LAI[a]	$CD4^+$ HeLa	0.06	0.18	4

a. Personal communication, D. Wakefield, Triangle Pharmaceuticals

b. [8]

c. [11]

d. Defined as the quotient of EC_{50} (3TC)/EC_{50} (FTC)

The sensitivity of HIV-1 clinical isolates to inhibition by anti-HIV drugs is assessed *in vitro* to gain insight into the variation in activity that might be encountered in a clinical setting. The results of one such study conducted with emtricitabine in human PBMCs are presented in Table 3. Schinazi et al. tested two low passage clinical isolates; J6 and 2:DR2, in phytohemagglutinin-stimulated PBMCs isolated from uninfected donors [8]. The EC_{50} values are similar to those calculated using laboratory strains of virus in PBMCs. The sensitivities to emtricitabine reported for two additional wild type clinical isolates, WT-pre-AZT (obtained from D. Richman, Veterans Affairs Medical Center, San Diego, CA) and WT-MKC09-day 29 (obtained from a Phase I Emivirine trial, Triangle Pharmaceuticals, Inc.), were similar to those determined by Schinazi et al. against J6 and 2:DR2. In the single experiment in which a direct comparison was made between the activity of emtricitabine and lamivudine, emtricitabine demonstrated the same fivefold potency advantage seen using laboratory strains of virus.

The potency of emtricitabine has also been determined using a coculture assay [12] and compared directly to the potencies of lamivudine, zalcitabine, didanosine, zidovudine, and the non-nucleoside RT inhibitor TIBO. In this study, PBMCs from HIV-infected patients were cocultured with PBMCs isolated from uninfected donors. The naturally infected PBMCs served as a source of a diversified population of virus not selected for by *in vitro* propagation. At the end of the coculture period, the degree of viral replication was measured by HIV-1 p24 ELISA. Results from this study expressed as mean EC_{50}, EC_{90}, and EC_{99} values are given in Table 4. A potency ranking (based on EC_{90} values) showed emtricitabine to be the most potent compound, followed by zalcitabine, lamivudine, zidovudine, TIBO, and didanosine. The low potency ranking for zidovudine compared to that observed in laboratory strains may be the result of inclusion of PMBCs from AZT-experienced patents in the coculture.

Table 3. Inhibition of HIV-1 clinical isolates by emtricitabine

Virus	EC_{50} (μM)	
	emtricitabine	lamivudine
J6[a]	0.002	0.01
2:DR2[a]	0.002	ND
WT-pre-AZT[b]	0.008	ND
WT-MKC09-day 29[b]	0.02	ND

a. [8]

b. Personal communication, K. Borroto-Esoda, Triangle Pharmaceuticals

ND. Not Determined

Table 4. Comparative potency of RT inhibitors in HIV-1-infected PBMCs using a cocultured method [a]

Inhibitor	EC_{50} (μM)	EC_{90} (μM)	EC_{99} (μM)
Emtricitabine	0.0085	0.055	0.43
3TC	0.11	0.3	0.85
ddC	0.011	0.074	0.6
ddI	0.76	6.4	65.8
AZT	0.055	0.53	6.4
TIBO R82913	0.17	0.67	2.95

a. [12]

To determine if the antiviral activity of emtricitabine varied in different subtypes of HIV-1, activity was evaluated against HIV-1 group M and group O in MAGI-CCR5 cells and PBMCs. Table 5 shows the results. EC_{50} values were also obtained for lamivudine, zidovudine, and didanosine. Emtricitabine was more active than lamivudine and didanosine, and had activity comparable to that of zidovudine.

Table 5. EC_{50} values of NRTIs against HIV-1 group M and O in PBMCs and MAGI cells [a]

Isolate	Subtype	Host Cell	AZT	3TC	ddI	FTC
Group M						
UG/92/024	D	PBMCs	0.003	0.026	0.21	0.007
BR/92/025	C	PBMCs	0.035	0.027	0.49	0.017
RW/92/008	A	PBMCs	0.008	0.054	0.26	0.012
Tha/92/019	E	PBMCs	0.039	0.069	0.5)	0.028
Br/930/20	F	PBMCs	0.003	0.022	0.34	0.009
RU570	G	PBMCs	0.008	0.090	0.34	0.030
Group O						
BCF02 O	O	PBMCs	0.028	2.5	4.75	0.14
Group M						
RW/92/008	A	MAGI	0.085	0.20	3.0	0.055
BR/92/025	C	MAGI	0.033	0.17	0.95	0.032
UG/92/024	D	MAGI	0.035	0.11	1.70	0.030
Tha/92/019	E	MAGI	0.080	0.15	1.50	0.065
Br/930/20	F	MAGI	0.045	0.15	1.50	0.050
RU570	G	MAGI	0.150	0.18	2.50	0.075
Group O						
BCF03 O	O	MAGI	0.09	0.20	2.20	0.065

a. Personal communication, D. Wakefield and S. Fleming, Triangle Pharmaceuticals

Anti-HBV activity

The *in vitro* anti-HBV activity of emtricitabine has been studied extensively using the stably HBV-transfected cell line HepG2 2.2.15. In this system, emtricitabine decreases levels of extra- and intracellular HBV DNA in a dose-dependent manner. EC_{50} values determined by various investigators using extracellular HBV DNA levels range from 0.01 ± 0.005 to 0.04 ± 0.001. The emtricitabine EC_{50} value based on intracellular DNA reported by Schinazi et al. [13] is somewhat higher, 0.16 ± 0.01 μM, than the EC_{50} values based on extracellular DNA (Table 6) [14]. For comparison EC_{50} values of other nucleoside analogues currently under development as anti-HBV agents are presented along with those of emtricitabine and lamivudine in Table 6. In contrast to HIV, the EC_{50} values for emtricitabine and lamivudine are similar against HBV.

Table 6. Anti-HBV activity in HepG2 2.2.15 of compounds approved and under development for HBV infection

Compound	EC_{50} values		
Emtricitabine	0.01 ± 0.005 μM[a]	0.075 ± 0.009 μM[d]	0.04 ± 0.006 μM[b, f]
Lamivudine	0.008 ± 0.003 μM[a]	0.05 ± 0.01 μM	
Adefovir	0.03 ± 0.01 μg/ml[c]		
Clevudine	0.1 ± 0.06 μg/ml[c]	0.38 ± 0.25 μM[d]	0.296 ± 0.036 μM[e]
Tenofovir	0.04 ± 0.02 μg/ml[c]		
Lobucavir	0.1 ± 0.1 μg/ml[c]		
Penciclovir	3.5 ± 0.2 μg/ml[c]		
Amdoxovir	13 ± 2.1 μg/ml[c]		
Entecavir	0.004 μM[g]		
Epavudine (L-dT)	0.19 ± 0.09 μM		
Epcitabine (L-dC)	0.24 ± 0.08 μM[f]		
β-L-Fd4C	<0.1 μM[f]		

a. [14]
b. [13]
c. [15, 16]
d. Personal communication W. Nicholson, Triangle Pharmaceuticals
e. Personal communication B. Korba, Division of Molecular Virology and Immunology, Georgetown University
f [17]
g. [18]

Condreay et al. examined the effect of emtricitabine on HBV replication in primary human hepatocytes [19]. Although EC_{50} values were not calculated, emtricitabine at 2 μM completely inhibited the production of intracellular HBV DNA, even when added 24 hours after infection. The EC_{50} value calculated from inhibition of extracellular virus production is <0.02 μM, a value that is comparable to that determined in HepG2 2.2.15 cells (Table 6).

Mechanism of action

Cellular uptake

Transport studies were conducted in confluent cultures of HepG2 2.2.15 cells to determine the route(s) of cellular uptake of emtricitabine [20]. Assays were performed at room temperature (20°C) using a modified rapid, cold buffer stop method. The influx of emtricitabine into the cells did not depend on the concentration of emtricitabine or the presence of a Na^+ gradient, and was only partially inhibited by competing nucleosides and nucleoside transport inhibitors (Table 7). The negligible impact of the protein modification agents N-ethylmaleimide, 4,4'-diisothiocyanato-2, 2'-stilbenedisulfonic acid and 4-aceamido-4'-isothiocynatostilbene-2, 2'-disulfonic acid on emtricitabine uptake suggests that a component of emtricitabine entry into HepG2 2.2.15 cells was not transporter mediated, but possibly results from non-facilitated diffusion.

Table 7. Inhibition of emtricitabine influx into cells by nucleoside transport inhibitors, competing nucleosides, and adenine[a, b]

Agent	Concentration (μM)	Inhibition (%)	Experiments (#)
NBMPR	10	45	6
Dipyridamole	10	48	6
Dilazep	10	35	6
Cytidine	500	37	3
Uridine	500	69	2
Inosine	500	60	2
Adenine	500	14	3

a. [20]

b. Experiments were performed in HepG2 2.2.15 cells in the presence of 10 μM emtricitabine

Anabolism

Emtricitabine is efficiently phosphorylated in HepG2 2.2.15 cells to the corresponding 5'-mono, 5'-di and 5'-triphosphates. A time course showed that the nucleotides of emtricitabine were formed rapidly and reached a steady-state intracellular concentration by three to six hours [20]. The concentration of emtricitabine 5'-diphosphate was somewhat higher than the concentration of the 5'-mono and 5'-triphosphate derivatives [7, 14, 20, 21], as shown in Figure 2. When the intracellular concentrations of the phosphorylated forms were measured as a function of the extracellular concentration (concentrations ranged from 0.01 to 10 μM), the concentration of the 5'-phosphorylated derivatives of emtricitabine increased in a dose-dependent manner, indicating that the anabolic pathway was not saturated at the concentrations tested (Figure 2). An intracellular half-life of approximately 2.4 hours was determined for emtricitabine 5'-triphosphate in HepG2 cells [20]. This half-life is extremely short compared to the estimated 30 hours half-life seen in PBMCs taken from healthy human volunteers dosed orally with 200 mg emtricitabine QD [22].

In studies to determine which enzymes were responsible for phosphorylating emtricitabine to the 5'-triphosphate, 2'-deoxycytidine kinase was identified as the enzyme that catalyzes the phosphorylation of emtricitabine to the corresponding 5'-monophosphate [14, 21, 23]. Using calf thymus 2'-deoxycytidine kinase, the relative

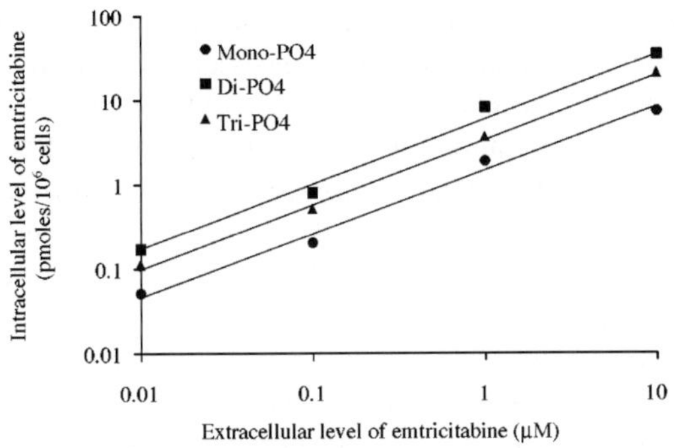

Figure 2. A $\log_{10}$ plot of the intracellular concentrations of emtricitabine 5'-phosphates as a function of extracellular emtricitabine ((●)-5'-monophosphate, (■)-5'-diphosphate, (▲) –5'-triphosphate) [20]. In this experiment HepG2 2.2.15 cells were incubated with emtricitabine for 24 hours.

rate of phosphorylation was 3.4% of that measured for 2'-deoxyguanosine and 40% of that observed for 2'-deoxycytidine. Shewach et al. demonstrated emtricitabine to be a good substrate for human deoxycytidine kinase [23]. An apparent K_m value of 11.8 μM and an apparent relative V_{max} of 9.3 nmol·mL^{-1}·hr^{-1} was determined when UTP was the phosphate donor. When ATP was the phosphate donor, an apparent K_m value of 7.4 μM and an apparent relative V_{max} of 3.8 nmol·mL^{-1}·hr^{-1} was obtained. Phosphorylation of the 5'-monophosphate was catalyzed by 2'-deoxycytidine monophosphate kinase [14, 21]. The efficiency with which the enzyme, purified from calf thymus, phosphorylates the 5'-monophosphate of emtricitabine was approximately 32% of that observed when using the natural substrate, 2'-deoxycytidine 5'-monophosphate. Emtricitabine 5'-monophosphate can also be phosphorylated by nucleoside monophosphate kinase purified from beef liver. However, the phosphorylation catalyzed by this enzyme is relatively inefficient. The formation of the 5'-triphosphate of emtricitabine from the 5'-diphosphate has been proposed to be catalyzed by nucleoside diphosphate kinase (NDP) [14], a cytosolic enzyme with a broad specificity for nucleoside 5'-diphosphates. However, Cheng et al. have recently suggested that the L-nucleotide 5'-diphosphates cannot be utilized as a substrate by NDP kinases but are selectively phosphorylated by 3-phosphoglyceride kinase. [24]

Inhibition of HIV-1 reverse transcriptase by the 5'-triphosphate of emtricitabine

Human immunodeficiency virus encodes a reverse transcriptase (HIV-RT) that synthesizes a double-stranded DNA copy of genomic RNA. Emtricitabine 5'-triphosphate serves as an alternative substrate inhibitor of HIV-RT and is incorporated into a growing chain of viral DNA. Incorporation results in the termination of nascent chain DNA synthesis due to the lack of a hydroxyl group in the 3'-position of the sugar moiety of emtricitabine, which in turn results in inhibition of viral replication.

Steady state kinetic experiments comparing emtricitabine 5'-triphosphate with the natural substrate dCTP showed the two substrates to have similar K_m values for HIV-RT (13 nM for emtricitabine 5'-triphosphate and 70 nM for dCTP). The K_i values for emtricitabine 5'-triphosphate inhibition of HIV-RT-catalyzed RNA-dependent DNA synthesis and DNA-dependent DNA synthesis were calculated to be 0.6 μM and 0.43 μM, respectively. In comparison, the K_i values for lamivudine 5'-triphosphate inhibition of HIV-RT-catalyzed RNA-dependent and DNA-dependent DNA synthesis were 0.97 and 0.7 μM, respectively.

Although a steady state kinetic analysis represents a useful beginning, it is insufficient to establish a detailed kinetic and mechanistic picture of the enzyme-catalyzed reaction [25]. A pre-steady-state kinetic analysis can provide a detailed picture of the events that occur at the enzyme active site. This includes binding of the nucleotide substrate to the enzyme-DNA complex to form an initial ternary complex (K_D), the maximum rate of incorporation of the single nucleotide 5'-monophosphate (k_{pol}), and the overall efficiency of incorporation, which is defined as the quotient k_{pol}/K_d. Using rapid quench techniques to carry out a pre-steady-state analysis, Feng et al. compared the pre-steady-state kinetics of single nucleotide incorporation of dCTP, lamivudine 5'-triphosphate and emtricitabine 5'-triphosphate opposite a template guanosine in RNA-dependent DNA synthesis with HIV-1 RT [26]. The results are shown in Table 8. The overall incorporation rate of the oxathiolane nucleoside analogs is significantly slower than that observed for the natural substrate dCTP, as evidenced by the values of k_{pol}.

Table 8. Incorporation of deoxycytidine 5'-triphosphate, emtricitabine 5'-triphosphate and lamivudine 5'-triphosphate into an RNA/DNA template/primer

Compound	Template/Primer	k_{pol} (s^{-1})	K_d (μM)	k_{pol}/K_d ($\mu M \cdot 1s^{-1}$)
2'-Deoxycytidine 5'-triphosphate	R44/D23[a]	9 ± 2	16 ± 5	-
	R45/D23[b]	23 ± 1	30 ± 4	0.76
Emtricitabine 5'-triphosphate	R44/D23[a]	0.240 ± 0.02	1.7 ± 0.3	-
	R45/D23[b]	0.082 ± 0.005	1.4 ± 0.4	0.06
Lamivudine 5'-triphosphate	R45/D23[b]	0.033 ± 0.002	5.0 ± 0.8	0.0067

a. [27]
b. [26]

The k_{pol} value of dCTP ranges from 280 to 700 times greater than the corresponding k_{pol} values for the oxathiolane nucleoside analogues. However, the K_d values reveal that the oxathiolane substrates bind much tighter to the enzyme-DNA complex than does the natural substrate, with the K_d values of the analogues being approximately six- to 30-fold lower than those of the natural substrate. Both the K_d and k_{pol} values reveal emtricitabine 5'-triphosphate to be a better overall substrate for the enzyme than is lamivudine 5'-triphosphate. The result of the k_{pol} and K_d advantage is increased efficiency for emtricitabine 5'-triphosphate relative to lamivudine 5'-triphosphate. Emtricitabine 5'-triphosphate is incorporated almost an order of magnitude more efficiently than is lamivudine 5'-triphosphate during RNA-dependent DNA synthesis. This efficiency advantage can account in part for the higher activity seen for emtricitabine compared to lamivudine in cell culture (Table 2).

Inhibition of HBV DNA polymerase by the 5'-triphosphate of emtricitabine

The replication cycle of hepadnavirus includes the reverse transcription of an RNA template [28]. This process is carried out by a polymerase that shares significant sequence homology with the RT of retroviruses, including HIV [29]. Since all attempts to date to purify the human HBV DNA polymerase have been unsuccessful, examination of the effect of emtricitabine 5'-triphosphate on HBV DNA polymerase was carried out using an endogenous polymerase assay. In this assay intact virus particles are treated with 1% Nonidet P40, a nonionic detergent that partially disrupts the virus particles and allows nucleotide substrates to enter the virus particle so that DNA synthesis can occur [14, 30]. HBV particles purified from culture supernatants and treated with detergent have been shown to incorporate the 5'-triphosphate of emtricitabine and to inhibit product formation in a dose-dependent fashion. Competition studies were performed to determine whether the 5'-triphosphate of emtricitabine competes only with dCTP for binding to the enzyme or with other 2'-deoxynucleoside 5'-triphosphate substrates as well. In these experiments, the ability of increasing concentrations of dCTP, dTTP or dGTP to block inhibition of DNA synthesis by emtricitabine 5'-triphosphate was examined. While increased concentrations of dTTP and dGTP had no effect on inhibition by emtricitabine 5'-triphosphate, a tenfold excess of dCTP completely blocked the ability of emtricitabine to inhibit DNA synthesis.

Davis et al., using the endogenous polymerase assay, demonstrated that the HBV DNA polymerase could incorporate [α-^{32}P] emtricitabine 5'-triphosphate into minus strand DNA [30]. In this study [α-^{32}P] emtricitabine 5'-triphosphate was incubated with HBV viral particles (2 x 10^{10}) isolated from HepG2 2.2.15 cell cultures, unlabeled dATP, dGTP, and dCTP. The radiolabeled DNA product was detected by autoradiography. A labeled 3.2 kb DNA was detected indicating that radiolabeled emtricitabine 5'-monophosphate was incorporated into the viral DNA. Endogenous polymerase assays using HBV virus particles isolated from cell cultures treated with emtricitabine 5'-triphosphate showed either reduced or no polymerase activity depending on the concentration of emtricitabine 5'-triphosphate used, even though they had detectable HBV minus strand DNA. Furthermore, the particles produced in emtricitabine 5'-triphosphate-treated cells did not contain any detectable HBV plus strand DNA, which is consistent with the incorporation and chain terminating activity of emtricitabine. Taken together, the results demonstrate that emtricitabine 5'-triphosphate serves as an alternative substrate inhibitor of the HBV DNA polymerase.

Selectivity at the enzyme level: effects on human DNA polymerases α, β, γ and ε

To gain further insight into the origins of the selective antiviral activity exhibited by emtricitabine, the inhibition of purified human HeLa cell DNA polymerases α, β, γ and ε by the 5'-triphosphate of emtricitabine was examined under steady-state conditions and compared to the inhibition of HIV RT [21]. Activated calf thymus DNA was used as the template for analysis of each enzyme. Under these conditions, emtricitabine 5'-triphosphate was a weak inhibitor of each of the human DNA polymerases when compared to HIV RT. Apparent K_I values were 6.0 μM for polymerase α, 17 μM for polymerase β, 6.0 μM for polymerase γ, and 150 μM for polymerase ε, compared to a K_I value of 0.17 μM for HIV-1 RT.

Long-term treatment with nucleoside analogues has been associated with various forms of toxicity. Inhibition of human DNA polymerase γ (Pol γ) is one of the proposed mechanisms for nucleoside analog-derived toxicity. The 5'-triphosphate form of many nucleoside analogs has been shown to serve as a substrate for Pol γ resulting in an inhibition of mitochondrial DNA synthesis. Therefore the potential for emtricitabine 5'-triphosphate and lamivudine 5'-triphosphate to serve as substrates for Pol γ was investigated (J. Feng, personal communication, Triangle Pharmaceuticals). For dCTP, emtricitabine 5'-triphosphate, and lamivudine 5'-triphosphate, the order of incorporation efficiency is dCTP > lamivudine 5'-triphosphate > emtricitabine 5'-triphosphate. The low rate of incorporation and poor binding affinity of emtricitabine 5'-triphosphate makes it the least favorable substrate for Pol γ.

The excision of 2', 3'-dideoxynucleoside 5'-monophosphate from the 3'-terminus of DNA by Pol γ-associated exonuclease activity can rescue mitochondrial DNA synthesis from the chain terminating effect of a nucleotide analog (J. Feng, personal communication, Triangle Pharmaceuticals). Unmodified primers terminated with the natural cytidine nucleotide (dCMP) have been shown to be the best substrates for the Pol γ-associated exonuclease, followed by emtricitabine 5'-monophosphate and lamivudine 5'-monophosphate. Little difference was observed in the ability of the Pol γ-associated exonuclease to excise emtricitabine 5'-monophosphate and lamivudine 5'-monophosphate from a terminated primer. Overall, these studies with DNA Pol γ demonstrated that emtricitabine has a lower inhibitory effect on the mitochondrial enzyme than does lamivudine, and therefore may be less likely to cause mitochondrial toxicity in the long term.

In vivo antiviral activity

Anti-HIV activity

The anti-HIV activity of emtricitabine has been tested in SCID (severe combined immunodeficient) mice. Mice were reconstituted with human PBMCs [31] and, after two weeks, infected with the HIV-1_{A1018} virus. Drug therapy was initiated one day before infection. Test compounds were administered intraperitoneally twice daily at 30 mg/kg. Viral inhibition was measured by quantitative coculture of infections HIV-1, and quantitative RNA viral load measurement on peritoneal wash cells, lymph nodes, spleen cells and plasma. At the concentration used in this study, emtricitabine completely inhibited viral infection.

Black and Furman (personal communication, Triangle Pharmaceuticals) evaluated the anti-HIV activity of orally administered emtricitabine and lamivudine side by side in the HuPBMC-SCID mouse model. Groups of 12 or 15 female C.N-17 SCID mice were reconstituted by the intraperitoneal (ip) injection of 1.3 x 10^8 human PBMCs. Two weeks later, the mice were infected ip with 2000 tissue culture infectious doses (TCID) of HIV-1_{A018}. After infection, mice were weighed and randomized to treatment or control groups. Mice in the treatment groups received a single ip-loading dose of drug. Drugs were then administered in drinking water, which contained 0.3 mg/ml emtricitabine. Water bottles were weighed at the beginning and the end of treatment, so that water consumption could be calculated. Seven days after infection, mice were anesthestized, weighed, and euthanized by exsanguination. Viral load in plasma was measured using a real-time reverse transcriptase-polymerase chain reaction (RT-PCR). Both emtricitabine and lamivudine were well tolerated during the seven days of the study with no evident toxicity. Average animal weights and daily water consumption for the three groups were similar. Thus average daily doses of the two drugs were similar, about 60 mg/kg. In the control group the geometric mean viral load was 2.5 x 10^4 copies/ml. Emtricitabine reduced plasma viral loads to below the limit of detection in all 12 treated mice, and lamivudine reduced plasma viral loads to below the limit of detection in 11 of the 12 treated mice. The reductions in viral loads in both treatment groups were statistically significant ($p<10^{-5}$) compared to control, but did not differ significantly from each other.

Anti-hepadnavirus activity

Chimeric mouse model

The *in vivo* anti-hepatitis activity of emtricitabine was first tested in a chimeric mouse model. NIH bg-nu-xid mice were subcutaneously injected with suspensions of 10^7 HepG2 2.2.15 cells. Subcutaneous injection of these cells resulted in the development of tumors of HepG2 2.2.15 cells producing HBV. HBV could be detected in serum samples from the tumor-bearing mice using an immunoaffinity system linked to quantitative PCR.

Beginning one week postinjection, mice were dosed orally with 0.9, 3.5, 18.4 and 88.8 mg/kg/day of emtricitabine. Comparison of tumor progression and human α-fetoprotein levels in control versus drugdosed mice indicated that emtricitabine did not have antitumor activity. However, emtricitabine at the 18.4 and 88.8 mg/kg/day doses did significantly reduce circulatory levels of HBV DNA. Examination of tumor extracts in these two dose groups revealed a marked reduction in intracellular levels of replication DNA HBV intermediates, including double-stranded linear DNA.

Transgenic SCID mice

Anti-HBV activity has also been reported for emtricitabine in HBV transgenic SCID mice [32]. A group of five mice was treated with emtricitabine at 100 mg/kg/day ip for six days, and observed for an additional six days posttreatment. By day three of treatment, two mice had undetectable HBsAg, and an additional two mice cleared HBsAg on day five. The remaining mouse cleared HBsAg on day eight. HBV DNA levels in blood were determined by semiquantitative PCR at days 3, 5, 8 and 12. By day three of treatment, PCR signals had dropped tenfold in all of the mice. By day eight none of the mice had detectable HBV DNA levels by PCR. In contrast to lamivudine, there were no signs of rebound in the levels of HBV DNA during the course of treatment.

DHBV

Duck hepatitis B virus has been used as a surrogate virus to test the *in vivo* activity of compounds under study as potential anti-HBV drugs. Although DHBV is in a different genus of hepadnaviridae than HBV (avihepadnavirus rather than orthohepadnavirus), it has significant enough structural and biological relatedness to HBV to support its use as an *in vivo* model. Emtricitabine was first tested against DHBV in a pilot study in which congenitally infected ducklings were treated orally with a dose of 50 mg/kg bid. This study established that emtricitabine inhibited viral replication and was well tolerated. In a longer-term study utilizing the 50 mg/kg bid. dosing regimen, four adult ducks were dosed for 12 weeks. Determination of the efficacy of emtricitabine was not a primary goal of this study, however the compound was described as being as effective as 2'-CDG, which reduced viremia by tenfold after four days of treatment and to nearly undetectable levels within a few weeks. Liver biopsies conducted two and six weeks into treatment revealed a significant decline in replicative forms of viral DNA, consistent with the ability of emtricitabine 5'-triphosphate to act as an alternative substrate inhibitor of DHBV polymerase. However, levels of cccDNA (circular covalently closed DNA) declined much more slowly, dropping 20%, 40% and 60% after two, six and 12 weeks of therapy, respectively.

WHV

The woodchuck hepatitis virus (WHV) and its natural host, the eastern woodchuck Marmota monax, are the most accepted and most frequently used model of hepatitis-induced disease. This is principally for three reasons: (1) WHV is more similar to HBV than the other hepadnaviridae available in animal model systems. Both HBV and WHV are members of the genus orthohepadnavirus and share approximately 70% nucleotide sequence homology [33]; (2) the range of hepatic injury produced by chronic infections in woodchucks closely resembles that seen in HBV-infected humans; (3) the relative *in vivo* effectiveness of antiviral agents is comparable against WHV and HBV. Four antiviral agents, which had previously been studied for anti-HBV activity in clinical trials, were studied in WHV and the results compared back to the clinical trial results [34]. This comparison showed parallel activity to that observed in the clinic and reinforced the utility of chronic WHV infection in woodchucks for *in vivo* evaluation of agents being developed for chronic HBV infection.

Emtricitabine has demonstrated profound anti-hepatitis virus activity in the woodchuck model. In an oral dosing study, five groups of chronically infected woodchucks were given emtricitabine QD. at one of five doses: 0.3, 1.0, 3.0, 10 or 30 mg/kg for four weeks [35]. At doses of 3.0 mg/kg and greater, emtricitabine induced a statistically significant reduction in both serum viremia and replicative intermediates. The largest reduction in viremia, approximately 4.9 $\log_{10}$, and in replicative intermediates, approximately 80-fold, was seen at the 30 mg/kg dose. No significant effect on the levels of intrahepatic RNA, serum levels of WHsAg, or the appearance of antibodies to WHsAg or WHcAg in the serum were observed. Viremia returned to pretreatment levels within one to two weeks following the end of treatment at all doses. This rapid rebound is consistent with a lack of significant impact on levels of WHV cccDNA.

These results are very similar to those obtained by the same group in a separate oral QD. dosing study of chronically infected woodchucks with lamivudine. The decreases in serum viremia and replicative intermediates in liver tissue produced by lamivudine are similar to those observed for emtricitabine at comparable exposures of drug. In addition, the rate and degree of viral rebound observed upon cessation of therapy was virtually identical for both compounds.

Cullen et al. have studied the effect of emtricitabine on WHV in naturally infected, wild-caught woodchucks [36]. Animals were dosed ip at either 20 or 30 mg/kg BID for four weeks. Administration of the 20 mg/kg dose suppressed WHV DNA levels from six- to 49-fold (average of 27-fold in the six animal groups). WHV DNA polymerase in serum was reduced in a similar fashion. Serum DNA polymerase activity was measured by the incorporation of [^{32}P] dCTP into WHV DNA. A more profound effect was seen at the 30 mg/kg dose. Serum WHV DNA levels were reduced from 20- to 150-fold (average of 56-fold) in the six animal groups. Serum DNA polymerase activity was similarly reduced. WHV DNA levels in the liver biopsy specimens were also reduced in all six of the animals in the 30 mg/kg-treatment group. Reductions ranged from 68% up to 98% of the pretreatment levels. The authors state that while the level of replicative intermediates remained close to those seen pretreatment, the WHV genome was being shifted toward shorter fragments. In this study, as in the study of Korba et al., levels of WHsAg or antibodies against WHsAg or WHcAg did not change [35].

In vitro resistance

HIV resistance

Because the emergence of drug-resistant virus is a major concern in anti-HIV chemotherapy and helps define the combinations within which a drug will be useful, the development of resistance to emtricitabine was examined by passaging virus *in vitro* in the presence of drug. In a study reported by Tisdale et al., the HXB2 strain of HIV-1 or the zidovudine-resistant mutant, HIV-1_{RTMC} (contains D67N, K70R, T215Y, and K219Q mutations), was passaged in MT4 cells in the presence of increasing concentrations of emtricitabine or lamivudine [11]. Rapid emergence of resistance occurred with both compounds. By the fourth passage of HXB2 and the second passage of HIV-1_{RTMC}, EC_{50} values exceeded 50 μM and by passage six, EC_{50} values were in excess of 250 μM. These variants were highly cross-resistant to lamivudine and emtricitabine, but showed no cross-resistance to zidovudine, didanosine, or nevirapine. DNA sequence analysis showed a change at codon 184, with methionine replaced by valine. Based on synergy data with zidovudine and the lack of cross-resistance, the authors suggested that combination of the oxathiolane analogues with zidovudine might slow the emergence of resistance to emtricitabine and/or lamivudine. Indeed, passaging virus in the presence of increasing concentrations of emtricitabine and 50 nM zidovudine was able to delay appreciably, but not prevent, the emergence of emtricitabine-resistant virus [11].

In experiments performed by Schinazi et al., the potential for HIV-1 resistance to develop to lamivudine and emtricitabine was evaluated by serial passage of the virus in human PBMCs in the presence of increasing drug concentrations [37]. Results presented in Figure 3 show that after two weeks of infection, 0.1 μM lamivudine was no longer able to inhibit virus replication, and drug-resistant variants dominated the replicating virus population. In contrast, using identical conditions, emtricitabine remained highly active, reducing virus replication by 80%. Emtricitabine was still able to inhibit virus replication by 50% at week three. At week four the concentration of lamivudine was increased 100-fold to 10 μM, and the concentration of emtricitabine was increased tenfold to 1 μM to produce the same level of inhibition. Emtricitabine retained up to a tenfold potency advantage over lamivudine after four weeks of passaging. These data in primary human cells suggest that emtricitabine may delay the breakthrough of resistant viruses relative to lamivudine.

DNA sequence analysis of the reverse transcriptase gene amplified from resistant viruses generated in these passaging experiments consistently identified mutations at codon 184, where methionine was changed to either valine or isoleucine. Resistant variants were cross-resistant to both emtricitabine and lamivudine, but remained sensitive to zalcitabine, didanosine, zidovudine, PFA, 3'-fluoro-3'-deoxythymidine (FLT), and two non-nucleoside reverse transcriptase inhibitors, the TIBO compound R82150 and the bis(heteroaryl) piperazine derivative U-87201E [37].

Biochemical studies were performed to quantify the change in susceptibility of HIV RT derived from virus resistant to emtricitabine 5'-triphosphate, lamivudine 5'-triphosphate, and the zalcitabine 5'-triphosphate [37]. Virus particle-derived RT was obtained from the supernatant of human PBMCs that were infected with M184V mutant virus. The mutated enzyme was 15-fold less sensitive to inhibition by emtricitabine 5'-triphosphate or lamivudine 5'-triphosphate than was wild type HIV_{LAI}-RT. However, only a threefold decrease in susceptibility was noted for zalcitabine 5'-triphosphate. Similar results were reported using a highly purified cloned RT containing the M184V mutation [27]. In these studies the K_i values for emtricitabine 5'-triphosphate and lamivudine 5'-triphosphate were increased 320- and 80-fold, respectively, compared to wild type HIV RT. Wilson et al. [38], using steady state and pre-steady-state kinetic analysis, examined the effect of the M184V mutation on HIV-1 RT catalytic function. These kinetic studies showed that the M184V mutation did not

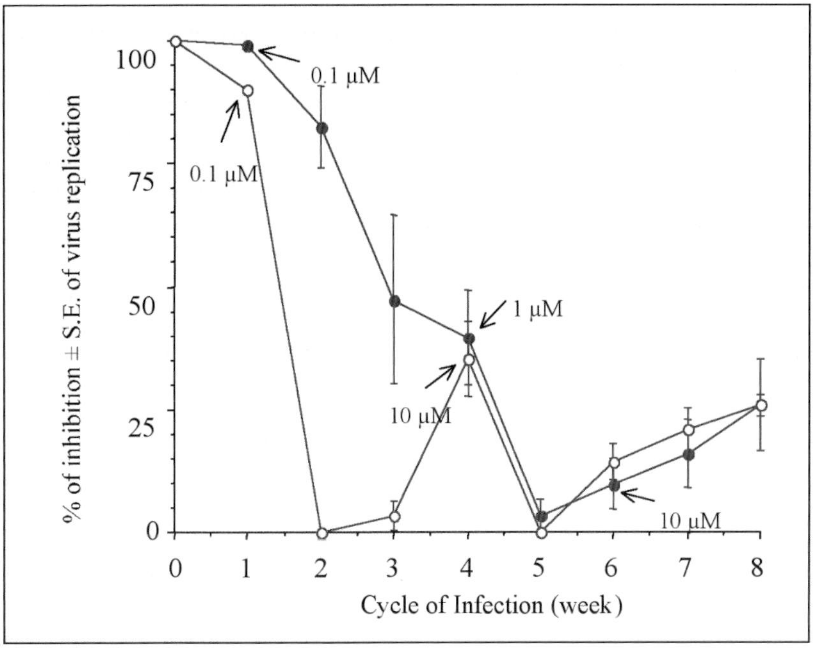

Figure 3. HIV-1 breakthrough in the presence of emtricitabine (●) and lamivudine (○) [37].

alter either the K_m or the k_{cat} values for the natural substrates, but did cause a 300-fold increase in the K_i for emtricitabine 5'-triphosphate.

The clinical emergence of the M184V virus was first reported by Schinazi et al. in a patient who had received lamivudine [37]. The M184V mutation was also found in recombinant virus prepared using RNA isolated from the plasma of three patients who had received emtricitabine monotherapy for two weeks. Phenotypic analysis in MT-2 cells demonstrated all three of these viruses to be resistant to emtricitabine and cross-resistant to lamivudine. The EC_{50} values of the recombinant virus for both emtricitabine and lamivudine increased greater than 50-fold relative to the EC_{50} value against wild type HIV-1_{LAI}. One of these isolates contained the M41L and T215Y mutations, but remained sensitive to inhibition by zidovudine. This observation is in keeping with a report by Schinazi et al. that the introduction of the M184V mutation against a zidovudine-resistant background can result in increased sensitivity to zidovudine [37].

Emtricitabine activity has been evaluated extensively against a panel of clinical isolates (Table 9). The panel consists of a series of recombinant wild type clinical isolates and 35 recombinant isolates containing anywhere from one to 12 mutations. Consistent with earlier passaging experiments, a high level of resistance is imparted by introduction of the M184V mutation against any mutation background. Moderate resistance to emtricitabine is seen for the highly mutated isolate (M41L, E44D, D67N, T69D, L74I, K101E, V108I, V118I, Y181C, G190A, L210W, T215Y) that contains the two mutations associated with moderate resistance to lamivudine (E44D, V118I).

Table 9. Phenotypic analysis of recombinant viruses generated from clinical isolates. analysis of emtricitabine resistance profile

Genotype	EC_{50} (μM)[a]		
	Emtricitabine	Lamivudine	Zidovudine
WT: LAI	0.619[b]	2.567[b]	0.487[b]
WT (n=16)	0.64[c]	2.998[c]	0.917[c]
L100I (A)	0.176	2.125	0.037
L100I (B)	0.595	2.350	0.160
G190A	0.220	0.900	0.205
G333E	1.350	1.265	0.260
M184V	>20.00	>50.00	0.140
K103T	0.330	1.100	0.140
V108I	0.205	0.650	0.135
K103N (A)	0.825	3.150	0.595
K103N (B)	0.680	4.000	0.250
K103N, M184V (A)	>20.00	>50.00	0.185
K103N, M184V (B)	>20.00	>20.00	3.02
E138K, M184V (A)	>20.00	>50.00	0.145
E138K, M184V (B)	>20.00	>50.00	0.130
E13Q, M184V	>20.00	>50.00	0.890
A98S, M184V	>20.00	>50.00	0.120
L74V, K103N	2.34	>2.26	1.87
K101Q, E138K	1.38	1.94	0.54
K103R, Y188C	1.13	1.16	0.72
K103N, Y181C	0.55	1.17	0.29
K70R, L74V, M184V	>20.00	>20.00	0.90
K103T, V106I, M184V	>20.00	>20.00	0.36
K101Q, E138K, K103N	0.55	0.48	0.67
K103N, V108I, M184V	>20.00	>20.00	0.31
T215Y, K103N, L210W	0.73	1.05	>2.00
M41L, K101R, M184V, T215Y	>20.00	>20.00	>2.00
A98S, F116Y, Q151M, T215Y	1.45	0.55	>2.00
T69N, K70R, M184V, K219Q	>20.00	>20.00	1.23
D67N, K70R, M184V, G190A	>20.00	>50.00	0.35
D67N, T69D, K103R, T219Q	2.58	2.92	5.75
A62V, A98S, K101D, K102Q, M184V	>20.00	>50.00	0.35
M41L, D67N, M184V, L210W, T215Y	>20.00	>20.00	>2.00
D67N, K70R, E138A, M184V, T215Y, K219E	>20.00	>20.00	>2.00
M41L, D67N, Y181C, M184V, L210W, T215Y	>25.00	>20.00	>2.00
M41L, D67N, T69D, V108I, M184V, T215Y	>20.00	>20.00	>2.00
A62V, V75M, K103N, F116Y, Q151M, M184V	>20.00	>20.00	>2.00
D67N, T69D, K70R, K103N, M184V, T215Y, K219Q	>20.00	>20.00	>2.00

Table 9. Continued

Genotype	EC_{50} (μM)[a]		
	Emtricitabine	Lamivudine	Zidovudine
M41L, D67N, A98G, K101E, K103N, M184V, G190A, L210W, T215Y, G333E	>20.00	>20.00	>2.00
M41L, E44D, D67N, T69D, L74I, K101E, V108I, V118I, Y181C, G190A, L210W, T215Y	7.27	6.63	1.85

[a] EC_{50} values are expressed as the median value of at least three replicates, unless otherwise noted.
[b] EC_{50} values is the average value of at least 10 replicates.
[c] EC_{50} values are the average of replicates from 16 different recombinants displaying a WT genotype.

HBV Resistance

Treatment of HBV-infected patients with lamivudine has been shown to be effective in suppressing virus replication and in reducing inflammatory activity. However, resistance to this agent has been documented that is associated with mutations in the YMDD motif in domain C of the viral DNA polymerase, analogous to changes seen in the YMDD motif of HIV-RT. Methionine 204 [39] had mutated to either isoleucine (M204I) or valine (M204V). The M204V mutation is almost always observed in conjunction with an additional mutation, L180M in the B domain. Because of the sequence homology between the active sites of HIV RT and the HBV DNA polymerase [29], the importance of the YMDD motif to the catalytic activity of both polymerases, and the role of the methionine in the resistance of HIV-1 to lamivudine and emtricitabine, it would be anticipated that HBV containing either the M204I or the M204V mutation is cross-resistant to emtricitabine. Inhibition assays performed using HepAD38 and HepAD79 cells, which replicate wild type and the M204V mutant HBV, respectively [40, 41], confirmed that the methionine-to-valine mutation conferred resistance to emtricitabine as well as to lamivudine. EC_{50} values for lamivudine and emtricitabine versus wild type and mutant HBV were 0.09 and 1.3 μM, and 0.04 and 1.25 μM, respectively. Interestingly, introduction of the M204V mutation into the HBV polymerase did not impart the same degree of resistance to emtricitabine or lamivudine seen upon introduction of the M184V mutation into the HIV polymerase.

Zoulim et al. (personal communication from F. Zoulim, INSERM, France) using a duck (DHBV) polymerase assay reported that mutations conferring resistance to lamivudine showed cross-resistance to emtricitabine. In their studies, mutations were made in the DHBV DNA polymerase at M204 and L180 that correspond to the M204 and the L180 mutations in HBV. The inhibitory activity of the 5'-triphosphates of lamivudine and emtricitabine was compared against wild type and mutant polymerases using enzyme expressed in a coupled transcription/translation rabbit reticulocyte lysate system. Both lamivudine 5'-triphosphate and emtricitabine 5'-triphosphate were inhibitors of viral minus-strand DNA synthesis, with IC_{50} values of 6.1 ± 3.5 μM and 8.5 ± 4.1 μM, respectively. When tested against the M204V-, M204I-, and M204V + L180M- containing mutants, the IC_{50} values for lamivudine 5'-triphosphate and emtricitabine 5'-triphosphate increased markedly (>100 μM). In cell culture assays using LMH cells transiently transfected with DHBV genomes containing mutations M204V, M204I, or M204V + L180M, neither lamivudine nor emtricitabine showed any antiviral activity.

Toxicological studies

Cytotoxicity

The cytotoxicity of emtricitabine has been evaluated extensively *in vitro* (Table 10). In all of the cell lines examined, cell growth was not affected at concentrations of emtricitabine up to and including 200 mM [7]. Similar results were obtained with lamivudine [8, 13, 42, 43].

Because of the apparent correlation between toxicity to bone marrow progenitor cells *in vitro* and bone marrow suppression *in vivo*, human bone marrow progenitor colony forming assays were performed. The concentration of emtricitabine required to inhibit the formation of granulocyte-macrophage (GFU-GM) colonies by 50% (CC_{50}) was 300 ± 40 μM (n = 6). The CC_{50} for erythroid colonies (BFU-E) was 220 ± 8 μM (n = 6). CC_{50} values for lamivudine are comparable with a value for GFU-GM of 260 ± 8 μM and a value for BFU-E of 180 ± 2 μM [8, 14, 42]. CC_{50} values of the (+) isomer of 3TC in the bone marrow progenitor cell assay were determined to be 10 ± 2 μM for GFU-GM and 4 ± 1 μM for BFU-E. It is interesting that the (+)-isomer of lamivudine shows bone marrow toxicity, while the (+)-isomer of emtricitabine has CC_{50} values comparable to those of the (-)-isomer.

Although the mechanism(s) responsible for the toxic side effects of the nucleoside antiviral agents is multifactorial, delayed mitochondrial toxicity is believed to be a major underlying contributor [44]. Previous studies on ddC-induced peripheral neuropathy [45] and AZT-induced myopathy [46] have revealed a depletion of mitochondrial DNA content in drug-treated cells. This depletion could account for toxicities observed in the clinic. In an effort to evaluate the potential for mitochondrial toxicity, human hepatoblastoma HepG2 cells were incubated with emtricitabine at concentrations ranging between 0.1 and 10 μM for two weeks [47] and up to 100 μM for up to eight weeks (J. Jeffrey, personal communication, Triangle Pharmaceuticals). Under these conditions, emtricitabine had no adverse effects on cell growth, mitochondrial DNA synthesis or lactic acid production. In a separate study conducted in HepG2 cells exposed to concentrations of emtricitabine ranging from 0.1 to 10 μM for eight days, no effects on mitochondrial morphology were observed by transmission electron microscopy.

Table 10. Cytotoxicity of emtricitabine in comparison to lamivudine and zidovudine

	CC_{50} (μM)		
Cells	emtricitabine	lamivudine	zidovudine
MT4	>100[a], >200[b]	>100[a], >33[b]	20[a], > 100[b]
PBMC	>100[a]	>100[a]	>100[a]
CEM	>100[a], >100[b]	>100[a], >100[b]	14.3[a], >6[b]
Vero	>100[a]	>100[a]	28.0[a]
IM9	>100[b]	>100[b]	70[b]
Molt 4	>100[b]	>100[b]	10[b]
HepG22.2.15	>200[b], >200[c]	>200[b]	>200[b]

a. [13]
b. [42]
c. [14]

In vivo toxicology

The preclinical toxicology profile of emtricitabine is extremely favorable [48]. In six-month mouse and one-year monkey studies, CD-1 mice were dosed orally up to 3000 mg/kg/day, and cynomolgus monkeys were dosed orally up to 500 mg/kg/day. Mild, reversible anemia was the only observed toxicity. Anemia occurred only at the highest doses tested, where plasma exposures (AUC_{0-24}) in mice were approximately 150-fold human exposures at the proposed dose of 200 mg/day, and in monkeys, where plasma exposures exceeded 25-fold human exposures. In accord with *in vivo* studies, mitochondria in liver, heart and skeletal muscle examined by transmission election microscopy were normal in mice given oral doses of emtricitabine at 3000 mg/kg/day for six months.

Emtricitabine had no effect on reproduction or development at exposures approximately 100 times human exposure. Reproductive toxicity studies consisted of fertility studies in CD-1 mice and in CD male rats. Developmental toxicology studies were conducted in pregnant mice and in pregnant New Zealand white rabbits.

Genetic toxicology studies consisting of an Ames assay, a mouse lymphoma assay and an assay using Chinese hamster ovary (CHO) cells to detect chromosomal aberrations were all negative.

Preclinical pharmacokinetics, metabolism and excretion

The pharmacokinetics, metabolism and excretion of emtricitabine have been investigated in mice, rats and cynomolgus monkeys after single and repeated dosing [49, 50]. Emtricitabine is rapidly and well absorbed after oral administration in all three species, with oral bioavailability ranging from 58% to 97%. Peak plasma emtricitabine concentrations occur between 0.5 to 2.5 hours post dose. Plasma concentrations of emtricitabine expressed as AUC increase linearly with dose over a wide dose range (up to 1500 mg/kg/day in mice and 500 mg/kg/day in monkeys). Plasma emtricitabine is eliminated with a half-life ($t_{1/2}$) of one to four hours and a total body clearance of ~1.5 L/kg/hr in rats and ~ 0.7 L/kg/hr in monkeys.

Emtricitabine has a volume of distribution (Vd_{ss}, 0.8 – 1.5 L/kg) slightly larger than the total body water in all species, suggesting that it is distributed into both the intracellular and extracellular fluid spaces. The fraction of protein-bound emtricitabine in plasma is <4% for all species.

Tissue distribution studies of ^{14}C-emtricitabine in rats and monkeys confirm that emtricitabine is widely distributed to all tissues [51]. The ^{14}C-radioactivity concentrations in tissues generally decline in parallel with those in plasma, with no indication of drug accumulation. Virtually no radioactivity remains in the body at 72 hours post-dosing. The ^{14}C concentrations in the kidneys, gut and liver exceed those in plasma, while concentrations in CNS tissues were <10% of those in plasma. Renal excretion of unchanged drug is the principal route of emtricitabine elimination. In rats, 91% of the ^{14}C-emtricitabine dose was recovered in the urine after an IV dose, and 74% after an oral dose. Approximately 67% and 41% of an oral ^{14}C dose was recovered in the urine of mice and monkeys, respectively. The majority of the dose recovered in the feces after an oral dose most likely represents unabsorbed drug. Renal clearance of emtricitabine generally exceeded the glomerular filtration rate, suggesting that emtricitabine is excreted by renal tubules. In all three species, metabolism is a minor route of emtricitabine elimination. Over 90% (mice) and 64% (monkeys) of radioactivity recovered in urine was unchanged drug. The principal metabolites, the isomeric 3'-sulfoxides, accounted for ~2% of the dose in mice, 2.6% in rats and 8% in monkeys. The only other metabolite detectable in monkey urine was a 2'-glucuronide metabolite, which accounted for 1.1% of the dose. In mice, very minor metabolites, the 2'-glucuronide, 5'-fluorouridine (all <1-2% of dose) were detected. No 5'-flurouracil was detected in any species.

Clinical development — HIV

Clinical pharmacology (human pharmacokinetic) phase I/II studies

The PK and disposition of emtricitabine following single- or multiple-dose administration have been extensively characterized. Emtricitabine is rapidly and well absorbed following oral administration, with steady-state plasma concentrations reaching levels several-fold above the mean *in vitro* EC_{90} value for anti-HIV activity (Figure 4). At 24 hours post-dose, plasma trough concentrations following a 200 mg QD dose exceeded the mean *in vitro* EC_{90} for anti-HIV activity by about fourfold. Based on extrapolation of this data, plasma emtricitabine concentrations are expected to be within the range of the EC_{90} at 48 hours post-dose, and within the range of EC_{50} at 72 hours post-dose.

Emtricitabine disposition follows linear kinetics with small inter-subject variability, predictable steady-state concentrations and dose proportionality over a wide dose range. The high concentrations and long half-lives of emtricitabine in plasma (8-9 hours) and emtricitabine-5'-triphosphate (>39 hours) in peripheral blood mononuclear cells (PBMCs) support once daily dosing. Renal excretion of unchanged drug is the principal route of emtricitabine elimination from plasma, and thus presents little potential for metabolic drug interactions. Plasma AUC and total body clearance appear to be correlated with creatinine clearance. A pediatric dose of 6 mg/kg QD has been identified and is under evaluation in phase II studies.

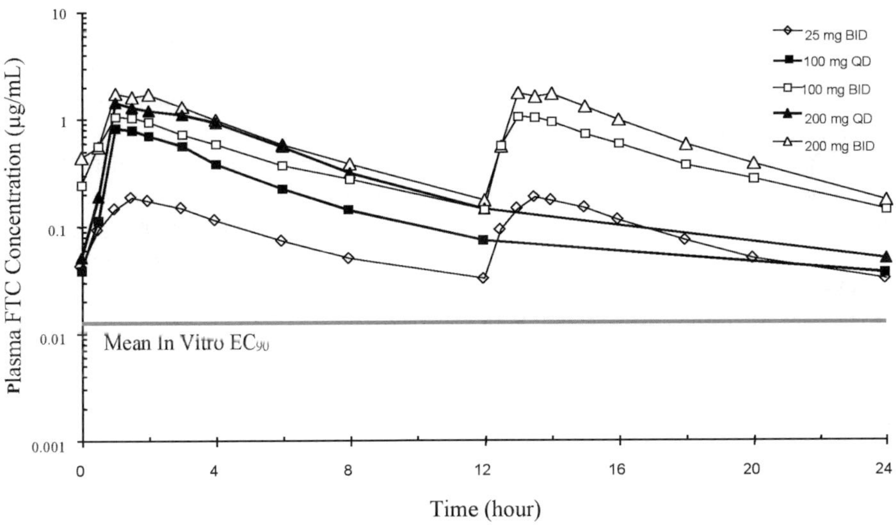

Figure 4. Mean steady-state plasma emtricitabine concentrations following a 25 mg, 100 mg QD, 100 mg BID, 200 mg QD or 200 mg BID dosing regimen.

Drug interaction studies

The PK of emtricitabine was not significantly affected when it was coadministered with either zidovudine (ZDV) or stavudine (d4T). A single dose of emtricitabine had no clinically significant PK effect on d4T, but did increase the AUC and C_{max} of ZDV by 26% and 66%, respectively. Due to large intersubject variability and the small sample size (n = 6), the actual extent of interaction may be less than that reported in this study.

In addition, the moderate increase in ZDV exposure observed would not be expected to be clinically significant. No clinically significant PK interactions between emtricitabine and the protease inhibitor indinavir, or the non-nucleoside reverse transcriptase inhibitor emivirine were observed following a single oral administration of emtricitabine to 12 subjects. In a study of nine treatment-naïve, HIV-infected patients enrolled in the ANRS091 trial, the simultaneous administration of FTC, ddI and efavirenz did not significantly affect the PK of any of these drugs.

Because emtricitabine is primarily eliminated as unchanged drug in urine, a study focusing on the potential interactions between emtricitabine and famciclovir at the site of urinary excretion was conducted. Famciclovir was chosen as a typical drug for this evaluation because its active form in plasma (penciclovir) is primarily eliminated in urine. No interactions were seen.

Dose selection trials

Two short-term monotherapy trials were conducted to define a dosage regimen for use in Phase III therapeutic trials, FTC-101 and FTC-102. Protocol FTC-101 was an open-label, sequential, dose-ranging trial evaluating the *in vivo* antiviral activity of emtricitabine in HIV-infected patients given 14 days of monotherapy at 25 mg BID, 100 mg QD, 100 mg BID, 200 mg QD, and 200 mg BID. A total of 41 patients (N = 8 or 9 per dose group) naïve to lamivudine and abacavir were enrolled. At screening, $CD4^+$ cell count ranged from 198 to 1071 cells/mm^3 and plasma HIV-1 RNA ranged from 3.9 to 5.9 log_{10} copies/mL. Plasma HIV-1 RNA was measured at baseline and frequently over the 14 days of treatment. The pharmacokinetics of emtricitabine in plasma and emtricitabine 5'-triphosphate levels in PBMCs were also evaluated.

Potent antiretroviral activity occurred in all dosage cohorts, with a strong trend towards greater activity at the higher doses (Figure 5). Viral suppression in the 200 mg QD group was comparable to that observed in the 200 mg BID group. The 200 mg QD dose group showed a median drop from baseline at day 15 of 1.9 log_{10}, as compared to 1.3, 1.5, 1.7, and 1.9 log_{10} for the 25 mg BID, 100 mg QD, 100 mg BID, and 200 mg BID dose groups, respectively. The onset of anti-HIV activity occurred within 48 hours of initiating emtricitabine dosing with the most rapid viral load decline occurring between days 3 and 8. Results of statistical analyses of HIV-1 RNA AAUCMB (average area under the curve minus baseline), change from baseline at day 15 (last day on study treatment), and maximum change from baseline, consistently supported the dose-response relationship and the maximal antiviral effect at the 200 mg QD and 200 mg BID doses.

Protocol FTC-102 was an open-label, randomized, parallel-group monotherapy trial comparing three once-daily dosage regimens of emtricitabine (25 mg, 100 mg and 200 mg QD) and the approved lamivudine regimen (150 mg BID) during 10 days of monotherapy. A total of 81 patients, naïve to lamivudine and abacavir, were randomized to one of the four treatment regimens. At screening, median $CD4^+$ cell count ranged from 350 to 431 cells/mm^3, and median plasma HIV-1 RNA ranged from 4.3 to 4.7 log_{10} copies/mL. Plasma HIV-1 RNA levels were measured at baseline and frequently over the 10 days of treatment.

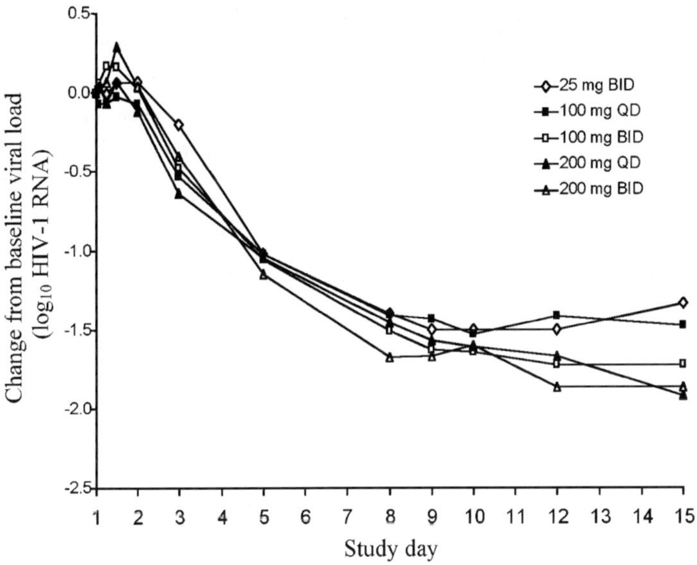

Figure 5. Study FTC-101: Median change in HIV-1 RNA from baseline.

This randomized, controlled study confirmed the dose-response results of FTC-101, with the most potent antiviral activity occurring in the emtricitabine 200 mg QD dose group (Figure 6). Median change from baseline at day 11 was 1.50, 1.58, and 1.69 log_{10} for the 25, 100 and 200 mg QD emtricitabine doses, respectively, and was 1.48 log_{10} for the 150 mg BID lamivudine dose. Results from statistical analyses of HIV-1 RNA AAUCMB, change from baseline at day 11 (last day on study treatment), and maximum change from baseline consistently distinguish 200 mg QD from the lower emtricitabine doses.

In addition to the greater activity of emtricitabine 200 mg QD based on change from baseline in HIV-1 RNA, there was also a greater proportion of patients who achieved the limit of assay detection (400 copies/mL) or who had a two log_{10} decrease from baseline on the FTC 200 mg QD dose (Figure 7).

The dose-response relationship was further evaluated by correlating HIV-RNA AAUCMB with emtricitabine daily dose using a pharmacological E_{max} model, $E = (E_{max} \cdot Dose)/(EC_{50} + Dose)$. The pharmacological dose-response curves show that the effect of emtricitabine on HIV-1 RNA suppression had reached the maximal effect at doses > 200 mg per day. Very little additional effect on HIV-1 RNA suppression was observed with increasing the dose from 200 mg to 400 mg per day.

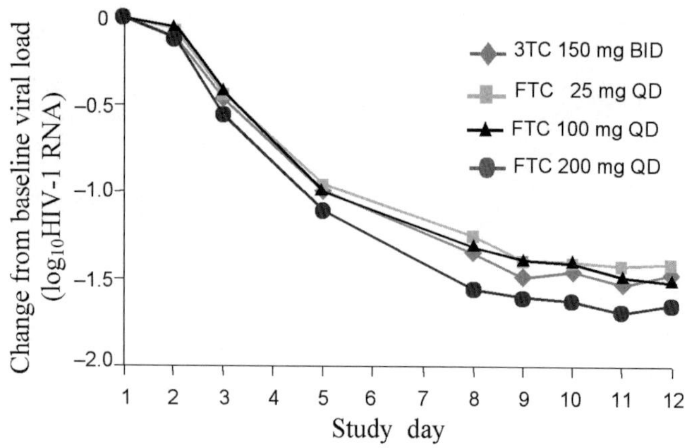

Figure 6. FTC-102 mean change from baseline in plasma HIV-1 RNA.

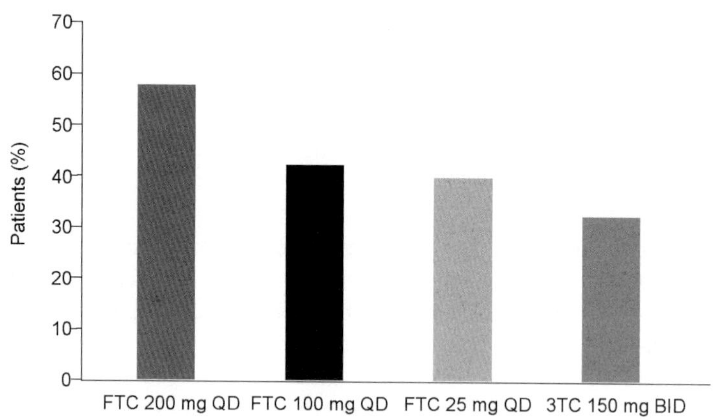

Figure 7. FTC-102: Proportion of patients with HIV-1 RNA < 400 copies/mL or >2 $\log_{10}$ decrease from baseline.

The steady-state plasma and intracellular pharmacokinetics of emtricitabine support the selection of a 200 mg QD dose. The steady-state intracellular emtricitabine 5'-triphosphate concentrations increased in a dose-related fashion, reaching an apparent plateau level at emtricitabine daily doses of 200 mg or greater. The clinical antiviral activity correlates well with the intracellular 5'-triphosphate levels in PBMCs (Figure 8). As the emtricitabine dose increased, intracellular emtricitabine 5'-triphosphate levels and viral load suppression increased, reaching an apparent plateau at daily doses of ≥200 mg.

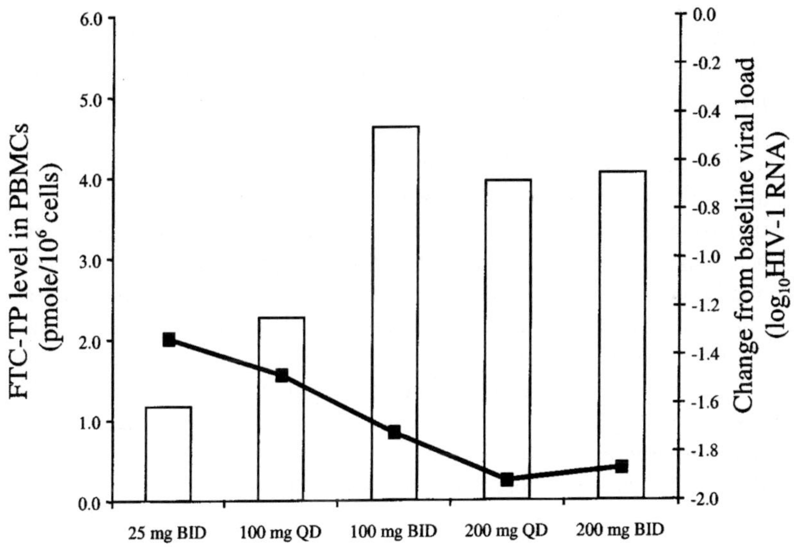

Figure 8. FTC-101: Correlation of antiviral activity of FTC with emtricitabine 5'-triphosphate levels of PBMCs.

Phase II/III clinical studies

A series of phase II/III clinical studies have been conducted with emtricitabine. An overview of each study is given below.

FTC-201: A Pilot Study Evaluating the Efficacy and Tolerance of the Combination Emtricitabine + ddI + efavirenz Administered Once Daily in the Treatment of HIV-1-Infected, Antiretroviral-Naïve Patients (ANRS091-Montana Study).

This Phase II study is being conducted by the ANRS (Agence Nationale de la Recherche sur le SIDA, Paris France) to evaluate a once-daily regimen of FTC + ddI + efavirenz. To date, 34 of 40 treatment-naive patients have completed 96 weeks. Results demonstrate durable antiviral and immunologic effects lasting for the 96-week period using a fully once-a-day regimen. Using a non-completer-equals-failure analysis at 96 weeks, 85% and 80% of patients maintained a plasma HIV RNA level below 400 and 50 copies/mL, respectively. There was a median $CD4^+$ cell count rise of 259 cells/μL at week 96. Overall, the regimen has been well tolerated. The most common treatment-related adverse events occurred during the first 24 weeks of the study, and were mild to moderate in severity.

FTC-303: A Randomized, Open-Label Equivalence Study of Emtricitabine Versus Lamivudine in Patients on a Stable Triple Antiretroviral Therapy Regimen Containing Lamivudine Plus Stavudine or Zidovudine, and a Protease Inhibitor or a Non-Nucleoside Reverse Transcriptase Inhibitor.

Study FTC-303 was a randomized (2:1), open-label, 48-week equivalence study of FTC vs. 3TC in 440 patients on a stable (HIV RNA ≤ 400 copies/mL) triple therapy regimen (≥12 weeks) containing 3TC. Patients were randomized to continue 3TC or switch to FTC by screening viral load (≤50 and >50-400 copies/mL) and by the presence of a protease inhibitor or non-nucleoside reverse transcriptase inhibitor in their regimens. At entry, the treatment groups were comparable with regard to race, gender, age, and baseline disease. Patients had a mean age of 41.5 (range 22-80) years, 64% were Caucasian, and 86% male. Median baseline $CD4^+$ cell count was 488 (range 37-1909) cells/mm^3 and median plasma HIV-1 RNA was 50 copies/mL. The median duration of previous antiretroviral therapy was 28 months.

Overall, 79% of patients completed the 48-week study. The reasons for early termination from the study were similar between treatment groups. Thirteen (4%) patients in the FTC group discontinued the study early due to an adverse event, while one patient (1%) died due to a heroin overdose in the 3TC group. Through 48 weeks of therapy, the proportion of patients who had confirmed virological loss of response was 7.8% in the FTC arm and 7.5% in the 3TC arm. These findings support the conclusion of equivalent safety and virologic efficacy of 200 mg once daily FTC compared to 150 mg 3TC administered twice daily.

FTC-302: A Randomized, Double-Blind Equivalence Trial Comparing Emtricitabine to Lamivudine within a Triple Combination Regimen in Antiretroviral-Drug-Naïve, HIV-1 Infected Patients.

Study FTC-302 was a randomized, double-blind equivalence study of FTC versus 3TC in combination with stavudine and either nevirapine (patients with HIV-1 RNA ≥100,000 copies/mL) or efavirenz (patients with HIV-1 RNA > 100,000 copies/mL) in 468 anti-retroviral-naïve patients. Of the 468 patients treated, 385 (82%) received FTC/3TC plus stavudine and nevirapine, while 83 (18%) received FTC/3TC plus stavudine and efavirenz. Seventy-four percent (74%) of the patients completed 48 weeks of therapy. The treatment groups were comparable with regard to race, gender, age, and baseline characteristics. Median age at entry was 32 years (range 18-63), 77% were black African, and 59% were female. Median screening $CD4^+$ cell count was 373 cells/mm^3 (range 140-1455), and median plasma HIV-1 RNA was 4.6 $\log_{10}$ copies/mL.

The majority of patients in both treatment arms achieved and maintained a plasma HIV-1 RNA ≤ 400 copies/mL through 48 weeks (65% receiving FTC and 71% receiving 3TC), with 60% (FTC) and 64% (3TC) of patients having a plasma HIV-1 RNA < 50 copies/mL at week 48.

Thirty-three FTC-treated patients (14%) and 23 3TC-treated patients (10%) were confirmed virological failures during the study. Interestingly, more of the FTC-treated virologic failures (13/33, 39%) had no genotypic changes associated with the medications used in the triple therapy regimen, compared to only three (18%) of the 3TC-treated patients. Seven (21%) and 11 (48%) of the FTC- and the 3TC-treated patients, respectively, had the M184V mutation at time of failure. The immunologic benefit observed through week 48 was comparable in each treatment arm, with a mean increase from baseline in absolute $CD4^+$ cell count of approximately 200 cells/mm^3 and a 10% increase in CD4%.

Eleven percent of the patients in each treatment arm discontinued blinded study medication due to an adverse event during the study, with the majority of these discontinuations associated with hepatotoxicities attributed to the use of nevirapine in the triple therapy regimen.

These results confirm that patients in both treatment arms of study FTC-302 derived significant virologic and immunologic benefit during the trial. Results from this trial compare favorably to other randomized, well-controlled, international clinical trials using standard-of-care triple therapy regimens and support the conclusion of equivalent efficacy and safety of FTC with 3TC [52].

Clinical development – HBV

FTCB-101 was a pilot dose-selection study designed to examine the pharmacokinetics and activity of emtricitabine for the treatment of chronic HBV infection [53]. Five once-daily doses of emtricitabine (25 mg, 50 mg, 100 mg, 200 mg and 300 mg) were evaluated sequentially for eight weeks in cohorts each consisting of at least eight patients with chronic HBV infection. Patients were positive for HBsAg and HBV DNA, and naïve to nucleoside analog therapy.

Pharmacokinetic analysis showed emtricitabine to be well absorbed after oral administration, with plasma concentrations reaching levels above the EC_{90} at all doses with once-daily administration. The elimination half-life of emtricitabine from plasma ranged from six to 10 hours, and the steady-state plasma concentrations increased nearly dose proportionally over the 25 mg to 300 mg dose range.

Suppression of HBV DNA depended on baseline viral load and assay sensitivity. On completion of dosing (day 56), HBV DNA suppression reached undetectable levels when assayed by the Digene Hybrid Capture Assay (lower limit of detection 145,000 copies/ml) at low and moderate baseline viral loads and showed a dose effect at high baseline viral load. Using the Chiron Amplicor® HBV Monitor assay (lower limit of detection 400 copies/ml), HBV suppression of greater than 4.0 $\log_{10}$ was observed. The absolute interpretation of dose response was complicated in this study by differing viral loads at baseline between cohorts and by sequential enrollment.

Consistent with what has been reported in HIV trials, emtricitabine was well tolerated. There were no serious adverse events, and no patient was intolerant to the drug. The only observed adverse event of grade II-III severity was headache, which occurred in more than 10% of patients (11% overall).

FTC-102 is a double-blind, randomized trial to evaluate three doses of emtricitabine, 25 mg, 100 mg and 200 mg qd [22, 54]. A total of 98 patients were enrolled, 32 in the

25 mg dose cohort and 33 each in the 100 and 200 mg dose cohorts. The mean age of the patients was 37 years; 70% were male and 88% were of Asian ethnicity. There were no important demographic differences among dose cohorts. The median baseline viral load ($\log_{10}$ c/ml) was 7.57, 7.68 and 7.42 in the 25 mg qd, 100 mg qd and 200 mg qd cohorts, respectively. The initial treatment period was set at 24 weeks, but was extended in a blinded fashion through 48 weeks.

Emtricitabine produced potent inhibition of HBV DNA in a dose-dependent manner. The median change from baseline in HBV DNA for the 25, 100 and 200 mg qd dose groups was 1.7, 3.1 and 3.2 $\log_{10}$, respectively. A similar dose response was seen in suppression of HBV DNA when analyzed by AAUCMB. However, differences between doses were pronounced when HBV suppression was viewed as the percentage of patients in whom viral load falls below the limit of detection (LOD). The percent of patients with HBV DNA below the LOD (4700/CmL) was 38% in the 25 mg qd dose cohort, 42% in the 100 mg qd dose cohort and 61% in the 200 mg qd dose cohort.

Based on this data the 200 mg qd dose was selected for evaluation in pivotal therapeutic trials, FTCB-301. FTCB-301 is a double-blind, randomized, placebo-controlled pivotal study designed to prove the safety and efficacy of the emtricitabine 200 mg qd dose for the treatment of chronic HBV infection.

Epilogue

It is apparent that emtricitabine represents one of the most potent anti-HIV agents identified to date, producing an almost two $\log_{10}$ drop in viral load as monotherapy at a 200 mg qd dose. In addition, the clinical profile of emtricitabine has demonstrated the following key features: 1) a plasma half-life of approximately eight to 10 hours with linear kinetics, 2) an intracellular emtricitabine 5'-triphosphate half-life of greater than 39 hours, which supports once daily dosing, 3) no significant drug – drug interactions which would limit the use of emtricitabine in combination therapy, 4) comparable safety and efficacy to lamivudine, 5) a low incidence of M184V mutations. This is an extremely important observation which suggests that emtricitabine could increase the durability of oxathiolane nucleoside analog-containing drug regimens.

Although the HBV clinical development program is just entering the pivotal phase, there are already data to suggest that at the same 200 mg qd dose selected for HIV development, there is a lower incidence of the rtM204V mutation than has historically been reported for lamivudine [55]. As with HIV, this observation holds out the possibility of more durable therapy for the treatment of chronic HBV infection. It also suggests that emtricitabine will be an extremely important drug for the treatment of patients coinfected with HIV and HBV.

Acknowledgement

This review would not have been possible without the expertise and dedication of numerous technicians, patients and scientific colleagues. We are indebted to all of them.

This work has been supported over the years, in part, by various grants from the NIH and the Department of Veterans Affairs (RFS). Finally, we would like to dedicate this manuscript to the memory of David Walter Barry, MD. His passion for finding drugs to treat serious viral disease has made millions of lives better. We miss him.

References

1. Anonymous. "Kaposi's sarcoma and pneumocystis pneumonia among homosexual men: New York City and California." *MMWR Morb. Mortal. Wkly. Rep.* 1981; 30.
2. Barre-Sinoussi F, Chermann J, Rey F, Nugeyre M, Chamaret S, Gruest J, Dauguet C, Axler-Blin C, Vezinet-Brun F, Rouzioux C, Rozenbaum W and Montagnier L. "Isolation of a T-lymphotropic retrovirus from a patient at risk for acquired immune deficiency syndrome (AIDS)." *Science* 1983;220: 868-871.
3. Gallo R, Sarin P, Gelmann E, Robert-Guroff M, Richardson E, Kalyanaraman V, Mann D, Sidhu R, Stahl R, Zolla-Pazner S, Leibowitch J and Popovic M. "Isolation of human T-cell leukemia virus in acquired immune deficiency syndrome (AIDS)." *Science* 1983;220: 865-867.
4. Carpenter C, Cooper D, Fischl M, Gatell J, Gazzard B, Hammer S, Hirsch M, Jacobsen D, Katzenstein D, Montaner J, Richman D, Saag M, Schechter M, Schooley R, Thompson M, Vella S, Yeni P and Volberding P. "Antiretroviral therapy in adults: Updated recommendations of the International AIDS society-USA panel." *JAMA* 2000;283: 381-390.
5. Beasley R. "Hepatitis B virus. The major etiology of hepatocellular carcinoma." *Cancer* 1988;61: 1942-1956.
6. Van Roey P, Panghorn W, Shinazi R, Painter G and Liotta DC. "Absolute configuration of the antiviral agent (-)-cis-5-fluoro-1-[2-hydroxymethyl-1,3-oxathiolane-s-yl] cytosine." *Antivir. Chem. Chemother.* 1993;4: 369-375.
7. Painter G, St. Clair MH, Chin S, Noblin J, Wang L and Furman PA. "524W91." *Drugs of the Future* 1995;20: 761-765.
8. Schinazi RF, McMillan A, Cannon D, Mathis R, Lloyd RMJ, Peck A, Sommadossi J-P, St. Clair MH, Wilson JE, Furman PA, Painter G, Choi W-B and Liotta DC. "Selective inhibition of human immunodeficiency viruses by racemates and enantiomers of *cis*-5-fluoro-1-[2-(hydroxymethyl)-1,3-oxathiolan-5-yl]cytosine." *Antimicrob. Agents Chemother.* 1992;36: 2423-2431.
9. Jeong LS, Schinazi RF, Beach JW, Kim HO, Nampalli S, Shanmuganathan K, Alves AJ, McMillan A, Chu CK and Mathis R. "A symmetric synthesis and biological evaluation of β-L-(2R,5S)- and α L-(2R,5R)-1,3-oxathiolane-pyrimidine and -purine nucleosides as potential anti-HIV agents." *Journal of Medicinal Chemistry* 1993;36: 181-195.
10. Gosselin G, Schinazi RF, Sommadossi J-P, Mathe C, Bergogne M-C, Aubertin A-M, Kirn A and Imbach J-L. "Anti-human immunodeficiency virus activities of the β-L enantiomer of 2',3'-dideoxycytidine and its 5-fluoro derivative *in vitro*." *Antimicrob. Agents Chemother.* 1994;38: 1292-1297.
11. Tisdale M, Kemp S, Parry NR and Larder B. "Rapid *in vitro* selection of human immunodeficiency virus type 1 resistant to 3'-thiacytidine inhibitors due to a mutation in the YMDD region of reverse transcriptase." *Proc. Natl. Acad. Sci. USA.* 1993;90: 5653-5656.
12. Mathez D, Schinazi RF, Liotta DC and Leibowitch J. "Infectious amplificatin of wild-type human immunodeficiency virus from patients' lymphocytes and modulation by reverse transcriptase inhibitors *in vitro*." *Antimicrob. Agents Chemother.* 1993;37: 2206-2211.

13. Schinazi RF, Gosselin G, Faraj A, Korba BE, Liotta DC, Chu CK, Mathe C, Imbach J.-L and Sommadossi J-P. "Pure nucleoside enantiomers of β-2',3'-dideoxycytidine analogs are selective inhibitors of hepatitis B virus *in vitro*." *Antimicrob. Agents Chemother.* 1994;38: 2172-2174.
14. Furman PA, Davis M, Liotta DC, Paff M, Frick LW, Nelson DJ, Dornsife RE, Wurster JA, Wilson LJ, Fyfe JA, Tuttle JV, Miller WH, Condreay L, Averett DR, Schinazi RF and Painter GR. "The anti-hepatitis B virus activities, cytotoxicities, and anabolic profiles of the (-) and (+) enantiomers of cis-5-fluoro-1-[2-(hydroxymethyl)-1,3-oxathiolan-5-yl]cytosine." *Antimicrob. Agents Chemother.* 1992;36: 2686-2692.
15. Ma TW, Lin J, Newton M, Cheng YC and Chu CK. "Synthesis and anti-hepatitis B virus activity of 9-(2-deoxy-2-fluoro-B-L-arabinofuranosyl)purine nucleosides." *Journal of Medicinal Chemistry* 1997;40: 2750-2754.
16. Ying C, De Clercq E, Nicholson W, Furman P and Neyts J. "Inhibition of the replication of the DNA polymerase m550v mutation variant of human hepatitis B virus with adefovir tenofovir, L-FMAU, DAPD, penciclovir and lobucavir." *J. Viral Hepat.* 2000;7: 161-165.
17. Shaw T, Mok S and Locarnini S. "Inhibition of hepatitis B virus DNA polymerase by enantiomers of penciclovir triphosphate and metabolic basis for selective inhibition of HBV replication by penciclovir." *Hepatology* 1996;24: 996-1002.
18. DeMan RA, Wotters L, Nevans F, Chuci D, Sherman M, Lai CL, Thomas N and Dettertogh D. *51st Annual American Association for the Study of Liver Desease Meeting,* 2000 Dallas, TX, USA.
19. Condreay LD, Condreay JP, Jansen RW, Paff MT and Averett DR. "(-)-cis-5-fluoro-1-[2-(hydroxymethyl)-1,3-oxathiolan-5-yl]cytosine (524W91) inhibits hepatitis B virus replication in primary human hepatocytes." *Antimicrob. Agents Chemother.* 1996;40: 520-523.
20. Paff MT, Averett DR, Prus KL, Miller WH and Nelson DJ. "Intracellular metabolism of (-)-and (+)-*cis*-5-fluoro-1-[2-(hydroxymethyl)-1,3-oxathiolan-5-yl]cytosine in HepG2 derivative 2.2.15 (subclone P5A) cells." *Antimicrob. Agents Chemother.* 1994;38: 1230-1237.
21. Furman PA, Wilson JE, Reardon JE and Painter G. "The effect of absolute configuration on the anti-HIV and anti-HBV activity of nucleoside analogues." *Antivir. Chem. Chemother.* 1995;6: 345-355.
22. Rousseau FS, Kahn JO, Thompson M, Mildvan D, Shepp D, Sommadossi JP, Delehanty J, Simpson JN, Wang LH, Quinn JB, Wakeford C and van der Horst C. "Prototype trial design for rapid dose selection of antiretroviral drugs: An example using emtricitabine (coviracil)." *J. Antimicrob. Chemother.* 2001;48: 507-13.
23. Shewach DS, Liotta DC and Schinazi RF. "Affinity of the antiviral enantiomers of oxothiolane cytosine nucleosides for human 2'-deoxycytidine kinase." *Biochem. Pharmacol.* 1993;45: 1540-1543.
24. Cheng Y-C, Krishnan, P, Chou KM, Liou JY, Lam W and Fu Q. "The role of 3-phosphoglycerate kinase and AP endonuclease for the action of antiviral L- nucleoside against hepatitis B and human immunodeficiency virus". *Hep. DART*, 2001; Maui, Hawaii, ELSEVIER.
25. Furman PA, Painter G and Anderson KS. "An analysis of the catalytic cycle of HIV-1 reverse transcriptase: Opportunities for chemotherapeutic intervention based on enzyme inhibition." Curr. Pharm. Des. 2000;5: 547-567.
26. Feng JY, Shi J, Schinazi RF and Anderson KS. "Mechanistic studies show that (-)-FTC-TP is a better inhibitor of HIV-1 reverse transcriptase than 3TC-TP." *FASEB J.* 1999;13: 1-7.
27. Wilson JE, Aulabaugh A, Caligan B, McPherson S, Wakefield JK, Jablonski S, Morrow CD, Reardon JE and Furman PA. "Human immunodeficiency virus type-1 reverse transcriptase." *J. Biol. Chem.* 1996;271: 13656-13662.
28. Ganem D and Varmus HE. "The molecular biology of the hepatitis B viruses." *Annu. Rev. Biochem.*

1987;56: 651-693.

29. Miller RH and Robinson WS. "Common evolutionary origin of hepatitis B virus and retroviruses." *Proc. Natl. Acad. Sci. USA* 1986;83: 2531-2535.
30. Davis MG, Wilson JE, Van Draanen NA, Miller WH, Freeman GA, Daluge SM, Boyd FL, Aulabaugh AE, Painter GR and Boone LR. "DNA polymerase activity of hepatitis B virus particles: Differential inhibition by L-enantiomers of nucleotide analogs." *Antiviral Res.* 1996;30: 133-145.
31. Ussery MA, Wood OL, Kunder SC, Bacho MA, Broud DD, Vona SF, Hall BE, Ciavarella A, Nielsen CJ, Hurwitz S and Schinazi RF. "Antiviral activity of six novel compounds [(-)-FTC, (+/-)-FTC, D-DAPD, D-D4FC, CS-92, and CS-87] in the HIV-infected HuPBMC SCID mouse model". 1998; *2nd International Workshop on HIV Drug Resistance and Treatment Strategies,* Lake Maggiore, Italy, International Medical Press.
32. Kamkolar M, Clayton MM, Zhang SM, Black PL, Schinazi RF and Feitelson MA. "Novel therapeutics for the hepatitis B and C; Evaluation of therapies for hepatitis B virus in the HBV transgenic SCID mouse model". 2002; *Frontiers in viral hepatitis.* ELSEVIER SCIENCE. Printed in the Netherlands. In Press.
33. Galibert F, Chen TF and Mandart E. "Nucleotide sequence of the cloned woodchuck hepatitis virus genome. Comparison with hepatitis virus B sequence." *J. Virol.* 1982;41: 51-65.
34. Tennant B, Peek SF, Tochkov IA, Baldwin BH, Hornbuckle WE, Korba B, Cote P and Guerin JL. "The woodchuck in preclinical assesment of therapy for hepatitis B infection." *Therapy for viral hepatitis.* 1998; RF Shinazi, JP Sommadossi and HC Thomas Eds. Atlanta, International Medical Press: 171-176.
35. Korba BE, Schinazi RF, Cote P, Tennant BC and Gerin JL. "Effect of oral administration of emtricitabine on woodchuck hepatitis virus replication in chronically infected woodchucks." *Antimicrob. Agents Chemother.* 2000;44: 1757-1760.
36. Cullen JM, Smith SL, Davis MG, Dunn SE, Botteron C, Cecchi A, Linsey D, Linzey D, Frick L, Paff MT, Goulding A and Biron K. "In vivo antiviral activity and pharmacokinetics of (-)-cis-5-fluoro-1-[2-(hydroxymethyl)-1,3-oxathiolan-5-yl]cytosine in woodchuck hepatitis virus-infected woodchucks." *Antimicrob. Agents Chemother.* 1997;41: 2076-2082.
37. Schinazi RF, Lloyd RMJ, Nguyen M-H, Cannon D, McMillan A, Ilksoy N, Chu CK, Liotta DC, Bazmi HZ and Mellors JW. "Characterization of human immunodeficiency viruses resistant to oxathiolane-cytosine nucleosides." *Antimicrob. Agents Chemother.* 1993;37: 875-881.
38. Wilson JE, Martin JL, Borroto-Esoda K, Hopkins S, Painter G, Liotta DC and Furman PA. "The 5' -triphosphates of the (-) and (+) enantiomers of cis-5-fluoro-1-[2-(hydroxymethyl)-1,3-oxathiolane-5-yl]cytosine equally inhibit human immunodeficiency virus type 1 reverse transcriptase." *Antimicrob. Agents Chemother.* 1993;37: 1720-1722.
39. Stuyver L, Locarnini S, Lok A, Richman D, Carman W, Dienstag J and Schinazi R. "Nomenclature for antiviral-resistant human hepatitis B virus mutations in the polymerase region." *Hepatology* 2001;33: 751-757.
40. Ladner S, Otto M, Barker C, Zaifert K, Wang G, Guo J, Seeger C and King R. "Inducible expression of human hepatitis B virus (HBV) in stably transfected hepatoblastoma cells: A novel system for screening potential inhibitors of HBV replication." *Antimicrob. Agents Chemother.* 1997;41: 1715-1720.
41. Ladner SK, Miller TJ and King RW. "The M539V polymerase variant of human hepatitis B virus demonstrates resistance to 2'-deoxy-3'-thiacytidine and a reduced ability to synthesize viral DNA." *Antimicrob. Agents Chemother.* 1998;42: 2128-2131.
42. Van Draanen NA, Tisdale M, Parry NR, Jansen R, Dornsife RE, Tuttle JV, Averett DR and Koszalka GW

"Influence of stereochemistry on antiviral activities and resistance profiles of dideoxycytidine nucleosides." *Antimicrob. Agents Chemother.* 1994;38: 868-871.

43. Richman DD. "Antiretroviral activity of emtricitabine, a potent nucleoside reverse transcriptase inhibitor." *Antiviral Therapy* 2001;6: 83-88.
44. Chen C, Vazquez-Padua M and Cheng Y. "Effect of anti-human immunodeficiency virus nucleoside analogs on mitochondrial DNA and its implication for delayed toxicity." *Mol. Pharmacol.* 1991;39: 625-628.
45. Chen C and Cheng Y. "Delayed cytotoxicity and selective loss of mitochondrial DNA in cells treated with the anti-human immunodeficiency virus compound 2',3'- dideoxycytidine." *J. Biol. Chem.* 1989;264: 11934-11937.
46. Dalakas M, Illa I, Pezeshkpour G, Laukaitis J, Cohen B and Griffin J. "Mitochondrial myopathy caused by long-term zidovudine therapy." *N. Engl. J. Med.* 1990;322: 1098-1105.
47. Cui L, Schinazi RF, Gosselin G, Imbach J-L, Chu CK, Rando RF, Revankar GR and Sommadossi J-P. "Effect of β-enantiomeric and racemic nucleoside analogues on mitochondrial functions in HepG2 cells." *Biochem. Pharmacol.* 1996;52: 1577-1584.
48. Grizzle TB, Wang LH, Walsh JP, Hart RW, Begley JA and Szczech GM. "Emtricitabine: Summary of toxicology and nonclinical pharmacology evaluations". 2000; *40th Interscience Conference on Antimicrobial Agents and Chemotherapy*, Toronto, Canada.
49. Frick L, Lambe C, St. John L, Taylor L and Nelson D. "Pharmacokinetics, oral bioavailability, and metabolism in mice and cynomolgus monkeys of (2'R,5'S-)-cis-5-fluoro-1-[2-(hydroxymethyl)-1,3-oxathiolan-5-yl] cytosine, an agent active against human immunodeficiency virus and human hepatitis B virus." *Antimicrob. Agents Chemother.* 1994;38: 2722-2729.
50. Frick L, St. John L, Taylor L, Painter G, Furman P, Liotta D, Furfine E and Nelson D. "Pharmacokinetics, oral bioavailability, and metabolic disposition in rats of (-)-cis-5-fluoro-1-[2-(hydroxymethyl)-1,3-oxathiolan-5-yl] cytosine, a nucleoside analog active against human immunodeficiency virus and hepatitis B virus." *Antimicrob. Agents Chemother.* 1993;37: 2285-2292.
51. Grizzle TB, Wang LH, Walsh JP, Song N and Szczech GM. "Adsorbtion, distribution, metabolism and excretion (adme) studies of ^{14}C-emtricitabine (Coviracil; FTC) in monkeys and rats." 2001; *Society of Toxicology Annual Meeting 2001*, San Franscisco, USA.
52. Bartlett JA, DeMasi R, Quinn J, Moxham C and Rousseau F. "Overview of the effectiveness of triple combination therapy in antiretroviral-naive HIV-1 infected adults." *AIDS* 2001;15: 1369-1377.
53. Gish RG, Leung NW, Schooley R, Sykes A, Turner HS, Wakeford C, Delahanty J and Rousseau F. "Emtricitabine (FTC): Activity against hepatitis B virus in a phase I/II clinical study". 1999; *39th Interscience Conference on Antimicrobial Agents and Chemotherapy.*
54. Gish RG, Wright TL, Wang C, Corey L, Leung NW, Chang F, Fried MW, Sacks S, Fang L, Wang LH, Rousseau FS and Delahanty J. "Emtricitabine (FTC): Results from 24-week dose selection trial in patients with chronic HBV infection (FTCB102)". 2000; *51th Annual American Association for the Study of Liver Desease Meeting.*
55. Rousseau F, Fang H, Sykes A, Rigney A and Mondou E. "Emtricitabine: Antiviral efficacy and lack of development of resistance in patients treated one year for chronic hepatitis B virus infection." 2001; *5th International workshop on HIV drug resistance and treatment strategies*, Scottsdale, AR, USA.

CD81 receptor expression in human cells: Implications for HCV therapeutics

PHILLIP M. THARNISH[1], AMY S. JUODAWLKIS[1], CRAIG L. HILL[2], and RAYMOND F. SCHINAZI[1]

[1] *Emory University School of Medicine/VA Medical Center, Decatur, GA, 30033, USA*
[2] *Emory University, Department of Chemistry, Atlanta GA, 30322, USA*

Abstract

Background

It was reported that the HCV envelope protein E2 binds to human CD81, a tetraspanin expressed on hepatocytes and lymphocytes. Inhibitors of this binding could prevent HCV transmission.

Objectives

The objectives were to determine the level of expression in continuous cell culture systems and primary human cells to develop therapeutic modalities that prevent the binding of HCV to the CD81 receptor, and to determine which of nine cell systems (PBM, human peripheral blood mononuclear cells; CEM, human T-cell lymphoma cells; Vero, African green monkey kidney cells; SK-MES-1, human lung squamous carcinoma cells; SK-MEL-28, human melanoma cells; HepG2, human liver carcinoma cells; JY, human B-cells; BL41, human B-cells; and 9L, rat glioma cells) had the highest CD81 expression using flow cytometric analysis. Using the best cell system (CEM cells), 23 polyoxometalates, a bicyclam, and three sulfated alkyl oligosaccharides were evaluated for their ability to inhibit CD81 binding.

Methods

Single cell suspensions were prepared of each cell line. Cells were washed with PBS and then incubated with either an isotype control or CD81-PE. Cells were washed with PBS and fixed with 1% paraformaldehyde, then analyzed on a FACScalibur cell sorter. The cells were incubated for one hour with the compounds (100 μM), washed and processed as above.

Frontiers in Viral Hepatitis Ed. by RF Schinazi, J-P Sommadossi and CM Rice. 485 — 492

Results

The order of percent increase in fluorescence of R-Phycoerythrin conjugated anti-human CD81 compared to isotype control was found to be CEM (99%) = Vero (99) = JY (98) = BL-41 (98) = PBM (98) = SK-MEL-28 (97) > SK-MES-1 (88) >> 9L (1) > HepG2 (0). Since CEM expressed a high level of CD81 receptors, studies were initiated to determine if polyoxometalates, a bicyclam, and sulfated alkyl oligosaccharides could specifically prevent binding to the receptor. None of the 27 compounds evaluated demonstrated inhibition of greater than 50% at 100 μM.

Conclusions

The lack of CD81 receptors on human HepG2 cells may explain the inability to infect these cells with HCV. The results indicate that the capacity to mediate or inhibit HCV attachment by CD81 should be studied in primary human lymphocytes (such as CEM cells), B cells or Vero cells. Certain compounds that were known to inhibit HIV-1_{LAI} modestly inhibited CD81 binding.

Introduction

Hepatitis C virus (HCV) is a medically important human pathogen. This virus infects approximately 170 million people worldwide, yet there is no vaccine available [1]. Treatment of HCV with alpha interferon alone or in combination with ribavirin is only efficacious in a small portion of infected individuals [2]. The need is great for more effective antiviral drugs that are orally bioavailable for HCV. Specific antiviral agents are needed to block direct viral replication, prevent ongoing infection of normal hepatocytes, and progression to hepatocellular carcinoma [3]. Research has identified and characterized new targets for HCV, such as the HCV serine protease [4], helicase [5] and HCV RNA-dependent RNA polymerase (RDRP) [6]. Additional targets for antiviral studies are core and envelope proteins, the internal ribosomal entry site, and most recently CD81 [7].

It was reported that the HCV envelope protein E2 binds to human CD81, a tetraspanin expressed on hepatocytes and lymphocytes [7]. The CD81 protein is a member of the tetraspanin family, which contains four transmember domains with two extracellular loops [8, 9]. CD81 forms many molecular complexes across different species and cell types. The CD81 large extracellular loop (LEL) domain is highly conserved among primates, yet humans and chimpanzees are the only primates susceptible to HCV infection. The CD81 receptor on the cells of these two mammals can also bind HCV-E2 [7]. Similar studies in other primates, including the African green monkeys and tamarins, have shown that these species are naturally resistant to HCV infection [10, 11]. This is thought to be due to a species-specific form of CD81 in these animals, rendering them resistant by not permitting the requisite HCV-E2 interaction [12].

Inhibitors of binding HCV-E2 to CD81 could prevent or reduce HCV transmission. To develop a high throughput screening system for discovering antiviral agents that can prevent the binding of HCV to the CD81 receptor, the level of CD81 expression in continuous cell culture systems and primary human cells was first determined. The results indicated that most mammalian cells expressed high levels of CD81 and were readily accessible. The next step was to evaluate compounds known to inhibit the binding and fusion process for other viruses including HIV, such as polyoxometalates [13], a bicyclam, and sulfated alkyl oligosaccharides [14] for inhibition of antibody binding to CD81. Nine cell systems (PBM, human peripheral blood mononuclear cells; CEM, human T-cell lymphoma cells; Vero, African green monkey kidney cells; SK-MES-1, human lung squamous carcinoma cells; SK-MEL-28, human melanoma cells; HepG2, human liver carcinoma cells; JY, human B-cells transformed with Epstein Barr virus (EBV); BL41, human Burkitt's lymphoma cells; and 9L, rat glioma cells) were investigated for CD81 expression using flow cytometric analysis.

Determination of levels of CD81 expression in cell culture systems

Human PBM cells were obtained from the American Red Cross, and cell lines CEM, Vero, SK-MES-1, SK-MEL-28, HepG2, and 9L were originally obtained from the American Type Culture Collection (Rockville, MD). The two other cell lines (JY and BL41) were obtained from Dr. J. Fingeroth, Beth Israel Deaconess Medical Center (Boston, MA). Single cell suspensions were washed with phosphate-buffered saline (PBS) and resuspended in a 10% inactivated human serum (Sigma)/PBS solution. The cells were incubated at room temperature for 15 min, then washed once with PBS and resuspended at a concentration of 5×10^5 cells in 200 μl PBS. The cells were stained with R-phycoerythrin-conjugated anti-human CD81 (BD Pharmingen, San Diego, CA) for 30 min at room temperature, washed and resuspended in 1% paraformaldehyde. The stained cells were then analyzed using a FACScalibur (Becton Dickinson, San Jose, CA) flow cytometer. Two data points were obtained: mean channel number (fluorescence intensity) and percent positive cells. Mean channel number (MCN) data were then calculated as a percent of CEM CD81 fluorescence intensity, as these cells expressed the highest mean channel number (highest intensity). To determine the percent positive cells, a region was selected around the cell population that was stained with the PE-conjugated isotype control IgG1 (BD Pharmingen, San Diego, CA). Cells stained with R-phycoerythrin-conjugated anti-human CD81 outside the identical region were labeled positive for CD81 expression.

Determination of the inhibition of anti-human CD81 binding on CEM cells by various antiviral agents

CEM cells were washed with PBS and resuspended in a 10% human serum/PBS solution (Sigma). The cells were incubated at room temperature for 15 min, then were washed once with PBS and resuspended at a concentration of 5×10^5 cells in 100 μl PBS. To determine the optimum concentration for a binding inhibition negative control, the following concentrations of the purified human CD81 antibody (positive inhibition control) were selected: 0.5, 0.05, 0.025, 0.0125, and 0.00625 μg/ml. The optimum concentration was determined to be 0.025 μg/ml. Polyoxometalates were obtained from Dr. C. Hill, Department of Chemistry, Emory University, and sulfated alkyl oligosaccharides were obtained from Dainippon Ink and Chemicals, Chiba, Japan. AMD3100 was obtained from Dr. G. Henson, AnorMED, Langley, BC, Canada. Stock solutions were prepared in water and then the compounds in solution were added to the CEM cells at 100 μM final concentrations. The cells were then incubated at room temperature for one hour, and then processed as described as above.

Determination of anti-HIV activity in human PBM cells

Assays were performed in activated primary human PBM cells infected with HIV-1 (strain LAI) as previously described [13].

Table 1. CD81 expression in different cells stained with R-phycoerythrin (R-PE)-conjugated mouse anti-human monoclonal antibody to CD81, as determined using a FACScalibur flow cytometer.

Cells	MCN[a] (% of CEM)	% positive cells
CEM[b]	100	98.7
Vero[c]	96.1	98
HepG2[d]	0.1	0
9L[e]	0.1	1
SK-MES-1[f]	9.5	90.8
SK-MEL-28[g]	72.4	98.7
JY[h]	40.8	94.1
BL41[i]	57.9	98.7
PBM[j]	79.2	99.1

[a] MCN: mean channel number
[b] CEM: Human T-cell lymphoma
[c] Vero: African green monkey kidney
[d] HepG2: Human liver carcinoma cell
[e] 9L: Rat glioma
[f] SK-MES-1: Human lung squamous carcinoma
[g] SK-MEL-28: Human melanoma
[h] JY: Human Burkitt's lymphoma, EBV+
[i] BL41: Human Burkitt's lymphoma, EBV-
[j] PBM, Human peripheral blood mononuclear cell

Results

As shown in Table 1, CEM cells expressed CD81 at the highest intensity of the nine cell systems tested. The CEM cell population also stained ≈ 99% positive for CD81. Other cell systems also stained well for CD81, but some cells, such as HepG2 and 9L, did not. The cell systems are listed below by decreasing fluorescence intensity (mean channel number) of CD81-PE staining (percent, compared to CEM): Vero (96%) > PBM (79) > SK-MEL-28 (72) > BL41 (58) > JY (41) > SK-MES-1 (10) > HepG2 (0) = 9L (0). Seven cell systems were found to have over 90% of cells stain positive for CD81. The human HepG2 and 9L (rat glioma) cell systems did not stain over 1% of the cells positive for CD81. Results obtained with HepG2 cells were unexpected, as these cells are derived from human liver carcinoma cells.

Table 2. Inhibition of CD81 binding by polyoxometalates, a bicyclam, and sulfated alkyl oligosaccharides (at 100 μM), as measured by reduction in fluorescent staining of PE-conjugated anti-CD81.

Competitor/Code	Treatment	% negative for CD81[1]	% reduction in fluorescence intensity[2]	HIV-1_{LAI} activity (EC_{50}, μM) tested in PBMC[3]
None, cells only (+ control)		0.0	0.0	-
Isotype (- control)		98.8	100.0	-
5 μg α-human CD81		95.6	99.0	-
0.5 μg α human CD81		96.7	97.2	-
0.25 μg α-human CD81		98.1	98.6	-
0.125 μg α-human CD81		39.1	84.0	-
0.0625 μg α-human CD81		8.7	68.8	-
HS-005	$(NH_4)_{17}Na[NaSb_9W_{21}O_{86}]$	3.8	27.1	0.2
HS-008	β-$H_4SiW_{12}O_{40}$	1.6	**49.7**	0.3
HS-010	α-$(NH_4)_6 P_2W_{18}O_{62}$	1.9	6.4	0.9
HS-026	$(NH_4)_{14}NaP_5W_{30}O_{110}$	7.6	**78.7**	0.3
HS-052	$Na_{16}P_4W_{30}Ni_4(H_2O)_2O_{112}$	0.2	7.8	0.1
HS-053	$Na_{16}P_4W_{30}Mn_4(H_2O)_2O_{112}$	0.0	0.0	0.3
HS-054	$Na_{16}P_4W_{30}Fe_4(H_2O)_2O_{112}$	0.0	0.0	0.4
HS-055	$K_{10}Zn_4(H_2O)_2(PW_9O_{34})_2$	0.0	15.5	1.6
HS-056	$K_{10}Ni_4(H_2O)_2(PW_9O_{34})_2$	0.0	22.7	4.5
HS-057	$K_{10}Mn_4(H_2O)_2(PW_9O_{34})_2$	0.0	29.0	1.3
HS-058	$K_{10}Fe_4(H_2O)_2(PW_9O_{34})_2$	7.8	37.4	1.7
HS-083[4]	$M_4SiW_{11}O_{39}O(Si(CH_2)_3CH_3)_2$	0.0	28.7	36.2
HS-091	$K_9Mn(II)P_2O_{17}O_{61}$	0.0	17.1	0.2
HS-105	$(Me_3NH)_7SiW_9Nb_3O_{40}$	0.0	22.8	0.9

Table 2. Continued.

Competitor/Code	Treatment	% negative for CD81[1]	% reduction in fluorescence intensity[2]	HIV-1_{LAI} activity (EC_{50}, μM) tested in PBMC[3]
HS-106	$(Me_3NH)_8Si_2W_{18}Nb_6O_{77}$	0.0	29.1	0.3
HS-122	$Li_7HSi_2W_{18}Nb_6O_{77}$	3.3	18.5	0.8
HS-126	$K_4H_3PV_4W_8O_{40}$	0.0	24.0	0.8
HS-131	$(Me_3NH)_5(NbO_2)SiW_{11}O_{39}$	0.0	16.2	0.8
HS-133	$(Me_3NH)_5(TaO_2)SiW_{11}O_{39}$	0.0	14.7	1.4
HS-136	$(Me_3NH)_7(NbO_2)_3SiW_9O_{37}$	0.0	18.0	2.0
HS-144	$(Me_3NH)_5TaSiW_{11}O_{40}$	0.0	11.8	0.2
HS-146	$K_7NbP_2W_{17}O_{62}$	0.0	9.7	0.2
HS-158	$K_{12}Nb_6P_2W_{12}O_{62}$	17.3	**70.3**	0.3
AMD-3100	Bicyclam	0.4	1.7	<0.1
DIC-002	*n*-dodecyl β-D-laminari-tetraoside sulfate	0.0	14.2	0.9
DIC-003	*n*-dodecyl β-D-laminari-trioside sulfate	0.0	10.7	7.2
DIC-008	4-t-octylphenyl β-D-laminari-pentaoside sulfate	0.0	3.0	0.1

1 All data were compared to cells that were only stained with a human CD81-PE, these data were then given a value of percent negative.

2 Measured by reduction in mean channel number compared to stained CEM cells. Compounds in **BOLD are active**, ≥ 50% decrease in MCN.

3 See reference 13 and 14. Other results were obtained in human PBM cells infected with HIV_{LAI}.

4. $M = Me_4N$

The inhibition of CD81 binding by three different classes of compounds are shown in Table 2. Three polyoxometalates (HS-008, HS-026, and HS-158) showed ≥50% reduction in fluorescence intensity at 100 μM. One compound (HS-158) also inhibited total CD81 binding by 17.3%. No sulfated alkyl oligosaccharides or bicyclam affected CD81 binding. All the compounds evaluated had activity against HIV-1 in primary human lymphocytes.

Discussion

Contrary to our initial hypothesis, there was no CD81 receptor expression on HepG2 cells. This could explain the poor success of infecting these cells with HCV. It appears that different clones of HepG2 may express different levels of CD81 [15]. Vero cells expressed CD81 receptors at a high intensity. This suggests that the dissociation process (trypsinization) of the anchored cells did not remove the receptor.

The most advantageous cell system to study CD81 binding inhibition is the CEM system. These cells are a suspension and continuous line, they are readily available in most laboratories, easy to grow, and ≥99% of the cells express CD81 at a high intensity. This not only allows the determination of the percent of cells that will not bind with anti-CD81 after drug presence, but also the reduction in fluorescence intensity. The ideal candidate for CD81 binding inhibition would be a compound that reduces not only the fluorescence intensity, but also the actual number of cells that test positive for these receptors.

The polyoxometalates that had an inhibitory effect on the binding of CD81 (HS-008, HS-026, and HS-158) have previously shown inhibition of other viruses. These three compounds had an EC_{50} of 0.3 μM against $HIV\text{-}1_{LAI}$ in human PBM cells [13].

The significance of the CD81 receptor in the pathogenesis of HCV remains to be confirmed. Alternately, a coreceptor may be needed in liver cells for virus entry and replication. The results in CEM cells demonstrated that certain antifusion/binding compounds could interfere with the CD81 receptor. The availability of a reliable virus-producing cell culture system for evaluating potential anti-HCV compounds would greatly accelerate this research [16].

Acknowledgment:

This work was supported in part by the Department of Veterans Affairs, Emory Center for AIDS Research, and NIH grant AI-49180.

References

1. World Health Organization. *Hepatitis C Weekly Epidemiol. Rec.* 1997;72:65-69.
2. McHutchinson JG, Gordon SC, Schiff ER, Shiffman ML, Lee WM, Rustgi VK, Goodman ZD, Ling MH, Cort S, Albrecht JK. Interferon alpha-2b alone or in combination with ribivarin as initial treatment for chronic hepatitis C. *N. Engl. J. Med.* 1998;339:1485-1492.
3. DiBisceglie AM. Hepatitis C--virology and future antiviral targets. *Am J Med* 1999;107(6B):45S-48S.
4. Love RA, Paige HE, Wickersham JA, et al. The crystal structure of hepatitis C virus NS3 proteinase reveals a trypsin-like fold and a structural zinc-binding site. *Cell* 1996;87:331-342.
5. Kim JL, Morgentern KA, Griffith JP, et al. Hepatitis C virus NS3 RNA helicase domain with a bound oligonucleotide: the crystal structure provides insights into the models of unwinding. *Structure* 1998;6:89-100.
6. Caselman WH, Eisenhardt S, Alt M. Synthetic antisense oligodeoxynucleotides as potential drugs against hepatitis C. *Intervirology* 1997; 40:394-399.
7. Pileri P, Uematsu Y, Campagnoli S, et al. Binding of hepatitis C virus to CD81. *Science* 1998;282:938-941.
8. Levy S, Todd SC, Maeker HT. CD81 (TAPA-1) : a molecule involved in signal transduction and cell adhesion in the immune system. *Annu Rev Immunol* 1998;16:89-109.
9. Maeker HT, Todd SC, Levy S. The tetraspanin superfamily: molecular facilitators. *FASEB J.* 1997;11:428-442

10. Abe K, Kurata T, Termoto Y, Shiga J, and Shikata T. Lack of susceptibility of various primates and woodchucks to hepatitis C virus. *J Med Primatol* 1993;22:433-434.
11. Garson JA, Whitby K, Watkins P, and Morgan AJ. Lack of susceptibility of the cottontop tamarin to hepatitis C infection. *J Med Virol* 1997;52:286-288.
12. Higgenbottom A, Quinn ER, and Levy S. Identification of amino acid residues in CD81 critical for interaction with hepatitis C virus envelope glycoprotein. *J Virol* 2000;74:3642-3649.
13. Rhule JT, Hill CL, Judd DJ, Schinazi RF. Polyoxometalates in medicine. *Chem Rev* 1998;98:327-357.
14. Nakashima H, Inazawa, Ichiyama, Ito M, Ikushima N, Shoji T, Katsuraya K, Uryu T, Yamamoto N, Juodawlkis AS, Schinazi RF. Sulfated alkyl oligosaccarides inhibit human immunodeficiency virus *in vitro* and provide sustained drug levels in mammals. *Antiviral Chem Chemother* 1995;6:271-280.
15. Abrignani S. Hepatitis C virus - CD81 interaction: pathogenetic affects. *3rd International Conference on Therapies for Viral Hepatitis*. Maui, HI. Dec. 12-16, 1999. Abstract 6.
16. Schinazi RF, Ilan E, Black PL, Yao X, Dagan S. Cell based and animal models for hepatitis B and C viruses. *Antiviral Chem Chemother* 1999;10(3):99-114.

PREVENTION AND TREATMENT OPTIONS FOR HEPATOCELLULAR CARCINOMA

Resolution of hepatic fibrosis as a consequence of interferon therapy for hepatitis C

YASUSHI SHIRATORI, HARUHIKO YOSHIDA
and MASAO OMATA

Department of Gastroenterology, University of Tokyo, 7-3-1 Hongo, Bunkyo-ku, Tokyo 113, Japan

The natural history of chronic hepatitis C virus (HCV) infection suggests that there is a sequential but slow progression from acute HCV infection to chronic infection and cirrhosis, leading to death from either liver failure or hepatocellular carcinoma (HCC) [1-11]. Although chronic hepatitis, cirrhosis, and HCC are now accepted sequelae, their frequency and the rate of development of decompensation and HCC by which they contribute to mortality are not well known yet. Current knowledge comes mainly from retrospective studies. In contrast, prospective studies with long-term observation are rare. Thus, the natural history of chronic HCV infection could only be made by the summation of short-term prospective studies as well as a variety of retrospective studies.

Natural course of disease progression

Development of cirrhosis

Chronic infection with hepatitis C virus is a major cause of cirrhosis and hepatocellular carcinoma worldwide [11-19]. Chronic hepatitis C is a disease with considerable mortality and morbidity when the disease stage reaches cirrhosis, and HCC and decompensation occur in a large proportion of patients with HCV-related cirrhosis [7-9]. Many previous retrospective studies show that HCC and decompensation occur in a large proportion of advanced-stage chronic hepatitis C patients and compensated cirrhotic patients with HCV infection. Fattovich et al. [12] and Niederau C et al. [13] demonstrated that chronic hepatitis C is a disease with considerable mortality and morbidity, particularly when cirrhosis is present at diagnosis. Furthermore, Bonis et al. [14] recently showed that history of decompensation and serum albumin are useful for predicting the development of HCC, the need for liver transplantation, and death due to liver disease.

Although data have been collected from selected cases or from studies with relatively short follow-up periods [7-19] (Table 1), Yano et al. clarified the slowly progressive change of liver fibrosis by evaluating a fibrosis stage using two to ten biopsies during a mean follow-up period of 8.8 years (range: 1-26 years) in 70 chronic hepatitis C patients. Furthermore, they revealed that cirrhosis developed at a rate of 5% yearly

Frontiers in Viral Hepatitis Ed. by RF Schinazi, J-P Sommadossi and CM Rice. 495 — 514

among these patients. These data suggest that it takes approximately 20 years before developing cirrhosis after the onset of chronic hepatitis C. Furthermore, Fattovich [12] and Serfaty [18] showed that chronic hepatitis C is a disease with considerable mortality and morbidity with decompensation, particularly when cirrhosis is present at diagnosis, and the rate of decompensation ranged from 3.6% to 5% yearly. In addition, patients with compensated cirrhosis also progressed slowly, but once decompensation develops, the disease will be more progressive and results in higher mortality [20].

Concerning progression, alcohol intake is an independent risk factor in the clinical and histologic progression of HCV infection, and the latter is associated with the age of the patient, HCV genotype and viral level [21-23]. However, a precise mechanism has not yet been clarified. A recent study also showed that HIV seropositivity, alcohol consumption, age at HCV infection and severe immunosuppression are also associated with an increase in the fibrosis progression rate [24].

Development of hepatocellular carcinoma

The yearly incidence of HCC is approximately 3% in the various retrospective series of Caucasian patients with HCV-related compensated cirrhosis, in contrast to a 5-7% yearly incidence in Japan (Table 1), and risk factors for HCC include age (more than 60 years old), gender (male), advanced fibrosis staging (F3/4 vs. F1/2), histologic activity score, high ALT level, and IFN therapy.

Recently, annual incidence of HCC development was precisely calculated by Yoshida et al. [19] in the study Japanese National Surveillance Program of Inhibition of Hepatocarcinogenesis by Interferon Therapy (IHIT) using a large number of patients (2,890 patients; 490 were untreated and 2,400 were IFN treated.) with a moderately long observation period (4.3 years), indicating that the incidence of HCC was different according to the stage of fibrosis (Table 4). They clearly showed that the annual incidence of HCC was 0.4% for patients with F1, 2% for F2, 5% for F3, and 8% for F4. This high incidence of HCC in Japan may be partly due to the prevalence of periodic screening for HCC, with accurate diagnosis of HCC using ultrasonograhy, dynamic CT, and MR imaging in outpatient clinics in Japan. However, although there may be a high frequency of prior HBV infection among these patients, the difference in annual incidence of HCC between Asian and European countries should be clarified on the basis of detection modalities and screening for HCC development, as well as HBV viral markers.

Histological evaluation

Histological approaches to the assessment of disease progression and interferon (IFN) response have several limitations; factors influencing the interpretation of histological findings include sample variation, different or inconsistent definitions of pathological findings, the intra- and inter-observer variations in evaluation of histology, and the evaluation of an ordinal scale with nonconstant intervals in the case of paired biopsies. In spite of these difficulties, histological changes have become an important indicator of disease progression and treatment effect using several simple scoring systems.

Table 1. Annual frequency of disease progression and HCC development in patients with HCV infection

Author (Ref) (year)		Cirrhosis progression	HCC development
Colombo M (7) (1991)	Cirrhosis (n = 189)		2.6% yearly
Nishiguchi S (15) (1995)			
Cirrhosis (n = 45)		6.9% yearly	
Yano M (10) (1996)	CH (n = 70)	5% yearly	
		(3% yearly; low-grade activity)	
Mazella G (16) (1996)	Cirrhosis (n = 92)		3.4% yearly
Fattovich G (12) (1997)	CH (n = 384)	3.6% yearly	1.4% yearly
	[Cirrhosis (n = 136)]	(decompensation)	
Bruno S (17) (1997)	Cirrhosis (n = 163)		2.7% yearly
Serfaty L (18) (1998)			
Cirrhosis (n = 103)	5% yearly	3.3% yearly	
		(decompensation)	
Niederau C (13) (1998)			
CH (n = 838)		0.5% yearly	
	[Cirrhosis (n = 130)]		
Bonis PAL (14) (1999)	CH (n = 256)		1.9% yearly
Yoshida H (19) (1999)	CH (n = 490)		
	F1		0.4% yearly
	F2		2.0% yearly
	F3 (Pre-cirrhosis)		5.3% yearly
	F4 (Cirrhosis)		7.9% yearly

CH: chronic hepatitis, HCC: hepatocellular carcinoma
(n =): number of patients
(decompensated): incidence of decompensated cirrhosis

Histological scoring system

Histologic assessment has been evaluated according to validated scoring systems, mostly using the semiquantitative score proposed by Knodell or Scheuer [25, 26] (Table 2). Four categories are assessed according to the scoring system of Knodell; piecemeal necrosis and bridging necrosis, intralobular necrosis, portal inflammation, and fibrosis. Three categories are assessed in the scoring system of Scheuer; portal/periportal activity, lobular activity and fibrosis. Instead of these complex scoring systems using several

Table 2. Histological scoring systems

(a) Knodell score

Piecemeal necrosis and bridging necrosis

0: non
1: mild PMN
3: moderate PMN (<50% of the most portal tract)
4: marked PMN (>50% of the most portal tract)
5: moderate PMN plus bridging necrosis
10: multilobular necrosis

Intralobular necrosis

0: non
1: foci of hepatocellular necrosis <1/3 of lobule
3: foci of hepatocellular necrosis 1/3-2/3 of lobule
4: foci of hepatocellular necrosis >2/3 of lobule

Portal inflammation

0: non
1: mild
3: moderate
4: marked

Fibrosis

0: non
1: fibrous portal expansion
3: bridging fibrosis
4: cirrhosis

(b) Scheuer score

Portal/periportal activity

0: absent
1: portal inflammation
2: mild piecemeal necrosis
3: moderate piecemeal necrosis
4: severe piecemeal necrosis

Lobular activity

0: absent
1: inflammation but no necrosis
2: focal necrosis or acidophil bodies
3: severe focal cell damage
4: bridging necrosis

Fibrosis

0; absent
1: enlarged, fibrotic portal tract
2: periportal or portal-portal septa, but intact architecture
3: fibrosis with aechitectural distortion, but no obvious cirrhosis
4: probable or definite cirrhosis

Table 2. continued

(c) METAVIR score
Activity grade
A0: non
A1: mild
A2: moderate
A3: severe
Fibrosis stage
F0: non
F1: portal fibrosis without septa
F2: few septa
F3: numerous septa without cirrhosis
F4: cirrhosis

categories, histological features of chronic hepatitis have recently been classified into two simple categories: necroinflammatory activity and fibrosis, based on the distinction between necroinflammatory activity (the grade of disease) and the fibrosis (the stage of disease) [27-30]. The simple scoring system proposed by the METAVIR group and by Desmet et al. offers more reproducibility than the use of a numerical index in terms of intra-observer and inter-observer variation.

Natural course of histologic activity grade and fibrosis progression

Several studies using untreated patients as controls in the randomized control studies revealed that the activity grade of untreated chronic hepatitis C patients was not changed during 24-72 weeks of observation [31-37] (Table 3). Progression of fibrosis could not be defined in the short-term observation (Table 3). Only a couple of studies by Yano [10] and Shiratori [38] showed changes in inflammation and fibrosis stage of the liver using more than a couple of biopsy specimens over one to 25 years, indicating a slow progression of fibrosis in chronic hepatitis C (Table 4). Histological activity grade sometimes correlates well with clinical and biochemical assessments, but precise correlation of biochemical tests and histological grading has not been defined.

Recently, by using an equation for suspected estimation of the fibrosis progression rate from the value of fibrosis score (estimated by using a simple semiquantitative scoring system of fibrosis stage from F0 to F4) and the suspected date of infection (blood transfusion or intravenous drug use) (Table 5-a), Poynard et al. [39] evaluated the natural course of fibrosis progression rate in patients with chronic hepatitis C as 0.133/year (Table 6). They also clarified that the fibrosis progression rate was much higher in patients who were alcohol drinkers (0.168 unit/year) and male. In contrast, Mathurin et al. [40] show that persistently normal ALT levels are correlated with a

Table 3. Short-term histological change in activity grade and fibrosis stage in HCV-infected patients

Author (year)		Activity Grade		Fibrosis Stage
(1.5 year interval)				
	Entry	78 weeks	Entry	78 weeks
Gomez-Rubio M (31) (1991) (n = 15)	7.6	8.0	1.5	2.1
(1 year interval)				
		Activity Grade		Fibrosis Stage
	Entry	52 weeks	Entry	52 weeks
Camps J (32) (1993) (n = 16)	7.4	7.5	1.8	2.1
De Alava E (33) (1993) (n = 28)	8.4	7.7	1.8	2.0
Castillo I (34) (1993) (n = 20)	6.9	7.5	1.9	2.0
Rumi MG (35) (1995) (n = 28)		Activity Grade + Fibrosis Stage		
		Entry	52 weeks	
		9.0	8.8	
(0.5 year interval)				
		Activity Grade		Fibrosis Stage
	Entry	24 weeks	Entry	24 weeks
Causse × (36) (1991) (n = 16)	7.3	5.7	2.9	3.3
Marcellin P (37) (1991) (n = 18)	6.9	5.6	1.8	1.8

Activity garde: summation of the values of periportal necrosis, intralobular necrosis, and portal inflammation
(n =): number of patients

Table 4. Long-term histological change in activity grade and fibrosis stage in HCV-infected patients

Author (year)	Activity Grade		Fibrosis stage	
Shiratori Y (38) (2000) (n = 106)	Entry	4.8 years	Entry	4.8 years
	1.6	1.8	1.8	2.3

Assessment of activity grade: A0 to A3
Assessment of fibrosis stage: F0 to F4
(n =): number of patients

Table 5. Assessment of fibrosis progression rate

a) Suspected estimate of fibrosis progression rate

$$= \frac{\text{F score}}{\text{Tb T susp}}$$

F score: fibrosis staging score

Tb: Date of biopsy

T susp: Date of suspected infection (blood transfusion, drug use, etc.)

b) Validated evaluation of fibrosis progression rate

$$= \frac{\text{F 2nd F 1st}}{\text{T b2 T b1}}$$

F 2nd, F 1st: fibrosis staging score of 2nd biopsy or 1st biopsy

Tb2, Tb1: Date of 2nd biopsy and 1st biopsy

slow progression rate of fibrosis (0.05 unit/year). These values are based upon single, not paired, biopsies, and suspected (rather than proven) duration of infection from the patient's history. Shiratori et al. [38] calculated fibrosis progression rates using paired biopsy samples which were obtained at a significant time interval (Table 5-b), indicating that the natural fibrosis progression rate, calculated as the change of fibrosis staging per year, is approximately 0.100 unit/year in untreated patients free from alcohol. This fibrosis progression rate value was similar to the data of Sobesky [41], although they calculated the rate using a short-term interval (20 months) (Table 6).

Factors contributing to fibrosis progression

Factors contributing to histological progression were age, duration of disease, high level of ALT, and high histological activity index. Fibrosis has a strong correlation with periportal necrosis as well as portal inflammation. In addition, several studies revealed that histological progression is associated with age, HCV genotype and viral level, and alcohol intake is an independent risk factor in the clinical and histologic progression of HCV infection. Furthermore, Benhamou et al. [24] demonstrated that the fibrosis progression rate in HCV-HIV coinfected patients was 0.153 unit/year, in contrast to 0.106 unit/year in HCV-infected patients (Table 6), and that HIV seropositivity, alcohol consumption, age at HCV infection and severe immunosuppression are found to be associated with an increase in the fibrosis progression rate.

Table 6. Fibrosis progression rate in relation to host factors

Author (year)	Factor	Fibrosis progression rate (unit/year)
Poynard Y et al. (39) (n = 2235)		
	all cases with HCV infection	0.133
	alcohol >50g/day	0.168
	alcohol <50g/day	0.143
	no alcohol	0.125
	male	0.154
	female	0.111
Mathurin P et al. (40) (n = 80)		
	patients with normal ALT	0.050
Shiratori Y et al. -	Using paired biopsy- (38) (n = 106)	
	no alcohol	0.100
Sobesky R et al. -	Using paired biopsy- (41) (n = 102)	
		0.103
Benhamou Y et al. -	Using paired biopsy- (24)	
	HIV-HCV coinfection (n = 12)	0.153
	Matched HCV infection (n = 12)	0.106

(n =): number of patients examined.

Interferon response

After the introduction of interferon (IFN) for chronic hepatitis C with beneficial effects in the 1980s [42, 43], factors predictive of sustained response to IFN have been studied extensively [44-46]. Early studies used biochemical response to assess the efficacy of IFN therapy. However, as biochemical response during and after IFN administration cannot predict sustained response, virological evaluation is superior to biochemical response in long-term follow-up studies [43]. Thus, the efficacy of IFN therapy is defined virologically as the loss of serum HCV RNA, which can be measured at > six months posttreatment (sustained response: SR).

Recent long-term follow-up studies revealed that patients who tested negative for HCV RNA six months after treatment remained in remission with normal liver function and improved histological features, and they may have been cured of infection [47-49]. In contrast, approximately 20% of patients who have a long-term decrease in serum ALT concentration have evidence of the presence of HCV RNA in serum, and ultimately may suffer later relapse. Thus, the stable disappearance of indicators of HCV infection and of necroinflammatory and fibrogenetic process in the liver is assumed to represent the cure of the disease, and it may be used as the best surrogate end point.

Histological response with interferon

Liver histology offers an important insight into disease progression, prognosis, and treatment response. Though questions may arise regarding the appropriateness of liver biopsy after treatment to evaluate the effects of therapy and to determine the progression/regression of liver disease, a repeated biopsy performed at a remote time interval from the completion of treatment may provide qualitative and quantitative information about long-term response and define the extent of progression or regression in responders and nonresponders. In fact, previous studies revealed that biochemical and virological responses to IFN therapy are associated with a significant improvement in liver histology during and shortly after IFN therapy. The short-term (less than two years after the end of IFN therapy) histological improvement indicates the changes in inflammatory activity grade, especially in sustained responders [32, 33, 51-56]. However, long-term effects on histological changes in fibrosis remained unclear, with the exception of some recent publications.

Change in activity grade

Short-term effect

Short term effects of IFN therapy on histological improvement have been previously examined by many authors, and most studies have shown that histological improvement is seen at treatment cessation and/or within one to two years of follow-up [32, 33, 37, 50-58] (Table 7). A decline in the three inflammatory components (piecemeal necrosis, lobular inflammation, and portal inflammation) was observed at the end of treatment, especially in patients who were responders, including relapse patients (PR) and sustained responders (SR). A recent metanalysis shows the correlation of biochemical response (normalization of serum ALT) to IFN with histological improvement of inflammatory activity (periportal necrosis, interlobular necrosis, portal inflammation) [59]. The reduction in inflammatory activity among sustained responders persisted for six to 12 months after completion of IFN therapy.

Long-term effect

In contrast to a large number of studies with short-term observation after IFN therapy, only five studies revealed that an improvement of activity grade in patients with sustained response persisted beyond the two-year follow-up [38, 48, 60-62] (Table 8]. They also showed that activity grade in nonresponders was not improved, but remained unchanged.

Table 7. Change in activity grade between the paired biopsy samples (short-term observation: < 2 years)

Author (year)	Interferon response	Pretreatment	End-of-Tx	12 months after Tx
Camma C (51) (1998)	SR (n = 35)	10.1	3.9	-
	PR (n = 14)	9.8	4.7	-
	NR (n = 18)	11.3	12.4	-
Schiffman M (52) (1997)	SR (n = 45)	9.6	5.0	-
	NR (n = 45)	9.6	7.7	-
Lindsay KL (53) (1996)	SR (n = 62)	9.1	5.7	-
	NR(n = 48)	8.7	7.0	-
Hiramatsu N (54) (1995)	SR, PR (n = 25)	6.8	2.4	-
	NR (n = 15)	6.6	4.9	-
Kasahara A (55) (1995)	SR (n = 16)	6.0	2.4	-
	PR (n = 10)	5.0	2.0	-
	NR (n = 8)	6.0	6.0	-
Craxi A (56) (1995)	SR (n = 17)	5.7	1.8	-
	PR (n = 14)	6.7	4.1	-
DeAlava E (33) (1993)	SR (n = 10)	9.7	4.2	4.6
Camps J (32) (1993)	SR (n = 15)	9.7	4.1	-
	PR (n = 8)	7.0	4.2	-
Yamada G (57) (1993)	SR (n = 12)	8.9	4.1	-
	PR (n = 7)	10.7	7.8	-
	NR (n = 10)	12.0	11.4	-
Sieck JQ (58) (1993)	NR (n = 19)	8.9	8.4	-
Marcellin P (37) (1991)	PR (n = 16)	7.8	4.4	-
	NR (n = 22)	7.4	7.2	-

Scores of necroinflammatory activity were evaluated using the histological scoring systems of Knodell or Scheuer et al.

(n =): number of patients. Tx: treatment

SR: Sustained response, PR: Partial response (Relapse), NR: Nonresponse

Table 8. Change in activity grade between the paired biopsy samples with IFN therapy (long-term observation: ≥ 2 years)

Author (year)	Interferon response	Pretreatment	End-of-Tx	Date after Tx
Reichard O (48) (1995)				2 year
	SR (n = 14)	3.0	0.5	0.4
Tsubota A (60) (1997)				2 year
	SR (n = 93)	6.6	1.6	1.2
				2-6 year
				1.1
Marcellin P (61) (1997)				1-7.6 years
	SR (N = 80)	8	4	3-4
Lau DTY (62) (1998)				5-11 years
	SR (n = 5)	10	4	3
	NR (n = 5)	10	8	10
Shiratori Y (38) (2000)				3.2 years
	SR (n = 183)	2.1		0.6
	PR, NR (n = 304)	1.9		1.7

SR: Sustained response, PR: Partial response (Relapse), NR: Nonresponse
(n =): number of patients. Tx: treatment

Change in fibrosis stage

Short-term effect

In contrast to the improvement in activity grade in patients with SR and PR after a short-term interval following IFN therapy, amelioration or aggravation of the fibrosis staging score could not be determined during or shortly after the end of IFN therapy, due to the short time interval between paired biopsy samples (Table 9). The impact of treatment on the history of such a slowly progressive disease cannot be ascertained by evaluating results at the completion of treatment in a short-term observation of less than two years.

Table 9. Changes in fibrosis staging between the paired biopsy samples with IFN therapy (short-term observation: < 2 years)

Author (year)	Interferon response	Pretreatment	End-of-Tx	12 months after Tx
Lindsay KL (53) (1996)	SR (n = 62)	2.6	2.4	-
	NR (n = 48)	3.3	3.1	-
Hiramatsu N (54) (1995)	SR, PR (n = 25)	1.9	1.1	-
	NR (n = 15)	2.1	2.0	-
Kasahara A (55) (1995)	SR (n = 16)	2.2	1.3	-
	PR (n = 10)	1.7	1.2	-
	NR (n = 8)	3.1	2.9	-
Craxi A (56) (1995)	SR (n = 17)	2.2	1.6	-
	PR (n = 14)	2.3	2.6	-
Gallorini A (63) (1994)	SR (n = 15)	1.9	1.7	-
	PR (n = 11)	1.8	1.9	-
	NR (n = 9)	2.3	2.6	-
Marzella G (64) (1994)	PR (n = 16)	2.4	2.5	-
	NR (n = 8)	2.4	2.2	-
DeAlava E (33) (1993)	SR (n = 10)	1.3	1.3	1.3
Camps J (32) (1993)	SR (n = 15)	2.1	1.5	-
	PR (n = 8)	1.9	1.9	-
Capra F (65) (1993)	PR (n = 12)	2.7	2.6	-
	NR (n = 8)	2.0	2.0	-
Marcellin P (37) (1991)	PR (n = 16)	2.0	2.1	-
	NR (n = 22)	1.8	1.8	-

Scores of fibrosis staging were evaluated using the histological scoring systems of Knodell or Scheuer et al. SR: Sustained response, PR: Partial response (Relapse), NR: Nonresponse. (n =): number of patients, Tx: treatment.

Long-term effect

The effect of treatment on fibrosis regression or progression should instead be evaluated on a long-term basis. For this reason, it is possible that repeated liver biopsies performed at remote time intervals from the completion of treatment may provide qualitative and quantitative information about long-term response and may serve to define the activity grade and the extent of progression or regression in responders and nonresponders. As indicated in Table 10, amelioration of the fibrosis staging score was observed more than two years after IFN therapy in sustained responders.

When the fibrosis regression or progression rate was calculated using a validated evaluation equation (Table 5-b), Sobesky et al. [41] showed the amelioration of the fibrosis progression rate in 185 IFN-treated patients (calculated as 0.000 unit/year) in comparison with 102 untreated patients (0.103 unit/year), especially in the IFN responders, but the interval between the paired biopsies was too short (20 months) to evaluate the long-term histological changes. Furthermore, using a large number of patients (593) with paired biopsy samples at a remote interval of one to 10 years, a recent study by Shiratori et al. [38] showed that fibrosis was found to be regressed in patients with virological SR at a rate of -0.282 units/year. Among the patients with virological SR, the fibrosis progression rate ranged from -0.152 to -0.374 units/year (regression), irrespective of the initial fibrosis stages. They clearly showed that the fibrosis progression rate was retarded at a rate of 0.024 units/year, even in patients with non-SR after IFN therapy (Figure 3).

Table 10. Change in fibrosis stage between the paired biopsy samples with IFN therapy (long-term observation: $\geq$ 2 years)

Author (year)	Interferon response	Pretreatment	End-of-Tx	Follow-up after Tx
Reichard O (48) (1995)				2 year
	SR (n = 14)	1.3	1.2	0.8
Tsubota (60) (1997)				2 year
	SR (n = 93)	2.3	1.7	1.4
				2 6 year
				1.3
Marcellin P (61) (1997)	1-7.6 years	SR (N = 80)	1.6	1.0 1.2
Lau DTY (62) (1998)				5-11 years
	SR (n = 5)	1.2	0.5	0
	NR (n = 5)	3	3	3.6
Shiratori Y (38) (2000)				3.2 years
	SR (n = 183)	2.2		1.5
	PR, NR (n = 304)	2.1		2.2

SR: Sustained response, PR: Partial response (Relapse), NR: Nonresponse
(n =): number of patients. Tx; treatment

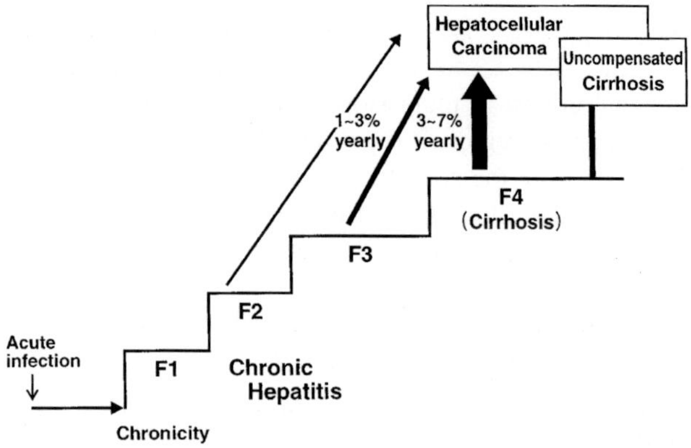

Figure 1. Scheme of natural course of HCV infection (fibrosis progression to cirrhosis and HCC development).

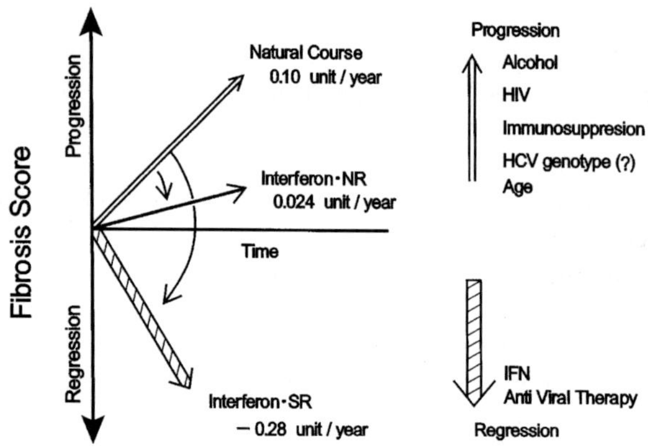

Figure 2. Effect of IFN therapy on fibrosis regression. Progression of fibrosis was different according to gender, alcohol drinking, and serum ALT levels (see in the text).

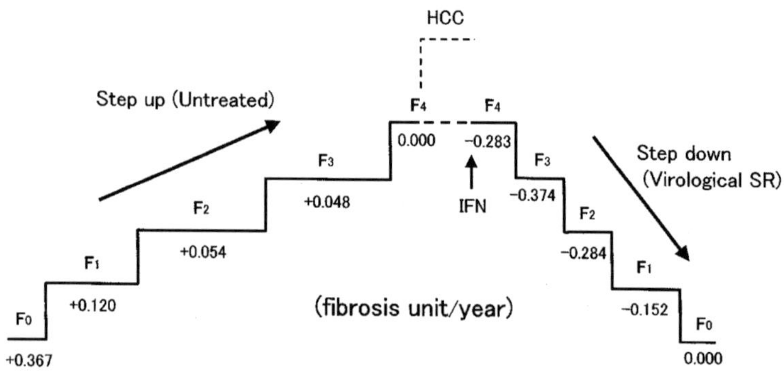

Figure 3. Progression of fibrosis in natural course of HCV infection and regression of fibrosis in patients with IFN therapy. SR; sustained virological responders, NR; nonsustained responders.

Table 11. Change in fibrosis progression/regression rate after interferon therapy

Shiratori Y et al. -	Using paired biopsies- (1-10 year observation) [38]	
	IFN-treated patients	fibrosis progression rate (fibrosis unit/year)
	Sustained responder (n = 183)	-0.282
	Nonsustained responder (n = 304)	0.024
Sobesky R et al. -	Using paired biopsies- (20 months observation) (41)	
	IFN-treated patients (n = 185)	0.000

+; progression of fibrosis, -; resolution of fibrosis

Correlation between improvement of histological activity and fibrosis regression after IFN therapy

The studies cited above show that the activity grade was markedly reduced after IFN therapy, especially in patients with sustained virological response. The reduction in activity grade in patients with sustained response could be observed soon after IFN therapy, and persisted thereafter. Fibrosis staging was regressed among these patients, and the change in fibrosis staging regressed stepwise and became dominant in association with the long term interval after IFN therapy. This phenomenon may be explained by the fact that the severity of hepatic inflammation may be a major factor driving progression of chronic hepatitis C to cirrhosis, and improving hepatic inflammation may be associated with regression or retardation of fibrosis.

Clinical improvement in natural course through IFN therapy

Delayed progression to cirrhosis

The benefit of therapy is remarkable, considering that cirrhosis is a major prognostic factor, and IFN prevents and delays these complications. Fattovich et al. [12] and Niederau C et al. [13] clearly showed the delay of decompensation, although IFN therapy did not reduce the risk of HCC, perhaps due to the small number of HCC cases in their studies. In addition to these studies, several retrospective cohort studies clearly showed that IFN therapy reduces the risk for disease progression (Table 9). From the results of these studies, more efficient therapy using IFN and ribavirin may have a strong impact on the improvement of the natural course of hepatitis C infection, since combination therapy is known to induce a higher eradication rate compared with IFN monotherapy.

Reduced risk of HCC development in relation to fibrosis stage with IFN therapy

In evaluating the effect of IFN therapy on inhibition of HCC development from published papers, the most important points that should be taken into account are that patients with advanced liver fibrosis are more likely to develop HCC, but are resistant to IFN therapy. The yearly incidence of HCC is 3% in the retrospective series of Caucasian patients with HCV-related compensated cirrhosis, in contrast to a yearly incidence of 5-7% in Japan [33-35].

There appears to be clear evidence of inhibition of HCC development after IFN therapy in a large number of patients with four to five years of follow up after IFN therapy [19, 66-72]. As the annual incidence of HCC development varies according to the fibrosis stage of the liver, the effect of IFN therapy was markedly demonstrated in patients with moderate fibrosis (F3 stage) in whom the risk of HCC development was high. On the other hand, the effect in patients with milder liver fibrosis (F0, F1) was low, because the annual incidence of HCC was low. In contrast, the difference between IFN-treated and untreated patients with liver cirrhosis did not attain statistical significance, due to low efficacy of IFN therapy among these patients.

These studies clearly showed that the reduced risk of HCC development seems to be associated not only with the disappearance of viremia, but with histological amelioration of hepatic inflammation. Yoshida [19] and Ikeda [70] adjusted the background features using multivariate analysis, indicating that an inhibition of HCC development with IFN was found in patients with persistent ALT normalization, indicating that the decreased risk of HCC development may be related to the suppression of inflammation and regeneration in the liver.

Conclusion

Chronic hepatitis C is a common disease that is often asymptomatic and mild, but which may slowly progress to cirrhosis and eventually to hepatocellular carcinoma (HCC). The data on delay of decompensation and inhibition of HCC development with IFN therapy shown in this chapter depend on the histological improvement in activity grade and regression of fibrosis stage with IFN therapy. The data shown in the recent retrospective studies may indicate that fibrosis may be improved even in cirrhotic patients after IFN therapy, and the viral eradication status of the cirrhotic patients may be similar to that in patients receiving liver transplantation.

References

1. Di Bisceglie AM, Goodman ZD, Ishak KG, Hoofnagle JH, Melpolder JJ, Alter HJ. Long-term clinical and histopathological follow-up of chronic posttransfusion hepatitis. Hepatology 1991; 14: 969-974
2. Seef LB, Buskell-Bales Z, Wright EG, et al. Long-term mortality after transfusion-associated non-A, non-B hepatitis. N Engl J Med 1992; 327: 1906-1911
3. Tong MJ, Neveen S, El-Farra NS, Reikes AR, Co RL. Clinical outcomes after transfusion-associated

hepatitis C. N Engl J Med 1995; 332: 1463-1466

4. Fattovich G, Giusta G, Degos F, et al. Morbidity and mortality in compensated cirrhosis type C: A retrospective follow-up study of 384 patients. Gastroenterology 1997; 112: 463-472
5. De Bisceglie AM, Goodman ZD, Ishak KG, Hoofnagle JY, Melpolder JJ, Alter HJ. Long-term clinical and histopathological follow-up of chronic posttransfusion hepatitis. Hepatology 1991; 14: 969-974
6. Roudot-Thoraval F, Bastie A, Pawlotsky JM, Dhumeaux D, and the study group for the prevalence and the epidemiology of hepatitis C virus. Epidemiological factors affecting the severity of hepatitis C virus-related liver disease: A French survey of 6664 patients. Hepatology 1997; 26: 485-490
7. Colombo M, de Franchis R, del Ninno E, Sangivanni A, De Fazio C, Tommasini M. Hepatocellular carcinoma in Italian patients with cirrhosis. N Engl J Med 1991; 325; 675-680
8. Tsukuma H, Hiyama T, Tanaka S, et al. Risk factor for hepatocellular carcinoma among patients with chronic liver disease. N Engl J Med 1993; 328: 1797-1801
9. Takano S, Yokosuka O, Imazeki F, Tagawa M, Omata M. Incidence of hepatocellular carcinoma in chronic hepatitis B and C: a prospective study of 251 patients. Hepatology 1995; 21: 650-655
10. Yano M, Kumada H, Kage M, et al. The long-term pathological evolution of chronic hepatitis C. Hepatology 1996; 23: 1334-1340
11. Kage M, Shimamatsu K, Nakashima F, Kojiro M, Inoue O, Yano M. Long-term evolution of fibrosis from chronic hepatitis to cirrhosis in patients with hepatitis C: morphometric analysis of repeated biopsies. Hepatology 1997; 25: 1028-1031
12. Fattovich G, Giustina G, Degos F, et al. Effectiveness of interferon alfa on incidence of hepatocellular carcinoma and decompensation in cirrhosis type C. J Hepatol 1997; 27: 201-205
13. Niederau C, Lange S, Heintges T, Erherdt A, Buschkamp M, Hurter D, et al. Prognosis of chronic hepatitis C: results of a large prospective cohort study. Hepatology 1998; 28: 1687-1695
14. Bonis PAL, Young MJ, Blatt LM, et al. A predictive model for the development of hepatocellular carcinoma, liver failure, or liver transplantation for patients presenting to clinic with chronic hepatitis C. Am J Gastroenterol 1999; 94: 1605-1612
15. Nishiguchi S, Kuroki T, Nakatani S, et al. Randomized trial of effects of interferon-alpha on incidence of hepatocellular carcinoma in chronic active hepatitis with cirrhosis. Lancet 1995; 346: 1051-1055
16. Mazella G, Accogli E, Sottili S, et al. Alpha interferon treatment may prevent hepatocellular carcinoma in HCV-related liver cirrhosis. J Hepatol 1996; 24: 141-147
17. Bruno S, Silini E, Crosignani A, et al. Hepatitis C virus genotypes and risk of hepatocellular carcinoma in cirrhosis: a prospective study. Hepatology 1997; 25: 754-758
18. Serfaty L, Aumatre H, Chazouileres O, Bonnan AM, Rosmorduc O, Poupon RE, Poupon R. Determinants of outcome of compensated hepatitis C virus-related cirrhosis. Hepatology 1998; 27: 1435-1440
19. Yoshida H, Shiratori Y, Moriyama M, Arakawa Y, Ide T, Sata M, et al. Interferon therapy reduces the risk for hepatocellular carcinoma: national surveillance program in Japan of cirrhotic and non-cirrhotic patients with chronic hepatitis C. Ann Intern Med 1999; 131:174-181
20. Hu KQ, Tong MJ. The long-term outcome of patients with compensated hepatitis C virus-related cirrhosis and history of parenteral exposure in the United Sates. Hepatology 1999; 29: 1311-1316
21. Wiley TE, McCarthy M, Breidi L, McCarthy M, Layden T. Impact of alcohol on the histological and clinical progression of hepatitis C infection. Hepatology 1998; 28: 805-809
22. Tassopoulos NC, Papatheodoridis GV, Katsoulidou A, et al. Factors associated with severity and disease progression in chronic hepatitis C. Hepatogastroenterology 1998; 45: 1678-1683
23. Pozzato G, Kanoko S, Moretti M, et al. Different genotypes of hepatitis C virus are associated with different severity of chronic liver disease. J Med Virol 1994; 43: 291-296

24. Benhamou Y, Bochet M, Di Martino V, et al. Liver fibrosis progression in human immunodeficiency virus and hepatitis C virus coinfected patients. Hepatology 1999; 30: 1054-1058
25. Knodell RG, Ishak KG, Black WC, et al. Formulation and application of a numerical scoring system for assessing histologic activity in asymptomatic chronic active hepatitis. Hepatology 1981; 1: 431-435
26. Scheuer C. Chronic hepatitis. In: Liver biopsy interpretation. Church Hills: London, 1988; 113-146
27. Desmet VJ, Gerber M, Hoofnagle JH, Manns M, Scheuer PJ. Classification of chronic hepatitis: Diagnosis, grading and staging. Hepatology 1994; 19: 1513-1520
28. Bedossa P, Poynard T for the METAVIR. An algorithm for the grading of activity in chronic hepatitis C. Hepatology 1996; 24: 289-293
29. The French METAVIR cooperative study group. Intraobserver and interobserver variations in liver biopsy interpretation in patients with chronic hepatitis C. Hepatology 1994; 20: 15-20
30. Kaserer K, Fiedler R, Steindl P, et al. Liver biopsy is a useful predictor of response to interferon therapy in chronic hepatitis C. Histopathology 1998; 32: 454-461
31. Gomez-Rubio M, Porres JC, Castillo I, et al. Prolonged treatment of chronic hepatitis C with recombinant alfa-interferon in comparison with a control group. J Hepatol 1990; 11: s63-s67
32. Camps J, Gaicia-Granero M, Riezu-Boj JI, et al. Prediction of sustained remission of chronic hepatitis C after a 12-month course of alfa interferon. J Hepatol 1994; 21: 4-11
33. De Alava E, Camps J, Pardo-Mindan J, et al. Histological outcome of chronic hepatitis C treated with a 12-month course of lymphoblastoid alfa interferon. Liver 1993; 13: 73-79
34. Castillo I, Bartolome J, Navas S, et al. Virological and biochemical long-term follow up of patients with chronic hepatitis C treated with interferon. Hepatology 1994; 19: 1342-1346
35. Rumi MG, del Ninno E, Parravicicni ML, et al. Long-term titrated recombinant interferon-alfa2a in chronic hepatitis C: a randomized control trial. J Viral Hep 1995; 2: 73-76
36. Causse X, Godinot H, Chevallier M, et al. Comparison of 1 or 3 MU of interferon alfa2b and placebo in patients with chronic non-A, non-B hepatitis. Gastroenterology 1991; 101: 497-502
37. Marcellin P, Boyer N, Giostra E, et al. Recombinant human alfa-interferon in patients with chronic non-A, non-B hepatitis: a multicenter randomized controlled trial from France. Hepatology 1991; 13: 393-397
38. Shiratori Y, Imazeki F, Moriyama M, et al. Histological improvement of fibrosis in patients with hepatitis C who have sustained response to interferon therapy. Ann Intern Med 2000; 132: 517-524
39. Poynard T, Bedossa P, Oplon P, for the OBSTIRC, METAVIR, CLINIVIR, and DOSVIRC groups. Natural history of liver fibrosis progression in patients with chronic hepatitis C. Lancet 1997; 349: 825-832
40. Mathurin P, Moussalli J, Cadranel JF, Thibault V, Charlotte F, Dumouchel P, Cazier A, et al. Slow progression rate of fibrosis in hepatitis C virus patients with persistently normal alanine transaminase activity. Hepatology 1998; 27: 868-872
41. Sobesky R, Mathurin P, Charlotte F, Moussalli J, et al. Modeling the impact of interferon alfa treatment on liver fibrosis progression in chronic hepatitis C: A dynamic view. Gastroenterology 1999; 116: 378-386
42. Hoofnagle JH, Di Bisceglie AM. The treatment of chronic viral hepatitis. New Engl J Med 1997; 336: 347-356
43. Lindsay KL. Therapy of hepatitis C: overview. Hepatology 1997; 26 (Suppl 1); 71s-77s
44. Lau JYM, Davis GL, Kniffen J, et al. Significance of serum hepatitis C virus RNA levels in chronic hepatitis C. Lancet 1993; 341: 1501-1504
45. Shiratori Y, Kato N, Yokosuka O, et al. Predictors of the efficacy of interferon therapy in chronic

hepatitis C virus infection. Gastroenterology 1997; 113: 558-566
46. Poynard T, Leroy V, Cohard M, et al. Meta-analysis of interferon randomized trials in the treatment of viral hepatitis C: effects of dose and duration. Hepatology 1996; 24: 778-789
47. Chemello L, Cavalletto L, Casarin C, et al. Persistent hepatitis C viremia predicts late relapse after sustained response to interferon-alpha in chronic hepatitis C. Ann Intern Med 1996; 124: 1058-1060
48. Reichard O, Glaumann H, Fryden A, et al. Two-year biochemical, virological, and histological follow-up in patients with chronic hepatitis C responding in a sustained fashion to interferon alpha-2b treatment. Hepatology 1995; 21: 918-922
49. Manesis EK, Papaioannou C, Gioustozi A, Kafiri G, Koskinas J, Hadziyannis SJ, Biochemical and virological outcome of patients with chronic hepatitis C treated with interferon alpha-2b for 6 or 12 months: A 4-year follow-up of 211 patients. Hepatology 1997; 26: 734-739
50. Camma C, Giunta M, Linea C, Pagliaro L. The effect of interferon on the liver in chronic hepatitis C: a quantitative evaluation of histology by meta-analysis. J Hepatol 1997; 26: 1187-1199
51. Camma C, Di Marco V, Iacocno OL, et al. Log-term course of interferon-treated chronic hepatitis C. J Hepatol 1998; 28: 531-537
52. Shiffmann M, Hoofmann CM, Thompson EB, et al. Relationship between biochemical, virological, and histological response during interferon treatment of chronic hepatitis C. Hepatology 1997; 26: 780-785
53. Lindsay KL, Davis GL, Schiff ER, et al. Response to higher doses of interferon alfa2b in patients with chronic hepatitis C: a randomized multicenter trial. Hepatology 1996; 24: 1034-1040
54. Hiramatsu N, Hayashi N, Kasahara A, et al. Improvement of liver fibrosis in chronic hepatitis C patients treated with natural interferon alpha. J Hepatol 1995; 22: 135-142
55. Kasahara A, Hayashi N, Hiramatsu N, et al. Ability of prolonged interferon treatment to suppress relapse after cessation of therapy in patients with chronic hepatitis C: a multicenter, randomized controlled trial. Hepatology 1995; 21: 291-297
56. Craxi A, Di Marco V, LoIanoco O, et al. Transfusion associated chronic hepatitis C: alfa interferon for 6 vs. 12 months. J Hepatol 1996; 24: 539-546
57. Yamada G, Takahashi M, Endo H, et al. Quantitative hepatitis C virus RNA and liver histology in chronic hepatitis C patients treated with interferon alfa. Gut 1993; suppl: S133-S134
58. Sieck JO, Ellias ME, Alfurayh O, et al. Histologically advanced chronic hepatitis C treated with recombinant alfa-interferon: a randomized placebo-controlled double-blind crosss over study. J Hepatol 1993; 19: 418-423
59. Bonis PA, Ioannidis JPA, Cappelleri JC, Kaplan MM, Lau J. Correlation of biochemical response to interferon alfa with histological improvement in hepatitis C: A meta-analysis of diagnostic test characteristics. Hepatology 1997; 26: 1035-1044
60. Tsubota A, Kumada H, Chayama K, et al. Time course of histological changes in patients with a sustained biochemical and virological response to interferon-alfa therapy for chronic hepatitis C virus infection. J Hepatol 1997; 27: 49-55
61. Marcellin P, Boyer N, Gervais A, Martinot M, Pouteau M, Castelnau C, et al. Long-term histologic improvement and loss of detectable intrahepatic HCV RNA in patients with chronic hepatitis C and sustained response to interferon-alfa therapy. Ann Intern Med 1997; 127: 875-881
62. Lau DTY, Kleiner DE, Ghany MG, Park Y, Schmid P, Hoofnagle JH. 10-year follow-up after interferon-alfa therapy for chronic hepatitis C. Hepatology 1998; 28: 1121-1127
63. Gallorini A, Plebani M, Pontisso P, et al. Serum markers of hepatic fibrogenesis in chronic hepatitis type C treated with alfa-2a interferon. Liver 1994; 14: 125-134

64. Mazella G, Salzetta A, Casanova S, et al. Treatment of chronic sporadic type non-A, non-B hepatitis with lymphoblastoid interferon. Dig Dis Sci 1994; 39: 866-870
65. Capra F, Casarii M, Gabrielli GB, et al. Alfa-interferon in the treatment of chronic viral hepatitis: effects on fibrogenesis serum markers. J Hepatol 1993; 18: 112-118
66. Kuwana K, Ichida T, Kamimura T, Ohkoshi S, Ogata N, Harada T, et al. Risk factors and the effect of interferon therapy in the development of hepatocellular carcinoma: a multivariate analysis in 343 patients. J Gastroenterol Hepatol 1997; 12: 149-155
67. International interferon-alfa hepatocellular carcinoma study group. Effect of interferon-alfa on progression of cirrhosis to hepatocellular carcinoma: a retrospective cohort study. Lancet 1998; 351: 1535-1539
68. Kasahara A, Hayashi N, Kochizuki K, Takayanagi M, Yoshioka K, Kakumu S, et al. Risk factors for hepatocellular and its incidence after interferon treatment in patients with chronic hepatitis C. Hepatology 1998; 27: 1394-1402
69. Imai Y, Kawata S, Tamura S, Yabuuchi I, Noda S, Inada M, et al. Relation of interferon therapy and hepatocellular carcinoma patients with chronic hepatitis C. Ann Intern Med 1998; 129: 94-99
70. Ikeda K, Saitoh S, Arase Y, Chayama K, Suzuki Y, Kobayashi M, et al. Effect of interferon therapy on hepatocellular carcinogenesis in patients with chronic hepatitis type C: a long-term observation study of 1643 patients using statistical bias correction with proportional hazard analysis. Hepatology 1999; 29: 1124-1130
71. Okanoue T, Itoh Y, Minami M, Sakamoto S, Yasui K, Sakamoto M, Nishioji K, Murakami Y, Kashima K. Interferon therapy lowers the rate of progression to hepatocellular carcinoma in chronic hepatitis C, but not significantly in an advanced stage: a retrospective study in 1148 patients. J Hepatol 1999; 30: 653-659
72. Shindo M, Ken A, Okuno T. Varying incidence of cirrhosis and hepatocellular carcinoma in patients with chronic hepatitis C responding differently to interferon therapy. Cancer 1999; 85: 1943-1950

Symptomatic therapies for prevention of hepatocellular carcinoma developing in chronic hepatitis C

HIROSHI YOTSUYANAGI[1], YUZO MIYAKAWA[2] and SHIRO IINO[1]

[1] *Division of Gastroenterology and Hepatology, Department of Internal Medicine, St. Marianna University School of Medicine, 2-16-1 Sugao, Miyamae-Ku, Kawasaki, Kanagawa 216-8511, Japan*
[2] *Miyakawa Memorial Research Foundation, 2-19-8 Minami-Aoyama, Minato-Ku, Tokyo 107-0062, Japan*

Ever since interferon (IFN) was found effective in clearing hepatitis C virus (HCV) from the circulation, it has become the mainstay for the treatment of chronic hepatitis C. In early clinical trials with IFN monotherapy, complete response with normalization of liver enzymes and clearance of detectable HCV RNA from serum, however, was achieved in only 5-30% of patients with chronic hepatitis C who received it. Response rates have been improved to 30-40% by long-term therapy with IFN alone or combined IFN and ribavirin. Development of pegylated IFN with a longer half-life and fewer side effects, especially when combined with ribavirin, is expected to increase the response rate to higher than 50%. Even with such an increase in response rate, however, attending physicians are left with the remaining ~50% of patients with chronic hepatitis C who fail to respond to the combined therapy and who continue to have HCV in the circulation.

Chronic hepatitis C in nonresponders can evolve to liver cirrhosis and eventually into hepatocellular carcinoma. Remarkable success with IFN and combined therapies averted, however, the general attention from nonresponders. It has become a pressing concern how to treat nonresponders to retard the progression of their liver disease, thereby preventing hepatocellular carcinoma. Fortunately, several lines of evidence have pointed to the possibility that the development of hepatocellular carcinoma can be retarded or aborted by suppressing necroinflammatory processes in the liver and keeping normal or low transaminase levels for many years. By so doing, the appearance of hepatocellular carcinoma would be postponed, hopefully, beyond the life expectancy of patients calculated as if they had no liver disease. Drugs for suppressing inflammation in the liver and lowering aminotransferase levels for symptomatic therapy of patients with chronic hepatitis C are reviewed, with a discussion of some clinical examples of their application.

Frontiers in Viral Hepatitis Ed. by RF Schinazi, J-P Sommadossi and CM Rice. 515 — 530

Introduction

In Japan, almost all patients who developed elevated levels of alanine aminotransaminase (ALT) in serum following a diagnosis of non-A, non-B hepatitis post-blood transfusion, have turned out to be infected with hepatitis C virus (HCV) by serological and molecular biological tests after HCV was discovered. Because the pathology in the liver does not progress rapidly, and remains mild even in patients with posttransfusion hepatitis having persistently elevated ALT levels for as long as 20 years, it may appear as if they have a favorable outcome. In individuals who have been infected with HCV for more than 20 years, however, liver pathology continues to progress. As time goes by, histology deteriorates from chronic hepatitis through liver cirrhosis (LC) to eventual hepatocellular carcinoma (HCC) at constant rates. Hence, posttransfusion HCV infection gradually lapses into serious morbidity with a poor prognosis.

HCV infection in Japan primarily spread in the community through illicit intravenous injection with methamphetamine just after the end of the World War II. A secondary transmission of HCV occurred by transfusion of blood units donated by drug addicts who were infected. Thirdly and probably most significantly, the pool of HCV increased in size through medical and paramedical practices with the use of insufficiently sterilized needles and syringes. Such a stepwise spread of HCV has resulted in more than two million people who are infected in Japan today [1].

As the most dreadful sequel of HCV infection in the past, the incidence of HCC has kept increasing yearly since 1975. As we reported earlier, the causality rate in Japan due to HCC gradually increased from 10 per 100,000 in 1975 to 35 per 100,000 in 1999. In addition, deaths due to liver cirrhosis number 10-20 per 100,000 yearly, and this has stayed rather constant [2].

This background obligates hepatologists in Japan to prevent a rapid increase in mortality due to HCV-associated chronic liver disease. Fortunately, the treatment of chronic hepatitis C patients with interferon (IFN) can reduce the development of HCC by half, as we reported previously [2]. In addition, we have found that IFN decreases the development of HCC not only in the patients with chronic hepatitis C who respond by clearing HCV RNA from the circulation (virological responders), but also in those in whom ALT levels are normalized or suppressed (complete or partial biochemical responders), despite the continuation of HCV infection after IFN. Our observations have been corroborated by subsequent reports [3, 4].

A six-month IFN monotherapy with a high initial dose, which has been given in Japan, induces sustained virological response in 30% of the recipients, of whom 70% were infected with HCV genotype 1b [2]. The response rate is similar to those achieved by a six-month combined therapy with IFN and ribavirin in many other countries. Large-scale clinical trials with combined IFN and ribavirin have been completed in the United States and Europe [5, 6]; the recipients are being followed for long-term outcome, with hopes for achieving great success. With the most optimistic projections, however, the rate for sustained virological response would not exceed 50% of the combined IFN and ribavirin recipients.

The use of pegylated IFN combined with ribavirin is presently under evaluation, which may further increase the response rate. Even with this regimen, however, approximately 40% of the recipients are not expected to clear HCV from the circulation and will continue to have progressive liver disease. Accordingly, clinical hepatologists are burdened with nonresponders to the optimal therapeutic regimen of combined IFN and ribavirin, as well as the patients with chronic hepatitis C who can not receive it for various reasons. Hence, of utmost concern to attending physicians is how to decrease morbidity and mortality in these unfortunate groups of patients.

Symptomatic therapies for chronic HCV-associated liver diseases

In general, treatment of patients with chronic disease has been conducted with medications that have long-lasting, alleviating effects on symptoms, which has been the measure of their long-term efficacy (for example, drugs for normalizing hyperlipidemia in coronary heart disease, reduction of blood glucose levels in diabetes mellitus and reduction of blood pressure in hypertension). Symptomatic therapies with these drugs have been evaluated for their capacity to improve the prognosis. As to the results, they all have been found efficient in decreasing the morbidity and mortality associated with the respective diseases in the long run.

In the case of HCV-associated chronic liver diseases, some symptomatic clues have surfaced during long-term follow-up of patients. In patients who have been followed for a long time with checkups at regular intervals, those with low mean ALT levels did better, with reduced rates of progression to LC or HCC. Arase et al. [7] found in their clinical trial with a symptomatic therapy that HCC developed less often in the patients in whom ALT levels had been lowered artificially, and there was amelioration of inflammatory process in the liver. Their observations suggest, also, that lowered mean ALT levels during a long period would accompany a reduced rate of progression, from chronic hepatitis C to LC, and a decreased incidence of hepatic failure.

It has to be pointed out that medications for symptomatic therapy of chronic hepatitis have not been licensed. This rejection is based on the failure to achieve histological improvements during a short period spanning only one to two years, despite the fact that symptomatic drugs do lower ALT levels and, therefore, are thought to suppress necroinflammatory processes in the liver. The authorities may have been too hasty with their decisions on this issue.

Let's look at chronic hepatitis B, as an example. Individuals persistently infected with HBV who seroconvert to HBeAg (anti-HBe) either spontaneously or through treatment, and in whom hepatitis ameliorates, rarely show histological improvement, especially in the stage of hepatic fibrosis, within a short period of only 1-2 years. They still harbor HBV, and as a result probably continue to have slight to moderate inflammation in the liver.

This is actually the case with chronic hepatitis C. The patients with chronic hepatitis C who clear HCV from the circulation improve the histopathology in the liver during a follow-up of one to two years. Those who achieve sustained biochemical response with continuously normal ALT levels, but fail to respond virologically by clearing HCV RNA from serum, however, do not achieve improvement in hepatic fibrosis within a matter of one to two years [8], probably because slight inflammation goes on in the liver; it takes five to 10 years for these patients with sustained biochemical response to have their liver histology improved. Fibrosis may not be lessened in degree for these patients; its rate of progression may be halted, however. Nonetheless, sustained normal or lowered ALT levels in serum, reflecting suppressed inflammatory processes in the liver, could prevent the evolution of chronic hepatitis to LC, and eventually into HCC, or retard this process, at least. Should this be achieved, mortality due to hepatic failure or HCC as sequelae of LC would be reduced substantially.

Hence, although killing and eradicating HCV is the principal goal in treatment of chronic hepatitis C, normalizing or lowering ALT levels accompanied by suppression of hepatic inflammation should not be taken lightly, especially in patients who do not respond to IFN virologically by clearing HCV RNA from serum. From this viewpoint, symptomatic treatment of chronic hepatitis C at present would deserve much more attention than ever.

1. Reduction of iron load

Di Biceglie et al. [9] reported that in chronic hepatitis, of type C in particular, serum levels of iron, ferritin and saturation of transferrin are increased frequently, while few cases exhibit increased iron in the liver. Their observations led them to suggest that liver injuries would be responsible for increased iron and ferritin levels in serum. Takikawa et al., however, found an iron load in the liver higher in chronic hepatitis C than B, and on that basis, have implicated hepatic iron deposition in elevated serum ALT levels in chronic hepatitis C. They went on to report a correlation between serum levels of ferritin and ALT in male donors positive for anti-HCV [10]. On the premise that iron overload would be involved in liver injuries associated with HCV infection, Hayashi et al. [11] evaluated the effect of maintaining ferritin levels $\leq$10 ng/ml by weekly or biweekly phlebotomy on serum ALT. The mean ALT decreased from pretreatment levels of 152 $\pm$ 49 to 55 $\pm$ 32 IU/L after therapeutic phlebotomy, with five of ten patients normalizing serum ALT levels. They found phlebotomy more efficient in the patients with higher activity of hepatitis [12].

Recently, the effect of increasing iron load on hepatitis was examined in chimpanzees by Bassett et al. [13] Chimpanzees infected with HCV, when they were placed on a high iron load, accumulated more iron in the liver than noninfected controls, accompanied by aggravation in histological pictures of chronic hepatitis. Thus, they have validated phlebotomy as a means of decreasing iron load and improving liver pathology in chronic hepatitis C.

Methods for reducing iron load are not restricted to phlebotomy, per se. An iron-deficient diet, as well as deferoxamine, a chelator of iron, are capable of reducing serum ALT levels in patients with chronic hepatitis. Kaltwasser et al. [14] gave black tea to patients with genetic hemochromatosis. Intriguingly, they observed that tannate in black tea reduced the absorption of iron, thereby reducing iron load in the liver. Their experience may be extended to patients with chronic hepatitis C for the purpose of reducing iron load.

Despite strong evidence for correlation between hepatic iron load and serum ALT levels, the mechanism is not fully explained. Farinati et al. [15], Sergent et al. [16] and

Weiss et al. [17] have tackled this issue to shed light on how iron disturbs hepatocytes and, conversely, why iron-reducing therapies work on chronic hepatitis. The present state of knowledge on these issues is summarized in the review by Bonkovsky et al. [18], as follows.

It is generally accepted that iron increases the formation of hydroxyl radicals and other highly reactive oxidizing molecules in biological systems. Secondary reactions and indirect effects lead to lipid peroxidation, oxidative damage to proteins and nucleic acids, and to a net increase in collagen and ground substance formation. In iron-loaded livers, such changes produce defects in organelle function (lysosomes, mitochondria, endoplasmic reticulum) and chronic deposition of scar tissue, and eventually hepatocellular carcinoma.

In addition, iron would have to be evaluated for the capacity to influence viral replication and mutagenesis, as well as for its direct or indirect effects on immune responses of the host.

Another practical aspect of an iron-reducing strategy relates to IFN therapy on chronic hepatitis C. van Thiel et al. [19] reported finding lower iron contents in the liver of responders to IFN. Their observations have been reproduced in studies that followed [20, 21], and point to the possible influence of iron reduction on increasing response rates to IFN. Some misunderstandings of 'response to IFN' may mar the judgement on the effect of iron reduction, however, which needs to be taken into consideration.

We have repeatedly discussed criteria for defining the efficacy of IFN on chronic hepatitis C [8, 22]. Our criteria have not achieved general consensus, mainly because the concept of 'response' differs widely depending on the doctors who use it, which has created much confusion. In the early days, when liver function tests were the only means of diagnosing non-A, non B hepatitis, the response was judged by normalization of ALT levels during or at the completion of IFN therapy. Discovery of HCV has made it possible to detect HCV RNA in serum, and now it is increasingly used for evaluating the response to IFN therapy. Hence, 'response to IFN' has dual connotations at the present time, one of which is biochemical (normalization of serum ALT), while the other is virological (loss of HCV RNA from serum). These two distinct kinds of responses can create misjudgement in evaluating the efficacy of IFN therapy, because they do not associate.

Patients with low pretreatment values of serum iron and ferritin have lower baseline ALT levels than those with high values. Hence, they are predisposed already to normalizing ALT levels after receiving IFN, which does not necessarily correlate with the loss of HCV RNA by IFN. Likewise, the implied effects of iron reduction prior to IFN therapy, to increase efficacy, need to be taken with caution; they can simply reflect ramifications of reduced iron load, as such, that may have been erroneously counted in for overestimating the true 'response' to IFN. Despite these serious reservations, the overall effect of iron reduction has been estimated impartially in previous studies, regardless of the judgement of 'response,' either by normalized ALT or loss of HCV RNA, which has produced deep confusion. To help answer this question, a randomized placebo-controlled clinical trial was conducted to evaluate the net effect of iron reduction on increasing the rate of sustained response (SR) in IFN therapy [23].

One can expect little, if any, influence of iron reduction on SR inducible by IFN, and it has been borne out by the actual results [23].

2. Interferon (IFN)

The SR rate to IFN increases in parallel with the duration of therapy, extending from six through 12 to 18 months [24]. Although longer treatment times with IFN increases SR, the patients who respond to long-term IFN are restricted to those who clear HCV RNA from serum while they are on IFN.

It has to be pointed out that there are patients who fail to archieve SR, but in whom ALT levels continue to be normalized despite persistent high titers of HCV RNA during IFN. ALT levels in these patients elevate after the withdrawal of IFN. As long as they are continued on IFN, however, ALT levels stay normalized, accompanied by improved histopathology in the liver. Long-term use of low-dose IFN, for suppressing necroinflammatory processes in the liver, is proposed by Shiffmann et al. [25].

Kasahara et al. [26] and Okanoue et al. [27] have reported a decreased incidence of HCC in transient responders to IFN, in whom ALT normalized and HCV RNA was cleared only while they were on IFN, in long-term follow-ups after the completion of IFN therapy. The effect of IFN in this situation is produced by its ability to retard the development of HCC by a time span of three to five years [26]; transient responders develop HCC at a rate comparable to that of nonresponders beyond that time point. Based on these observations, it may be possible to postpone the development of HCC in transient responders by placing them on IFN regularly at intervals of a few years.

3. Glycyrrhizin

Glycyrrhizin is the active substance in extracts of the root of *Glycyrrhiza glabra* (licorice root). Glycyrrhizin is composed of one molecule of glycyrrhetinic acid coupled with two molecules of glucuronic acid. It has been used for ages as an anti-allergic drug in China, and as a substitute for sucrose and an anti-ulcer drug in Europe [28]. In Japan, glycyrrhizin is supplied as an intravenous drug for the past 60 years, principally for treatment of urticaria and dermatitis. The indication for glycyrrhizin has been extended to chronic hepatitis, on the premise that hepatitis would be induced by allergic reactions.

Encouraged by the early success of glycyrrhizin in reducing ALT levels in sporadic cases of chronic hepatitis, Suzuki et al. conducted a randomized double-blind trial of glycyrrhizin in 1977 in patients with chronic hepatitis, most of whom turned out to be infected with HCV. The results were introduced by them to Western societies of medicine in 1983 [29]. They showed that glycyrrhizin can lower ALT levels significantly. Since then, glycyrrhizin has been used for symptomatic treatment of patients with chronic hepatitis in Japan. Hino et al. [30] went on to demonstrate that glycyrrhizin not only lowers ALT levels, but also suppresses inflammation in the liver. As mentioned above, Arase et al. [7] have shown that long-term use of glycyrrhizin for more than 15 years can significantly decrease the incidence of HCC in patients with chronic hepatitis C.

Although glycyrrhizin evidently suppresses necroinflammatory processes in the liver, the mechanism is not certain despite many studies focusing on it. Glycyrrhizin in large doses can induce pseudoaldosteronism in a few patients, which is easily controlled by regular tests for serum electrolytes and prescribing spinorolactone to the patients with critically low K^+ levels. The reproducible and reliable activity of glycyrrhizin to reduce ALT levels with minimal side effects has resulted in many clinical trials with it in patients with chronic hepatitis C in a number of European and Asian countries.

4. Ursodeoxycholic acid (UDCA)

UDCA represents one of the hydrophilic bile acids, originally identified in the bile of bears. It is contained in human bile in small amounts as a secondary bile acid. UDCA has been used for a long time in China as a drug for bowel disturbances and for stimulating secretion of bile.

In 1976, Yamanaka et al. [31] conducted a randomized controlled trial in patients with chronic hepatitis using placebo, 150 and 600 mg/day of UDCA, and found that 600 mg/day UDCA significantly decreased the levels of ALT, aspartate aminotransferase and γ-glutamyl transpepitidase. Their results were corroborated by Buzzelli et al. in 1991 [32].

Trauner et al. [33] reviewed in detail the effect of UDCA on chronic hepatitis; it has not been fully explained, as yet. The present understanding of the pharmaceutical effects of UDCA on chronic hepatitis includes: (1) replacement of endogenous toxic bile acids; (2) cytoprotective effects on hepatocytes and bile duct cells; and (3) immonomodulatory activity. UDCA stimulates the alimentary tract as a side effect, an effect which is circumvented by timing the intake to just before each meal.

5. Ribavirin

Ribavirin is an antiviral drug that has been in use for many years. By virtue of its ability to enhance the capacity of IFN to eradicate HCV, combined use of IFN and ribavirin has become the first therapeutic choice in the treatment of chronic hepatitis C. Ribavirin by itself, however, has a high activity to suppress ALT levels, although it does not prohibit the replication of HCV. Monotherapy with ribavirin was started by Richard et al. [34] in 1991, and followed by several groups of investigators thereafter. On the grounds that ribavirin cannot clear HCV from serum, even though it suppresses ALT, ribavirin monotherapy has been proposed to be ineffective for treatment of chronic hepatitis C [35]. Ribavirin has side effects represented by hemolytic anemia, and cholelithiasis is reported in recipients who have received long-term treatment. Due to the capacity of ribavirin for suppressing serum ALT, it is hard to dismiss ribavirin monotherapy from the list of symptomatic therapies for chronic hepatitis C.

6. Corticosteroids (CS)

Persistent HCV infection elicits a variety of autoantibodies [36], typified by antinuclear antibodies, and accompanies many extrahepatic diseases such as cryoglobulinemia, in which HCV proteins are involved, along with IgM rheumatoid factors [37]. Although

CS have not been evaluated for long-term efficacy in symptomatic therapy of chronic hepatitis C, Fong et al. [38] and Thiele et al. [39] refer to the effect of CS on patients with chronic hepatitis C. Their results agree on the capacity of CS for lowering serum ALT levels; the reduction is accompanied by increased HCV RNA titers in serum, however. CS are expected to lower ALT levels by means of a cytoprotective activity or immunosuppressive capacity, or both. Hence, CS would be particularly effective in patients with chronic hepatitis C who have stigmata of autoimmune hepatitis represented by high-titered autoantibodies.

7. Cyclosporine A (CsA)

CsA suppresses cell-mediated immune responses and, therefore, has been widely used for preventing graft-versus-host disease and allograft rejection in recipients of transplants, as well as for treatment of autoimmune diseases. Although the exact mechanism of hepatocyte injury in chronic hepatitis C is not clear, as yet, the involvement of cellular immunity mediated by lymphocytes is strongly suspected.

Kakumu et al. [40] placed ten patients with chronic hepatitis C on daily 1.5-4.0 mg/kg of CsA. They found a significant decrease in ALT levels while the patients were given CsA, with minimal side effects inclusive of renal injuries.

8. Interleukin-10 (IL-10)

Frequent suppression or normalization of serum ALT levels has been reported by McHuchison et al. [41], who gave 4 or 8 μg/kg/day of IL-10 to 16 patients with chronic hepatitis C for 28 days. This was also verified by Nelson et al. [42], who prescribed the same doses of IL-10 to 24 patients for 90 days. Significant changes in HCV RNA were not seen during IL-10 in either trial, however. ALT returned to pretreatment levels after withdrawal of IL-10. Nelson et al. [42] compared paired biopsy specimens, taken before and after IL-10 therapy, and recognized significant suppression of fibrosis in the liver following treatment. All in all, IL-10 may be another promising candidate for symptomatic therapy of chronic hepatitis C.

Application of symptomatic therapies to patients with chronic hepatitis C

Optimal doses are not determined for any drugs for the symptomatic therapies of chronic hepatitis C reviewed above. In terms of practical care for patients with chronic hepatitis C, therefore, many issues remain unsolved, including long-term side effects of these drugs.

We have gained experience on symptomatic therapies during the past 15 years, starting when chronic hepatitis C was called non-A, non-B hepatitis. Optimal therapeutic doses have been worked out for some of these drugs and will be presented with some examples.

Of our series of 300 patients with chronic hepatitis C, with or without compensated LC, who have received symptomatic therapy for 10 years or longer, HCC developed in only six (2%). The outcome is biased in that only the patients who received symptomatic therapies for a long while have been selected and followed, without appropriate controls. Even with such reservations, the incidence of HCC in them (2% in 10 years) would be very low by any standards and in comparison with historical controls.

1. UDCA

To the patients with serum ALT levels less than 60-70 IU/L, 600 mg of UDCA daily in three divided doses is given with the goal of maintaining ALT below 40 IU/L. As shown in Table 1, ALT levels decrease by one rank or more by this therapeutic regimen. When ALT decreases to around 30 IU/L, the dose of UDCA is reduced to 300 mg. An example is shown in Figure 1 for a case in whom ALT levels were controlled for three years using UDCA.

Table 1. Average ALT levels before and during the administration of daily 600 mg ursodeoxycholic acid (UDCA) in 52 patients with chronic hepatitis C

Mean ALT levels during 6 months or longer (IU/L)	Pretreatment	During UDCA[a]
>100	6 (12%)	6 (12%)
70-100	22 (42%)	9 (17%)
50-70	17 (33%)	12 (23%)
32-50	7 (13%)	17 (33%)
<32	0	8 (15%)

[a] Lower than pretreatment levels ($p < 0.05$).

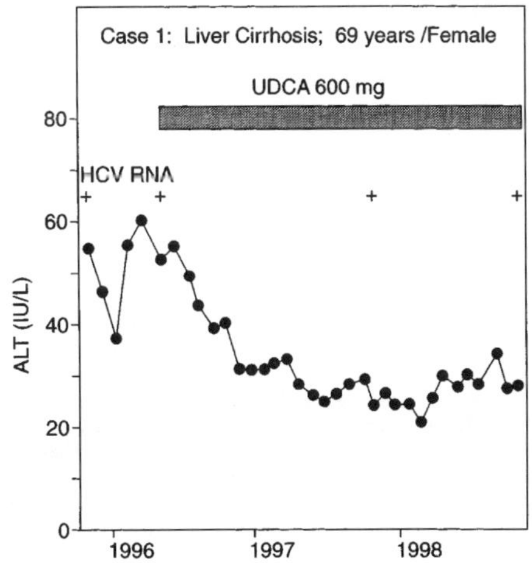

Figure 1. Symptomatic therapy with ursodeoxycholic acid alone.

2. Glycryrrhizin

For patients with serum ALT levels higher than 50-60 IU/L, Stronger Neo-Minophagen C (SNMC; Minophagen Pharmaceutical Company, Tokyo Japan) is used. One ampoule of SNMC contains 40 mg of glycyrrhizin in a 20-ml solution, supplemented with 20 mg/ml glycine and 1 mg/ml cysteine. With constraints for being an intravenously administered drug, SNMC does reduce ALT levels and has been used in tens of thousand patients with chronic hepatitis for more than 20 years in Japan, with minimal side effects. Patients are started on two ampoules, or 40 ml, of SNMC per day (equivalent to 80 mg of glycyrrhizin), and if they fail to respond by lowering ALT below 60 IU/L, the dose can be increased to five ampoules, or 100 ml, of SNMC per day (equivalent to 200 mg of glycyrrhizin). The dose of SNMC is gradually reduced, once a low ALT level is archieved, to the maintenance dose of two or four ampoules per day (equivalent to 80 or 160 mg of glycyrrhizin) (Figure 2).

When SNMC alone cannot suppress serum ALT below 50 IU/L, or if a decreased dose of SNMC is desired, UDCA may be combined for controlling ALT. Conversely, when UDCA alone cannot reduce serum ALT below 50 IU/L, SNMC may be added for suppressing ALT levels below 50 IU/L (Figure 3).

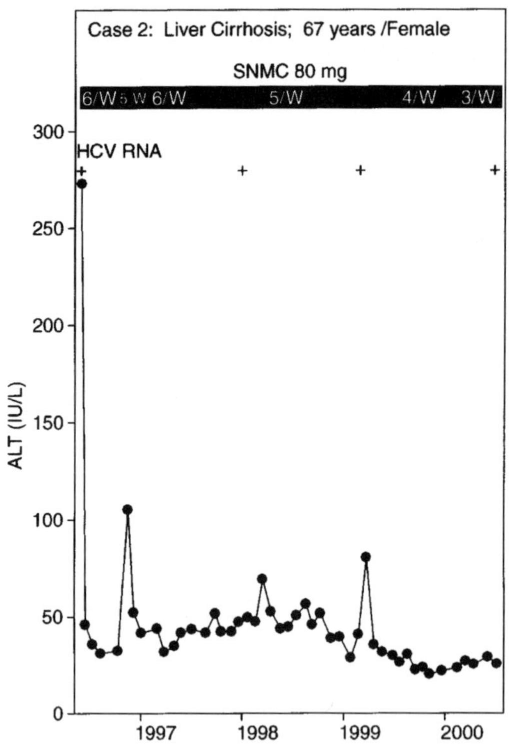

Figure 2. Symptomatic therapy with varying doses of Stronger Neo-Minophagen C.

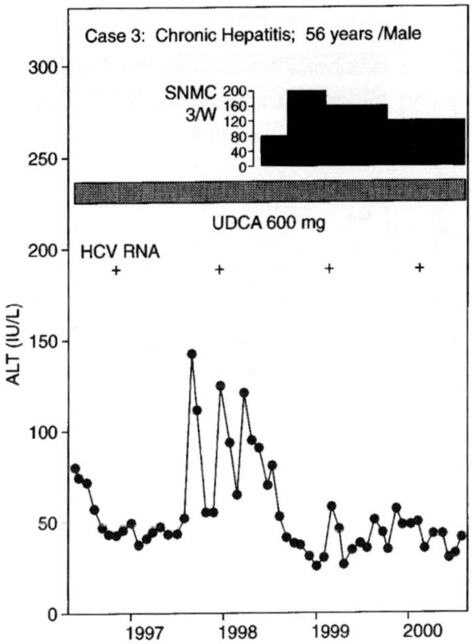

Figure 3. Treatment with Stronger Neo-Minophagen C superimposed on ursodeoxycholic acid.

3. Phlebotomy

Biweekly phlebotomy of 400 ml is repeated until serum ferritin decreases to 10-20 ng/ml. Usually, the target level of ferritin is reached within five to seven cycles of phlebotomy. If and when ALT increases thereafter, phlebotomy of 400 ml is performed for controlling ferritin levels. In most cases, a phlebotomy every four to six months suffices to maintain low ALT levels.

One patient received phlebotomy when SNMC and UDCA could not suppress ALT levels below a desired level (Figure 4). Phlebotomy was effective in controlling ALT levels.

4. IFN

In many clinical trials reported in the literature, IFN at a dose of 3 MU three times a week normalizes ALT in 50-60% of the recipients. Sporadic cases are observed which achieve continued normal ALT levels, even though they keep serum HCV RNA (albeit in somewhat lowered titers) and fail to clear it from serum. A case is presented in Figure 5 in which SNMC and UDCA failed to sufficiently suppress ALT levels. Additional IFN-α at a dose of 3 MU three times a week normalized ALT, whereupon SNMC and UDCA were withdrawn. IFN-α was curtailed to two times a week; ALT was maintained for longer than three years.

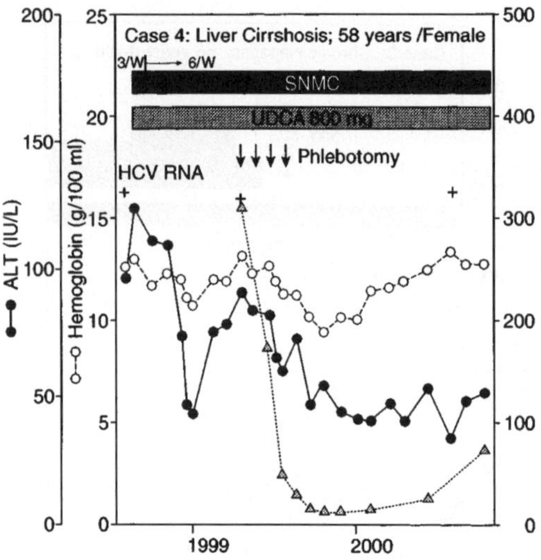

Figure 4. Triple treatments with Stronger Neo-Minophagen C, ursodeoxycholic acid and occasional phlebotomies.

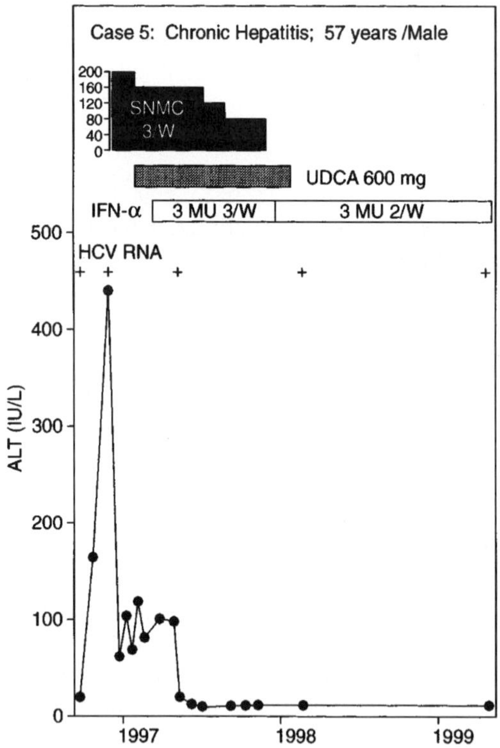

Figure 5. Induction with Stronger Neo-Minophagen C, followed by urosdeoxycholic acid and maintenance with low-dose interferon-α.

5. CS

CS at a dose of 5-10 mg/day can keep serum ALT levels low in some patients with chronic hepatitis C. Most of these patients have antinuclear antibodies in high titers in serum. An example is shown in Figure 6 for a case with antinuclear antibody in a titer of 1:1,280 before the patient was placed on IFN. It went up to 1:260 during IFN treatment, accompanied by increased ALT levels. On the withdrawal of IFN, ALT decreased, but HCV RNA turned positive. For control of ALT levels, 5 mg/day CS was given to the patient, which was effective in lowering ALT to within the normal range.

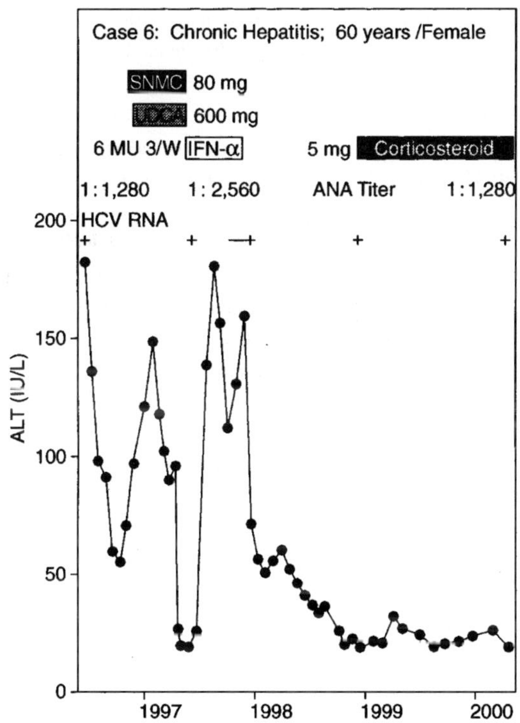

Figure 6. Normal ALT levels attempted by a triple therapy with Stronger Neo-Minophagen C, ursodeoxycholic acid and interferon-α. Levels were successfully maintained by a low-dose corticosteroid in a female patient with chronic hepatitis C who was seropositive for antinuclear antibodies.

References

1. Moriya T, Koyama T, Tanaka J, Mishiro S & Yoshizawa H. Epidemiology of hepatitis C virus in Japan. *Intervirology* 1999;42:153-158.
2. Iino S. Relationship between infection with hepatitis C virus and hepatocellular carcinoma in Japan. *Antiviral Therapy* 1998;3:143-146.
3. Ikeda K, Saitoh S, Arase Y, Chayama K, Suzuki Y, Kobayashi M, Tsubota A, Nakamura I, Murashima N, Kumada H and Kawanishi M. Effect of interferon therapy on hepatocellular carcinogenesis in patients with chronic hepatitis type C: A long-term observation study of 1, 643 patients using statistical bias correction with proportional hazard analysis. *Hepatology* 1999;29:1124-1130.
4. Yoshida H, Shiratori Y, Moriyama M, Arakawa Y, Ide T, Sata M, Inoue O, Yano M, Tanaka M, Fujiyama S, Nishiguchi S, Kuroki T, Imazeki F, Yokosuka O, Kinoyama S, Yamada G, Omata M and for the IHIT Study Group. Interferon therapy reduces the risk for hepatocellular carcinoma: national surveillance program of cirrhotic and noncirrhotic patients with chronic hepatitis C in Japan. IHIT Study Group. Inhibition of Hepatocarcinogenesis by Interferon Therapy. *Annals of Internal Medicine* 1999;131:174-181.
5. McHutchison JG, Gordon SC, Schiff ER, Shiffman ML, Lee WM, Rustgi VK, Goodman ZD, Ling MH, Cort S, Albrecht JK and for the Hepatitis International Therapy Group. Interferon alpha-2b alone or in combination with ribavirin as initial treatment for chronic hepatitis C. *New England Journal of Medicine* 1998;339:1485-1492.
6. Poynard T, Marcellin P, Lee SS, Niederau C, Minuk GS, Ideo G, Bain V, Heathcote J, Zeuzem S, Trepo C, Albrecht J and for the International Hepatitis Therapy Group (IHIT). Randomised trial of interferon alpha2b plus ribavirin for 48 weeks or for 24 weeks versus interferon alpha2b plus placebo for 48 weeks for treatment of chronic infection with hepatitis C virus. *Lancet* 1998;352:1426-1432.
7. Arase Y, Ikeda K, Murashima N, Chayama K, Tsubota A, Koida I, Suzuki Y, Saitoh S, Kobayashi M and Kumada H. The long term efficacy of glycyrrhizin in chronic hepatitis C patients. *Cancer* 1997;79:1494-1500.
8. Iino S, Hino K and Yasuda K. Current state of interferon therapy for chronic hepatitis C. *Intervirology* 1994;37:87-100.
9. Di Bisceglie AM, Axiotis CA, Hoofnagle JH and Bacon BR. Measurements of iron status in patients with chronic hepatitis. *Gastroenterology* 1992;102:2108-2113.
10. Takikawa T, Hayashi H, Nishimura N, Yano M, Isomura T and Sakamoto N. Correlation between serum levels of alanine aminotransferase and ferritin in male blood donors with antibody to hepatitis C virus. *Journal of Gastroenterology* 1994;29:593-597.
11. Hayashi H, Takikawa T, Nishimura N, Yano M, Isomura T and Sakamoto N. Improvement of serum aminotransferase levels after phlebotomy in patients with chronic active hepatitis C and excess hepatic iron. *American Journal of Gastroenterology* 1994;89:986-988.
12. Hayashi H, Takikawa T, Nishimura N and Yano M. Serum aminotransferase levels as an indicator of the effectiveness of venesection for chronic hepatitis C. *Journal of Hepatology* 1995;22:268-271.
13. Bassett SE, Di Bisceglie AM, Bacon BR, Sharp RM, Govindarajan S, Hubbard GB, Brasky KM and Lanford RE. Effects of iron loading on pathogenicity in hepatitis C virus-infected chimpanzees. *Hepatology* 1999;29:1884-1892.
14. Kaltwasser JP, Werner E, Schalk K, Hansen C, Gottschalk R and Seidl C. Clinical trial on the effect of regular tea drinking on iron accumulation in genetic haemochromatosis. *Gut* 1998;43:699-704.
15. Farinati F, Cardin R, De Maria N, Della Libera G, Marafin C, Lecis E, Burra P, Floreani A, Cecchetto A

and Naccarato R. Iron storage, lipid peroxidation and glutathione turnover in chronic anti-HCV positive hepatitis. *Journal of Hepatology* 1995;22:449-456.

16. Sergent O, Griffon B, Morel I, Chevanne M, Dubos MP, Cillard P and Cillard J. Effect of nitric oxide on iron-mediated oxidative stress in primary rat hepatocyte culture. *Hepatology* 1997;25:122-127.
17. Weiss G, Umlauft F, Urbanek M, Herold M, Lovevsky M, Offner F and Gordeuk VR. Associations between cellular immune effector function, iron metabolism, and disease activity in patients with chronic hepatitis C virus infection. *Journal of Infectious Diseases* 1999;180:1452-1458.
18. Bonkovsky HL. Therapy of hepatitis C: other options. *Hepatology* 1997;26:S143-151.
19. Van Thiel DH, Friedlander L, Fagiuoli S, Wright HI, Irish W and Gavaler JS. Response to interferon alpha therapy is influenced by the iron content of the liver. *Journal of Hepatology* 1994;20:410-415.
20. Clemente MG, Congia M, Lai ME, Lilliu F, Lampis R, Frau F, Frau MR, Faa G, Diana G, Dessi C and et al. Effect of iron overload on the response to recombinant interferon-alfa treatment in transfusion-dependent patients with thalassemia major and chronic hepatitis C. *Journal of Pediatrics* 1994;125:123-128.
21. Olynyk JK, Reddy KR, Di Bisceglie AM, Jeffers LJ, Parker TI, Radick JL, Schiff ER and Bacon BR. Hepatic iron concentration as a predictor of response to interferon alfa therapy in chronic hepatitis C. *Gastroenterology* 1995;108:1104-1109.
22. Iino S. Problems in the treatment of hepatitis C with interferon. *Intervirology* 1999;42:166-172.
23. Di Bisceglie AM, Bonkovsky HL, Chopra S, Flamm S, Reddy RK, Grace N, Killenberg P, Hunt C, Tamburro C, Tavill AS, Ferguson R, Krawitt E, Banner B and Bacon BR. Iron reduction as an adjuvant to interferon therapy in patients with chronic hepatitis C who have previously not responded to interferon: a multicenter, prospective, randomized, controlled trial. *Hepatology* 2000;32:135-138.
24. Poynard T, Bedossa P, Chevallier M, Mathurin P, Lemonnier C, Trepo C, Couzigou P, Payen JL, Sajus M, Costa JM, Vidaud M, Chaput JC and the Multicenter Study Group. A comparison of three interferon alpha-2b regimens for the long-term treatment of chronic non-A, non-B hepatitis. *New England Journal of Medicine* 1995;332:1457 1462.
25. Shiffman ML, Hofmann CM, Contos MJ, Luketic VA, Sanyal AJ, Sterling RK, Ferreira-Gonzalez A, Mills AS and Garret C. A randomized, controlled trial of maintenance interferon therapy for patients with chronic hepatitis C virus and persistent viremia. *Gastroenterology* 1999;117:1164-1172.
26. Kasahara A, Hayashi N, Mochizuki K, Takayanagi M, Yoshioka K, Kakumu S, Iijima A, Urushihara A, Kiyosawa K, Okuda M, Hino K, Okita K and the Osaka Liver Disease Study Group. Risk factors for hepatocellular carcinoma and its incidence after interferon treatment in patients with chronic hepatitis C. *Hepatology* 1998;27:1394-1402.
27. Okanoue T, Itoh Y, Minami M, Sakamoto S, Yasui K, Sakamoto M, Nishioji K, Murakami Y, Kashima K and the Viral Hepatitis Therapy Study Group. Interferon therapy lowers the rate of progression to hepatocellular carcinoma in chronic hepatitis C but not significantly in an advanced stage: a retrospective study in 1148 patients. *Journal of Hepatology* 1999;30:653-659.
28. van Rossum TG, Vulto AG, de Man RA, Brouwer JT and Schalm SW. Review article: glycyrrhizin as a potential treatment for chronic hepatitis C. *Alimentary and Pharmacological Therapy* 1998;12:199-205.
29. Suzuki H, Ohta Y, Takino T, Fujisawa K and Hirayama C. Effects of glycyrrhizin on biochemical tests in patients with chronic hepatitis. *Asian Medical Journal* 1983;26:423-438.
30. Hino S, Miyakawa H, Takahashi A, Kumada H, Ikdeda K, Yoshiba A, Ohta Y and Suzuki H. Large-dose administration of Stronger Neo-Minophagen C (SNMC) for the treatment of chronic active hepatitis. *Hepatology Research*, in press.
31. Yamanaka M, Ohtou M, Obata H, Shimizu M, Sugata F, Hatta Y, Dohi Y and Miyahara H. Double

blind trial of therapeutic effects of ursodeoxycholic acid on chronic hepatitis (in Japanese). *Diagnosis and Treatment* 1976;64:2150-2157.

32. Buzzelli G, Moscarella S, Focardi G, Dattolo P, Giusti A, Relli P, Rusticali AG and Gentilni P. Long-term treatment with ursodeoxycholic acid in patients with chronic active hepatitis. *Current Therapeutic Research* 1991;50:635-642.
33. Trauner M and Graziadei IW. Review article: mechanisms of action and therapeutic applications of ursodeoxycholic acid in chronic liver diseases. *Alimentary Pharmacology and Therapeutics* 1999;13:979-996.
34. Reichard O, Andersson J, Schvarcz R and Weiland O. Ribavirin treatment for chronic hepatitis C. *Lancet* 1991;337:1058-1061.
35. Di Bisceglie AM, Conjeevaram HS, Fried MW, Sallie R, Park Y, Yurdaydin C, Swain M, Kleiner DE, Mahaney K and Hoofnagle JH. Ribavirin as therapy for chronic hepatitis C. A randomized, double-blind, placebo-controlled trial. *Annals of Internal Medicine* 1995;123:897-903.
36. Zauli D, Cassani F and Bianchi FB. Auto-antibodies in hepatitis C. *Biochemical Pharmacology* 1999;53:234-241.
37. Cacoub P, Renou C, Rosenthal E, Cohen P, Loury I, Loustaud-Ratti V, Yamamoto AM, Camproux AC, Hausfater P, Musset L, Veyssier P, Raguin G, Piette JC and for the GERMIVIC. Extrahepatic manifestations associated with hepatitis C virus infection. A prospective multicenter study of 321 patients. *Medicine (Baltimore)* 2000;79:47-56.
38. Fong TL, Valinluck B, Govindarajan S, Charboneau F, Adkins RH and Redeker AG. Short-term prednisone therapy affects aminotransferase activity and hepatitis C virus RNA levels in chronic hepatitis C. *Gastroenterology* 1994;107:196-199.
39. Thiele DL, DuCharme L, Cunningham MR, Mimms LT, Cuthbert JA, Lee WM and Combes B. Steroid therapy of chronic hepatitis: characteristics associated with response in anti-hepatitis C virus-positive and -negative patients. *American Journal of Gastroenterology* 1996;91:300-308.
40. Kakumu S, Takayanagi M, Iwata K, Okumura A, Aiyama T, Ishikawa T, Nadai M and Yoshioka K. Cyclosporine therapy affects aminotransferase activity but not hepatitis C virus RNA levels in chronic hepatitis C. *Journal of Gastroenterology and Hepatology* 1997;12:62-66.
41. McHutchison JG, Giannelli G, Nyberg L, Blatt LM, Waite K, Mischkot P, Pianko S, Conrad A and Grint P. A pilot study of daily subcutaneous interleukin-10 in patients with chronic hepatitis C infection. *Journal of Interferon and Cytokine Research* 1999;19:1265-1270.
42. Nelson DR, Lauwers GY, Lau JY and Davis GL. Interleukin 10 treatment reduces fibrosis in patients with chronic hepatitis C: a pilot trial of interferon nonresponders. *Gastroenterology* 2000;118:655-660.

Mutations of the core gene sequence of HCV from patients with hepatocellular carcinoma in China

TOSHIHIRO OMOYA[1], ICHIRO SHIMIZU[1*], CHIYO HORIE[1], TAKAHIRO HORIE[1], DENG-FU YAO[2], MINA ITONAGA[1], YOSHIHIRO OKAMURA[3], HIROHITO HONDA[1] and SUSUMU ITO[1]

[1] *Second Department of Internal Medicine, Tokushima University School of Medicine, Tokushima 770-8503, Japan*
[2] *Nantong Medical College, Nantong, Jiangsu Province, China*
[3] *General Laboratory for Medical Research, Tokushima University School of Medicine, Tokushima 770-8503, Japan*

Summary

We investigated the association between hepatocellular carcinoma (HCC) and the genomic characteristics of the hepatitis C virus (HCV) isolated from residents of the inshore region of the Yangtze River. This area of China has one of the highest incidences of HCC. Our data revealed that nucleotide substitutions are unevenly scattered along the HCV genome, with a cluster of missense mutations in the region encoding the second hydrophilic domain of the core protein, and that the number of these mutations in the clustering variable region (CVR) is significantly higher in isolates from HCC patients than in those from individuals with chronic hepatitis. Moreover, we determined the sequence divergence of the CVR in HCV isolates from cancerous and noncancerous liver tissues in Japanese patients with HCC. The number of nucleotide substitutions giving rise to changes in amino acid residues in the CVR was significantly greater in liver tissues than in sera from HCC patients. The number of amino acid residues in the CVR that differed from the representative clone from cancerous liver portions was significantly higher than the number differing from noncancerous portions in each patient. An amino acid alteration from Gly to Ser at core codon 45 in the CVR was dominant in noncancerous portions, rather than in cancerous portions and sera from HCC patients. These findings suggest that a large number of mutations, including biologically important amino acid sequence changes in the HCV core gene from liver tissue, might be related to hepatocarcinogenesis.

Introduction

Epidemiological studies [1-4] indicate that the inshore region of the Yangtze River, including Nantong, in eastern China, is a high-risk area for hepatocellular carcinoma

Frontiers in Viral Hepatitis Ed. by RF Schinazi, J-P Sommadossi and CM Rice. 531 — 545

(HCC), with hepatitis B virus (HBV) having been identified as a risk factor. Hepatitis C virus (HCV) is a more important cause of HCC than HBV in Japan and Western countries [5-7]. Our preliminary studies [1-3] indicated that the prevalence of antibodies to HCV (anti-HCV) and HCV RNA is low in patients with chronic liver disease and HCC in Nantong. Comparative analyses of complete or partial genomic sequences of HCV isolates from Taiwan (HCV-T) [8], Beijing (HCV-PRC1) [9], Japan (HCV-J [10] and HCV-BK [11]), and the United States (HCV-1) [12] have indicated that the Chinese isolates (HCV-T and HCV-PRC1) are more similar to those from Japan than to those from the United States. All known HCV isolates are assigned to at least four genotypes on the basis of variation in the nucleotide sequence of restricted regions of the HCV core gene [13]. Genotype 1b was detected in 86% of HCV infections in Beijing [14], and 60% of individuals with non-A, non-B (NANB) liver disease in Japan [15]. Genotype 2a, a minor type in Beijing and Japan, appears to be more sensitive to interferon treatment than genotype 1b [15, 16]. Thus, knowledge of the heterogeneity of the HCV genome is important for developing prophylactic and treatment strategies for HCV-associated liver disease. However, detailed data on the association between HCC and the genomic characteristics of HCV isolates from this high-risk region for HCC have not been available.

Long-term studies of nucleotide sequence changes in HCV-infected humans and chimpanzees have suggested that the HCV genome is highly susceptible to mutation [17, 18]. Furthermore, a high degree of HCV sequence variation has been proposed as a possible mechanism for escape from the host immune system [19]. However, previous studies focused primarily on the hypervariable region at the 5' end of the envelope [2] or nonstructural 1 (E2/NS1) glycoprotein gene of HCV [20, 21], despite the fact that the core protein of HBV has been suggested to be a target for cytotoxic T lymphocytes (CTLs) [22, 23]. Because studies on endogenously processed viral peptides from a nucleocapsid protein indicated that a peptide as small as eight amino acids could be recognized by CTLs [24, 25], it might be possible to detect alterations in deduced amino acid sequence in a restricted segment of the HCV core gene in response to pressure from CTLs.

To investigate the possible role of the HCV core gene in hepatocarcinogenesis, we compared the sequence divergences of the genomic core gene isolated from serum samples in Chinese patients with and without HCC living in Nantong. Our data revealed that nucleotide (nt) substitutions are unevenly scattered along the HCV genome, with a cluster of missense mutations in the region encoding the second hydrophilic domain from the 5' end of the core gene in Nantong patients [26]. The clustering variable region (CVR) was located in a small segment of 38 amino acids (AAs), codons 39-76 from the start of the core gene. Moreover, we determined the genomic heterogeneity of HCV and the sequence divergence of the CVR in HCV isolates from cancerous and noncancerous liver tissues in Japanese patients with HCC, as well as those from serum samples in chronic hepatitis (CH), liver cirrhosis (LC), and HCC subjects [27].

Sequence diveregence of the HCV core gene isolated from serum samples in Chinese patients with HCC

Serum samples were obtained from 10 subjects with NANB liver disease (five with CH and five with HCC and LC) [26] at the Affiliated Hospital of Nantong Medical College in China. The sera of all patients were positive for HCV RNA with genotype 1b, and were negative for hepatitis B surface antigen (HBsAg) and hepatitis B core antibodies (HBcAb). The clinical and laboratory data of these patients are summarized in Table 1 (patients 1-10). We also obtained serum samples as pooled sera positive for HCV RNA with genotype 1b from NANB CH patients in Nantong. The HCV cDNA clones propagated from the pooled sera and the 10 individual sera from Nantong were designated as Nantong prototype HCV-N and isolates HCV-N-1 to HCV-N-10, respectively; isolates HCV-N-1 to HCV-N-5 were from patients 1 to 5 with CH, and isolates HCV-N-6 to HCV-N-10 were from patients 6 to 10 with HCC and LC. Five HCV cDNA clones were obtained from each Nantong patient with the exception of patients 2, 3, and 6, from each of whom one cDNA clone was isolated.

Analysis of the sequence homology of the HCV core gene of HCV-N isolates with that of other isolates revealed that the Nantong prototype HCV-N was 94.6, 95.2, and 89.7% identical at the nt level with the Chinese (HCV-T and HCV-PRC1), Japanese (HCV-J and HCV-BK), and United States (HCV-1) isolates, respectively; the corresponding values for identity of the deduced AA sequence were 93.5, 93.7, and 92.1%, respectively. Thus, the nt sequence of the Nantong HCV prototype was more homologous to those of the genotype 1b isolates from China and Japan than to that of the genotype 1a isolate from the United States. Moreover, the nt sequence of HCV-N isolates from Nantong patients with CH (HCV-N-1 to HCV-N-5) or HCC (HCV-N-6 to HCV-N-10) showed a higher degree of homology to those of the Chinese and Japanese isolates than to that of the United States isolate. The homology with other isolates was greater for HCV-N isolates from CH patients than for those from patients with HCC at both the nt and deduced AA levels [26].

As shown in Table 2, nt and deduced AA residues differing from those of the Nantong prototype HCV-N were identified in the core gene of the 38 HCV cDNA clones obtained from the 10 Nantong patients with CH or HCC. A total of 238 nt substitutions was detected in the 17 HCV cDNA clones from the five patients with CH, with a mean of 14.0 substitutions per clone, and 481 substitutions were detected in the 21 clones from the five HCC patients, with a mean of 22.9 substitutions per clone. For clones from patients with CH, the substitution rate at each nt position was 0.024, and the alteration rate at AA position was 0.034; of the 238 substitutions, 121 were missense mutations, with a mean of 7.1 per clone. Clones from HCC patients showed higher rates of nt substitutions and AA alterations (0.040 and 0.050, respectively) than those from CH patients. Of the 481 substitutions in clones from HCC patients, 244 were missense mutations, with a mean of 11.6 per clone, a value significantly higher than that for clones from CH patients.

The 314 AA alterations detected in the two groups were located in the core gene region, and 189 (60%) of these changes were clustered in a small segment of 38 AA (codons 39 to 76 from the start of the core gene, corresponding to 20% of the core peptide).

Table 1. Clinical and laboratory data for the 10 Chinese patients (numbers 1 to 10) with NANB liver disease from the inshore region of the Yangtze River and the 22 Japanese patients (numbers 11 and 32) with NANB liver disease from Japan from whom HCV cDNA clones were isolated

Samples		Patient			HCV		HBV*		Diagnosis of noncancerous liver
		Number	Age (years)	Gender	Genotype	Number of clones	HBsAg	HBcAb	
Chinese sera									
	CH	1	42	M	1b	5	Negative	Negative	
		2	39	M	1b	1	Negative	Negative	
		3	53	M	1b	1	Negative	Negative	
		4	47	M	1b	5	Negative	Negative	
		5	31	F	1b	5	Negative	Negative	
	HCC	6	50	M	1b	1	Negative	Negative	LC
		7	67	M	1b	5	Negative	Negative	LC
		8	75	F	1b	5	Negative	Negative	LC
		9	56	M	1b	5	Negative	Negative	LC
		10	42	M	1b	5	Negative	Negative	LC
Japanese sera									
	CH	11	50	F	1b	8	Negative	Negative	
		12	43	M	1b	8	Negative	Negative	
		13	43	M	1b	7	Negative	Negative	
		14	58	M	1b + 2a	10	Negative	Negative	
		15	60	M	1b	10	Negative	Negative	
	LC	16	58	M	1b	9	Negative	Negative	
		17	59	M	1b	8	Negative	Negative	
		18	66	F	1b	7	Negative	Negative	
		19	59	M	1b	9	Negative	Negative	
		20	46	M	1b + 2a	10	Negative	Negative	
	HCC	21	65	F	1b	9	Negative	Negative	LC
		22	78	M	1b	10	Negative	Negative	LC
		23	63	M	1b	9	Negative	Negative	LC
		24	49	M	1b + 2a	10	Negative	Negative	LC
		25	70	M	1b	7	Negative	Negative	LC

Table 1. continued

Samples		Patient			HCV		HBV*		Diagnosis of noncancerous liver
		Number	Age (years)	Gender	Genotype	Number of clones	HBsAg	HBcAb	
Japanese liver tissues									
	HCC	26	58	M	1b + 2a	7 (non)	Negative	Negative	LC
		27	73	M	1b + 2a	8 (non)	Negative	Negative	LC
		28	49	M	1b	6 (non)	Negative	Negative	LC
		29	64	M	1b	10 (non) + 9 (can)	Negative	Negative	LC
		30	61	M	1b	11(non) + 12 (can)	Negative	Negative	LC
		31	55	M	1b + 2a	11 (non) + 10 (can)	Negative	Negative	LC
		32	57	M	1b	7 (non) + 9 (can)	Negative	Negative	LC

* HBV markers in serum samples in all patients, numbers 1-32.
(non), HCV cDNA clones from noncancerous liver tissues in patients with HCC; (can), HCV cDNA clones from cancerous liver tissues in patients with HCC.

Table 2. Nt substitutions and alterations in deduced AA residues in the core gene of HCV-N isolates from Chinese patients (numbers 1 to 10) with CH or HCC

Samples		Nt	AA	Nt substitution	AA alteration	Substitution/ nt × 10^{-2}	Alteration/ AA × 10^{-2}	Missense mutation/ Nt substitutions × 10^{-2}
CH	CVR	114	38	6.5 ± 1.4	3.6 ± 1.3	5.7 ± 1.2**	9.4 ± 3.4**	59.8 ± 3.1**
	Other	459	153	7.5 ± 1.3	3.0 ± 1.1	1.6 ± 0.3	2.0 ± 0.7	42.6 ± 2.1
HCC	CVR	114	38	11.3 ± 3.0*	6.1 ± 1.2*	9.9 ± 2.6*, **	16.2 ± 3.2*, **	62.8 ± 3.2**
	Other	459	153	11.6 ± 2.3*	3.5 ± 1.8	2.5 ± 0.5*	2.3 ± 1.2	38.8 ± 2.1

* $P < 0.05$ vs. corresponding value for CH.

** $P < 0.05$ vs. corresponding other core gene sequence (two-tailed Mann-Whitney U test).

The 17 HCV cDNA clones from five patients with CH (HCV-N-1 to HCV-N-5) and 21 clones from five patients with HCC (HCV-N-6 to HCV-N-10) were examined for nt substitutions and alterations of deduced AA residues in the entire core gene sequence (nt 1 to 573, codons 1 to 191 from the start of the core gene), as well as in the clustering variable region (CVR) (nt 115 to 228, codons 39 to 76) and the remaining (Other) sequence. Data are means ± SD.

This CVR in clones from patients with CH or HCC showed a significantly higher rate of missense mutations per nt substitution and a higher rate of nt substitutions than the other core gene sequence (Table 2). The numbers of nt substitutions, AA alterations, and missense mutations in the CVR were significantly greater for clones from HCC patients than in those from CH.

The hydrophilicity profiles of the products of the core gene of HCV-N-6, from an HCC patient and the HCV-N prototype, are shown in Figure 1. At least three domains of high local hydrophilicity and two hydrophobic domains were recognized in the upstream region (codons 1 to 120) and downstream region (codons 115 to 144 and 157 to 186), respectively. Of the three hydrophilic domains, the second, containing the CVR, showed the greatest divergence of hydrophilicity scores between HCV-N-6 and the prototype, whereas the scores of the two hydrophobic domains were virtually identical for the HCV-N-6 and HCV-N isolates.

Like Nantong [1-3], Taiwan is also a high-risk region for HCC, with a low prevalence of HCV infection but a high prevalence of HBsAg [28]. However, in a case-control study of pairs of HCC patients and control subjects matched for age and sex, Yu et al. [29] showed that HCV infection is associated with an increased risk of HCC and has a synergistic interaction with HBV infection in Taiwan. Our study revealed the predominance of genotype 1b in HCV infections in Nantong and the similarity of the HCV-N isolates to those of genotype 1b from Taiwan (HCV-T), Beijing (HCV-PRC1), and Japan (HCV-J and HCV-BK). Moreover, a study showed that HCV is the major agent responsible for HBsAg-negative HCC, and also plays a role in HBsAg-positive

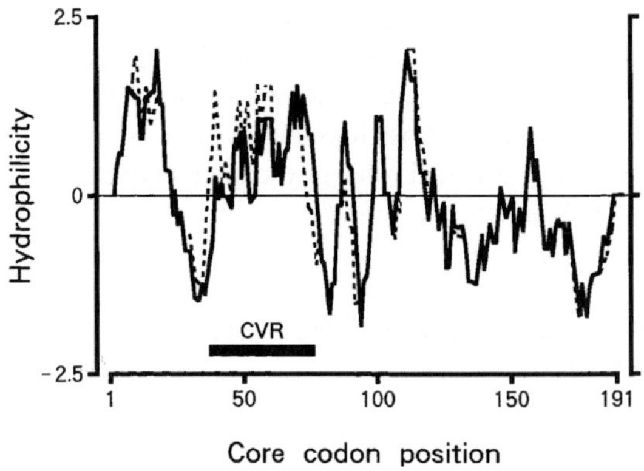

Figure 1. Relative hydrophilicity profiles of the products of the core gene of the HCV-N prototype (dotted line) and the HCV-N-6 isolate. The hydrophilicity score, corresponding to a window of six consecutive AA residues, is indicated along the core gene sequence of 191 AAs. The horizontal solid bar indicates the clustering variable region (CVR) (codons 39 to 76).

HCC, in the inshore area of the Yangtze River (Yao et al., unpublished data). Thus, HCV may participate in the pathogenesis of HCC in HBV-hyperendemic areas such as Nantong and Taiwan.

Virus specific CTLs protect against virus infection *in vivo* and contribute to the development of disease by direct or indirect mechanisms [30]. In HBV infection, the core protein is thought to be an immunological target of CTLs [22, 23]. Clustered missense mutations in some regions of the HBV core gene have been shown to be related to liver damage in individuals with chronic HBV infection [31, 32], consistent with our data on HCV infection. A study in which recombinant vaccinia viruses were used to express HCV proteins showed that HCV-specific, human leukocyte antigen (HLA) class I-restricted, $CD8^+$ CTLs recognized epitopes in variable regions of the virus [33]. Furthermore, antibody-epitope binding experiments revealed HCV-specific linear epitopes located in the hypervariable region at the NH_2-terminus of the E2/NS1 glycoprotein [19]. The core, NS3, NS4, and NS5 proteins exhibit greater sequence conservation in isolated genotypes than the E1 and E2/NS1 glycoproteins [17, 18]. The hypervariability of the HCV envelope protein suggests that HCV may escape the host immune system by rapid mutation, and that mutations may stimulate new CTL responses, which are followed by further nt substitutions, as in infection with the human immunodeficiency virus [34]. Nevertheless, the relatively conserved epitopes in the core and NS5 regions, whose AA sequences show 94 to 100% identity within the same genotype [14, 35], have also been shown to be recognized by $CD8^+$ CTLs in a patient with chronic HCV infection [36] and in mice after immunization with a vaccinia-HCV recombinant virus [37], respectively. In our study, the rates of nt substitutions, alterations of deduced AA residues, and missense mutations per nt change in the CVR were significantly greater than in the remaining region of the

HCV core gene. In addition, the number of nt substitutions that gave rise to changes in deduced AA residues in the CVR was significantly greater in HCC than in CH. These observations suggest that missense mutations in the CVR may be subject to higher selection pressure from the host immune system as liver disease progresses to HCC, and that they may play the dual roles of escape mutations and targets for CTLs in patients with chronic HCV infection.

Comparison of sequence diveregences of HCV isolates between Chinese and Japanese patients with HCC

To compare the genomic sequences of HCV isolates from Nantong with those of isolates from Japanese individuals with NANB chronic liver disease, we obtained serum samples from 15 Japanese patients (five with CH, five with LC, and five with HCC and LC) and liver tissues from seven patients [27] undergoing surgical resection of HCC at the University of Tokushima in Japan. For liver tissue specimens, the center part of the tumor was sampled as the cancerous portion, and the surrounding liver tissue clearly separated from the tumor was sampled as the noncancerous portion. All 22 sera were positive for HCV RNA with genotype 1b and were negative for HBsAg and HBcAb (Table 1; patients 11-32). None had been treated with interferon-α or -β. In addition, we obtained serum samples as pooled sera positive for HCV RNA with genotype 1b and negative for HBsAg and HBcAb from 10 CH patients in Tokushima.

From six to 12 independent clones were isolated from the 15 HCV RNA-positive sera and the noncancerous and cancerous liver tissues of seven patients with HCC, and a total of 231 clones were sequenced. A major representative clone in 12 clones obtained from pooled sera positive for HCV RNA from CH patients in Tokushima was sequenced and designated as Tokushima prototype (Figure 2): out of 12 clones, nine clones had an alteration of deduced AA residue to serine at codon 110 from threonine conserved in the genotype 1b sequences of HCV-J [10] and HCV-BK [11].

Figure 2 shows the differences in deduced AA residues of the core gene (codons 1 to 125) between the Tokushima prototype [27] and HCV isolates from serum samples of Japanese and Nantong patients with HCC. Whereas few alterations of the deduced AA residues, either inside or outside the CVR, were evident in the Japanese HCV isolates, the increased number of AA alterations apparent in the Nantong isolates were unevenly clustered in the CVR.

As far as we are aware, the existence of the CVR in the core region of HCV isolates has not been previously described. The nt mutation rate of the HCV genome is about 10^6 times that of the human genome in the absence of immune pressure [17]. However, the HCV genotype 1b isolates obtained from serum samples of Japanese HCC patients in the present study did not show mutation clustering in the CVR. The reason for the difference in mutation rate in the core region between Japanese and Nantong HCV isolates is unknown, but it may be attributable to differences in the distribution of HLA types between Japanese and Chinese [38, 39].

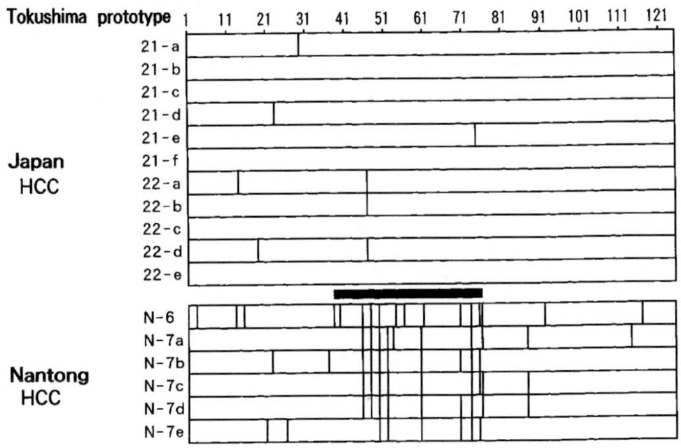

Figure 2. Comparison between deduced AA residues of the core gene (codons 1 to 125) of HCV isolates from Japanese and Nantong patients with HCC. Ten deduced AA sequences of 11 HCV cDNA clones from Japanese patients 21 and 22 and six HCV cDNA clones from Nantong patients 6 and 7 were compared with that of Tokushima prototype [27]; differences are indicated by vertical solid lines. Core codons are numbered from the start of the core gene of the prototype. The horizontal solid bar indicates the CVR (codons 39 to 76).

Comparison of sequence diveregences of HCV isolates from noncancerous and cancerous liver portions in Japanese patients with HCC

As shown in Table 3, nt sequences and deduced AA residues differing from those of the Tokushima prototype were identified in the core gene of the 152 HCV cDNA clones obtained from the sera of 15 patients with CH, LC, or HCC, and the noncancerous tissues of three HCC patients. Clones from CH patients showed significantly lower frequencies of nt substitutions and AA alterations (1.7×10^{-2} and 0.4×10^{-2}, respectively) than those from LC and HCC patients. In all of the 109 examined clones from LC and HCC patients, there was no significant difference among the frequencies of nt substitutions and AA alterations, with the exception of the frequency of AA alterations in the CVR in clones from noncancerous tissue samples. The number (3.6×10^{-2}) of AA alteration frequencies in the CVR was significantly greater than that (1.5×10^{-2}) in the remaining region in clones from the noncancerous liver tissues, although the frequency of nt substitutions in the CVR was not significantly different from that in the remaining sequence. This finding clearly indicated that the number of nt substitutions giving rise to changes in deduced AA residues in the CVR was significantly greater in liver tissues than in sera from HCC patients. Moreover, at codon 45 in the core gene, an AA alteration from Gly to Ser with an nt substitution from G to A at the nt 133 was observed in 47 out of 88 (53%) clones isolated from serum samples in patients with

Table 3. Nt and deduced AA sequences differing from those of Tokushima prototype in the core gene of HCV isolates from Japanese patients (numbers 11 to 28) with CH, LC, or HCC

Samples		Nt	AA	Nt substitution	AA alteration	Substitution/ nt × 10^{-2}	Alteration/ AA × 10^{-2}
Sera							
CH	CVR	114	38	1.2 ± 0.7	0.4 ± 0.5	1.1 ± 0.6	1.1 ± 1.3
	Other	234	78	4.7 ± 0.9	0.1 ± 0.6	1.2 ± 0.4	0.1 ± 0.7
LC	CVR	114	38	2.5 ± 0.7	0.3 ± 0.4	2.2 ± 0.6*	0.8 ± 1.1
	Other	234	78	7.7 ± 0.8*	1.3 ± 0.4*	3.3 ± 0.3*	1.5 ± 0.5*
HCC	CVR	114	38	2.8 ± 0.9	0.5 ± 0.7	2.5 ± 0.8*	1.3 ± 1.8
	Other	234	78	8.4 ± 0.5*	1.1 ± 0.3*	3.6 ± 0.2*	1.3 ± 0.3*
Liver tissues							
HCC	CVR	114	38	3.8 ± 0.9*	1.4 ± 0.5*	3.3 ± 0.8*	3.6 ± 1.6*, *, ***
	Other	234	78	8.3 ± 1.0*	1.2 ± 0.5*	3.6 ± 0.4*	1.5 ± 0.6*

* $P < 0.05$ vs. corresponding value for serum samples in CH.

** $P < 0.05$ vs. corresponding value for serum samples in HCC.

*** $P < 0.05$ vs. corresponding value for the remaining (Other) core gene sequence (two-tailed Mann-Whitney *U*-test with Bonferroni correction).

HCV cDNA clones were examined for nt substitutions and alterations of deduced AA residues in a part (nt 1 to 348, codons 1 to 116 from the start of the core gene) of the entire core gene sequence, as well as in the CVR (nt 115 to 228, codons 39 to 76) and the remaining (Other) sequence. Data are means ± SD.

LC and HCC, and in 19 out of 21 (90%) clones from noncancerous liver tissues in HCC patients, whereas no changes were found at this position in any of the clones from serum samples in CH patients.

There has been a similar report that HCV clones obtained from sera are different than those from liver tissues: a sequence analysis of the hypervariable region (HVR) at the 5' end of the envelope 2 or nonstructural 1 (E2/NS1) glycoprotein gene of HCV revealed that nt sequences of HVR in noncancerous, cancerous, and serum samples were different in the same patient [40]. On the other hand, single-strand conformation polymorphism (SSCP) analysis of HVR indicated that viral populations differed in noncancerous and cancerous portions, but were the same in the serum and the noncancerous portion in the same patient [41]. It is unclear whether or not the constitution of viral populations isolated from sera and liver tissues is the same. However, an analysis of the HCV core gene sequence by multiple fluorescence-based PCR SSCP demonstrated that different populations of HCV quasispecies proliferate in cancerous and noncancerous liver portions [42]. In this study, a deduced AA alteration from Gly to Ser at the core codon 45 accompanied by an nt substitution from G to A was observed dominantly in noncancerous portions rather than in cancerous portions and sera from HCC patients. These findings suggest that HCV replication and populations may be heterogeneous among different regions in the liver tissue in the same patient with HCC, and may be supplied to sera, producing many quasispecies populations.

The nt sequences and deduced AA residues in the CVR were determined using seven to 12 clones each from the noncancerous and cancerous liver portions of four patients, numbers 29 to 32. The frequencies of nt sequences and deduced AA residues that were different from the representative clone in each case were compared between clones from noncancerous and cancerous portions. In two cases out of four, the mean number of nt substitution frequencies was significantly higher in the cancerous than the noncancerous portions. However, in all four cases, the mean number of deduced AA alteration frequencies was significantly higher than that in noncancerous portions (Figure 3), because most nt substitutions in cancerous portions gave rise to changes in deduced AA residues. Furthermore, the AA alteration from Gly to Ser at the core codon 45 with the accompanying nt substitution from G to A at nt 133 occurred more frequently in noncancerous (36 out of 39 clones, 92%) than in cancerous portions (12 of 40 clones, 30%).

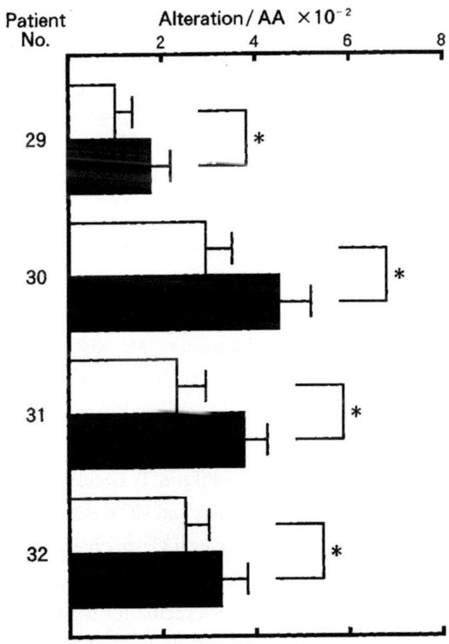

Figure 3. Comparison of deduced AA residues in clones from noncancerous (□) and cancerous (■) liver portions in Japanese patients (numbers 29 to 32) with HCC. The nt sequences and deduced AA residues in the CVR (codons 39 to 76) were determined using seven to 12 clones each from noncancerous and cancerous liver portions of four patients. The frequency of deduced AA residues that are different from the representative clone in each case was compared between clones from noncancerous and cancerous portions. *Two-tailed Mann-Whitney *U*-test ($p < 0.05$) was performed.

HCV core protein and hepatocarcinogenesis

Ravaggi et al. [43] and Suzuki et al. [44] showed that a truncated HCV core protein containing the residues of core codon from 38 to 43 without the hydrophobic COOH-terminus had translocated to the nucleus, whereas the intact core protein was localized in the cytoplasm. Whether such a truncated core protein is actually produced during the course of HCV replication remains to be determined. Moreover, whether a core protein with a cluster of mutations in the second hydrophilic domain binds to nucleic acids is also not known. The HCV core protein contains potential phosphorylation sites for protein kinase A (Ser^{53} and Ser^{116}) and for protein kinase C (PKC) (Ser^{53} and Ser^{99}). Shin et al. [45] showed that mutation of either of the two serine residues at codons 99 and 116 to alanine or aspartate resulted in a marked reduction in the inhibitory effects of the protein on HBV gene expression, whereas mutation of Ser^{53} had no effect on such activity. All serine mutants of the HCV core protein retained the ability to translocate to the nucleus. In addition, the AA alteration from Gly to Ser at codon 45 caused a phosphorylation site, AA sequence of Ser-Val-Arg for PKC [46]. Moreover, there are several myristoylation sites in the HCV core gene sequence. The mutation from Gly to Ser at codon 45 resulted in the loss of the myristoylation site. The protein myristoylation is associated with important biological processes, such as growth control and virus replication [47]. These observations indicate that mutations in the HCV core protein may affect the regulation of the expression of genes, possibly including that of cellular oncogenes. Although the mechanism of hepatocarcinogenesis induced by HCV is still far from clear, further analysis of the HCV core protein may increase our understanding of the pathogenesis of HCV infection and its contribution to the development of HCC.

References

1. Ito S, Yao DF, Nii C, Hibino S, Yano A, Kamamura M, Nishikado T, Honda H, Shimizu I and Meng X-Y. Epidemiological characteristics of the incidence of hepatitis C virus (C100-3) antibodies in patients with liver diseases in the inshore area of the Yangtze R -iver. J Gastroenterol Hepatol 1993; 8: 232-237.
2. Ito S, Yao DF, Nii C, Horei T, Kamamura M, Nishikado T, Honda H, Shibata H, Shimizu I and Meng X-Y. Incidence of hepatitis C virus (HCV) antibodies and HCV-RNA in blood donors and patients with liver diseases in the inshore area of the Yangtze River. J Gastroenterol Hepatol 1994; 3: 245-249.
3. Horie C, Horie T, Honda H, Shimizu I, Ito S and Yao DF. Virological features of hepatitis C virus infection in patients with liver diseases in a high risk region for hepatocellular carcinoma in the inshore area of the Yangtze River. Acta Hepatol Jpn 1995; 36: 76-84 (in Japanese).
4. Yeh FS and Shen KN. Epidemiology and early diagnosis of primary liver cancer in China. Adv Cancer Res 1986; 47: 297-329.
5. Saito I, Miyamura T, Ohbayashi A, Harada H, Katayama T, Kikuchi S, Watanabe Y, Koi S, Onji M and Ohta Y. Hepatitis C virus infection is associated with the development of hepatocellular carcinoma. Proc Natl Acad Sci USA 1990; 87: 6547-6549.
6. Di Bisceglie AM, Order SE, Klein JL, Waggoner JG, Sjogren MH, Kuo G, Houghton M, Choo QL and Hoofnagle JH. The role of chronic viral hepatitis in hepatocellular carcinoma in the United States.

Am J Gastroenterol 1991; 86: 335-338.

7. Colombo M, Rumi MG, Donato MF, Tommasini MA, Del Ninno E, Ronchi G, Kuo G and Houghton M. Hepatitis C antibody in patients with chronic liver disease and hepatocellular carcinoma. Dig Dis Sci 1991; 36: 1130-1133.
8. Chen PJ, Lin MH, Tai KF, Liu PC, Lin CJ and Chen DS. The Taiwanese hepatitis C virus genome: Sequence determination and mapping the 5' termini of viral genomic and antigenomic RNA. Virology 1992; 188: 102-113.
9. Liu K, Hu Z, Li H, Prince AM and Inchauspe G. Genomic typing of hepatitis C viruses present in China. Gene 1992; 114: 245-250.
10. Kato N, Hijikata M, Ootsuyama Y, Nakagawa M, Ohkoshi S, Sugimura T and Shimotohno K. Molecular cloning of the human hepatitis C virus genome from Japanese patients with non-A, non- B hepatitis. Proc Natl Acad Sci USA 1990; 87: 9524-9528.
11. Takamizawa A, Mori C, Fuke I, Manabe S, Murakami S, Fujita J, Onishi E, Andoh T, Yoshida I and Okayama H. Structureand organization of the hepatitis C virus genome isolated from human carriers. J Virol 1991; 65: 1105-1113.
12. Choo QL, Richman KH, Han JH, Berger K, Lee C, Dong C, Gallegos C, Coit D, Medina-Selby R and Barr PJ. Genetic organization and diversity of the hepatitis C virus. Proc Natl Acad Sci USA 1991; 88: 2451-2455.
13. Okamoto H, Tokita H, Sakamoto M, Horikita M, Kojima M, Iizuka H and Mishiro S. Characterization of the genomic sequence of type V (or 3a) hepatitis C virus isolates and PCR primers for specific detection. J Gen Virol 1993; 74: 2385-2390.
14. Wang Y, Okamoto H, Tsuda F, Nagayama R, Tao QM and Mishiro S. Prevalence, genotypes and an isolate (HC-C2) of hepatitis C virus in Chinese patients with liver disease. J Med Virol 1993; 40: 254-260.
15. Okamoto H, Sugiyama Y, Okada S, Kurai K, Akahane Y, Sugai Y, Tanaka T, Sato K, Tsuda F and Miyakawa Y. Typing hepatictis C virus by polymerase chain reaction with type-specific primers: application to clinical surveys and tracing infectious sources. J Gen Virol 1992; 73: 673-679.
16. Kanai K, Kato M and Okamoto H. HCV genotypes in chronic hepatitis C and response to interferon. Lancet 1992; 339: 1543.
17. Ogata N, Alter HJ, Miller RH and Purcell RH. Nucleotide sequence and mutation rate of the H strain of hepatitis C virus. Proc Natl Acad Sci USA 1991; 88: 3392-3396.
18. Okamoto H, Kojima M, Okada S, Yoshizawa H, Iizuka H, Tanaka T, Muchmore EE, Peterson DA, Ito Y and Mishiro S. Genetic drift of hepatitis C virus during an 8.2-year infection in a chimpanzee: variability and stability. Virology 1992; 190: 894-899.
19. Weiner AJ, Geysen HM, Christopherson C, Hall JE, Mason TJ, Saracco G, Bonino F, Crawford K, Marion CD and Crawford KA. Evidence for immune selection of hepatitis C virus (HCV) putative envelope glycoprotein variants: potential role in chronic HCV infections. Proc Natl Acad Sci USA 1992; 89: 3468-3472.
20. Hijikata M, Kato N, Ootsuyama Y, Nakagawa M, Ohkoshi S and Shimotohno K. Hypervariable regions in the putative glycoprotein of hepatitis C virus. Biochem Biophys Res Commun 1991; 175: 220-228.
21. Weiner AJ, Brauer MJ, Rosenblatt J, Richman KH, Tung J, Crawford K, Bonino F, Saracco G, Choo QL and Houghton M. Variable and hypervariable domains are found in the regions of HCV corresponding to the flavivirus envelope and NS1 proteins and the pestivirus envelope glycoproteins. Virology 1991; 180: 842-848.
22. Mondelli M, Vergani GM, Alberti A, Vergani D, Portmann B, Eddleston AL and Williams R. Specificity

of lymphocyte cytotoxicity to autologous hepatocytes in chronic hepatitis B virus infection: evidence that T cells are directed against HBV core antigen expressed on hepatocytes. J Immunol 1982; 129: 2773-2778

23. Vento S, Hegarty JE, Alberti A, O'Brien CJ, Alexander GJ, Eddleston AL and Williams R. T lymphocyte sensitization to Hbs Ag and T cell-mediated unresponsiveness to HBsAg in hepatitis B virus- related chronic liver disease. Hepatology 1985; 5: 192-197.
24. Van Bleek GM and Nathenson SG. Isolation of an endogenously pr ocessed immunodominant viral peptide from the class I H- 2Kb molecule. Nature 1990; 348: 213-216.
25. Rotzschke O, Falk K, Deres K, Schild H, Norda M, Metzger J, Jung G and Rammensee HG. Isolation and analysis of naturally processed viral peptides as recognized by cytotoxic T cells. Nature 1990; 348: 252-254.
26. Shimizu I, Yao D-F, Horie C, Yasuda M, Shiba M, Horie T, Nishikado T, Meng X-Y and Ito S. Mutations in a hydrophilic part of the core gene of hepatitis C virus from patients with hepatocellular carcinoma in China. J Gastroenterol 1997; 32: 47-55.
27. Horie T, Shimizu I, Horie C, Yogita S, Tashiro S and Ito S. Mutations of the core gene sequence of hepatitis C virus isolated from liver tissues with hepatocellular carcinoma. Hepatol Res 1999; 13: 240-251.
28. Chen DS, Kuo GC, Sung JL, Lai MY, Sheu JC, Chen PJ, Yang PM, Hsu HM, Chang MH and Chen CJ, et al. Hepatitis C virus infection in an area hyperendemic for hepatitis B and chronic liver disease: the Taiwan experience. J Infect Dis 1990; 162: 817-822.
29. Yu MW, You SL, Chang AS, Lu SN, Liaw YF and Chen CJ. Association between hepatitis C virus antibodies and hepatocellular carcinoma in Taiwan. Cancer Res 1991; 51: 5621-5625.
30. Pasternack MS. Cytotoxic T-lymphocytes. Adv Intern Med 1988; 33: 17-44.
31. Ehata T, Omata M, Yokosuka O, Hosoda K and Ohto M. Variations in codons 84-101 in the core nucleotide sequence correlate with hepatocellular injury in chronic hepatitis B virus infection. J Clin Invest 1992; 89: 332-338.
32. Chuang WL, Omata M, Ehata T, Yokosuka O, Ito Y, Imazeki F, Lu SN, Chang WY and Ohto M. Precore mutations and core clustering mutations in chronic hepatitis B virus infection. Gastroenterology 1993; 104: 263-271.
33. Koziel MJ, Dudley D, Wong JT, Dienstag J, Houghton M, Ralston R and Walker BD. Intrahepatic cytotoxic T lymphocytes specific for hepatitis C virus in persons with chronic hepatitis. J Immunol 1992; 149: 3339-3344.
34. Phillips RE, Rowland-Jones S, Nixon DF, Gotch FM, Edwards JP, Ogunlesi AO, Elvin JG, Rothbard JA, Bangham CR and Rizza CR. Human immunodeficiency virus genetic variation that can escape cytotoxic T cell recognition. Nature 1991; 354: 453-459.
35. Houghton M, Weiner A, Han J, Kuo G and Choo QL. Molecular biology of the hepatitis C viruses: implications for diagnosis, development and control of viral disease. Hepatology 1991; 14: 381- 388.
36. Kita H, Moriyama T, Kaneko T, Kaneko T, Harase I, Nomura M, Miura H, Nakamura I, Yazaki Y and Imawari M. HLA B44-restricted cytotoxic T lymphocytes recognizing an epitope on hepatitis C virus nucleocapsid protein. Hepatology 1993; 18: 1039-1044.
37. Shirai M, Akatsuka T, Pendleton CD, Houghten R, Wychowski C, Mihalik K, Feinstone S and Berzofsky JA. Induction of cytotoxic T cells to a cross-reactive epitope in the hepatitis C virus nonstructural RNA polymerase-like protein. J Virol 1992; 66: 4098-4106.
38. Kumagai M. Genetic factors (HLA) and cellular immunity in the pathogenesis of asymptomatic HBsAg carriers. Acta Hepatol Jpn 1979; 20: 339-345 (in Japanese).

39. Lin DY, Liaw YF, Chu CM and Chen GH. Histocompatibility profile of hepatoma in Taiwan. J Formosan Med Assoc (Taiwan I Hseuh Hui Tsa Chih) 1982; 81: 1126-1131.
40. Paterlini P, Driss F, Nalpas B, Pisi E, Franco D, Berthelot P and Brechot C. Persistence of hepatitis B and hepatitis C viral genomes in primary liver cancers from HBsAg-negative patients: a study of a low-endemic area. Hepatology 1993; 17: 20-29.
41. Kurosaki M, Enomoto N, Sakamoto N, Tanaka Y, Tang L, Hoshino Y, Izumi N, Marumo F and Sato C. Detection and analysis of replicating hepatitis C virus RNA in hepatocellular carcinoma tissues. J Hepatol 1995; 22: 527-535.
42. Horie C, Iwahana H, Horie T, Shimizu I, Yoshimoto K, Yogita S, Tashiro S, Ito S and Itakura M. Detection of different quasispecies of hepatitis C virus core region in cancerous and non-cancerous lesions. Biochem Biophys Res Commun 1996; 218: 674-681.
43. Ravaggi A. Natoli G, Primi D, Albertini A, Levrero M and Cariani E. Intracellular localization of full-length and truncated hepatitis C virus core protein expressed in mammalian cells. J Hepatol 1994; 20: 833-836.
44. Suzuki R, Matsuura Y, Suzuki T, Ando A, Chiba J, Harada S, Saito I and Miyamura T. Nuclear localization of the truncated hepat -itis C virus core protein with its hydrophobic C terminus deleted. J Gen Virol 1995; 76: 53-61.
45. Shin C-M, Chen C-M, Chen S-Y and WuLee Y-H. Modulation of the transsuppression activity of hepatitis C virus core protein by phosphorylation. J Virol 1995; 69: 1160-1171.
46. Kennelly PJ and Krebs EG. Consensus sequences as substrate specificity determinants for protein kinases and protein phosphates J Biol Chem 1991; 266: 15555-15558.
47. David-Pfeuty T, Bagrodia S and Shalloway D. Differential localizaon patterns of myristoylated and nonmyristoylated c-Src protein interphase and mitotic c-*Src* overexpresser cells. J Cell Sci 1993; 105: 613-628.

Characterization of hepatitis B virus X variants that are integrated and expressed in human hepatocellular carcinomas

WEI NING CHEN and CHONG JIN OON

Hepatitis and Liver Cancer Research Unit,
Department of Clinical Research, Singapore General Hospital,
Singapore 169608, Republic of Singapore

Abstract

Hepatitis B virus X protein (HBX) has been implicated in the transactivation of diverse cellular genes, and possibly also the pathogenesis of human hepatocellular carcinoma (HCC). We report the characterization of HBX variants from HBV-related human hepatocellular carcinoma (HCC). Mutations and deletions were identified in well-defined functional domains of HBX essential for transactivation and Kunitz-like serine protease inhibitor activities. Genomic Southern blot analysis revealed that HBX sequences were integrated into the host chromosomes of HCC tissues. Analysis using reverse transcriptase-based polymerase chain reaction (RT-PCR) indicated that these integrated HBX genes were expressed in the HCC tissues. We also report a novel *in vitro* HBX activity assay based on color changes that were indicative of the β-galactosidase enzyme activity. Conducted in wheat germ lysates, the transactivating function of either wild type or mutant HBX protein was measured through its interaction with the Early Growth Response factor 1 (Egr-1) that controls the β-galactosidase gene. Further analysis of these HBX deletion mutants using this assay may shed new insights on the significance of various mutations occurring in HCC-associated HBX.

Introduction

Persistent infection by hepatitis B virus (HBV) has been closely associated with the pathogenesis of human hepatocellular carcinoma (HCC) [1-3]. Moreover, HBV genomes have been found integrated in the host genomes of most HBV-related HCC [4]. The involvement of these integrated HBV DNA in hepatocarcinogenesis has been suggested by the formation of transformed foci in transfected mammalian cells [5]. While the *in vivo* oncogenic potential of the whole HBV genome has so far not been demonstrated in transgenic mice [6], overexpression of individual viral gene products including HBX protein may also contribute to the development of HCC in carrier mice [7]. Although the ability of HBX in inducing HCC has been seen in only one line of transgenic mice, an increased susceptibility to carcinogens and progression to HCC

Frontiers in Viral Hepatitis Ed. by RF Schinazi, J-P Sommadossi and CM Rice. 547 — 555

in other lines suggest a synergistic role of HBX in interacting with other oncogenes involved in the pathogenesis of HCC [8, 9].

Consisting of 154 amino acid residues, HBX has been reported to interact with a wide range of cellular proteins [10], among them transcription activators that are involved in the activation of proto-oncogenes (c-*jun*) and growth control (Egr-1) [11, 12]. In addition to the domains that are important for the transactivation and *in vitro* transforming activities [13, 4], there is also a split but functional Kunitz-like serine protease inhibitor domain [15]. The function of HBX as a protease inhibitor has been further strengthened by the recent identification of proteasome as its new target [16, 17]. These findings suggest a more general role for HBX in inhibiting cellular processes of protein degradation.

Mutations and deletions have been identified in the integrated HBX sequences [18-21]. In contrast to mutations occurring in the immunogenic HBsAg that are characteristic of vaccine escape mutants [22, 23], the effects of these HCC-integrated HBX mutants on hepatocarcinogenesis remains unclear, although some 3' truncated HBX genes are shown to retain their activity [24, 25].

Identification of HBX variants in HCC

To investigate the significance of HBX in HBV-related hepatocarcinogenesis, five patients who tested positive for both HBsAg and anti-HBc IgG were selected and designated as G1 to G5, respectively (Table 1). The serological profile of a healthy person without HBV infection (G6, Table 1) was included as a control.

Table 1. Serological profile of patients

Patient	HBV DNA (pg/ml)	HBsAg (µg/ml)	anti-HBs (mIU/ml)	anti-HBc IgG
G1	-	0.56	2	+
G2	-	0.28	-	+
G3	-	0.90	-	+
G4	-	2.80	-	+
G5	-	4.30	-	+
G6 (Control, Non HCC)	-	-	-	-

Serological markers tested by commercial kits (Abbott Laboratories, North Chicago, USA)

Serum DNA was isolated from HCC patients and used for amplification of the HBX gene. Whereas HBsAg was amplified from G1, G2, G3 and G5 in a separate PCR (*data not shown*), HBX was detected in G2, G3 and G5. No HBV DNA was amplified from G4 and the control sample G6. The deletions in the 3' part of the coding region were observed and resulted in C-terminal deletions of the predicted amino acid sequences of both G2 (residues 143 to 154) and G5 (residues 117 to 154), as shown in Figure 1.

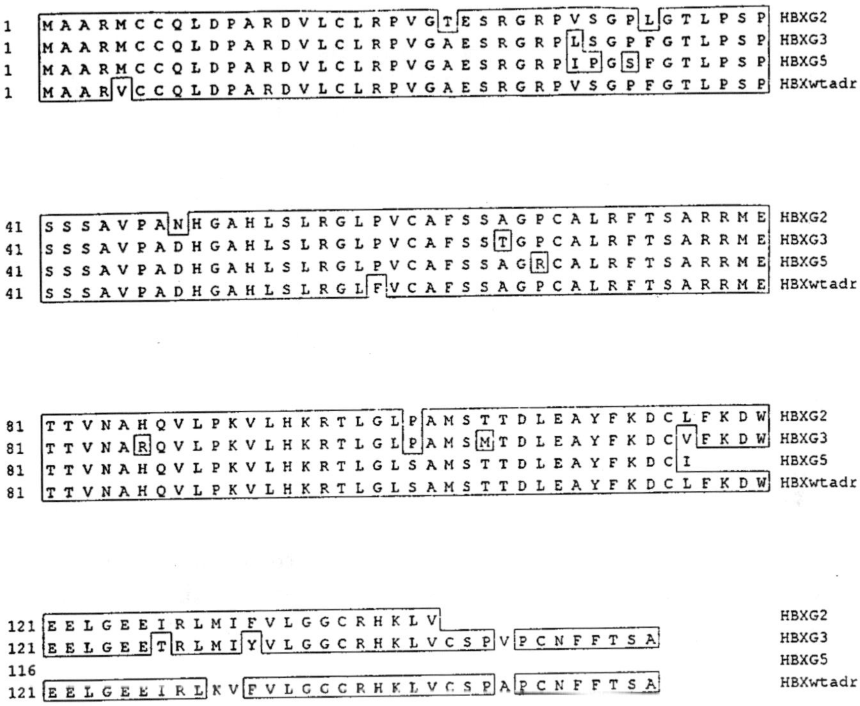

Figure 1. Multialignment of HBX protein sequences. Amino acid sequences G2, G3 and G5 were predicted from the serum HBX isolated in this study, while that of the wild type HBX (HBXwtadr) was derived from Genbank. Identical amino acid residues were *boxed*. Reference numbering was that of HBXwtadr.

Genomic integration of HBX in HCC tissues

To investigate whether the detected HBX mutants were also integrated into the genome of the HCC tissues, genomic DNA was extracted and restricted by EcoRI prior to Southern blot analysis. Results shown in Figure 2 revealed bands of variable sizes that hybridized with the digoxigenin-labeled HBX probe. These include the two bands in G1 (approximately 20 and 13 kb), four bands in G2 (approximately 18, 14, 9 and 7 kb), one band in G3 (approximately 16 kb) and two bands in G5 (19 and 14 kb).

None of the integrated HBX sequences appear to have the complete coding region, as shown by PCR analysis on DNA extracted from the hybridizing agarose gel slices. The deletions encompassed the DR1 element, a 11 bp direct repeat sequence that is the initiation site for DNA minus-strand synthesis and also the preferred site on the HBV DNA during integration into the host genome [26].

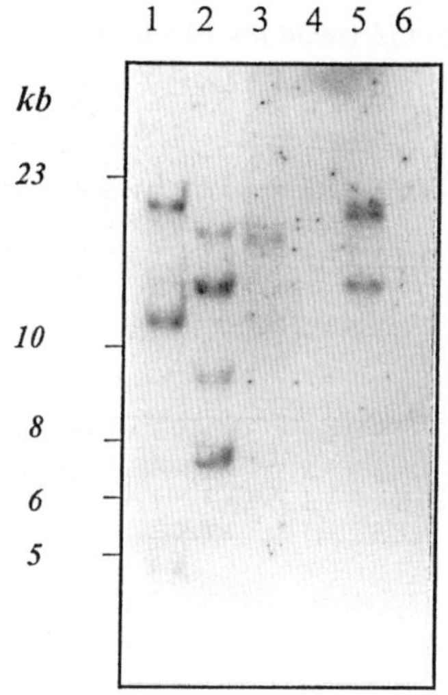

Figure 2. Detection of integrated HBX sequences in HCC tissues. 10 μg of genomic DNA were digested by EcoRI restriction enzyme prior to Southern blot analysis, using the digoxigenin-labeled HBX coding region as probe. Samples in lanes corresponded to the order of patients in Table 1 and were as follows: *lane 1*: G1; *lane 2*: G2; *lane 3:* G3; *lane 4:* G4; *lane 5:* G5 and *lane 6:* G6. Sizes of DNA molecular marker were shown on the left side of the figure. Hybridizing fragments were seen in all lanes except *lane 6*.

RNA expression of HCC-integrated HBX

To investigate the RNA expression of the integrated HBX in HCC tissues, a two-step nested PCR was carried out. The total RNA was extracted from both the serum and the frozen liver tissues of the patients, and treated with Dnase I to remove the coexisting HBV DNA as the selected patients were tested positive for HBsAg. Results of the nested-PCR shown in Figure 3 showed the amplification band of the expected size (210 bp) in all the HCC-integrated HBX. No PCR band was seen in the control amplification involving the RNA samples that were not reverse transcribed (*data not shown*).

To rule out the possibility that the HBX RNA detected in HCC tissues was derived from RNA of serum HBV, similar nested-PCR was carried out using Dnase I-treated serum RNA as template. No PCR products were amplified (*data not shown*). It was therefore likely that integrated HBX was expressed in the respective HCC tissue.

In vitro assay for HBX activity in wheat germ lysates

To determine the significance of the *in vivo* expression of the HCC-integrated HBX mutants in the pathogenesis of HCC, a novel activity assay was developed on the basis of the synergistic interaction between HBX and Egr-1 in stimulating the expression of TGF-β1 [12]. Because the extent of deletion for each integrated HBX remained to be

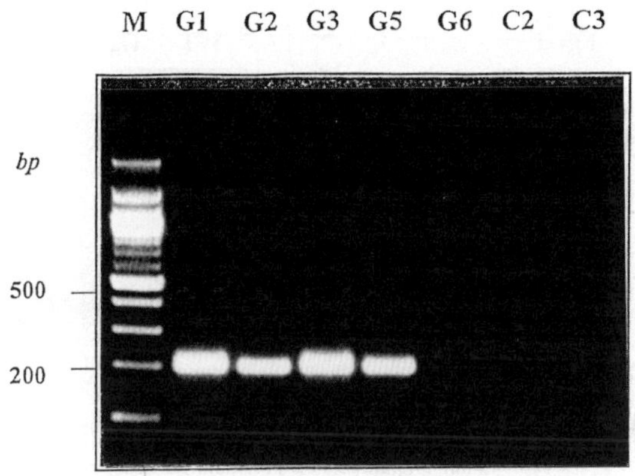

Figure 3. Analysis of RNA expression of HBX variants in HCC by RT-PCR. Total RNA was extracted from either serum or HCC tissues and treated with DNAse. Results of RT-PCR were shown in four *panels*. Sizes of DNA molecular marker were shown in *lane M* and indicated on the left side of each *panel*. *Panel A,* RNA samples from HCC tissues were reverse transcribed and the two-step PCR carried out. Amplification bands were seen in G1, G2, G3 and G5, but not in G6 and controls. The controls included H_2O for reverse transcription (C2) and H_2O for PCR (C3).

determined, the serum HBX mutants (G2, G3 and G5) that displayed identical amino acid sequences as their integrated counterparts were used in the activity assay.

In this study, the mammalian CMV promoter on the pCMV-β plasmid was replaced with the fragment of TGF-β1 promoter that contains two copies of the Egr-1 binding site. Wild type and HCC-integrated HBX mutants were amplified with a 5' primer containing a SP6 viral promoter prior to the *in vitro* translation of individual proteins in wheat germ lysates. The Egr-1 protein of the expected size of 80 kDa [27] that has no reported homologue in plant cells was synthesized (in the presence of [^{35}S]Methionine) from the cDNA cloned in pGEM-T plasmid (*panel A*, Figure 4). Likewise, the wild type and mutant HBX proteins were translated similarly from linear DNA containing the coding region of the corresponding HCC-integrated HBX gene (*panel B*, Figure 4). The *in vitro*-translated HBX proteins also showed the expected sizes (Figure 4). Specifically, G3 without deletion in the coding region shared the same size as wild type HBX (17 kDa), whereas a size shift was seen in G2 (15 kDa) and G5 (14 kDa), due to deletions in their C-terminus (Figure 4).

The modulation of bacterial β-galactosidase activity by HBX (either wild type or HCC-integrated mutants) and Egr-1 was measured, after effective inactivation of the endogenous eukaryotic β-galactosidase activity [28]. A time course of the inactivation indicated that a four-hour incubation at 55°C was the most effective in inactivating the endogenous enzyme activity (*data not shown*). Under these conditions, the wild type HBX protein displayed the highest stimulation of the enzyme activity, with an increase of eightfold as compared with basal level that was assayed with either Egr-1 or wild type HBX protein alone (Figure 5). In contrast, decreases of stimulation were observed when G2, G3 and G5 were assayed. While G2 and G5 with C-terminal deletions

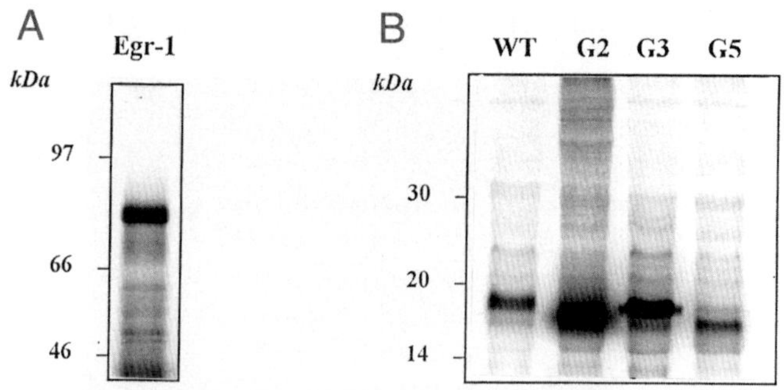

Figure 4. *In vitro* translation of Egr-1 and HBX proteins. The proteins were synthesized in wheat germ lysates in the presence of [^{35}S]Methionine. The translated products were separated on SDS-PAGE gel, dried, and exposed to autoradiogram overnight at ambient temperature. *Panel A*, translation product of expected 80 kDa Egr-1. Sizes of *rainbow* protein migration markers (Amersham, USA) were indicated on the left. *Panel B*, translation products of HBX from wild type (WT), as well as mutants G2, G3 and G5. Expected sizes were seen as 17 kDa (WT), 16 kDa (G2), 17 kDa (G3) and 15 kDa (G5). Sizes of *rainbow* protein migration markers (Amersham, USA) were indicated on the left.

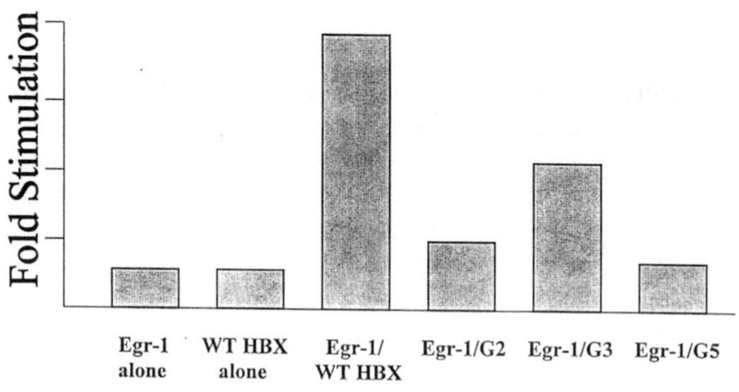

Figure 5. Novel activity assay for HBX. The bacterial β-galactosidase was placed under the control of the TGF-β1 promoter containing Egr-1 binding sites. Stimulation of the bacterial β-galactosidase by synergistic action of Egr-1 and HBX (either wild type or mutants) on the upstream TGF-1 promoter was measured in wheat germ lysates by color changes. Mean value of four independent experiments was shown in bars, and represented the relative activity of the bacterial β-galactosidase.

displayed a significant loss of stimulation, a detectable stimulation by G3 was seen. The significance of this assay was further strengthened by the increasing stimulation of the bacterial enzyme activity with an increasing amount of wild type HBX protein (*data not shown*).

The activity assay developed in our study has provided a simple and fast (within one day) method of measuring HBX activity and appears particularly useful in differentiating functional effects of various mutations detected in HBX. The choice of TGF-β1 promoter that controls the expression of the bacterial β-galactosidase gene is also relevant in assessing the role of HBX in hepatocarcinogenesis, as high levels of TGF-β1 are closely associated with the development of human HCC [29, 30].

Summary

HBX mutants with deletions and mutations are identified in serum and host genomes of HBV-related human HCC. A role of the integrated HBX genes in the hepatocarcinogenesis is suggested by their active expression in the tumor tissues. Effects of the deletions/mutations detected in the HBX variants are assessed by a simple and novel *in vitro* activity assay, by measuring the co-stimulation of HBX with Egr-1 on TGF-β1 promoter. Application of this assay on more HBX variants, either those integrated in HCC or others circulating in serum, should provide more information on the significance of various mutations occurring in HCC-associated HBX.

Acknowledgments

We thank the National Medical Research Council of Singapore and the Ministry of Health Liver Cancer Endowment Singapore for their support. We also thank Ai Lin Leong, Shiuan Koh, Siaw Wei Teng and Yi Zhao for technical assistance and helpful discussion.

References

1. Tiollais P, Pourcel C and Dejean A. The hepatitis B virus. *Nature* 1985; 317: 489-495.
2. Breasley RP. Hepatitis B virus: the major etiology of hepatocellular carcinoma. *Cancer* 1988; 61: 1942-1956.
3. Oon C-J and Friedman MA. Primary hepatocellular carcinoma, present state of the disease and prospects for the future. *Cancer Chemotherapy and Pharmacology* 1982; 8: 231-235.
4. Brechot C, Pourcel C, Louise A, Rain B and Tiollais P. Presence of integrated hepatitis B virus DNA sequences in cellular DNA of human hepatocellular carcinoma. *Nature* 1980; 286: 533-535.
5. Hohne M, Schaefer S, Seifer M, Feitelson MA, Paul D and Gerlich WH. Malignant transformation of immortalized transgenic hepatocytes after transfection with hepatitis B virus DNA. *EMBO Journal* 1990; 9: 1137-1145.
6. Araki K, Miyazaki JI, Hino O, Tomita N, Chisaka O, Matsubara K and Yamamura KI. Expression and replication of hepatitis B virus genome in transgenic mice. *Proceedings of the National Academy of Sciences*, USA 1989; 86: 207-211.
7. Koike K, Moriya K, Iino S, Yotsuyanagi H, Endo Y, Miyammmura T and Hurakawa K. High level expression of hepatitis B virus HBx gene and hepatocarcinogenesis in transgenic mice. *Hepatology*

1994; 19: 810-819.

8. Slagle B, Lee T, Medina D, Finegold M and Butel J. Increased sensitivity to the hepatocarcinogen diethylnitrosamine in transgenic mice carrying the hepatitis B virus X gene. *Molecular Carcinogenesis* 1996; 15: 261-269.
9. Terradillos O, Billet O, Renard C, Levy R, Molina T, Briand P and Buendia M. The hepatitis B virus X gene potentiates c-myc induced liver oncogenesis in transgenic mice. *Oncogene* 1997; 14: 395-404.
10. Feitelson MA and Duan L-X. Hepatitis B virus X antigen in the pathogenesis of chronic infections and the development of hepatocellular carcinoma. *American Journal of Pathology* 1997; 150: 1141-1157.
11. Twu J-S, Lai M-Y, Chen D-S and Robinson WS. Activation of protooncogene c-*jun* by the X protein of hepatitis B virus. *Virology* 1993; 192: 346-350.
12. Yoo YD, Ueda H, Park K, Flanders KC, Lee YI, Jay G and Kim S-J. Regulation of transforming growth factor-1 expression by the hepatitis B virus (HBV) X transactivator, role in HBV pathogenesis. *Journal of Clinical Investigation* 1996; 97: 388-395.
13. Runkel L, Fischer M and Schaller H. Two-codon insertion mutations of the HBx define two separate regions necessary for its trans-activation function. *Virology* 1993; 197: 529-536.
14. Gottlob K, Pagano S, Levrero M and Graessmann A. Hepatitis B virus X protein transcription activation domains are neither required nor sufficient for cell transformation. *Cancer Research* 1998; 58: 3566-3570.
15. Koike K, Takada S. Biochemistry and functions of hepatitis B virus X protein. *Intervirology* 1995; 38: 89-99.
16. Fischer M, Runkel L and Schaller H. HBx protein of hepatitis B virus interacts with the C-terminal portion of a novel human proteasome alpha-subunit. *Virus Genes* 1995; 10: 99-102.
17. Huang J, Kwong J, Sun EC-Y and Liang TJ. Proteasome complex as a potential cellular target of hepatitis B virus X protein. *Journal of Virology* 1996; 70: 5582-5591.
18. Takeuchi M, Fujimoto J, Niwamoto H, Yamamoto Y and Okamoto E. Frequent detection of hepatitis B virus X-gene DNA in hepatocellular carcinoma and adjacent liver tissue in hepatitis B surface antigen-negative patients. *Digestive Diseases and Sciences* 1997; 42: 2264-2269.
19. Hsia CC, Nakashima Y and Tabor E. Deletion mutants of the hepatitis B virus X gene in human hepatocellular carcinoma. *Biochemical and Biophysical Research Communications* 1997; 241: 726-729.
20. Hsia CC, Hao Y and Tabor E. Hot-spot mutations in hepatitis B virus X gene in hepatocellular carcinoma. *Lancet* 1996; 348: 625-626.
21. Chen WN and Oon CJ. Human hepatitis B virus mutants: significance of molecular changes. *FEBS Letters* 1999; 453: 237-242.
22. Carman WF, Zanetti AR, Karayiannis P, Waters J, Manzillo G, Tanzi E, Zuckerman AJ and Thomas HC. Vaccine-induced escape mutant of hepatitis B virus. *Lancet* 1990; 336: 325-329.
23. Oon CJ, Chen WN, Koh S and Lim GK. Identification of hepatitis B surface antigen variants with alterations outside the 'a' determinant in immunized Singapore infants. *Journal of Infectious Diseases* 1999; 179: 259-63.
24. Takada S and Koike K. Trans-activation function of a 3' truncated X gene-cell fusion product from integrated HBV DNA in chronic hepatitis tissue. *Proceedings of the National Academy of Sciences, USA* 1990; 87: 5628-5632.
25. Poussin K, Dienes H, Sirma H, Urban S, Beaugrand M, Franco D, Schirmacher P, Brechot C and Brechot PP. Expression of mutated hepatitis B virus X genes in human hepatocellular carcinomas. *International Journal of Cancer* 1999; 80: 497-505.
26. Dejean A, Sonigo P, Wain-Hobson S and Tiollais P. Specific hepatitis B virus integration in

hepatocellular carcinoma DNA through a viral 11-base-pair direct repeat. *Proceedings of the National Academy of Sciences, USA* 1984; 81: 5350-5354.

27. Cao XM, Koski RA, Gashler A, McKiernan M, Morris CF, Gaffney R, Hay RV and Sukhatme VP. Identification and characterization of the Egr-1 gene product, a DNA-binding zinc finger protein induced by differentiation and growth signals. *Molecular and Cell Biology* 1990; 10: 1931-1939.
28. Young DC, Kingsley SD, Ryan KA and Dutko FJ. Selective inactivation of eukaryotic β-galactosidase in assays for inhibitors of HIV-1 TAT using bacterial β-galactosidase as a reporter enzyme. *Analytical Biochemistry* 1993; 215: 24-30.
29. Shirai Y, Kawata S, Tamura S, Ito N, Tsushima H, Takaishi K, Kiso S and Matsuzawa Y. Plasma transforming growth factor-β1 in patients with hepatocellular carcinoma. *Cancer* 1994; 73: 2275-2279.
30. Tsai J-F, Jeng JE, Chuang LY, Yang ML, Ho MS, Chang WY, Hsieh MY, Lin ZY and Tsai JH. Clinical evaluation of urinary transforming growth factor-β1 and serum α-fetoprotein as tumour markers of hepatocellular carcinoma. *British Journal of Cancer* 1997; 75: 1460-1466.

SUBJECT INDEX

Frontiers in Viral Hepatitis Ed. by RF Schinazi, J-P Sommadossi and CM Rice. 557 — 565

cccDNA, 208, 234-237, 283-285, 296, 383-384, 464-465

AUTHOR INDEX

Frontiers in Viral Hepatitis Ed. by RF Schinazi, J-P Sommadossi and CM Rice. 567 — 567